Ficin 249

NEVILLE J. BRYANT

A.R.T., F.A.C.B.S.

Technical Director
Serological Services Ltd., Toronto;
President, Serological Serums, Ltd.,
Toronto, Ontario, Canada

An Introduction to IMMUNOHEMATOLOGY

Second Edition

W. B. SAUNDERS COMPANY

Philadelphia   London   Toronto   Mexico City   Rio de Janeiro   Sydney   Tokyo

W. B. Saunders Company: West Washington Square
Philadelphia, PA   19105

1 St. Anne's Road
Eastbourne, East Sussex BN21 3UN, England

1 Goldthorne Avenue
Toronto, Ontario M8Z 5T9, Canada

Apartado 26370 – Cedro 512
Mexico 4, D.F., Mexico

Rua Coronel Cabrita, 8
Sao Cristovao Caixa Postal 21176
Rio de Janeiro, Brazil

9 Waltham Street
Artarmon, N.S.W. 2064, Australia

Ichibancho, Central Bldg., 22-1 Ichibancho
Chiyoda-Ku, Tokyo 102, Japan

Library of Congress Cataloging in Publication Data

Bryant, Neville J.

An introduction to immunohematology.

1. Immunohematology.   2. Blood groups – ABO system.
   3. Immunohematology – Technique.   I. Title. [DNLM:
   1. Antigen-antibody reactions.   2. Blood groups.
   3. Immunity. QW 570 B915i]

RB145.B75 1982   612'.11822   81–51193

ISBN 0–7216–2167–8   AACR2

An Introduction to Immunohematology   ISBN   0-7216-2167-8

Last digit is the print number: 9   8   7   6   5   4   3   2

For my wife,
Sheila,
who, in spite of everything, still puts up with me.

Preface

This second edition of *An Introduction to Immunohematology* has been expanded to encompass considerably more information than was contained in the first edition. It is hoped that the additional material will provide a source of reference for laboratories and will serve to whet the appetites of students whose curiosity requires a more detailed explanation of the science and its peculiarities.

Once again, objectives have been included—this time with each chapter—as have sets of examination questions so that the student may test his or her knowledge of each section. In this edition, answers to these questions have been provided at the end of the text.

In preparing this book, I have used the 8th edition of the *Technical Manual* of the American Association of Blood Banks (1981) as a constant source of reference. In the majority of cases, the techniques included are those recommended by the American Association of Blood Banks.

This new edition has been highly referenced with respect to authors of original papers, and it is hoped that this inclusion will prove useful to those requiring such references for the additional data they contain and to students in the preparation of reading assignments, papers or theses.

Despite these changes, the basic purpose of the book remains unchanged: to introduce the newcomer to the major information available and to provide, collected in one place, the essentials of the subject matter. As such, it is my hope that the book will continue to be used as a guide to the fascinating, intricate science that immunohematology has become.

NEVILLE BRYANT

Acknowledgments

I gratefully acknowledge the guidance and encouragement afforded me in the preparation of this book by many friends and colleagues.

In particular, my thanks go to Mrs. Theresia Decurtins, who typed the entire manuscript from often illegible script with great patience and precision, and also to Mrs. Mary Phillips, who typed the entire bibliography for the book on index cards so expertly that proofreading became unnecessary. Without the help of these people, this book would have taken another year to prepare, and I am immensely grateful to both of them. Special thanks also are due to Ms. Linda Stacey for her tireless assistance and constructive criticism with respect to both accuracy and content.

I would also like to acknowledge at this time the interest and encouragement (that seems without end) from the people of W. B. Saunders Company, in particular Mr. Baxter Venable, who has always been patient and has shown the kind of interest in my book that at times led me to believe that this was his only project.

To these and to all others who have helped in one way or another, I express my gratitude. The responsibility for the book's shortcomings and errors is, of course, exclusively my own.

A Brief History
of Blood Transfusion

The possibility of transferring blood from the vessels of one individual directly into those of another was considered, although not seriously, as early as the sixteenth century. The positive era of blood transfusion really began when William Harvey, at a lecture on anatomy at the College of Physicians, England, described the circulation of blood in 1616. Some years later, in 1665, the first animal-to-animal blood transfusions were successfully performed by an English physiologist, Richard Lower, who kept exsanguinated dogs alive by transfusion of blood from other dogs.

In 1667, Jean Baptiste Denys, a Montpellier philosopher, mathematician and personal physician to Louis XIV, successfully transfused nine ounces of blood from the carotid artery of a lamb into the vein of a young man. Subsequent transfusions using animal blood were also performed by Denys, but most of them were unsuccessful; in some cases, patients began to pass black urine. Finally, the wife of a patient who died following three transfusions took legal action against Denys, charging him with murder. A long legal battle ensued, and while Denys was exonerated, from this time on transfusions were prohibited except with the sanction of the Faculty of Medicine in Paris. Then, in 1678, an edict of the French Parliament declared transfusion unlawful, and this decision caused similar edicts to be passed in other countries.

During the next 150 years, little was written or done about transfusion until 1818. That year James Blundell, an English obstetrician and physiologist, advocated the use of blood transfusion as a means of furnishing blood to women who were exsanguinated at childbirth. In October 1818, Blundell gave the first transfusion from man to man. (This is, in fact, disputed by supporters of Philip Syng Physick, who, it is stated, transfused human beings with human blood before Blundell. Physick's aversion to publication may well have denied him the distinction of having been the first to successfully perform person-to-person transfusions.)

The immunologic era was introduced in 1900, when Karl Landsteiner discovered the blood groups by noting the agglutinating properties of the erythrocytes of some persons with the serum of others. This agglutination phenomenon had, in fact, already been noted by S. G. Shattock in 1899 but was interpreted to be the result of rheumatic fever. Other diseases were subsequently held responsible for agglutination by the same investigator.

Landsteiner isolated three groups, which he called 1, 2 and 3. Decastello and Sturli, his pupils, discovered the group we now call AB in 1902, yet considered it exceptional because it lacked agglutinins. Only in 1906 did Jansky recognize that it, too, was physiologic and representative of the fourth blood group.

Jansky recommended the use of roman numerals to signify the blood groups. The numeral "I" was used for the group we now call "O," "II" represented the group we now call "A," "III" represented the group we now call "B" and "IV" was used for the group discovered by Decastello and Sturli. In 1910, Moss, unaware of Jansky's report, independently classified the groups but reversed groups I and IV, which led to confusion. In 1921, the American Medical Association recommended the adoption of the Jansky classification on the basis of priority. This decision held only until 1928, when the League of Nations adopted the present international ABO classification.

Up until 1914, there was no knowledge of how to store blood. When a patient required a transfusion, it was necessary for the donor to lie next to the patient and for the blood to be directly transferred. Various anticoagulants, such as phosphate, hirudin and peptone, were tried; blood was defibrinated and oxalated, yet in all cases poor results were obtained. Agote, in 1915, introduced sodium citrate as an anticoagulant, and soon afterward it was independently introduced for the same purpose in the United States by Lewisohn. This considerably simplified transfusion practices, since it allowed for the collection and storage of blood prior to transfusion. In 1916, Rous and Turner published studies on the preservation of stored blood. Their results were applied by Oswald Robertson, who conceived of and operated the first blood bank in France during World War I.

Hektoen (1907a, 1907b) is credited with being the first to suggest the tremendous importance of blood grouping for transfusion (a surprising fact in retrospect, since this was the first practical application of Landsteiner's discovery). Ottenberg (1911) was probably the first to actually select compatible blood for transfusion, and Moss published his suggested compatibility test method in 1914. Biologic pretransfusion tests, however, were still carried out as late as 1931. Various techniques were applied, including the infusion of 10 to 20 ml of blood 15 minutes prior to transfusion; the blood was considered "compatible" if no untoward reaction occurred.

In 1908, Ottenberg and Epstein suggested that the blood groups were inherited, and this was established beyond doubt by von Dungern and Hirszfeld in 1910. The exact manner of inheritance was explained by Bernstein in 1925. Blood grouping had now spilled over into the field of genetics, and had also become of significance in forensic medicine in cases of disputed paternity.

In 1927, Landsteiner and Levine discovered the MN system and the P system through the direct immunization of animals with human red cells. While these systems did not affect the transfusion of blood, they were of tremendous genetic and anthropologic significance.

The second most important contribution to the history of the blood groups was made by Levine and Stetson (1939) and Landsteiner and Weiner (1940) through the discovery of the Rh system and its role in the disease known as erythroblastosis foetalis (hemolytic disease of the newborn). Knowledge of this system increased rapidly in the early 1940's and, indeed, continues to increase today.

The period of 1944 through 1946 saw the introduction of three important new tests that allowed for the detection of antibodies that were capable of red cell sensitization yet were incapable of causing agglutination. Bovine albumin was first used for this purpose in 1945. Later in the same year,

Coombs, Mourant and Race introduced the antiglobulin test, which was based on a method described by Moreschi (1908). In 1946 it was shown that certain proteolytic enzymes could also be used to detect these sensitizing antibodies. The use of these tests resulted in the discovery of several new blood group systems. In 1946, the Kell system was discovered by Coombs, Mourant and Race, and the Lewis system was described by Mourant. The Duffy system (Cutbush, Mollison and Parkin) and the Kidd system (Allen, Diamond and Niedziela) were described in 1950 and 1951, respectively. The Lutheran system, also described in this time period, was detected by means of direct agglutination tests (Callender, Race and Paykoc, 1945).

Since 1951, the literature on these and other blood group systems has expanded to encyclopedic proportions. Each major system has been found to be increasingly complex, with seemingly endless red cell polymorphism. Blood transfusion, once considered to be of use only in cases of dire emergency, is now commonplace—yet there are still innumerable problems to surmount. While radical surgical procedures are now possible, the hazard of alloimmunization remains. While we have learned to recognize some of the factors involved, there is little doubt that the best *in vitro* tests are poor mimics of what happens *in vivo*. Other hazards, including those resulting from bacterial contamination, circulatory overload and disease transmission, although reduced, still remain with us. Perhaps most important, however, is the sobering fact that blood transfusion, being in effect a tissue transplantation, is a surgical operation of a special nature, and once performed is virtually impossible to undo.

In spite of these and other risks, blood transfusion is the most frequently employed form of clinical therapy, and it is clearly evident that because of it, millions of lives have been saved or at least extended.

Contents

Contents

Section One

BASIC GENETICS

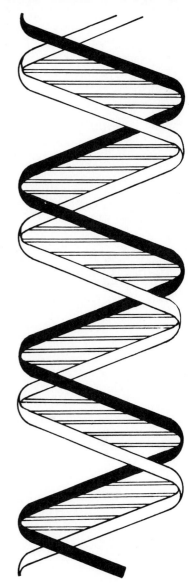

Our main purpose is to provide blood for transfusion that is as safe as our knowledge and technical ability can make it. To this end, we apply the principles of *immunology* to a study of *hematologic* disorders. Thus, ours is an allied science — aptly named *immunohematology*.

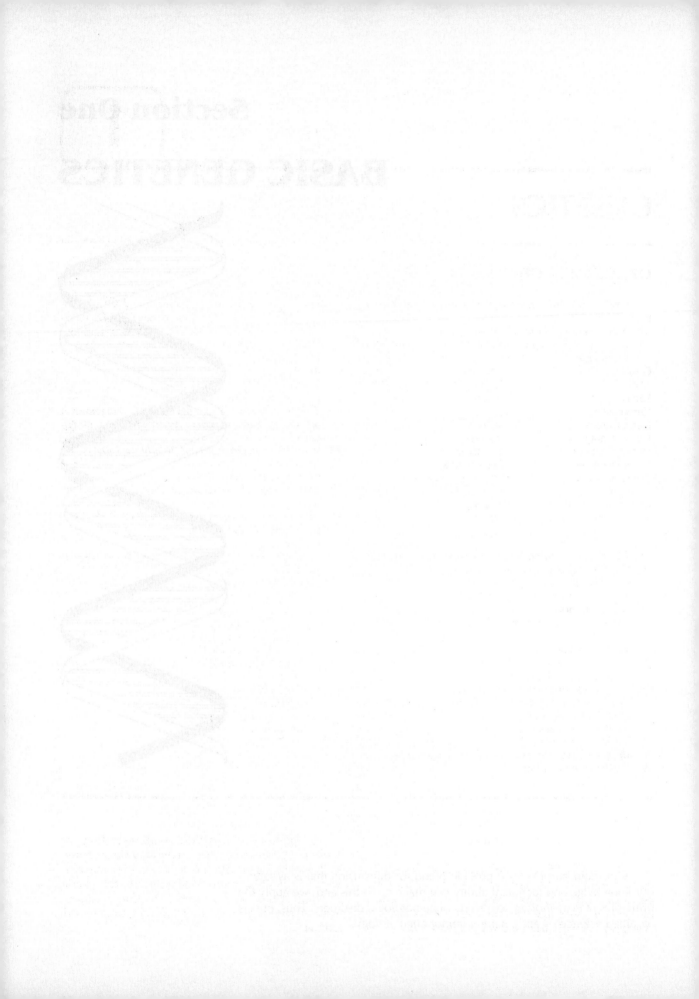

GENETICS

OBJECTIVES — GENETICS

The student shall know, understand and be prepared to explain:

1. A brief history of the science of genetics
2. The terms that apply to the science of genetics, specifically:

Gene	DNA
Allele	RNA (mRNA, tRNA, sRNA,
Locus	rRNA)
Chromosome	Codon
Homozygous	Meiosis
Heterozygous	Mitosis
Dominant gene	Autosome
Recessive gene	Gene product
Co-dominance	Propositus (proposita)
Amorph	Somatic cell
Genotype	Haploid
Phenotype	Diploid
	Zygote

3. The physical and chemical characteristics of DNA
4. The method of performing a family study
5. The symbols used in pedigree charts
6. The sex chromosomes with relation to the determination of an individual's sex
7. The sequence of events governing protein synthesis, including:
   (a) DNA replication
   (b) The role of RNA
   (c) The role of the ribosome
8. The process of meiosis, including:
   (a) The four main stages: prophase, metaphase, anaphase, telophase
   (b) The five stages of prophase
   (c) The first meiotic division of gametogenesis
   (d) The second meiotic division of gametogenesis
9. The process of fertilization
10. The process of mitosis, including:
    (a) The four main stages: prophase, metaphase, anaphase, telophase
11. The mitotic (cell) cycle, to include:
    (a) G_1 period
    (b) S period
    (c) G_2 period
    (d) Duration of the cycle
12. The mendelian laws: segregation, independent assortment and dependent assortment (unit inheritance)
13. Variation of mendelian laws with respect to:
    (a) Mutation
    (b) Crossing over
14. The process of chromosome classification (karyotyping)
15. Chromosomal aberrations, specifically to include:
    (a) Numerical aberrations:
    Nondisjunction
    Terms used in numerical aberrations, specifically:

    Euploid
    Polyploid
    Aneuploid
    Trisomic aneuploid
    Monosomic aneuploid
    Heteroploid
    (b) Structural aberrations:
    Deletion
    Duplication
    Inversion
    Translocation
    Insertion
    Isochromosomes

Introduction

The study of immunohematology logically begins with an understanding of the basic concepts of inheritance and heredity — the science of genetics — since the human blood factors discussed in this text are subject to its laws.

A somewhat detailed understanding of these concepts is of ever-increasing importance to the immunohematologist; therefore, the material presented here will include the basic principles and a discussion of the relationship of these principles to the human blood groups.

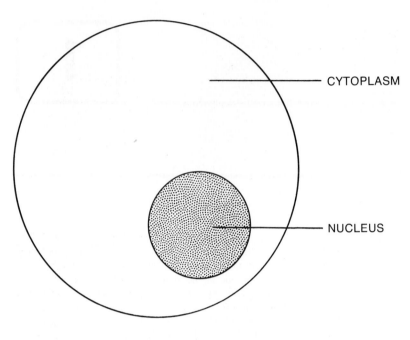

Figure 1-1 Typical somatic (body) cell.

CYTOPLASM

NUCLEUS

History

The term "genetics" was coined by William Bateman, an Englishman, in 1905 from a Greek word meaning "to generate." The original descriptions of the science, however, were made in 1865 by an Augustinian monk, Gregor Mendel, who postulated that all bodily characteristics (color of eyes, hair and so forth) were derived from a combination of characteristics, some of which were inherited from one parent and the remainder from the other parent. (In this, Mendel differed from other researchers of the time, who believed that an offspring was a "blend" of characteristics from both parents.)

Because so many glaring "exceptions" were noted, Mendel's theories and experimental results were largely ignored until early in the twentieth century, when the discovery of the human blood groups revealed an aspect of human biology that fully obeyed Mendel's original principles. Since that time, genetics has become a science in its own right and an essential component part of many subspecialties; yet the basic concepts as stated by Mendel have remained for the most part unaltered and are fully accepted today as being correct.

CHROMOSOMES

In order to appreciate the concepts of human genetics, it is necessary to begin with a basic study of somatic (body) cells.

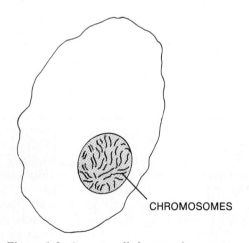

CHROMOSOMES

Figure 1-2 Somatic cell showing chromosomes.

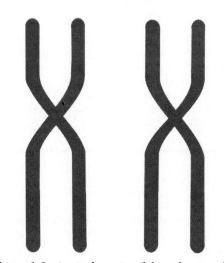

Figure 1-3 A single pair of homologous chromosomes.

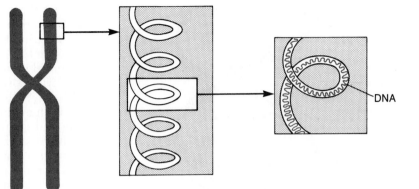

Figure 1-4 Portion of the chromosome showing DNA strands. (Modified from Gardner, E. J.: Principles of Genetics, 5th Ed. John Wiley & Sons, Inc., New York, 1975.)

The human body is entirely made up of cells, the majority of which (the major exception being the red cells of the blood) consist of two distinct parts — a dark, almost circular area in or near the center, known as the *nucleus,* surrounded by a rambling lighter area, known as the *cytoplasm* (Fig. 1–1).

While the cell cytoplasm is responsible for a number of different functions including oxidative processes, phagocytosis and the addition of carbohydrates to synthesized protein, the cell nucleus is primarily concerned with *body growth* and *cell division.*

Within the nucleus are 23 pairs of long, rodlike structures, known as chromosomes (Fig. 1–2). These *pairs* of *chromosomes* are said to be "homologous," a term which means "identical in terms of structure, position, character and so forth" (Fig. 1–3). The number of chromosomes in any one species is usually constant. In man, a full complement consists of 46 single chromosomes (i.e., 23 pairs).

The Chemical Basis of Inheritance: DNA

Chromosomes are composed of long strands (molecules) of *deoxyribonucleic acid* (DNA) on a protein framework (Fig. 1–4). Nucleic acid, first called *nuclein* because it was obtained from the cell nucleus, was isolated by Miescher in 1869. DNA (deoxyribonucleic acid), the nucleic acid component of the reproductive cell, was shown to be genetic mate-

rial through investigations on pneumococcus bacteria beginning in the 1920's. While several attempts were made to explain the physical and chemical nature of DNA, it was not until 1953 that Watson and Crick proposed a model for DNA that today has gained wide acceptance.

On the basis of the Watson-Crick model, the *basic physical* structure of DNA is seen as two long polynucleotide chains forming a double spiral (helix), with each chain running in the opposite direction (Fig. 1–5). The strands that form the spirals around the axis are made up of phosphates and pentose sugars. Crosswise, the strands are less rigidly connected by *organic bases* through hydrogen (H) bonds. The chains are therefore composed of nucleotides, each nucleotide being composed of one pentose sugar, one phosphate and one organic base. The length of one spiral is 34 Angstrom units (Å), and the distance between the crosswise bonds is 3.4 Å (Fig. 1–6).

Four kinds of nucleotides exist in DNA, each including a different nitrogenous base — adenine (A) and guanine (G), which are purine bases, and thymine (T) and cytosine (C), which are pyrimidine bases.

Chemical analyses used by Watson and Crick were those of Chargaff and his associates. These analyses showed a 1:1 relation between adenine and thymine and between cytosine and guanine, through the observation that the total amount of purine always equaled the total amount of pyrimidine. It was therefore conclud-

Figure 1-5 The basic physical structure of DNA. (See also Figure 1-4.) (Modified from Gardner, E. J.: Principles of Genetics, 5th Ed. John Wiley & Sons, Inc., New York, 1975.)

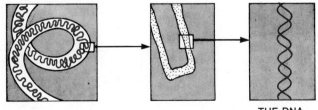

THE DNA DOUBLE HELIX

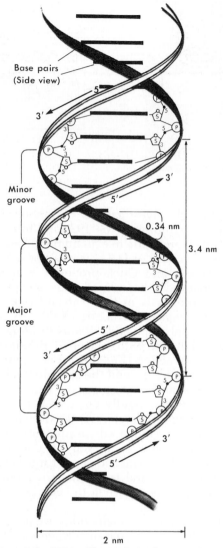

Figure 1-6 DNA (deoxyribonucleic acid). (From DeRobertis, Sarz, and DeRobertis, Cell Biology. W. B. Saunders Co., Philadelphia, 1980.)

ed that the adenine base (a purine) must *pair* with the thymine base (a pyrimidine) and that the guanine base (a purine) must pair with the cytosine base (a pyrimidine). The model for the chemical structure of DNA proposed by Watson and Crick is seen as organic base *pairs*, connected by hydrogen (H) bonds, adenine and guanine being connected by two H bonds and cytosine and guanine being connected by three. In each crosslink, therefore, the bases are arranged in such a way that a certain purine is bound to a certain pyrimidine, adenine-thymine and cytosine-guanine (Fig. 1–7).

GENES

William Roux, in 1883, postulated that chromosomes within the nucleus of the cell are the bearers of hereditary factors. While the concept of the "gene" as a discrete unit of inheritance had been implicit in Mendel's visualization of a physical element or factor as the foundation for the development of a trait, it was not until 1902 that experiments by Boveri and Sutton brought evidence that a gene is, in fact, part of a chromosome.

It is now known that genes are arranged in *linear* (i.e., in lines) order on the chromosomes and that each gene occupies a specific position on the DNA chain (known as the *locus*). Segments of the DNA molecule, therefore, compose the genes, which are coded for by *three-base sequences*, known as *triplets* or *codons*. Each codon, depending on the type and sequence of the three bases involved, codes for a particular amino acid. A series of codons determine the amino acid sequence on a polypeptide chain, and a *gene* is a sequence of triplets (codons) that contains the code for one polypeptide (Fig. 1–8).

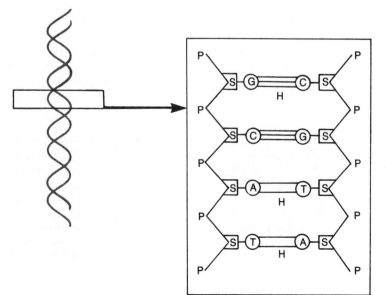

Figure 1-7 Linear sequence of nucleotides as proposed in the DNA model of Watson and Crick. P = Phosphate, S = Sugar, A = Adenine, T = Thymine, C = Cytosine, G = Guanine, H = Hydrogen Bonds.

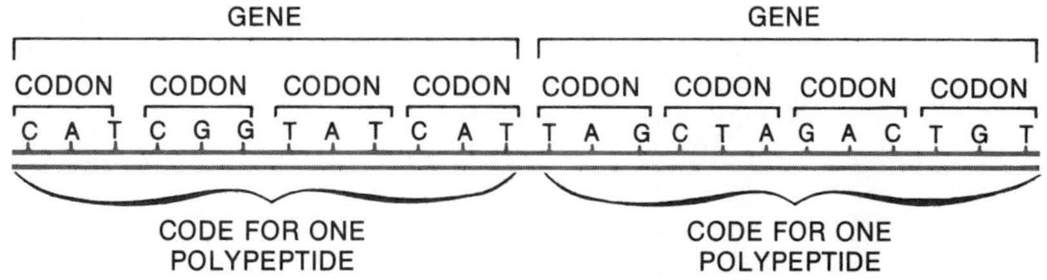

GENE | GENE

| CODON | CODON | CODON | CODON | CODON | CODON | CODON | CODON |

C A T | C G G | T A T | C A T | T A G | C T A | G A C | T G T

Figure 1–8 A single strand of DNA (one part of the double helix) illustrating the concept of a codon and a gene.

CODE FOR ONE POLYPEPTIDE | CODE FOR ONE POLYPEPTIDE

A particular locus may be occupied by several different forms of the gene, and these alternatives are known as *alleles.* When these allelic genes on a pair of homologous chromosomes are identical (i.e., the individual has inherited a gene coding for the same characteristic from both parents), the individual is said to be *homozygous* for that factor or characteristic; when the alleles are different, the individual is said to be *heterozygous* (Fig. 1–9).

As Mendel and others showed, genes carry from generation to generation the information that specifies the characteristics of a particular species. At the present time we are unable to detect a gene on a chromosome by direct testing; however, in some cases we are able to detect its *product.* The product of a gene is the characteristic that it produces (e.g., the blue of an individual's eyes can be considered as the product of the particular gene determining that characteristic.)

An individual obtains his chromosomes (and therefore his genes) by each parental sex cell (gamete) donating 23 single chromosomes (see under the heading Fertilization). If we consider for the purpose of this discussion that eye color is a result of simple (single-gene) inheritance, a child may inherit the gene for blue eyes from his father and the gene for brown eyes from his mother. The two genes are alleles. In this case, the child will almost certainly have brown eyes, since the gene for brown eyes is a *dominant* gene — the term indicating that the gene is always expressed (always produces a product) regardless of whether it occurs in a homozygous or heterozygous state. The gene for blue eyes is termed *recessive* since it can produce a product only when it occurs in the homozygous state. If two dominant genes are inherited, the products of both genes are detectable and the situation is termed *codominance.*

It is well to note at this point that certain blood group genes appear to produce no product, even when present in a homozygous state. Such "silent alleles" are known as *amorphs* or *amorphic* genes. (See Inheritance of ABO Groups, Chapter 3).

Genotypes and Phenotypes

The term "genotype" refers to the total sum of genes present on the chromosomes (with respect to one or more than one characteristic), regardless of whether or not they produce detectable products. In a sense, the genotype is based totally on deduction and assumption as a result of direct testing of gene products and family studies.

The term "phenotype" refers to the detectable products only, demonstrated through direct testing.

The following example may clarify the distinction:

Consider the hypothetical gene Q and its allele q. (Note: gene symbols are always printed in *italics.)* Let us assume that we have the means of detecting the products of both genes, and that both are dominant. Upon testing, the product of Q is revealed, yet the product of q is not. The individual's "phenotype" is Q, since this is the only gene product that we can detect. Since we have the means to detect the product of the allelic gene q yet it cannot be demonstrated, we assume that it is not present in the individual and that the gene Q is present in a homozygous state. The individual's genotype is therefore assumed to be QQ (Fig. 1–10).

In the same example, if, upon testing, the products of both the Q and q genes were re-

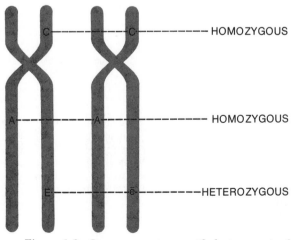

HOMOZYGOUS

HOMOZYGOUS

HETEROZYGOUS

Figure 1–9 Genes occupying specific loci on a pair of homologous chromosomes, illustrating the concept of homozygosity and heterozygosity.

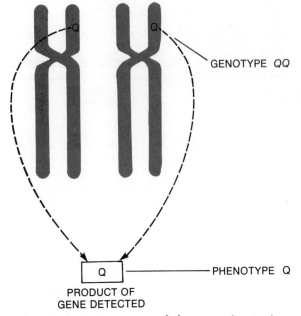

GENOTYPE *QQ*

Q ————— PHENOTYPE Q

PRODUCT OF
GENE DETECTED

Figure 1–10 Genotypes and phenotypes (see text).

Family Studies

In certain instances in which it is necessary to determine the exact genotype of an individual, or in which it is necessary to show the mode of inheritance of a particular trait, factor or characteristic, a family study can often prove helpful. A family study merely indicates the testing of all available immediate family of an individual. In cases such as this, the family member through whom the family comes to be studied is known as the *propositus* (male) or *proposita* (female).

Family data can be summarized in a *pedigree chart* for easy reference. The symbols used in drawing up a pedigree chart vary somewhat, and special symbols may be invented to demonstrate special situations. Those symbols that are in most common use are shown in Figure 1–11.

An example of how a family study can help in the determination of a genotype is given in Figure 1–12. In this example, we can deduce that the grandparents (Generation I) are both heterozygous, since child 3 (Generation II) is of phenotype O, and therefore must have inherited the *O* gene from both parents. Child 1 (Generation II) has inherited the *A* gene from his mother and since he did not inherit the *B* gene from his father, he must have inherited the *O* gene, making his genotype *AO*. The same principle is applied to child 4 (Generation II), who has inherited the *B* gene from her father and the *O* gene from her mother. Both children in Generation III are of phenotype A and of genotype *AO*, since their mother is of phenotype O (genotype *OO*) and must therefore pass the *O* gene to all of her children.

vealed, then the phenotype would be Qq. The genes are now known to be present in a heterozygous state, and the genotype is therefore given as *Qq*.

If we have no means of detecting the product of *q*, then in all cases the genotype would be *QQ* or *Qq*, yet it could not be determined exactly — except occasionally through a family study (see below).

Another term often used in referring to genetic make-up is *genome*. This term refers to a complete set of chromosomes (and therefore of genes), inherited as a unit from one parent.

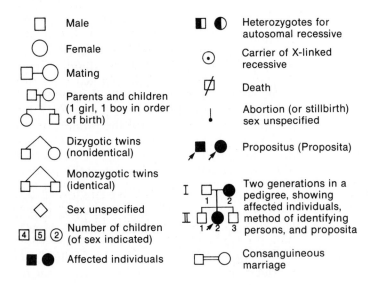

Figure 1–11 Symbols used in pedigree charts. (Data from Thompson, J. S. and Thompson, M. W.: Genetics in Medicine, 3rd ed. W. B. Saunders, Philadelphia, 1980.

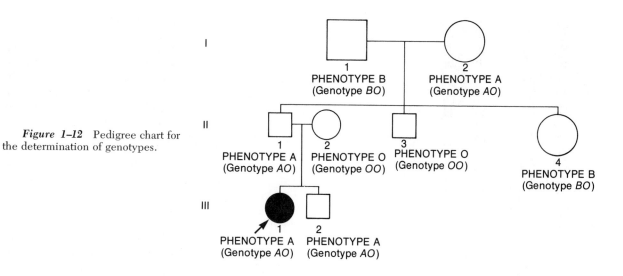

Figure 1-12 Pedigree chart for the determination of genotypes.

I
1 PHENOTYPE B (Genotype *BO*)
2 PHENOTYPE A (Genotype *AO*)

II
1 PHENOTYPE A (Genotype *AO*)
2 PHENOTYPE O (Genotype *OO*)
3 PHENOTYPE O (Genotype *OO*)
4 PHENOTYPE B (Genotype *BO*)

III
1 PHENOTYPE A (Genotype *AO*)
2 PHENOTYPE A (Genotype *AO*)

As can be seen, therefore, from the study of eight individuals, the genotypes of all have been accurately determined.

SEX CHROMOSOMES

Twenty-two of the 23 pairs of chromosomes present in all body cells are known as *autosomes*. The sex chromosomes are the twenty-third pair, and it is these chromosomes that determine whether an individual is male or female. Both sex chromosomes in the female are termed "X" and they are equal in size. In males, however, one chromosome is an X, and the other, which is much smaller, is called "Y" (Fig. 1–13).

Almost all blood group genes are carried on the autosomes. (The term simply means any chromosome that is not a sex chromosome.) The major exception is the genes of the Xg blood group system, which are carried on the X chromosome. Males, having only one X chromosome, can only be Xg^a or (Xg) and are said to be *hemizygous*. Females, however, can be heterozygous or homozygous for Xg^a (see the heading Xg Blood Group System in Chapter 13).

THE SEQUENCE OF EVENTS GOVERNING PROTEIN SYNTHESIS

DNA Replication

Living things perpetuate their kind through *duplication* or *reproduction*. Duplication of the organism is preceded by replication of DNA molecules. A DNA molecule uses its own structure as a model *(template)* and takes from its immediate environment the necessary materials for replication.

Each of the two DNA strands in the double helix is the complement of the other. When duplication occurs, the hydrogen bonds between the bases break and the strands replicate as they unwind, with each strand acting as a model for the formation of a new complementary chain. Two *pairs* of chains now exist, with each chain being a complement of the one from which it was specified, carrying genetic qualities determined by the original structure (Fig. 1–14).

RNA

Ribonucleic acid (RNA) is a single-stranded molecule, similar to DNA, that plays an important role in the synthesis (production) of protein. In RNA, however, the pentose sugar is "ribose" and uracil (U) replaces thymine (T) (Fig. 1–15).

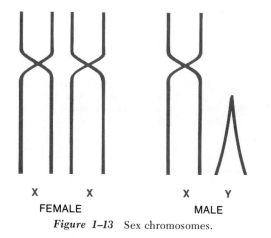

X   X   X   Y
FEMALE   MALE
Figure 1–13 Sex chromosomes.

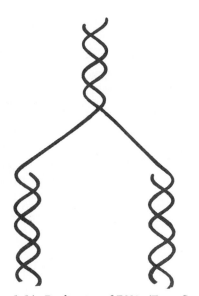

Figure 1–14 Replication of DNA. (From Gardner, E. J.: *Principles of Genetics*, 5th Ed. John Wiley & Sons, New York, p. 58, 1975.)

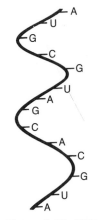

Figure 1–15 RNA.

Three kinds of RNA take part in protein synthesis: (1) messenger RNA (mRNA), (2) transfer RNA (tRNA—also known as soluble RNA, or sRNA) and (3) ribosomal RNA (rRNA).

Messenger RNA (mRNA) is produced by transcription from DNA, which is much like DNA replication except that uracil replaces thymine and that the RNA transcripts do not remain bonded to the DNA template. Synthesis of RNA molecules involves only one of the two strands of the double helix and is initiated at close intervals, producing copies of *individual genes* for immediate and short-term use in protein synthesis. The enzyme DNA-dependent polymerase (also known as RNA polymerase) aids in the reaction by attaching to the DNA molecule and opening up a section of the dou-

ble helix, thereby allowing free bases on one of the DNA strands to attract complementary bases and thus provide a *transcription* of the base sequence (Fig. 1–16). On messenger RNA, thymine (T) of DNA is represented by adenine (A), cytosine (C) is represented by guanine (G), guanine (G) by cytosine (C) and adenine (A) by uracil (U) (Fig. 1–17). As the RNA polymerase moves along its DNA template, the newly assembled mRNA bases are joined in tandem by an enzymatic reaction.

Once the mRNA has received the genetic code, it peels off the DNA template, passes from the nucleus of the cell to the cytoplasm and becomes attached to a *ribosome*, which is a minute granule consisting of two subunits, one small and the other large (Fig. 1–18). Ribosomes are composed largely of nucleic acid, protein and ribosomal RNA (rRNA) and are found in the cytoplasm attached to the membranes of the endoplasmic reticulum.

Ribosomes are *manufacturing centers* for protein. The granules are inactive until they make contact with a molecule of mRNA, and their action is nonspecific (i.e., they produce

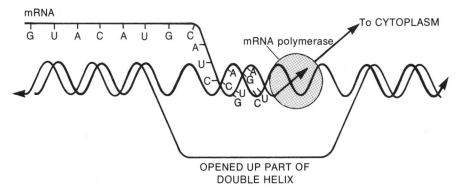

Figure 1–16 Transcription of DNA by mRNA. (Modified from Gardner, E. J.: Principles of Genetics, 5th Ed. John Wiley & Sons, Inc., New York, 1975, p. 71.)

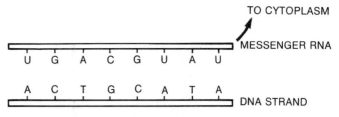

Figure 1-17 Genetic code representation on mRNA from the DNA template.

whatever kind of protein they are directed to produce by mRNA). Once contact is made between the mRNA and the ribosome, protein synthesis takes place as follows:

1. The smaller subunit of the ribosome adheres to a "sticky spot" on the mRNA. The necessary *amino acids*, which are dispersed in the cell, are brought to the ribosomes by *transfer RNA* (tRNA), which is a single-stranded molecule like mRNA, but much smaller. A specific tRNA exists for each amino acid, one part of the molecule being bound to the amino acid and the other part containing the anti-codon for pairing with a particular part of the mRNA transcript. (Fig. 1–19).

2. The ribosome proceeds along the mRNA, "reading" the code and placing the appropriate amino acids in a predetermined position (Fig. 1–20). In this way, the ribosome and its attendant protein *translate* the nucleotide sequences of DNA into protein. The amino acids that form the protein are held together by *peptide bonds*, which are formed through the action of an enzyme in the ribosome (Fig. 1–20).

3. Once this peptide bond is formed, the polypeptide chain begins to pull away from the ribosome, and the tRNA molecule goes free (Fig. 1–21).

The ribosome takes about ten seconds to read a length of mRNA, and a single mRNA molecule may be read by several ribosomes at the same time.

4. Once the reading of the mRNA molecule is complete, the polypeptide, having an exact and predetermined amino acid sequence, goes free. This molecule may be an enzyme (a biological catalyst), hemoglobin, etc. (Fig. 1–22).In

turn, the enzymes produced control virtually all of the numerous chemical processes performed in living systems. Genes therefore act by *synthesizing* (producing) proteins, and proteins represent the chemicals through which inherited traits are expressed.

MEIOSIS AND MITOSIS

The processes of reproduction are governed by two separate cell alterations known as *meiosis* and *mitosis*. The first, meiosis, is concerned with the production of sperm or ovum cells (known as *gametes*), which is termed spermatogenesis in the male and oögenesis in the female. The second, mitosis, is the process of cell division by which the body grows and replaces discarded cells.

The Process of Meiosis

The sex (or "germ") cells, unlike virtually all other normal cells that can reproduce themselves, are responsible for the initiation of re-

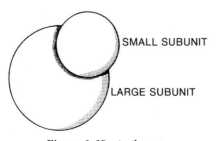

Figure 1-18 A ribosome.

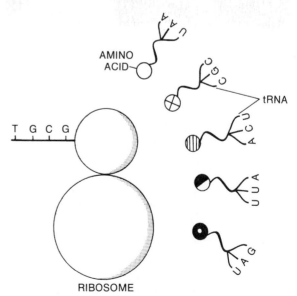

Figure 1-19 The smaller subunit of the ribosome attached to mRNA, surrounded by tRNA.

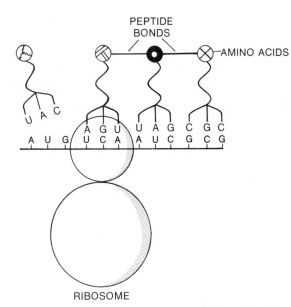

Figure 1–20 Appropriate amino acids are placed in a predetermined position as the ribosome "reads" the code on the mRNA.

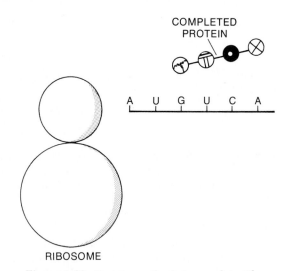

Figure 1–22 Protein synthesis is complete. The completed protein, possessing an exact and predetermined amino acid sequence, goes free.

production of the entire organism. The production of sperm and ovum is known as *gametogenesis*, a process that results in the production of a cell possessing only half the number of chromosomes present in a normal

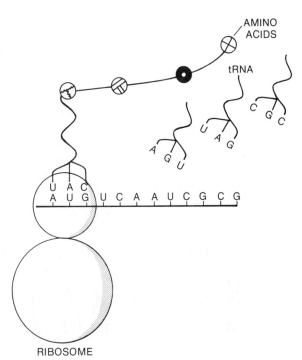

Figure 1–21 The polypeptide chain of amino acids breaks away from the ribosome, and the tRNA molecules go free.

somatic cell. Gametogenesis includes meiosis (from the Greek, meaning "to reduce"), the process by which the chromosome number is changed from the *diploid* or *2n* number (indicating a full set of chromosomes) to the *haploid* or *n* number (indicating half of a set of chromosomes).

Four main stages of meiosis have been distinguished and are known as *prophase, metaphase, anaphase* and *telophase*. A cell that is not actively dividing is said to be in interphase, during which chromosomes are elongated and not individually distinguishable (see under the heading The Cell Cycle).

During *prophase,* homologous chromosomes within the nucleus arrange themselves in pairs (so-called bivalents). Five major prophase stages are distinguishable, known as *leptonema, zygonema, pachynema, diplonema* and *diakinesis.* (Note: the ending -tene, though strictly speaking adjectival, is sometimes used instead of -nema.)

Leptonema.   The leptotene stage is characterized by the first appearance of the chromosomes as thin threads or filaments. The DNA has already duplicated prior to this stage, although on microscopic examination the threads still appear single (Fig. 1–23).

Zygonema.   The zygotene stage is characterized by pairing of the homologous chromosomes. The pairing process, known as *synapsis* (from the Greek, meaning "conjunction" or "union"), brings together maternal and paternal members of the same pair of chromosomes (Fig. 1–23).

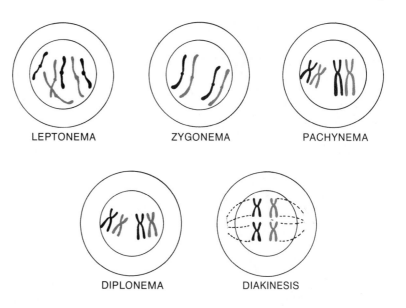

LEPTONEMA   ZYGONEMA   PACHYNEMA

DIPLONEMA   DIAKINESIS

Figure 1-23 The stages of the first meiotic prophase.

Pachynema. The pachytene stage is that of chromosomal thickening, with the paired chromosomes (bivalents) in close association. Each chromosome is now seen to consist of two *chromatids* (i.e., two parallel strands held together by a small mass of heterochromatin known as the *centromere)* so that each bivalent consists of four strands (Fig. 1–23).

Diplonema. During diplonema, the paired chromosomes separate (i.e., the two components of each bivalent). The centromeres remain intact, however, so that although the two chromosomes of each bivalent separate, the two chromatids of each individual chromosome remain together. Separation of the bivalents is usually not complete, for they are normally held together at one or several points called *chiasmata*, which may represent the visible expression of genetical "crossing over" (i.e., when homologous chromosomes exchange genetic material (Fig. 1–23).

Diakinesis. This is the final stage of prophase, characterized by further contraction of the chromosomes, which also become more widely separated from one another, owing to their migration toward the periphery of the nucleus. Toward the end of diakinesis, the nuclear membrane disappears and the spindle begins to form. The bivalents are now at their maximal state of contraction (Fig. 1–23).

This initial stage is known as the *first meiotic division of gametogenesis* and includes the phenomenon called *crossing over*. This is the process in which genetic material is exchanged between maternal and paternal chromosomes and allows for the reshuffling of genes, giving rise to enormous possibilities of variation in the offspring (Fig. 1–24).

METAPHASE I

The stage between the dissolution of the nuclear membrane and the arrival of the bivalents at the center of the spindle is often referred to as *prometaphase*. At full metaphase, the bivalents have moved to the equatorial plate and are arranged in such a way that the two homologous centromeres lie on either side of it at an equal distance. The centromeres are attached to the fibers of the spindle, pointing toward the opposite poles (Fig. 1–25).

ANAPHASE I

Once the chromosomes are in line along the equatorial plate, the two centromeres move toward their respective poles, each pulling its two attached chromatids after it. This stage is known as *anaphase*. The resulting half bivalents are sometimes referred to as *dyads*. If crossing-over has occurred, each chromatid of the two dyads will possess one chromatid that was solely of either maternal or paternal origin

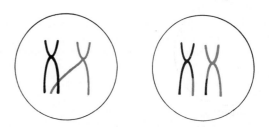

Figure 1-24 An example of crossing-over, illustrated using one of the 23 pairs of chromosomes. The phenomenon occurs during the diplotene stage of prophase (see text).

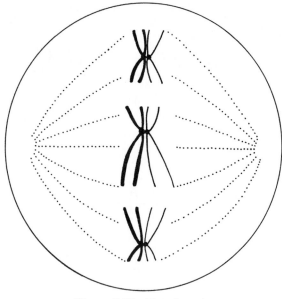

Figure 1–25 Metaphase 1.

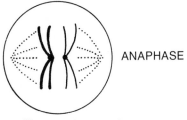

Figure 1–26 Anaphase 1.

and one chromatid that possessed a genetic contribution from both parental types. At the termination of this stage, the daughter nuclei possess a chromosome number that has been reduced to the haploid condition (i.e., 23 single chromosomes) (Fig. 1–26).

TELOPHASE

When the chromatids have reached their respective poles, the nuclear membrane may be reconstituted and two interphase nuclei be formed. Generally, however, there is no true reconstitution phase, and after a short period of time the cells proceed into the second meiotic division (Fig. 1–27).

It should be noted that during telophase I each chromosome consists of two chromatids, and therefore still contains the diploid amount of DNA. The cells enter prophase II without DNA synthesis.

THE SECOND MEIOTIC DIVISION

The second meiotic division basically resembles an ordinary mitosis (see below) in which only one of a pair of chromosomes is present.

PROPHASE II

At prophase II the nuclear membrane disappears and the spindle is formed. The chromosomes move toward the equatorial plate.

METAPHASE II AND ANAPHASE II

At metaphase II, the centromeres have reached the equatorial plate. The chromosomes are contracted and the constituent chromatids are widely separated. At anaphase II, the centromeres divide and the two halves move toward the opposite poles of the spindle. As a result, four nuclei are formed, each possessing the haploid chromosome number as well as the haploid amount of DNA.

The second meiotic division is illustrated in Figure 1–28. Four daughter cells are formed by one doubling of chromosomal material. In males, these four haploid cells are spermatozoa; in females only one of the four daughter cells is a viable ovum. The other three fail to develop and are discarded as what are termed *polar bodies*.

The sex cells (spermatozoa and ova) are known as *gametes*.

Fertilization

When the gametes unite in the process of fertilization, a *zygote* (a fertilized ovum) is formed, which receives half its chromosomes from the sperm and half from the ovum, making a full complement of 46 chromosomes (23 pairs). It is now referred to as a *somatic cell* (*soma* = body). This is the term used to describe any cell that possesses a full complement of chromosomes and that is said to be diploid in nature, the term meaning "doubled."

Fertilization, resulting in the formation of a zygote, also results in the fusion of the two nuclei, so that a single nucleus is formed (Fig. 1–29).

From this point, the somatic cell now formed undergoes the process known as *mitosis*.

The Process of Mitosis

Although mitosis is a continuous process, like meiosis it is usually divided into four stages, known also as prophase, metaphase, anaphase and telophase, which show characteristic features. The process of mitosis is

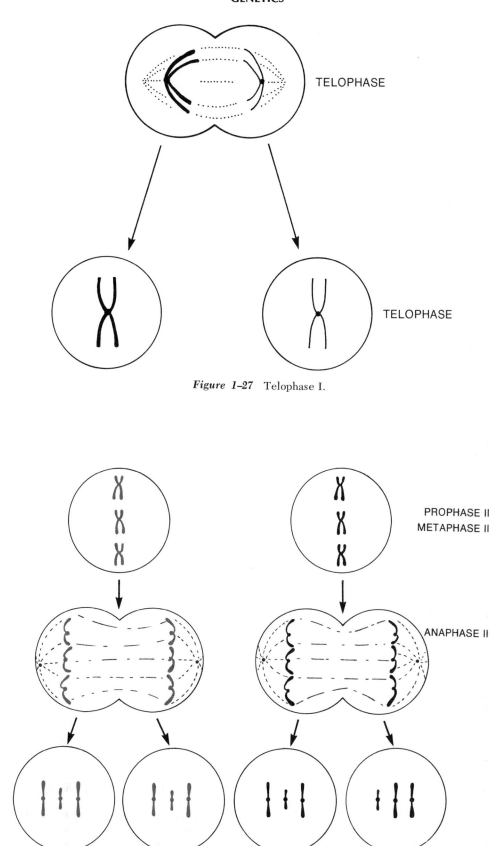

Figure 1-27 Telophase I.

Figure 1-28 The second meiotic division. Four daughter cells are produced, each being haploid in nature.

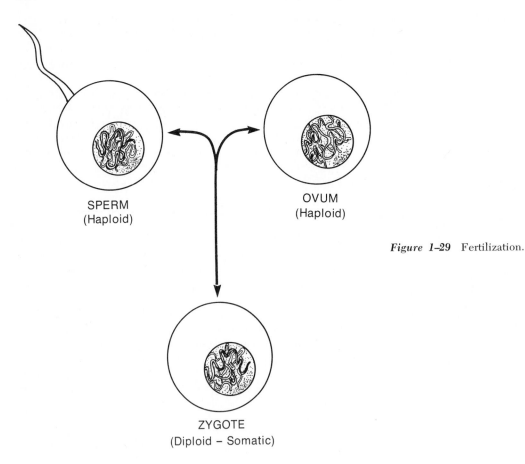

SPERM
(Haploid)

OVUM
(Haploid)

Figure 1-29 Fertilization.

ZYGOTE
(Diploid – Somatic)

shown diagrammatically in Figure 1–30, and is described as follows.

PROPHASE

As a cell prepares to divide, the chromosomes begin to condense by coiling up and thus becoming deeply staining bodies. As soon as the appearance of the nucleus changes and the chromosomes begin to be distinguishable, the cell has entered prophase. The DNA content of the cell has already doubled (see under the heading The Cell Cycle) and each chromosome therefore consists of two chromatids, held together at the centromere (also known as the *kinetochore*).

In addition to the contraction of the chromosomes, three other processes occur during prophase: the nuclear membrane loses its rigidity, the cell becomes polarized and the mitotic spindle is formed.

METAPHASE

During metaphase, the chromosomes move toward the center of the nucleus with each centromere taking up a position on the equatorial plate (also known as the metaphase plate), which is circumscribed by the equator of the spindle. By now the chromosomes have thickened and have become even more densely staining bodies. This is the stage at which individual chromosomes are most easily studied, since the chromatids have reached their most contracted state and the chromosomes are arranged in a more or less two-dimensional metaphase plate (see under the heading Karyotyping).

ANAPHASE

At the beginning of anaphase, the centromeres divide lengthwise. The two halves move in opposite directions toward the two poles, each one pulling a chromatid with it. The chromatids travel toward the poles as if drawn by the spindle, though the exact mechanism of movement of the chromosomes is unknown. The result of anaphase is that two identical sets of chromosomes arrive at the two opposite poles, where they reconstitute two daughter nuclei.

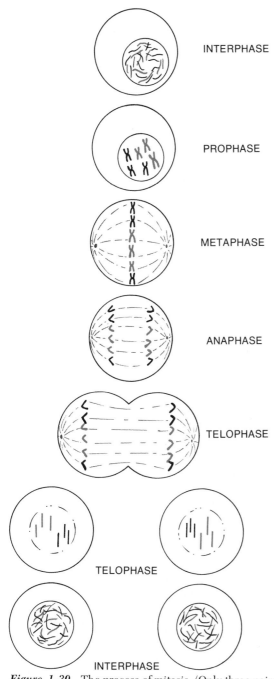

Figure 1–30 The process of mitosis. (Only three pairs of chromosomes are shown.)

TELOPHASE

The arrival of the chromosomes at the poles of the cell signifies the beginning of telophase, which may be regarded in many ways as the *reverse* of prophase. At the same time, the division of the cytoplasm begins by the formation of a furrow near the equatorial plate. Eventually a complete membrane is formed across the cell, which therefore becomes two cells,

each with the same number of chromosomes. These chromosomes unwind, become less densely staining bodies and eventually no longer stain as separate entities. The area in which they are located becomes enclosed by a nuclear membrane, which grows by the imbibition of water and by synthesizing protein and RNA. No DNA is synthesized unless the cell is to divide again. Each daughter cell therefore becomes a typical interphase cell, with the chromosomes actively participating in its metabolism.

THE MITOTIC (CELL) CYCLE

Before a cell divides, it must double its DNA content. This replication of DNA is known not to occur during mitosis, and therefore it was postulated that it must occur while the cell is in interphase (i.e., resting). In 1953, Howard and Pelc, in studying the root tip cells of the bean, *Vicia faba*, discovered that the cells incorporate radioactive phosphorus, P^{32}, *only* during a circumscribed period during the interphase prior to mitosis. Based on this information, they divided the intermitotic period into three phases, as follows:

1. G_1 or Gap_1: After division, the new cell enters a postmitotic period during which there is no DNA synthesis. This is known as G_1 or Gap_1.

2. S: The period of DNA synthesis follows, known as the "S" period.

3. G_2 or Gap_2: This is a premitotic nonsynthetic period, which is relatively short. During it the cells contain the duplicated amount of DNA and it is ended by the beginning of mitosis. Mitosis is of relatively short duration in comparison to the remainder of the cycle. Studies of human cells have shown that the complete cycle has a duration of 12 to 24 hours, whereas mitosis requires about one hour.

The stages of the mitotic cycle are shown diagrammatically in Figure 1–31.

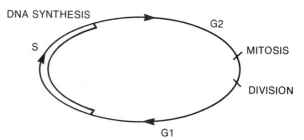

Figure 1–31 The mitotic (cell) cycle. (Modified from Stanners, C. P. and Till, J. E.: DNA synthesis in individual L-strain mouse cells. Biochim. Biophys. Acta 37:406, 1960.)

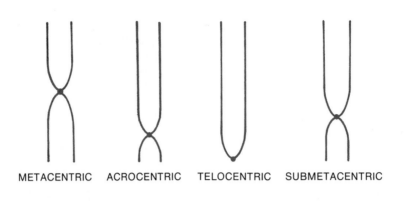

METACENTRIC   ACROCENTRIC   TELOCENTRIC   SUBMETACENTRIC

Figure 1–32   Chromosome classification according to
centromere position.

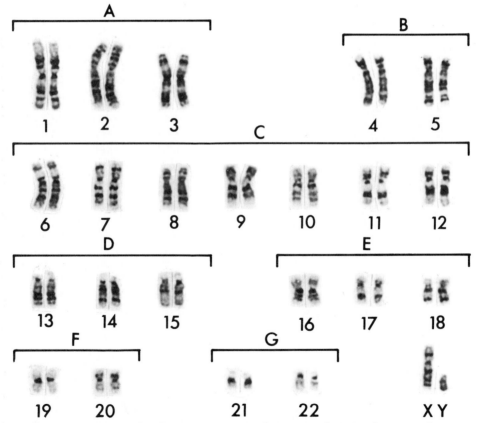

Figure 1–33   Human chromosome classification (From J. S. Thompson and M. W. Thompson: Genetics in Medicine.
3rd ed., W. B. Saunders Co., Philadelphia, p. 24, 1980.)

THE MENDELIAN LAWS

The growth of the body is therefore governed by the division of individual cells, which produce "daughter cells" containing precisely the same genetic information as the original parent cell.

The processes of cell division are covered by three laws devised by Mendel, and which, with certain exceptions, remain valid. These are *segregation, independent assortment* and *dependent assortment* (or *unit inheritance*).

Segregation. The segregation law states that the two members of a single pair of genes are never found in the same gamete but always segregate and pass to different gametes. This reduction division occurs once in the life of the sex cells, during meiosis.

Independent Assortment. Which one of a pair of chromosomes will end up in the sex cell at the reduction division is simply a matter of chance. The genes for different characteristics, therefore, segregate independently from one another in a completely random manner. This explains the variability between individuals.

Dependent Assortment (Unit Inheritance). Genes on the same chromosomes whose loci are within measurable distance of one another are usually inherited together as a unit and are said to be "linked."

Variation of the mendelian laws can occur as a result of two main processes: crossing over and mutation.

Crossing Over. This is the exchange of genetic material between homologous chromosomes (see Meiosis).

Mutation. If a quantitative or qualitative change occurs in a gene, a new gene may be formed. This new mutant gene occupies the locus of the gene it replaces and is passed to future generations. Its partner will often be a "normal" (i.e., unmutated, unchanged) gene. It should be noted that mutation is an extremely rare phenomenon among blood group genes, with a frequency of less than one in a million.

KARYOTYPING (CHROMOSOME CLASSIFICATION)

A group of cytogeneticists meeting at Denver, Colorado, in 1960 adopted a system for classifying and identifying human chromosomes on the basis of length and centromere position as seen during meiotic metaphase. Three chromosome classes were recognized:

metocentric, in which the centromere is situated in the center of the longitudinal axis; *acrocentric,* in which the centromere is very close to but not quite at one end; and *telocentric,* in which the centromere is at the very end. In 1962, Hamerton added the classification *submetocentric,* in which the centromere is placed in an intermediate position between that of the acrocentric and metacentric types (i.e., some distance from the end but not quite central) (Fig. 1–32).

In spite of this classification standard, it was still impossible to consistently identify every chromosome pair, and the 22 pairs of autosomes were therefore divided into seven *groups,* identified with the letters A to G in order of decreasing length. In this way, all chromosomes could be placed satisfactorily with a group, although the numbering within the groups was more or less tentative (Fig. 1–33).

In 1970, Caspersson *et al* demonstrated that when chromosomes are stained with quinacrine mustard or related substances and examined by fluorescence microscopy, each pair stains in a specific pattern of dark and light bands. The use of these banding techniques, along with other methods of identification, finally distinguished all 46 human chromosomes. Refinements in staining techniques now permit not only all human chromosomes but parts of chromosomes to be identified (Fig. 1–34).

If the chromosomes are to be analyzed, somatic cells (usually the white cells of the blood) are encouraged to undergo mitosis through stimulation with an agent known as *phytohemagglutinin,* which is an extract of red bean. The culture is incubated until the cells are dividing well, which usually takes about 72 hours.

A dilute solution of *colchicine* is then added, which stops mitosis at metaphase. A hypotonic solution is added to swell the cells and separate the chromatids while leaving their centromeres intact; the cells are then fixed, spread on slides and stained. A photograph is taken of the chromosomes through a microscope (Fig. 1–35), then individual chromosomes are cut from the photographic print, arranged in order in accordance with the Denver classification and mounted as shown in Figure 1–33. The process is called *karyotyping* and the complete picture is a *karyotype.*

When the chromosomes of a cell have been karyotyped, it is possible to determine whether they are normal in number and structure. The number is determined simply by counting,

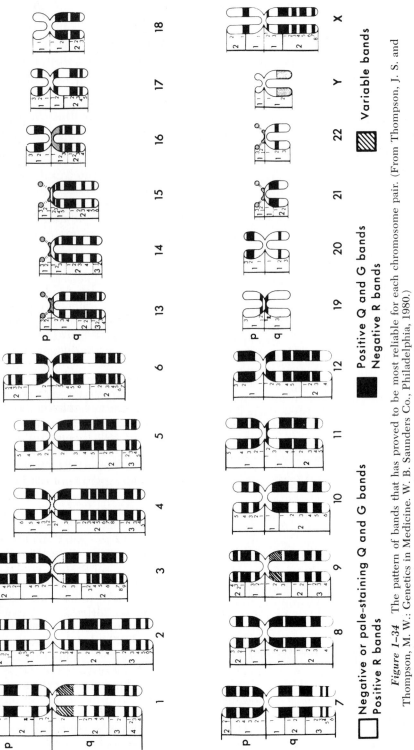

Figure 1-34 The pattern of bands that has proved to be most reliable for each chromosome pair. (From Thompson, J. S. and Thompson, M. W.: Genetics in Medicine. W. B. Saunders Co., Philadelphia, 1980.)

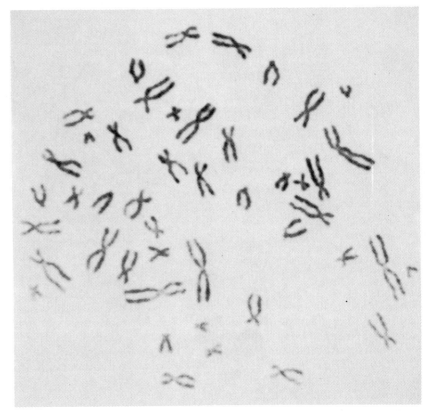

Figure 1–35 Human chromosomes in mitotic metaphase. (From Fraser, G. and Mayo, O.: Textbook of Human Genetics. J. B. Lippincott Co., Philadelphia, p. 213, 1975.)

though structural abnormalities are sometimes difficult to detect, especially if they are small. Banding techniques, however, greatly increase the probability of identifying specific chromosomal aberrations.

CHROMOSOMAL ABERRATIONS

Numerical Aberrations

Abnormalities of the chromosomes may be numerical or structural, and may affect autosomes, sex chromosomes or (rarely) both. In this section, only the more common types of chromosomal aberrations will be briefly discussed. The interested reader is referred to the general references at the end of this chapter for more detailed information.

Nondisjunction. This is the most common type of numerical aberration and results from the failure of paired chromosomes or sister chromatids to disjoin at anaphase either in a *mitotic* division, or in the first or second *meiotic* division (Fig. 1–36). The result of nondisjunction therefore is that two members of a chromosome pair, or two sister chromatids, end up in the same cell, resulting in an imbalance of chromosome or chromatid number.

The chromosome number in any one spe-

cies is usually constant. In humans, the characteristic diploid number is 46 *(2n)* and the characteristic haploid number is 23 *(n)*. Certain terms are used to describe a chromosome number that deviates from the normal, as follows:

Euploid. Any chromosome number that is an exact multiple of the haploid number is said to be *euploid*.

Polyploid. Chromosome numbers that are exact multiples of *n* but greater than 2n are said to be *polyploid*. Polyploidy can arise from a number of mechanisms, but 3n (triploidy) probably results from failure of one of the maturation divisions, either in the ovum or sperm, and 4n (tetraploidy) results from failure of completion of the first cleavage division of the zygote. Only a few triploids *(3n)* have been born alive and tetraploids *(4n)* have only been seen in early abortuses.

Aneuploid. Any chromosome number that is not an exact multiple of *n* is said to be *aneuploid*.

Trisomic Aneuploid. This type of aneuploid possesses 2n + 1 chromosomes and three members of one particular chromosome (as, for example, in Down's syndrome).

Monosomic Aneuploid. This type of aneuploid possesses 2n − 1 chromosomes and

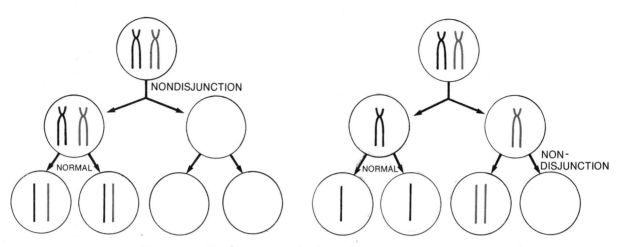

Figure 1-36   Nondisjunction at the first and second meiotic division.

therefore only one member of a particular chromosome pair.

In addition, double trisomics $(2n + 1 + 1)$ have an extra member of each of two chromosome pairs and so forth.

Heteroploid. Any number that deviates from the characteristic n and $2n$ is said to be *heteroploid,* whether it is euploid or aneuploid.

Structural Aberrations

Changes in chromosome structure usually result from chromosome breakage, which may be capable of passing through cell division unaltered (stable) or incapable of passing through cell division unaltered (unstable). The stable types include *deletions, duplications, inversions, translocations, insertions* and *isochromosomes.* These terms will be briefly defined here and shown diagrammatically. For more detailed information, consult the General References given at the end of this chapter.

Deletion. Deletion is the loss of part of a chromosome, which may involve one or more genes. The deleted portion, if it lacks a centromere, will fail to move on the spindle and will eventually be lost in a subsequent cell division. The affected chromosome lacks whatever genetic information was present in the lost fragment (Fig. 1-37).

Duplication. Duplication is the presence of an extra piece of chromosome, which usually originates from unequal crossing over. The reciprocal product is a deletion (Fig. 1-38). This results in the occurrence of a segment more than once in the same chromosome or genome.

Inversion. Inversion is the *rearrangement* of a group of genes in a chromosome in such a way that their order in the chromosome is reversed. This usually involves fragmentation of a chromosome by two breaks followed by reconstitution with inversion of the section of the chromosome between the break (Fig. 1-39).

Translocation. Translocation involves the transfer of part of one chromosome to another nonhomologous chromosome. If there is an exchange of parts between the two chromosomes, this is referred to as *reciprocal translocation.* The mechanism requires breakage of both chromosomes, with repair in an abnormal arrangement (Fig. 1-40).

Insertion. This is a type of translocation in which a broken part of a chromosome is *inserted into* a nonhomologous chromosome. The mechanism requires three breaks, with subsequent abnormal repair (Fig. 1-41).

Isochromosomes. This aberration occurs when, during cell division, the centromere of a chromosome separates transversely rather than longitudinally (Fig. 1-42).

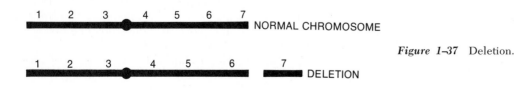

Figure 1-37   Deletion.

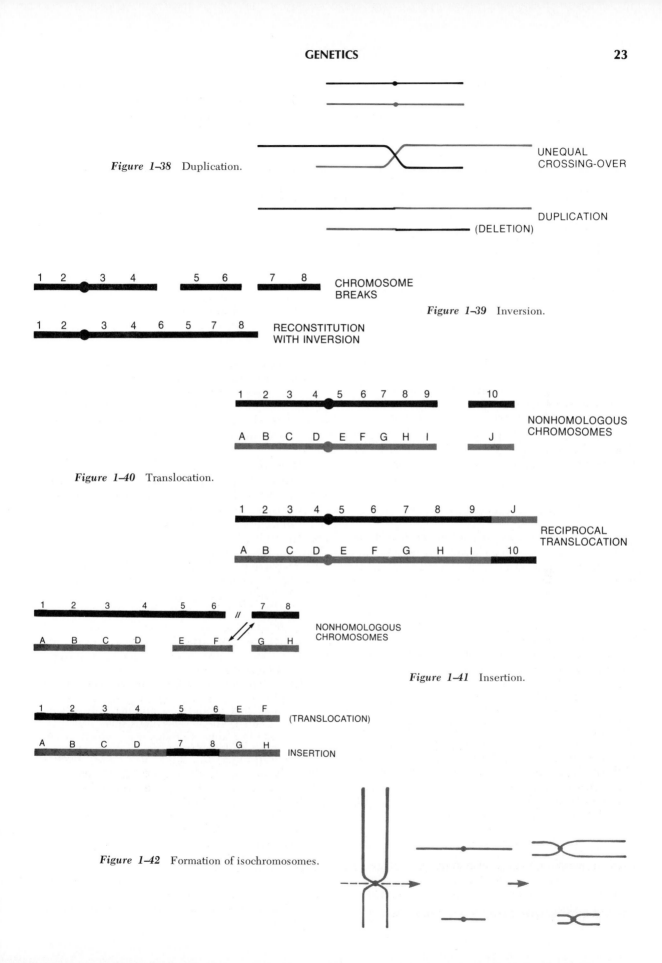

Figure 1-38 Duplication.

UNEQUAL CROSSING-OVER

DUPLICATION (DELETION)

CHROMOSOME BREAKS

RECONSTITUTION WITH INVERSION

Figure 1-39 Inversion.

NONHOMOLOGOUS CHROMOSOMES

Figure 1-40 Translocation.

RECIPROCAL TRANSLOCATION

NONHOMOLOGOUS CHROMOSOMES

Figure 1-41 Insertion.

(TRANSLOCATION)

INSERTION

Figure 1-42 Formation of isochromosomes.

Conclusion

The material presented in this chapter represents the basic principles of the science of genetics. The interested student will find many worthwhile texts on this fascinating subject, some of which have been listed under General References.

TYPICAL EXAMINATION QUESTIONS

The questions in this book are presented as an aid to students who wish to test their understanding of the various sections of study. The heading in parentheses given after each question refers to the section in which the question is discussed in the text. The answers to the questions can be found at the back of the book.

SECTION 1

Select the phrase, sentence of symbol that answers the question or completes the statement. Only one answer is considered correct in each case.

1. The original description of the science of genetics was made in
   (a) 1865 by Karl Landsteiner
   (b) 1865 by Gregor Mendel
   (c) 1900 by Gregor Mendel
   (d) The origins of genetics are unknown
   (History)

2. The number of single chromosomes in a somatic cell is
   (a) 24
   (b) 23
   (c) 46
   (d) 48
   (Chromosomes)

3. The nucleic acid component of the reproductive cell is known as
   (a) deoxyribonucleic acid
   (b) ribonucleic acid
   (c) nuclein
   (d) none of the above
   (The Chemical Basis of Inheritance — DNA)

4. The strands of DNA are *crosswise* connected by
   (a) organic bases through hydrogen (H) bonds
   (b) organic bases through nitrogen (N) bonds
   (c) phosphates
   (d) pentose sugars
   (The Chemical Basis of Inheritance — DNA)

5. The following are purine bases:
   (a) Thymine and cytosine
   (b) Adenine and guanine
   (c) None of the above
   (d) (a) and (b) are all purine bases
   (The Chemical Basis of Inheritance — DNA)

6. The base *guanine* in DNA always pairs with
   (a) cytosine
   (b) adenine
   (c) thymine
   (d) uracil
   (The Chemical Basis of Inheritance — DNA)

7. The specific position occupied by a gene on a chromosome is known as:
   (a) gene position
   (b) gene location
   (c) DNA position
   (d) locus
   (Genes)

8. A codon is a
   (a) two-base sequence of organic bases
   (b) four-base sequence of organic bases
   (c) three-base sequence of organic bases
   (d) sequence of bases not limited by number
   (Genes)

9. Alleles are
   (a) genes that occur in the homozygous state only
   (b) different *forms* of a gene at a given locus
   (c) different genes at different loci but on the same chromosome
   (d) genes that occur in the heterozygous state only
   (Genes)

10. When genes at a given locus on a pair of homologous chromosomes are identical, the individual is said to be
    (a) heterozygous
    (b) homozygous
    (c) hemizygous
    (d) None of the above
    (Genes)

11. A dominant gene is
    (a) a gene not producing a product in an individual
    (b) one that produces a product only when it occurs in the heterozygous state
    (c) one that always produces a product, regardless of whether it occurs in the homozygous or heterozygous state
    (d) one that produces a product only when it occurs in the homozygous state
    (Genes)

12. A female family member through which the family comes to be studied is known as the
    (a) propositus
    (b) proposita
    (d) Neither of the above
    (Family Studies)

13. An autosome is
    (a) any chromosome that is not a sex chromosome

(b) a sex chromosome
(c) a chromosome aberration
(d) any chromosome of human origin
(Sex Chromosomes)

14. With respect to the Xg blood group system, males can only be
    (a) heterozygous for Xg^a
    (b) homozygous for Xg^a
    (c) hemizygous for Xg^a
    (Sex Chromosomes)

15. The pentose sugar in RNA is
    (a) deoxyribose
    (b) uracil
    (c) thymine
    (d) ribose
    (RNA)

16. In RNA
    (a) thymine replaces uracil
    (b) uracil replaces thymine
    (c) adenine replaces uracil
    (d) uracil replaces guanine
    (RNA)

17. Ribosomes are composed of
    (a) nucleic acid
    (b) protein
    (c) ribosomal RNA (rRNA)
    (d) all of the above
    (RNA)

18. A cell that is not actively dividing is said to be in
    (a) interphase
    (b) prophase
    (c) metaphase
    (d) anaphase
    (The Process of Meiosis)

19. The final stage of prophase is known as
    (a) leptonema
    (b) diakinesis
    (c) diplonema
    (d) zygonema
    (The Process of Meiosis)

20. Four daughter cells are formed by one doubling of chromosomal material in meiosis. In females
    (a) only one of the four is a viable ovum
    (b) two of the four are viable ova
    (c) three of the four are viable ova
    (d) all four are viable ova
    (The Process of Meiosis)

21. A gamete is
    (a) a somatic cell
    (b) a blood cell
    (c) a sex cell
    (The Process of Meiosis)

22. A somatic cell is said to be
    (a) haploid in nature
    (b) diploid in nature
    (c) a sex cell
    (d) none of the above
    (Fertilization)

23. Immediately after division, a new cell enters a postmitotic period known as
    (a) gap 1
    (b) synthesis period

(c) gap 2
(d) none of the above
(The Mitotic Cycle)

24. Two members of a single pair of genes are never found in the same gamete, but always pass to different gametes. This mendelian law is known as
    (a) dependent assortment
    (b) unit inheritance
    (c) independent assortment
    (d) segregation
    (The Mendelian Laws)

25. In a *telocentric* chromosome
    (a) the centromere is close to but not quite at one end
    (b) the centromere is in the middle
    (c) the centromere is some distance from the end but not quite central
    (d) the centromere is at the very end
    (Karyotyping)

26. When two members of a chromosome pair or two sister chromatids fail to disjoin and end up in the same cell, resulting in an imbalance in chromosome or chromatid number, this is known as
    (a) deletion
    (b) translocation
    (c) nondisjunction
    (d) insertion
    (Chromosomal Aberrations)

27. Any chromosome number that is not an exact multiple of *n* is said to be
    (a) euploid
    (b) aneuploid
    (c) heteroploid
    (d) polyploid
    (Chromosomal Aberrations)

ANSWER TRUE OR FALSE

28. *Inversion* is the rearrangement of a group of genes in a chromosome in such a way that their order within the chromosome is reversed.
    (Chromosomal Aberrations)

29. The human cell possesses 23 pairs of autosomal chromosomes.
    (Chromosomes)

30. The basic physical structure of RNA is that of a double helix.
    (The Chemical Basis of Inheritance DNA)

31. An amorphic gene produces no detectable product.
    (Genes)

32. The male chromosome is known as the X chromosome.
    (Sex Chromosomes)

33. A ribosome is the manufacturing center for protein.
    (RNA)

34. The first stage of meiosis is known as prophase.
    (The Process of Meiosis)

35. A fertilized ovum is known as a zygote.
    (Fertilization)

GENERAL REFERENCES

The following texts were used as a source of reference in the preparation of this chapter, and will prove useful to students who wish to expand on their knowledge of the subject.

1. Gardner, E. J.: Principles of Genetics, 5th Ed. John Wiley and Sons, Inc., New York, 1975. *(This clear, well-written, excellently illustrated text provides both basic and advanced genetics in a way that is easy to understand and a pleasure to read.)*

2. Fraser, G. and Mayo, O. (eds.): Textbook of Human Genetics. Blackwell Scientific Publications, Oxford, 1975. *(A comprehensive text, well-illustrated and easy to understand. The chapter on Cytogenetics is particularly good.)*

3. Raphael, S. S.: Lynch's Medical Laboratory Technology, 3rd Ed. W. B. Saunders Co., Philadelphia, 1976. *(The chapter on Cytogenetics [Chapter 47, p. 1352] discusses the basic and the clinical aspects of the science. Considered excellent.)*

4. Thompson, J. S. and Thompson, M. W.: Genetics in Medicine, 3rd Ed. W. B. Saunders Co., Philadelphia, 1980. *(Probably the best basic text currently available. Should be part of every student's library.)*

Section Two

IMMUNOLOGY

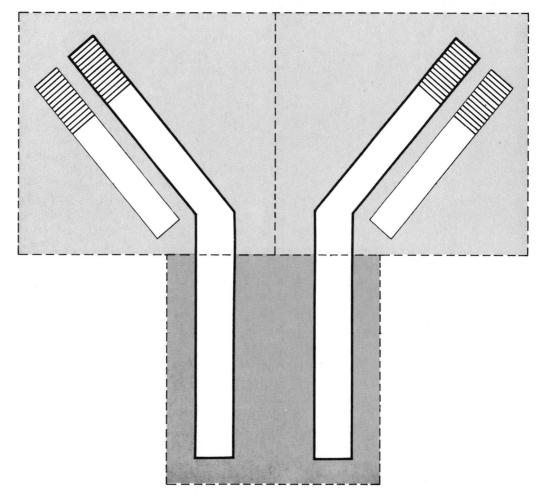

The human body does not distinguish between "harmful" and "non-harmful" foreign substances. All foreign substances that gain entry into the body are considered harmful and are labeled for destruction.

IMMUNOLOGY

OBJECTIVES — IMMUNOLOGY

The student shall know, understand and be prepared to explain:

1. A basic history of the science of immunology
2. The basic principles of humoral defense, specifically to include an understanding of the terms:
   Antigen
   Antibody
   Specificity
3. The basic principles of acquired immunity to include:
   (a) Natural acquired active immunity
   (b) Natural acquired passive immunity
   (c) Artificial acquired active immunity
   (d) Artificial acquired passive immunity
4. The composition of blood, with respect to
   (a) Cellular components (formed elements)
   (b) Plasma fractions
   (c) The difference between serum and plasma
5. The principles of the genetic inheritance of red cell antigens
6. The chemical characteristics of red cell antigens
7. The basic essentials for antigenic substances, specifically
   (a) Foreign substances
   (b) Size of molecules
   (c) Antigenicity
8. The factors that affect red cell antigens, specifically
   (a) Sex hormones
   (b) Enzymes
9. The stimulation of blood group antibodies by transfusion or pregnancy or both
10. Non-red cell–immune antibodies
11. Immunoglobulins, to include:
    (a) Structure of the basic molecule
    (b) The amino acid sequence of the chains with respect to
       (1) Variable portions of the molecule
       (2) Constant portions of the molecule
    (c) Site of antigen binding
    (d) Treatment with proteolytic enzymes papain, pepsin, and trypsin and fragments produced
    (e) Function
    (f) Domains
    (g) Types, to include:
       (1) IgG — structure, concentration, placental transfer, effects of enzymes, subclasses, production in fetus and newborn; also characteristics

       (2) IgM — structure, concentration, J chain, flexibility to bind complement, ability to cross the placenta, effects of enzymes, subclasses, production in newborns; also characteristics
       (3) IgA — structure, concentration, J chain, secretory piece (component), ability to bind complement, ability to cross the placenta, subclasses, effects of enzymes, production in newborns; also characteristics
12. The immune response, with reference to
    (a) The epithelial barriers
    (b) Inflammation
    (c) Phagocytosis
    (d) Complement
    (e) Antibody production
    (f) B-cells and T-cells—production and stimulation
13. The production of blood group antibodies, specifically to include:
    (a) Primary and secondary responses
    (b) Immunological memory
    (c) Tolerance
14. Antibody activity *in vivo* — extravascular and intravascular destruction
15. Complement, specifically to include:
    (a) The classical pathway of complement activation; sequence of events
    (b) The alternative pathway
    (c) Destruction of complement *in vitro* by
       (1) Anticoagulants
       (2) Heating
       (3) Zymosan
       (4) Normal serum inhibitor
       (5) Storage
16. Antibody activity *in vitro*, to include:
    (a) Sensitization
    (b) Agglutination and hemagglutination
    (c) Hemolysis
    (d) Precipitation
    (e) Inhibition (neutralization)
    (f) Complement fixation
17. Factors influencing antigen-antibody reactions, specifically to include:
    (a) "Reduced" IgG
    (b) Antibody size
    (c) Electrical repulsion between red cells (zeta potential)

(d) Enzymes
(e) Colloids
(f) Ionic strength
(g) Antigen characteristics — number of sites projecting from the cell membrane, proximity of sites
(h) Number of antibody molecules

(i) Serum or plasma (enhancing effect)
(j) pH
(k) Temperature
(l) Centrifugation
(m) Time
(n) Dosage
18. The Matuhasi-Ogata phenomenon

Introduction

The science of immunology concerns the study of resistance to infection and the rejection of "foreign" substances. Basically, it is a study of "immunity," which can be defined as the condition of a living organism whereby it overcomes infection or disease.

Humans (and all other living organisms) are equipped with an immune system to recognize and reject all substances foreign to themselves. Without this sytem, we would fall prey to all parasitic microorganisms that gain entry into the body, and inflammation, infection or disease would result.

The principles of immunology stem almost from the earliest written observations of mankind, in which it was realized that individuals who recovered from certain disease states rarely contracted the same disease again. This awareness prompted deliberate attempts to induce immunity through inoculation; in AD 1500 the Chinese developed a custom of inhaling crusts from smallpox lesions to prevent the development of smallpox in later life. This procedure was, of course, hazardous, yet its results probably led to the monumental work of Jenner, an English physician. In the late eighteenth century, he described a procedure of injecting pus from a lesion of an individual with cowpox into an individual free of disease and subsequently reinoculating the same individual with pus from a patient in the active state of smallpox. Individuals so treated were spared in subsequent smallpox epidemics, and the experiment was repeated several times with great success. The term *vaccination* (L. *vacca* = cow) was applied to the procedure, and referred specifically to the injection of smallpox "vaccine." The term is now generally used to mean an immunizing procedure in which vaccine is injected.

Jenner's work was extended almost 100 years later by Pasteur, who observed that the causative agent for chicken cholera induced immunity against that disease. These observations were soon applied to many other infectious diseases.

The general principles underlying vaccination were revealed by von Behring and Kitasato (1890), who demonstrated that induced immunity to tetanus was due to the appearance in the serum of a capacity to neutralize the toxin. This activity was noted to be so stable that it could be transferred to normal animals by infusions of blood or serum. This observation, along with others by Ehrlich at around the same time, opened the way to analysis of substances responsible for immunity. The term *antigen* (antibody + Gr. *gennan* = to produce) was used to describe the agent that conferred immunity on the host by the production of specific antibody, and it is on this principle that the modern science of *immunology* is based.

HUMORAL DEFENSE

When a foreign antigen gains entry into the body, specific antibodies may be produced by lymphocyte clones in the liver or spleen, which are released into the blood stream in the *globulin* portion of the plasma, and which are responsible in part for the destruction of the invading antigen. This is known as *humoral defense*, the term being defined as the response to invading substance that results in the production of specific antibody. It is important to note that the antibody formed is directed against that one specific invading substance. Any other foreign antigen that gains entry into the body will result in the production of a different antibody, which is specific for it.

Therefore, invading substances that cause the production of antibody are known by the general term *antigen*. In order to act as an antigen, however, the invading substance must be of sufficiently high molecular weight. Antigenic substances of low molecular weight (i.e., less than 5000) rarely stimulate the production of antibodies and are known as *haptens*. These haptens can, however, react with the antibody once formed, and can induce a strong immune response if coupled to a *carrier* protein of appropriate size (greater than 10,000). As a general rule, the more complex the molecule, the more effective it will be as an antigen. See under the heading Essentials for Antigenic Substances.

By definition, therefore, an "antigen" is a complex protein or polysaccharide substance of high molecular weight that, when introduced into a foreign circulation by infection or other means, stimulates the formation of antibodies that *specifically* combine with the antigen *in vivo* (within the body) or *in vitro* (outside the body).

An *antibody* is a substance found in the globulin portion of normal plasma or serum produced in response to the stimulation of an invading antigen and able to combine specifically with that antigen *in vivo* or *in vitro*.

Antibodies produced by an individual in response to antigens contained in the tissues of another of the same species are known as *alloantibodies*. Antibodies produced in one species that are active against antigens found in another species are known as *xenoantibodies* **or** *heterophile antibodies*. Antibodies produced by an individual in response to antigens possessed by that same individual are known as *autoantibodies*.

ACQUIRED IMMUNITY

Immunity to invading microorganisms may be acquired *naturally* or *artificially* and in an *active* or *passive* form. Active immunity indicates protection in the form of antibody produced by the host. Passive immunity indicates temporary protection not produced by the host (i.e., without the formation of antibody).

Natural Acquired Active Immunity. With this form, a disease state (e.g., measles) results in the production of specific antibody in the host, thus providing immunity to further attacks.

Natural Acquired Passive Immunity. This involves placental transfer of antibodies from mother to fetus, which provides temporary immunity (four to six months) from disease.

Artificial Acquired Active Immunity. This is defined as immunity against disease by the injection of virus or bacterium, resulting in the production of specific antibody by the host.

Artificial Acquired Passive Immunity. This is the injection of specific antibody (e.g., tetanus antitoxin) following injury or exposure, providing temporary immunity against disease.

Through these forms of immunity the body resists, copes with or is aided in combating the invasion of parasitic substances. In fact, the human body (as with all other living organisms) does not distinguish between so-called "harmful" and "nonharmful" foreign substances. *All* foreign substances that gain entry into the tissues are regarded as harmful and are labeled for destruction. This knowledge will help in the understanding of responses and protection provided by an individual's immune system against the invasion of foreign blood cells.

THE COMPOSITION OF BLOOD

Blood is a complex fluid tissue responsible for the supply of oxygen and food to the other tissues of the body and for the removal of carbon dioxide and waste products from them. Blood is made up of three formed elements, the cells, floating (suspended) in a protein and salt solution known as *plasma*. The cellular elements include erythrocytes (red cells), leukocytes (white cells) and thrombocytes (platelets). Each of these cells has its own function; they differ morphologically (i.e., in form and structure) and they have a characteristic life span. They are continually being destroyed, either because of old age or as a result of their functional activities, and replaced by newly formed cells. In healthy individuals there is a finely adjusted balance between the rates of formation and destruction, and thus the number of each cell type remains remarkably constant. In normal subjects, the red cells have an average life span in the circulation of between 100 and 120 days; white cells vary in their life span according to the *type* of white cell, and platelets have a life span of about 8 to 10 days.

The fluid plasma consists of a solution of 9 per cent solids in water. The main constituents are albumin, the chief protein constituent; fibrinogen, which is responsible in part for the clotting of blood; and globulins. Plasma also contains crystalloids, salts, buffers, hormones, proteins, enzymes and nutrient material. Under normal conditions, it constitutes 55 to 60 per cent of the total volume of blood.

It is important to understand that the cellular elements are held in suspension in the plasma. If blood is collected into a container with an *anticoagulant*, a substance that prevents the clotting of blood (see Chapter 17), the cellular elements will sink to the bottom of the container, because they are heavier than the plasma constituents, leaving the plasma as a translucent, straw-colored liquid on top.

We all know that when we cut ourselves, a clot eventually forms over the wound to prevent excessive bleeding. This is due to the action of

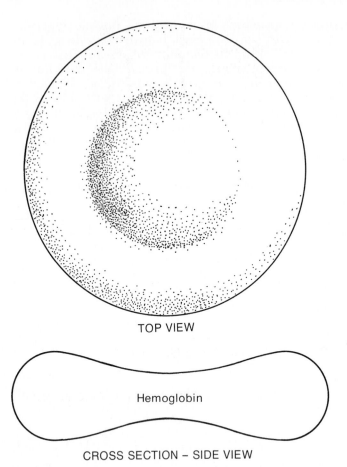

TOP VIEW

Hemoglobin

CROSS SECTION – SIDE VIEW

Figure 2–1 The red cell (erythrocyte).

fibrinogen, which converts to *fibrin* and forms a "mesh" over the wound. The same is true of blood collected into a "dry" tube (one that does not contain any anticoagulant). The fibrinogen is converted to fibrin, and the cells hold together in one large clot. The straw-colored fluid is now called *serum* because it lacks fibrinogen; that is, plasma without fibrinogen, or plasma from which fibrinogen has been removed, is called serum.

THE RED CELLS (ERYTHROCYTES)

Red cells in humans are small, *non-nucleated* (possessing no nucleus) biconcave discs that contain hemoglobin (an oxygen-carrying pigment responsible for the red color of fresh blood) (Fig. 2–1). The red cells number approximately 5 million per cubic millimeter in adults, ranging somewhat higher in men and lower in women. The red cell is flexible and can be readily distorted (e.g., in passage through the capillaries), but it quickly resumes its normal shape after distortion.

The red cell membrane (or outer cover) is composed of three layers: a bimolecular leaflet of phospholipids (the "hydrophobic" layer) covered internally and externally by layers of protein (the "hydrophilic" layers). *Note*: Hydrophobic = not readily absorbing moisture; hydrophilic = readily absorbing moisture (Fig. 2–2) (Singer and Nicolson, 1972).

The surface of the red cell carries a negative charge and thus repels other red cells. An important component of the red cell membrane

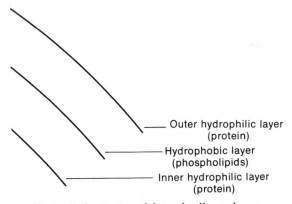

Outer hydrophilic layer (protein)
Hydrophobic layer (phospholipids)
Inner hydrophilic layer (protein)

Figure 2–2 Portion of the red cell membrane.

is the blood group antigens, which are situated largely on the external surface.

RED CELL ANTIGENS

Gene Products on the Red Cell

As discussed in Chapter 1, dominant genes in the homozygous and heterozygous state and recessive genes in the homozygous state express themselves through detectable products. Blood group genes express themselves through minute protein or glycolipid substances on or within the red cell membrane, (Fig. 2–3).

These cellular substances have specificity; that is, they are the products of specific genes. Because of their molecular size, they act as antigens. (They are capable of stimulating the production of specific antibody when introduced into a foreign circulation.) They are therefore known as *blood group antigens*.

When the two genes at allelic loci are identical (homozygous) the gene is said to be expressed in "double dose." When they are different (heterozygous), the gene is said to be expressed in "single dose." Amorphic genes, of which there are several examples among the blood groups, produce no product (Fig. 2–4).

The majority of blood group genes are dominant, allelic genes being co-dominant, and each particular gene is responsible for the production of many hundreds of *antigen receptors* on the red cell membrane. This is important, since it is necessary for many antibody molecules to combine with the appropriate antigen on each cell before agglutination, or

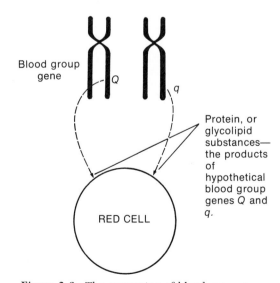

Figure 2–3 The expression of blood group genes on or within the red cell membrane.

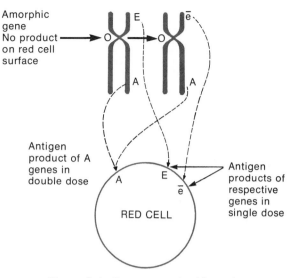

Figure 2–4 Gene expression (dosage).

"clumping," can occur (see under the heading Agglutination and Hemagglutination).

CHEMICAL CHARACTERISTICS OF BLOOD GROUP ANTIGENS

A great deal of work has been performed by various experts in attempts to understand the chemical characteristics of the red cell antigens — yet the facts remain somewhat sketchy. It is generally accepted, however, that red cell antigens are glycolipids or proteins. The specificity of the antigens is determined by the sequential addition of sugar residues to a common "precursor substance." This has proved to be the case in all blood group antigens studied so far.

The precursor substance is composed of four sugar molecules — two are known as D-galactose (GAL), one is N-acetyl-galactosamine (GAL NAc) and the last is N-acetyl-glucosamine (GNAc) (Fig. 2–5). Two types of precursor substance have been identified, known as Type 1 and Type 2 chains. These chains differ in the *linkage* of the terminal galactose molecule to the subterminal N-acetyl-glucosamine molecule. In Type 1 chains the linkage is beta (1 → 3), whereas in Type 2 chains the linkage is beta (1 → 4) (Chase and Morgan, 1961; Painter *et al*, 1963; Watkins, 1966) (Fig. 2–6A and *B*).

The addition of another sugar to this basic precursor determines the specificity of the antigen with the rest of the polysaccharide chain remaining unchanged.

Knowledge of the chemistry of blood group antigens has come mainly from work on body

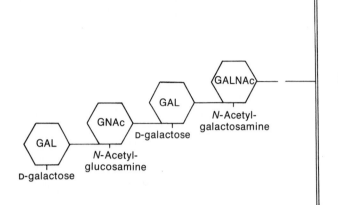

Figure 2–5 Precursor substance.

secretions (tears, semen, saliva and cyst fluids), since blood group *substances* on red cells are present in relatively small quantities and some of them are soluble only in alcohol. In *secretions,* these substances occur in much larger quantities and are soluble in water.

It has been established that the same sugars are present on the red cells, though on the red cells they are bound through sphingosine to fatty acid moieties. (Compounds of this type are known as *glycolipids.*)

The subject of the chemical nature of blood

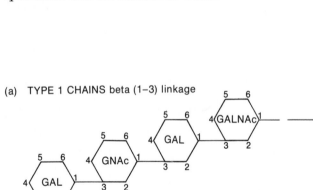

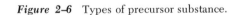

Figure 2–6 Types of precursor substance.

group antigens will be returned to in discussions of the individual blood group systems. The interested reader is also referred to the general references at the end of this chapter for more detailed information.

ESSENTIALS FOR ANTIGENIC SUBSTANCES

1. The first and most obvious essential for a substance to be antigenic is that it should present, at least in part, a configuration that is unfamiliar to the organism (i.e., that it should be a "foreign" substance).

2. The antigen molecule must have a sufficiently high molecular weight. The larger the molecule, the greater its likelihood of possessing unfamiliar determinant groups on its surface. The following may be taken as a guide:
(a) Molecules with a molecular weight below 5000 fail to act as antigens.
(b) Molecules with a molecular weight of 14,000 are poor antigens unless conjugated with adjuvants (enhancers).
(c) Molecules with a molecular weight of 40,000 or over are usually good antigens.
(d) High molecular weight molecules of 500,000 or more with complex protein or polypeptide-carbohydrate structures are the best antigens.

The lowest molecular weight limit for a substance to be a good antigen can be considered to be 40,000 to 50,000.

3. The *antigenicity* (the relative ability of a substance to stimulate the production of antibodies when introduced into a subject lacking the substance) is also dependent to some extent on both the *form* in which it is presented and the *route* of administration. Enzymes in phagocytic cells readily break down proteins. Enhancers (adjuvants) can help by prolonging effective contact; also, repeated administration may be of considerable significance. With respect to the route of administration, generally intravenous (into the vein) and intraperitoneal (into the peritoneal cavity) routes offer stronger stimulus than subcutaneous (beneath the skin) or intramuscular (into the muscle) routes.

FACTORS AFFECTING RED CELL ANTIGENS

Red cell antigens may be affected by sex hormones or enzymes. During pregnancy there is an apparent weakening of certain maternal antigens (see Chapter 4) and a fall in the level of A-specified transferase in the serum (Schachter *et al*, 1971; Tilley *et al*, 1978). Proteolitic en-

zymes remove sialopeptides from the red cell surface (Hubbard and Cohn, 1972), and inactivate or weaken several red cell antigens (see page 249). The effects appear to depend on the concentrations of the enzymes (Issitt *et al*, 1972). Red cells treated with enzymes take up certain antibodies at an increased rate, suggesting that the structures removed by enzyme treatment normally interfere with the access of the antibody to the corresponding antigen.

BLOOD GROUP ANTIBODIES

Stimulation of Blood Group Antibodies

As with the systems of natural and acquired immunity, red cells that present foreign antigenic configurations to the host are also considered harmful foreign substances, and specific antibody may be produced against them. Stimulation of blood group antibodies can occur by transfusion or through pregnancy.

By Transfusion. The transfusion of red cells possessing antigenic determinants foreign to the host may initiate an immune response.

Through Pregnancy. The placental transfer of red blood cells between infant and mother may initiate an immune response in the mother.

Red cell antibodies may occur in the serum of an individual who is not known to have had contact with the corresponding antigen. Such antibodies are referred to by some workers as *naturally occurring* (see Mollison, 1979), though the term probably holds an inaccurate connotation, since these antibodies are almost certainly the result of some sort of outside stimulus. The terms "non-red cell" and "non-red cell immune" have crept into modern usage, though even they may not reveal the whole story.

Note: A patient can only become immunized to a red cell antigen when that specific antigen is *lacking from the patient's own red cells*. Certain exceptions to this rule will be described later in this text.

Immunoglobulins

Antibodies belong to a family of proteins known as *immunoglobulins* (Ig) and occur in five different forms that possess two main features in common: (1) the basic *structure* of the molecule and (2) the *function* of the molecule (i.e., the ability to combine specifically with a corresponding antigenic determinant).

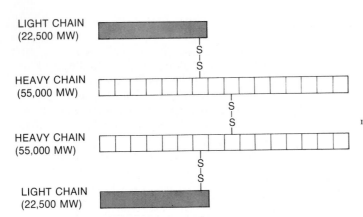

LIGHT CHAIN
(22,500 MW)

HEAVY CHAIN
(55,000 MW)

HEAVY CHAIN
(55,000 MW)

LIGHT CHAIN
(22,500 MW)

Figure 2–7 The basic structure of the immunoglobulin molecule.

Structure of the Molecule

The basic structural unit of the antibody molecule comprises a pair of larger polypeptide chains, so-called "heavy" (H) chains by virtue of their high molecular weight, coupled to a pair of smaller polypeptide chains, so-called "light" (L) chains by virtue of their lower molecular weight. The four chains are held together by covalent (disulphide) and noncovalent bonds. A model for the basic structure of the immunoglobulin molecule reveals a symmetrical, four-peptide unit consisting of two heavy chains and two light chains linked by interchain disulphide bonds (Fig. 2–7).

There are five *classes* of immunoglobulin, which are called IgG, IgA, IgM, IgD and IgE, with H chains γ, α, μ, δ or ϵ, respectively. In contrast, there are only two types of L chains — kappa (κ) and lambda (λ). Note that any H chains class may be combined with any L chain type. Therefore, there are 10 possible combinations of heavy and light chains, and all 10 are normally found in any individual. Whereas H chains are combined with any L chain type, it should be noted that in any immunoglobulin molecule the L chains will be *either* kappa or lambda, but never both together.

A general feature of the immunoglobulin chains is their *amino acid sequence*. The first 110 to 120 amino acids of both the heavy and light chains have a *variable* sequence and form the variable (V) region thought to determine antibody specificity. The rest of the light chains represent a constant (C) region with an amino acid sequence that is similar for each type and subtype. The rest of the heavy chain is also constant for each type and subtype and has a "hinge" region that gives the molecule flexibility (shown in Fig. 2–8).

The site of antigen-binding is believed to be located at the end of the heavy and light chains in the variable portion of the molecule (Fig. 2–8). Biological activities other than an-

tigen binding are the responsibility of the constant portion of the heavy chains (see following discussion).

Porter (1959) demonstrated that treatment of IgG (which consists of a single structural unit) with the enzyme papain splits the molecule into three fragments. Two of these fragments appeared to be identical and were shown to be capable of binding specifically with antigen, though they were not capable of causing agglutination or precipitation reactions, even in a high protein medium or with enzyme-treated cells (Fudenberg *et al*, 1964). These two fragments were called "Fab" (since the *f*ragments are capable of *a*ntigen *b*inding). Each of these fragments is composed of one light chain and one half of one heavy chain. The remaining fragment, in rabbit IgG, was found to crystallize upon purification and was therefore called Fc (*f*ragment *c*rystalline). This Fc fragment was found to be composed of two halves of two heavy chains and was further found to be involved in complement activation, fixation to the skin and placental transport (McNabb *et al*, 1976), though it does not have the ability to combine with antigen (see Fig. 2–8).

Treatment of IgG with the enzyme pepsin results in a slightly different Fab-type fragment that not only retains the ability to bind with antigen but also is capable of causing agglutination or precipitation reactions. This fragment is known as F(ab')$_2$. It has two halves of two heavy chains. The remainder of the molecule is split into many small fragments by pepsin digestion (Fig. 2–9).

The enzyme *trypsin* has also been employed in the fragmentation of immunoglobulins. Fragments produced by trypsin after short periods of digestion are the same as those produced by papain (i.e., two Fab(t) fragments and one Fc(t) fragment). Prolonged digestion with trypsin results in cleavage of the peptide chain and the production of so-called "tryptic peptides."

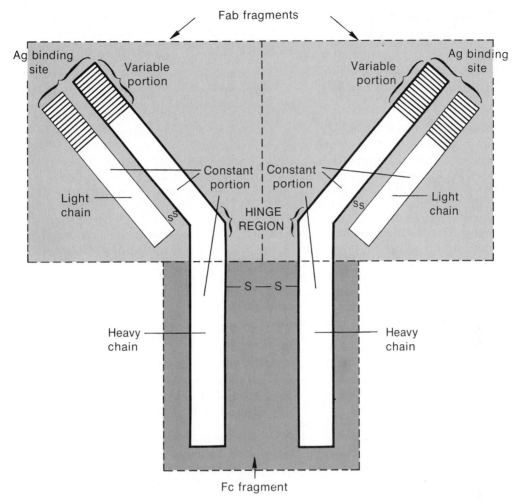

Fab fragments

Ag binding site

Variable portion

Constant portion

Light chain

Constant portion

Variable portion

Ag binding site

Light chain

HINGE REGION

S — S

Heavy chain

Heavy chain

Fc fragment

Figure 2–8 Antibody molecule—the basic structural unit.

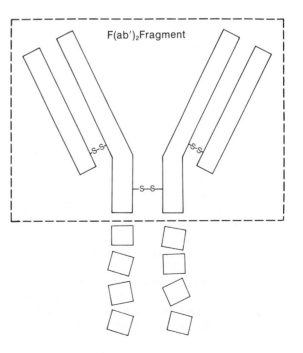

F(ab')₂Fragment

Figure 2–9 Cleavage of antibody molecule by pepsin.

These findings provided the following information: (1) The Fc portion of the molecule directs the *biological activity* of the antibody (e.g., placental transfer, complement fixing). (2) The Fab portion of the molecule is involved in antigen binding.

The Function of Immunoglobulin

For each molecule of foreign antigen, millions of specific antibody molecules may be produced and secreted into body fluids. The function of these immunoglobulin molecules is to *combine* with antigens on cellular surfaces, which then results in the destruction of the cells either extravascularly (outside the blood vessels) within the reticuloendothelial system or intravascularly (within the blood vessels) through the action of complement. Immunoglobulin molecules are also responsible for the neutralization of toxins (poisonous substances) and the facilitation of phagocytosis.

Immunoglobulin Domains

In addition to *interchain* disulphide bonds, which form the *connecting links*, the heavy and light chains of each immunoglobulin molecule

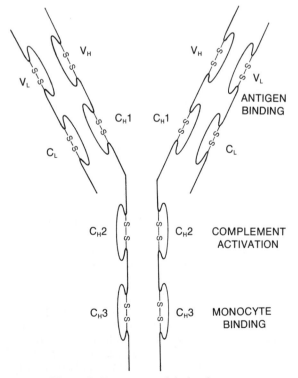

Figure 2–10 Immunoglobulin domains.

have *internal* disulphide links. These latter bonds form loops in the peptide chains that are compactly folded to form globular "domains" (Edelman, 1971) (Fig. 2–10). Each of these domains appears to serve a separate function. The variable region domains (V_L and V_H) are responsible for the formation of a specific antigen-binding site; the C_H2 region in IgG binds C1q, initiating the classic complement sequence; the C_H3 region is responsible for adherence to the monocyte surface. The variable part of the Ig heavy chain (V_H) occurs in three different forms, subgroups V_HI, V_HII and V_HIII, each of which can be recognized in IgG, IgM and IgA with appropriate antisera. Particular red cell alloantibodies tend to be made predominantly of one subgroup (Natvig et al, 1976 [b]) (Førre et al, 1977). Note that V_H restriction is independent of IgG subclass (see the heading IgG) or L-chain type.

Types of Immunoglobulin

The three classes of immunoglobulin that concern immunohematologists are IgG, IgM and IgA. Very little is known of the function of IgD, and IgE is known to carry reaginic antibody activity (i.e., it behaves like an antibody in complement fixation and similar reactions), has an extra domain and may have a role as a line of defense in respiratory allergies. Since these latter immunoglobulins are not applicable to the study of immunohematology, this discussion will be confined to the study of IgG, IgM and IgA.

The immunoglobulin classes are distinguished and categorized on the basis of their physiochemical, antigenic or biological properties, as summarized in Table 2–1.

IgG

Of the major classes of immunoglobulins, IgG, accounting for approximately 85 per cent of the total immunoglobulin with a plasma concentration of 800 to 1680 mg per 100 ml (or approximately 7.3 to 23.7 grams per liter), is the most important in humans. Most bacterial antibodies, virus-neutralizing antibodies, precipitating antibodies, hemagglutinins and hemolysins are IgG.

The IgG molecule consists of one basic structural unit known as a *monomer* (as shown in Fig. 2–8) possessing two heavy chains (γ) and two light chains that may be kappa or lambda, but not both. The molecule is capable of chang-

Table 2–1 PROPERTIES OF THE MAIN IMMUNOGLOBULINS IN SERUM

Characteristic	IgG	IgM	IgA
Heavy chains	γ	μ	α
Light chains	κ or λ	κ or λ	κ or λ
Molecular formula	$\gamma_2\kappa_2$ or $\gamma_2\lambda_2$	$(\mu_2\kappa_2)_5$J or $(\mu_2\lambda_2)_5$J	$\alpha_2\kappa_2(\alpha_2\kappa_2)_2$* $\alpha_2\lambda_2(\alpha_2\lambda_2)_2$*
Molecular weight	150,000	900,000	160,000 330,000*
Sedimentation coefficient	7S	19S	7S, 105S*
Percentage carbohydrate (serum)	3	11.8	7.5
Normal serum concentration (mg/100 ml)	1275(±280)	125(±45)	225(±55)
g/l adult range	7.3–23.7	0.47–1.47	0.61–3.3
g/l newborn	Slightly higher than adult	±0.1	Undetectable
Catabolic rate (T$^{1/2}$(d))	23	5	6
Percentage intravascular	44	80	40
Fractional catabolic rate (%/d)	7	18	33
Crosses placenta	Yes	No	No
Usual serologic behavior	"Incomplete" antibody	Agglutinin ("complete" ab)	Agglutinin ("complete" ab)
Serologic behavior after heating to 56° C for 3 hours	Unaffected	Reduced	Unaffected
Effect of alkylating agents on serologic behavior	May develop agglutinating activity	No longer agglutinates	Partially inactivated
Turnover rate (synthesis, mg/kg/d)	28	5–8	8–10
Complement fixation	Yes	Yes	No
Presence in colostrum	Yes	No	Yes
Usual temperature of reaction	37° C	20° C	37° C
Usual antigenic stimulus of red cell antibodies	Transfusion or pregnancy	Often "naturally occurring"	
Isoelectric points	6.2–8.5	5.5–7.4	4.8–6.5
Electrophoretic migration	Slow gamma	Slow gamma	Slow beta
Water solubility	Soluble	Insoluble	Soluble
Gm specificity (on gamma chains)	Yes	No	No
Km specificity (on kappa chains)	Yes	Yes	Yes
Antibody activity	Yes	Yes	Yes
External secretions	No	No	Yes
Effect of 2-ME and DTT	Not affected	Inactivated	Partial inactivation

*In serum, 10 per cent of IgA is in the form of dimers.

ing its shape: free IgG is usually Y-shaped, whereas antigen-bound IgG may adjust its shape to accommodate the antigen or to expose hidden sites responsible for various functions such as complement fixation (Edelman, 1971). This shape change is facilitated by the so-called "hinge" region (shown in Fig. 2–8) where the chains are uncoiled, allowing for considerable flexibility.

IgG is the only immunoglobulin to be transferred from mother to fetus, a fact that explains its role in the etiology of hemolytic disease of the newborn (see Chapter 16). This placental transfer is facilitated by a site on the Fc portion of the molecule that allows for attachment to placental tissue (McNabb et al, 1976).

Effects of Enzymes on IgG. Digestion with papain splits the IgG molecule into two Fab fragments and one Fc fragment (shown in Fig. 2–8). This attack generally takes place around the hinge region of the molecule.

Digestion with pepsin splits the molecule into an F(ab′)₂ fragment consisting of two Fab′ fragments joined together by a variable number of disulphide bonds. Pepsin degrades the Fc fragment (shown in Fig. 2–9).

Subclasses of IgG. Four subclasses of IgG have been recognized on the basis of structural and serological differences and are known as IgG1, IgG2, IgG3 and IgG4. We know IgG1 is the most abundant in normal adult serum and IgG4 is the least abundant (Morrell et al, 1971).

The number of interheavy chain disulphide bonds in the hinge region varies in the different subclasses — there are two such bonds in IgG1 and IgG4, there are four in IgG2 (Nisonoff et al, 1975) and eleven in IgG3 (Michaelsen et al, 1977) (Fig. 2–11).

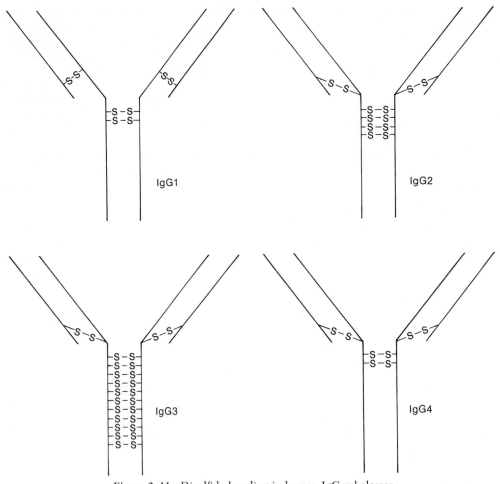

Figure 2–11   Disulfide bonding in human IgG subclasses.

Differences in IgG subclasses are recognized by antisera against polymorphic antigenic determinants on gamma chains, known as *Gm allotypes*. In addition, there are differences between the subclasses with respect to binding of macrophages, activation of complement, reactivity with dextrans and half-life, so that biological activity depends on the subclass of an antibody. Some characteristics of IgG subclasses are given in Table 2–2.

Production of IgG in the Fetus and Newborn. At birth, a small amount of IgG in the serum is of fetal origin (Mårtensson and Fuden-berg, 1965); the majority, however, is derived from the mother by placental transfer. Immunoglobulin levels start to increase between three and six weeks after birth, and antibodies are first demonstrable at about two months by which time the immunoglobulin level has reached 2 g/l (Zak and Good, 1959). Changes in immunoglobulin levels in the first year of life are shown graphically in Figure 2–12.

IgM

The IgM molecule is made up of five basic structural units in a circular arrangement. It

Table 2–2   SOME CHARACTERISTICS OF IgG SUBCLASSES

	IgG1	*IgG2*	*IgG3*	*IgG4*
Concentration in normal serum (% total IgG)	65	25	6	4
Average concentration in normal serum (g/l)	6.63	3.22	0.58	0.46
Half-life (days)	22	22	9	22
Complement fixation	Yes	Yes	Yes	No
Cryoprecipitation	Yes		Yes	
Reactivity with Dextrano	Yes	Yes	Yes	No

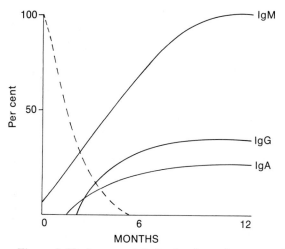

Figure 2–12 Immunoglobulin levels in first year of life. Dotted line indicates maternal IgG. (From Mollison, 1979, based on data of West *et al*, 1962.)

therefore possesses ten heavy chains and ten light chains. The heavy and light chains are linked to each other by disulphide bonds in the same general way as IgG, but there are additional disulphide bonds linking the Fc portions of alternate heavy chains so as to produce a molecule with a central circular portion and five radiating arms (Fig. 2–13).

Electron micrographs of IgM molecules show them to be about 300 Å (Å = angstrom, a unit of measurement equal to 10^{-7} mm) in diameter, the arms being 25 to 30 Å wide and 100 Å long, the length of the branched sections being 55 to 70 Å. The molecular weight of the molecule is about 900,000.

The average concentration of IgM in normal serum is about 1.0 g/l, of which about 80 per cent is intravascular, and 15 to 18 per cent is catabolized per day (Cohen and Freeman, 1960;

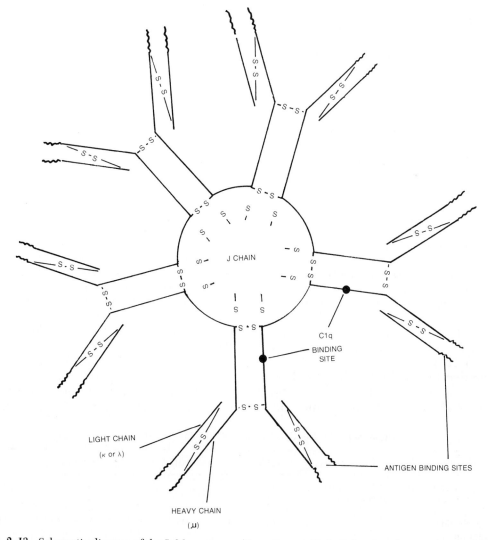

Figure 2–13 Schematic diagram of the IgM pentamer. (From Bryant, N. J.: Laboratory Immunology and Serology. W. B. Saunders Co., Philadelphia, 1979.)

Schultze and Heremans, 1966; Brown and Cooper, 1970).

The heavy chains of the IgM molecule are mu (μ) chains; the light chains, as in IgG, are either kappa or lambda but not both. A third type of chain is invariably found in association with intact IgM (and with polymerized IgA). (*Note: polymerization* is the act of forming a compound, usually of high molecular weight by the combination of simpler molecules.) This third type of chain is thought to function in the joining or linking together of the molecule's subunits. This chain is known as the *J chain* (J = joining), has a molecular weight of 15,000 and is a polypeptide that contains about 10 per cent carbohydrate. The structure and precise function of the J chain in relation to IgM and IgA are not fully elucidated.

Like IgG, the IgM molecule appears to be quite flexible in the region of the "hinge." It is capable of assuming numerous different shapes from the fully extended form shown in Figure 2–13 to a dumpy "crablike" form in Figure 2–14.

The IgM antibody may appear after primary antigenic stimulus (see following discussion) and in most cases is the first to appear in phylogeny (i.e., in a given species of animal) and the last to leave in senescense (the condition of growing old, i.e., deterioration). During the "primary response" (discussed later), synthesis of IgM usually diminishes as the concentration of IgG increases.

There is some doubt whether all IgM molecules are capable of binding complement, although when the immunoglobulin is involved in complement activation, the response is usually powerful (see discussion of Complement).

IgM is not transported across the human placenta.

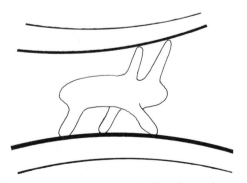

Figure 2–14 One of the possible shape changes of IgM. (From Bryant, N. J.: Laboratory Immunology and Serology. W. B. Saunders Co., Philadelphia, 1979.)

Effects of Enzymes on IgM. Treatment of IgM with papain splits the molecule into F(ab')$_2$ fragments with a molecular weight of about 90,000, or further into Fab' fragments with a molecular weight of about 40,000. These Fab' fragments retain the capacity to combine with antigen. Shorter periods of digestion with trypsin produces fragments similar to those derived by papain hydrolysis. In addition, the disulphide bonds linking the Fc portions can be broken by reducing agents (e.g., 2-mercaptoethanol).

Subclasses of IgM. No subclasses of IgM are recognized.

Production of IgM in Newborns. Since IgM is not transferred across the placenta, all IgM in "cord" serum (obtained from the umbilical cord) is of fetal origin. In general, the concentration in cord serum is between 5 and 10 per cent of that found in adult serum (Franklin and Kunkel, 1958; Polley *et al*, 1962).

Several IgM antibodies can be found in cord serum (e.g., anti-I, anti-A and anti-B occasionally and anti-λ chain, in about 90 per cent) (Epstein, 1965).

The concentration of IgM starts to rise within two to three days after birth, reaches 50 per cent of the adult level in two to three months and 100 per cent at about nine months (see Fig. 2–12).

IgA

The main serum component of IgA has been found to have a sedimentation constant of about 7, with minor components at 10, 13, 15 and 17 to 18: this suggests that the molecule can be found in varying degrees of polymerization, ranging from a single structural unit (monomer) to a double structural unit (dimer). In serum 90 per cent of IgA occurs as monomer (e.g., $\alpha_2 \lambda_2$) and 10 per cent as dimer, e.g., $(\alpha_2 \kappa_2)_2$. The heavy chains of the molecule are alpha (α) and the light chains, as in IgG and IgM, may be either kappa or lambda, but not both.

IgA is the main immunoglobulin in various body secretions such as saliva, colostrum, tears and secretions of the bronchial and gastrointestinal tracts, where it serves as the first line of defense against microorganism invasion. It is believed that the presence of IgA in secretions is due almost entirely to *local production* rather than to transport from plasma.

IgA, with a molecular weight of 160,000, constitutes 10 to 15 per cent of the total human immunoglobulin, with an average serum concentration of 225 mg/100 ml (2.2 g/l) of which about 40 per cent is intravascular. After equilibration with the total IgA space, injected IgA disappears with a half-life of about six days (Tomasi *et al*, 1965).

Following synthesis (production), some IgA finds its way into the systemic circulation, but most of it passes through or between the epithelial cells to be secreted. This last is referred to as *secretory IgA* (SIgA), of which about 90 per cent is found as dimer, coupled to a small "secretory" component. The SIgA molecule, therefore, is made up of two basic structural units, with a J chain similar to that found in IgM. This J chain is also found in polymeric forms of serum IgA. The glycoprotein secretory component (MW 60,000), which is linked to the respective heavy chains of the molecule by disulphide bonds, is thought to make the molecule more resistant to enzyme attacks and may protect it from intracellular degradation during transit through the epithelial cell cytoplasm or in the secretions (Fig. 2–15).

IgA does not fix complement and is not transported across the human placenta.

Subclasses of IgA. Two subclasses of IgA are known to exist — a major component, IgA1, and a minor component, IgA2. They are distinguished on the basis of antigenic differences in the alpha chain (Kunkel and Prendergast, 1966; Vaerman and Heremans, 1966, Jerry *et al*, 1970) as well as because of striking structural differences (Gray, 1970).

Effects of Enzymes on IgA. An enzyme produced by *enteric streptococci* has been found to have proteolytic activity specific for the IgA1 subclass. This enzyme cleaves IgA1 molecules in the hinge region and produces fragments quite similar in size to the Fab and Fc fragments of IgG. IgA2 is impervious to the enzyme.

Treatment of IgA with 2-mercaptoethanol usually weakens the *serological* activity of the antibodies. IgA monomers (7S) are apparently unaffected, but polymers (9S, 11S etc.) are inactivated (Tomasi, 1965).

Production of IgA in Newborns. IgA cannot be detected in cord serum. By the age of 2 months, the amount of IgA in the serum has reached about 20 per cent of the adult level (West *et al*, 1962).

THE IMMUNE RESPONSE

The immune response in man can be thought of conveniently as a series of related defenses. The first, referred to as "natural" or "innate" immunity, is the process by which the invasion of foreign or potentially harmful microorganisms is resisted by "natural" means (i.e., without the production of protective antibodies). This includes the following concepts:

Susceptibility and Nonsusceptibility. Certain animal species are resistant to particular disease states, whereas other species are highly susceptible to them. This phenomenon is not clearly understood, yet would appear to be controlled to some extent by hereditary or genetic influences. With respect to the blood groups, the Duffy antigens have been shown to be involved in susceptibility and nonsusceptibility to the malarial parasite (see Chapter 7). These concepts are not confined to species differences; they have been evident in different members of the *same species*, as seen in differences among various human groups and in those due to the effects of age and the influence of hormones.

The Epithelial Barriers. The skin and mucous membranes act as a *physical barrier* against parasite penetration and, in addition, possess certain active mechanisms for the killing of bacteria and other organisms. Lactic acid in sweat and fatty acids in sebaceous secretions are thought to be responsible for this bactericidal activity. The mucous membranes, by contrast, are protected primarily by a so-called "slime layer," which has been shown to possess antibodies of the IgA class and other antiviral and antimicrobial substances.

Inflammation. When microorganisms gain entry into the tissues, a series of *cellular* changes occur that cause an increase in the number of leukocytes at the site of injury, the formation of fibrin in the tissue to prevent blood loss, increased blood and lymph flow that dilutes and flushes away toxic substances, general or local rise in temperature, redness, swelling and pain. This is known as the *inflammatory process*. Inflamed areas, when studied microscopically, show heavy infiltration of polymor-

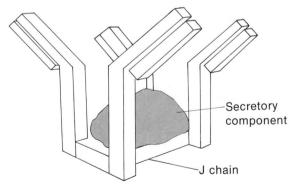

Figure 2–15 Secretory IgA (SIgA).

phonuclear phagocytes (neutrophils and eosin-
ophils) and also mononuclear phagocytes
(monocytes and macrophages). These two
groups of phagocytes are scavenger cells, serving to engulf and carry away debris introduced
into the tissues (see under the heading Phagocytosis.)

Phagocytosis. Early descriptions of the remarkable phenomenon of phagocytosis are attributed to Elie Metchnikoff (1907), a Russian-
born biologist, who recognized that specialized
phagocytic (eating) cells provide a defense
mechanism against invasion by engulfing
foreign particulate matter that they then attempt
to destroy enzymatically. Metchnikoff observed
that the process is a very general one and can be
observed in animals of all stages of evolution.
When injected microorganisms are engulfed by
phagocytes, no disease follows, whereas inoculation of microbes that resist the phagocytic
attack results in a disease state.

The ingestion of foreign particles occurs as
follows: Once the phagocyte has recognized
that a particle is foreign, engulfment occurs by
active ameboid motion (resembling an ameba in
movement). The phagocyte extends its cyto-
plasmic membrane around the invading organism, which is eventually surrounded and completely enclosed. The final structure containing
the phagocytized particle is known as a phagocytic *vacuole* or *phagosome* (Fig. 2–16).

Complement. Complement (see later discussion) is involved in defense through a
number of mechanisms that either involve the
full activation of the complement system to
destroy the membrane of invading organisms or
partial activation, which makes the microorganism more susceptible to phagocytosis.

The second and third events in the immune
response are far more specific and involve a
direct response to a *particular* invading substance. These stages are mounted by cells responsible for immunologic function (T-cells
and B-cells; see later discussion). The final
event involves "immunologic memory," described later. Immunohematology is primarily
concerned with the products of B-cells — the
circulating antibodies present in the serum.

Types of Immunity Involving Antibody

When foreign antigen gains entry into the
body, two types of immunological reactions
may occur. These fundamentally similar mechanisms are known as *humoral* and *cell-
mediated* immunity. Humoral immunity refers
to the synthesis and release of free antibody
into the blood and other body fluids, which is
capable of combining with specific foreign antigen. Cell-mediated immunity refers to the
production of "sensitized" lymphocytes, which
takes part in such reactions as the rejection of
skin transplants and the delayed hypersensitivity to tuberculin seen in persons immune to
tubercle bacilli.

B-Cells and T-Cells

The "parent" cell of all erythroid, myeloid
and lymphoid cells is known as the pluripotent
hemopoietic "stem cell." It migrates from the
yolk sac through the fetal liver, spleen and bone
marrow. From these sites, *lymphoid* stem cells
migrate to the thymus where further differentiation occurs, resulting in the production of
thymus-derived cells, known as T-cells. Other
lymphoid stem cells are independent of the
thymus. In birds they come under the influence
of the bursa of Fabricius; in man and other
mammals, a mammalian equivalent such as the
fetal liver, bone marrow or gut-associated lymphoid tissue appears to be involved. These
lymphoid stem cells differentiate to become
bursa- or *bone marrow–derived* cells, known as
B-cells.

Both B- and T-lymphocytes, on appropriate
stimulation by antigen, proliferate and undergo
morphological changes. The T-lymphocytes become *lymphoblasts*, which are involved in *cell-
mediated immunity*, and the B-lymphocytes become plasma cells, which are involved in humoral antibody synthesis (Fig. 2–17).

About 90 per cent of lymphocytes in the
thoracic duct and 70 to 80 per cent in the
peripheral blood show T-cell characteristics.
Most of these circulating T-cells are known as

PHAGOCYTE

VACUOLE OR
PHAGOSOME

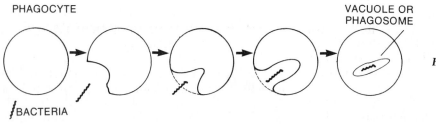

Figure 2–16 Phagocytosis.

BACTERIA

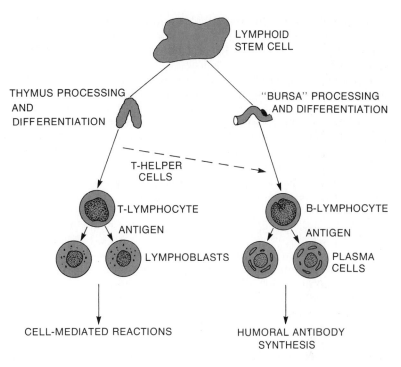

Figure 2–17 Production of B- and T-lymphocytes, and further transformation and proliferation to cells of the lymphoblast and plasma cell series.

"long-lived" lymphocytes, with an average half-life of 2.2 years. In contrast, short-lived lymphocytes, which are mostly B-cells, have a life span of only three days.

The actual mechanisms of the cell-mediated immune response are not well understood, and contrasting viewpoints have been reported by Unanue (1972) and by Feldman (1973). What *is* known is that lymphocyte transformations occur attendant to encounter with foreign antigen, and clonal proliferation of specific activated T-cells results. (*Note:* "clonal" refers to lymphocyte *clones*, which are a set of immunocytes of like hereditary constitution that are produced by a common precursor cell.) These events usually take place in the thymus-dependent zones of the lymph nodes and spleen. The antigenic receptors are probably immunoglobulins, though this has not been proved.

The antigens that elicit a cell-mediated immune response are ill understood, yet it has been reported that intracellular parasites, viruses and antigens incorporated into adjuvants (e.g., tubercle bacilli in mineral oil) all usually stimulate cellular immunity. The *route of administration* or *entry* into the host is also important. Antigens injected intradermally or subcutaneously are more likely to stimulate cell-mediated response than those injected intravenously.

About 10 to 20 per cent of peripheral blood lymphocytes have B-cell characteristics. They are produced in the bone marrow, where it appears that the microenvironment for antigen-independent B-cell differentiation is most similar to that of the avian bursa of Fabricius. B-cells circulate in a pattern similar to that of T-cells.

When B-cells encounter foreign antigen, a complex series of events is initiated that involves the interaction of B-cells with antigen, macrophages, T-cells and dendritic reticulum cells. The B-cells proliferate to form *memory cells* and to undergo differentiation into plasma cells, which secrete immunoglobulin. The antigenic receptors on B-cells are immunoglobulins.

It is important to understand that the induction of immune responses normally depends on collaboration between macrophages, which are believed to process the antigen in some way, T-lymphocytes (T-cells), which recognize DR antigens (i.e., *D*-related antigens of the HLA system; see Chapter 14) and B-lymphocytes, (B-cells), which recognize specific determinants and develop into cells which produce antibody.

THE PRODUCTION OF BLOOD GROUP ANTIBODIES

As discussed, macrophages, which ingest foreign, invading antigen, may present it in a "processed" form to B-lymphocytes. The B-lymphocyte clones then produce antibodies that are released into the blood stream in the *globulin* portion of the plasma and are responsible for the destruction of the invading antigen.

A single clone of B-cells produces antibody of *one specificity only*, though recent evidence suggests that a clone retains the ability to produce other antibodies. A single clone produces either kappa or lambda light chains, but not both. If antibody is produced that is composed of both types of light chain, it can be concluded that at least two clones of lymphocytes are involved in its production.

Primary and Secondary Responses

The *primary response* occurs after an animal first encounters a foreign antigen. Antibody production is usually slight and often relatively slow. The level of antibody produced (titer, or concentration of antibody molecules) depends on the dose of the challenging antigen; however, even when the dose is high, antibody concentration usually rises slowly, remains stable for a period of time and then declines.

Bauer and Stavitsky (1961) reported that in the primary response it is usual for IgM antibody to be formed initially and for production then to be "switched" to IgG antibody. With respect to red cell antibodies, however, this generalization is difficult to substantiate. Several red cell antibodies (e.g., anti-$Rh_o(D)$, anti-K, anti-Fy^a and anti-Jk^a) are in the primary response predominantly IgG, although in some individuals an IgM-IgG mixture is found (Abelson and Rawson, 1961; Polley *et al*, 1962; Adinolfi *et al*, 1962). Lutheran antibodies are often partly IgA. Although it is not clear, therefore, whether IgM is the first immunoglobulin to appear in the primary response, it *is* clear that in the majority of subjects IgG soon predominates and is often the only immunoglobulin that can be identified at any time. The *route of administration* may influence, to some extent, the class of immunoglobulin produced.

The *secondary response* (also known as the *anamnestic response* or *reaction*) is observed after second or subsequent encounter with the same specific antigen. Small doses of the challenging antigen (even as little as 0.1 ml) often result in brisk production of a relatively large amount of antibody; the antibody concentration may begin to rise at 48 hours after challenge and may reach a peak at 6 days. The concentration of antibody (which is usually predominantly IgG) remains stable for a long period of time and then declines very slowly (Fig. 2–18).

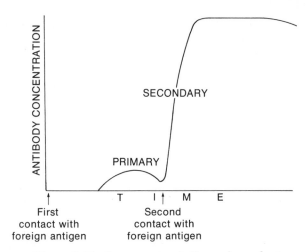

Figure 2–18 Response to challenge by a foreign antigen (primary and secondary).

Immunological Memory

The secondary response occurs as a result of "immunological memory," carried within the small lymphocytes. By this is meant that information is retained within the small lymphocytes regarding the challenging antigen. That such memory occurs has been verified by the fact that immunological memory can be transferred from one animal to another. For example, small lymphocytes from a rat that has already produced primary response to antigen challenge can be injected into another rat with no previous contact with that antigen. Subsequent challenge to the recipient rat with the antigen results in a secondary type of response with rapid production of high-strength antibodies.

Tolerance to Antigens

Tolerance to antigens (also referred to as "immune tolerance" refers to the situation in which a foreign antigen *fails* to elicit the formation of antibody in the recipient. Studies of immune tolerance stem from the work of Ehrlich (1900), who discovered that animals are tolerant of antigenic constituents of their own bodies, even though these same constituents make excellent antigens in other members of the same species. Ehrlich described this as a general law concerning the theories of "self" and "nonself" recognition and designated it "horror autotoxicus." The law has exceptions, as will be described later, yet for the most part it reflects a biological necessity.

Owen (1945) made the observation that

dizygotic twin cattle, which shared the same placental circulation and whose circulations were thereby "linked," progressed through life with appreciable numbers of each other's red cells in their blood. Conversely, if they had not shared the same circulation, red cells from one twin injected into the other rapidly provoked an immune response. This same phenomenon has been recognized several times in human dizygotic twins (Dunsford *et al*, 1953; Booth *et al*, 1957; Nicholas *et al*, 1957). Such individuals (those possessing dual populations of cells) are known as *chimeras*. Permanent chimerism may be due to exchange of tissue between twins *in utero*, as just described, or may be due to fusion of two ova (or ovum and polar body), which have been separately fertilized by two sperms (Gartler *et al*, 1962). Temporary chimerism may be observed in transfused patients or in patients who have received a graft of bone marrow.

On the basis of the "exchange of tissue" information, Burnet and Fenner (1949) postulated that an animal would be tolerant to antigens encountered during embryonic life, and in this way they explained the failure of an animal to produce antibodies against its own tissues. This hypothesis was put to the test by Billingham *et al* (1953), who injected embryonic mice with adult cells and, subsequent to birth, demonstrated tolerance in the infant mice toward skin from the same adult donors.

Lifelong tolerance can be secured by repeated injections throughout life of cells (Mitchison, 1959) or soluble antigens (Smith and Bridges, 1958) or by the introduction of a graft into the animal that survives. Transient exposure to antigens during fetal life is insufficient to secure lifelong tolerance (see review by Brent and Medawar, 1958).

It is now realized that tolerance can be induced in the adult as well as in the neonate by the administration of massive doses of the antigen concerned. Temporary tolerance can also be induced by giving very small doses of antigen (Mitchison, 1963). T-cells appear to be involved in tolerance at low antigen levels, whereas both B- and T-cells are made unresponsive at high antigen dose. The condition is known as *high dose tolerance* or *immunologic paralysis*.

Antibody response can also be suppressed by the administration of *passive* antibody. The practical aspects of this with respect to hemolytic disease of the newborn are discussed in Chapter 16. Experiments have also been performed with human red cells, in which cells carrying the antigens D and K were injected together with anti-K into volunteers, all of whom were D-negative and K-negative. It was observed in these experiments that the responses to both D and K were suppressed (Woodrow *et al*, 1975).

ANTIBODY ACTIVITY *IN VIVO*

At a convenient, basic level, we can think of the function of antibody *in vivo* as the ability to recognize and combine with specific foreign antigens and to cause them to be destroyed. With respect to cellular elements, the destruction of the antigen on the cell membrane also results in the destruction of the cell itself. Antibodies, it should be noted, do *not* damage cells carrying the corresponding antigens; however, they are instrumental in the destruction or removal of such cells from the blood stream through extravascular and intravascular destruction.

Extravascular Destruction. Once foreign cells become *coated* with antibody (i.e., "sensitized"), macrophages attempt to remove the antibody, and in the process cause irreversible damage to the red cell, which may be fragmented or deformed or may become spheroidal. (In this way they become "spherocytes," which are circular and inflexible.) The shape of the red cells is of extreme importance in normal circulation through the liver and spleen, where they are required to pass through "sinusoidal vessels" (minute holes in the splenic tissue). Red cells in their natural state are flexible and resilient and pass through the sinusoidal vessels by passing a flattened piece of their membrane through first, then allowing the fluid content of the cell to flow through into the membrane portion already past the constriction. Spherocytes are unable to effect this shape change and are thus trapped in the microcapillaries and removed from the circulation (Fig. 2–19). This is known as *extravascular destruction* (destruction outside the blood vessels).

Intravascular Destruction. The rate of phagocytosis is increased when a group of serum proteins, collectively known as *complement*, as well as antibody is attached to the red cell surface. (Note that not all antibodies cause the "binding" of complement. When complement is *not* bound, or when it is only *partially* bound, the sensitized cells undergo extravascular destruction.) Complement, in addition, can cause damage to the red cell membrane, thus disrupting the cell without the intervention of phagocytes. This is known as *intravascu-*

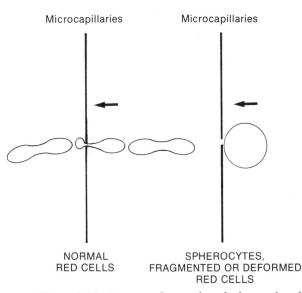

NORMAL   SPHEROCYTES,
RED CELLS   FRAGMENTED OR DEFORMED
                              RED CELLS

Figure 2–19 Passage of normal and abnormal red cells through the sinusoidal vessels. (Modified from Issitt and Issitt, 1975.)

lar destruction (destruction within the blood vessels).

Complement is activated by a very wide range of antibody molecules; that is to say, the majority of sensitized cells *in vivo* undergo intravascular destruction.

COMPLEMENT

The term "complement" refers to a complex set of nine distinct serum protein components that react with one another sequentially to form products with potent biological effects including immune adherence, phagocytosis and cell lysis. These products result from the activation of either of two pathways, known as the *classical* pathway and the *alternative* pathway. Complement is important to the immunohematologist in that it can cause hemolysis of sensitized cells *in vivo* or *in vitro* when certain "complement-binding" antibodies are involved. Activation of the complement system can occur with IgM or IgG, though the various subclasses of IgG vary widely in their ability to activate complement. IgG3 molecules are highly active, IgG1 moderately, IgG2 slightly and IgG4 not at all (Müller-Eberhard *et al*, 1967); Ishizaka *et al*, 1967).

A wealth of information is available on this vast subject. For comprehensive reviews, see Müller-Eberhard (1975, 1976); Götze and Müller-Eberhard (1976); Ward and Melean (1978) and Mollison (1979).

COMPLEMENT ACTIVATION

The Classical Pathway

C1. The complement activation site on the IgG molecule is in the C_H2 domain (refer to Fig. 2–10). This site binds (combines) with the first component of complement (C1), which is a macromolecular (19S) complex of three subcomponents known as C1q, C1r and C1s. C1q is the subcomponent that is actually fixed to the complement activation site in the C_H2 domain, thereafter binding C1r, which in turn activates and binds C1s. The C1 complex (C1qrs) is held together by ionized calcium (Ca^{++}). The presence of free Ca^{++} is therefore essential for the integrity of the complex and because of this, strong calcium-chelating agents (e.g., EDTA) inhibit C1 activation. C1r is a proteolytic enzyme and a beta globulin in its native state. When it has activated C1s, it develops esterase activity (Naff *et al*, 1964; Valet and Cooper, 1974). C1s, which is an alpha globulin, is also a proteolytic enzyme when free.

In order for the first component of complement to become activated, two antigen-bound Fc fragments are necessary. With IgG-coated red cells, therefore, two antibody molecules, each of which contributes one Fc fragment, must bind to *adjacent* antigen sites for complement to be activated. It has been calculated that if a cell has 600,000 binding sites for IgG molecules, about 800 molecules must be attached to antigen to provide an even chance that two will occupy closely adjacent sites and thus activate complement (Humphrey and Dourmashkin, 1965). If IgG molecules are attached to *nonadjacent* sites, it would appear that the Fc pieces are too far apart to initiate complement activation.

IgM, on the other hand, has five Fc fragments, and therefore one molecule of IgM is independently capable of causing complement to be bound (Humphrey and Dourmashkin, 1965; Borsos and Rapp, 1965), although when there are few antigen sites on a cell this may not occur, presumably because at least two of the binding sites on the antibody molecule must combine with antigen for complement to be bound (Ishzaka *et al*, 1963).

The actual mechanism by which C1 is converted to C1̄ (the bar over the number indicates that the component has been activated) by bound antibody is not yet established.

The activation of C1 is shown diagrammatically in Figure 2–20.

C4. The second component of complement to be involved in the reaction sequence is

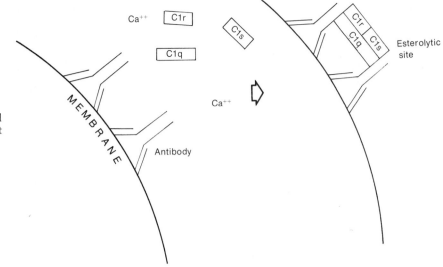

Figure 2-20 Fixation and activation of the first component of complement (C1).

The esterolytic site on C1s activates C4, causing it to split into two subunits, known as C4a and C4b. The C4a subunit is released and appears to play no further role in the reaction. Some C4b molecules attach to the cell membrane as well as to antibody molecules (Willoughby and Mayer, 1965; Müller-Eberhard and Lepow, 1965), although out of every hundred molecules activated only about five succeed in establishing a cellbound site and only about 5 per cent of these produce a site that is "effective" (Müller-Eberhard, 1968). This is probably due, at least in part, to the fact that there appear to be no specific C4 sites on the cell membrane, and the attachment is therefore probably a result of hydrophobic bonding (Dal-

called C4 — a fact that is unfortunate and is due simply to the order of discovery of the components. (C4 is the only one in the sequence that is out of order.)

masso and Müller-Eberhard, 1967). (*Note*: After a period of time C4b is acted upon enzymatically by C4b inactivator and split into subunits C4c and C4d. C4c is released into the body fluids, leaving C4d permanently affixed to the cell membrane).

Activation of C4 exposes a binding site on the C4d *segment* of C4b (Fig. 2–21).

C2. The third component to take part in the reaction sequence is C2—also activated by C1s, though probably only after the C1sC4 interaction has taken place. C2, like C4, splits into two subunits, termed C2a and C2b. This time it is the "b" piece (C2b) that is split off and released and appears to play no further role in the reaction. Most of the C2a, too, is released from the C1s activation site and floats free. The life span of free C2a is short (half-life of 7 minutes at 37° C) and in order to function, it must quickly complex with the activated C4b

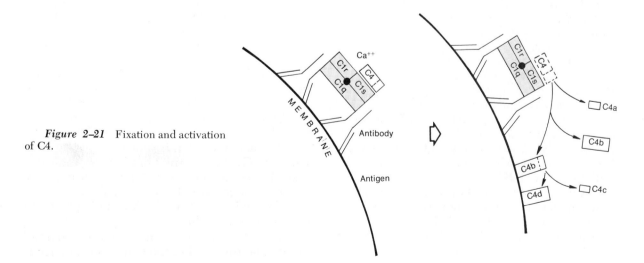

Figure 2-21 Fixation and activation of C4.

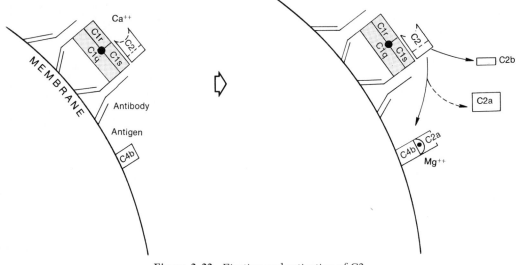

Figure 2–22   Fixation and activation of C2.

(C$\overline{4b}$) on the red cell membrane. The formation of the complex C$\overline{4b2a}$ depends on available magnesium ions (Mg^{++}) and even when formed is extremely unstable. C$\overline{2a}$ constantly disassociates from the complex and must be replaced by newly activated C$\overline{2a}$ in order for the complement sequence to continue (Fig. 2–22).

C3.   The C$\overline{42}$ complex functions as an enzyme (known as C3 convertase) acting on the next component of the sequence, C3. C3 convertase cleaves a small fragment, C3a, from native C3 (β_{1c} globulin) to produce C3b. C3a, which is a powerful anaphylatoxin (Bokisch *et al*, 1969) is not further involved in the reaction. C3b, however, which in itself is a complex of two

subcomponents, C$\overline{3c}$ (a β_{1A}-globulin) and C$\overline{3d}$ (an α_{2D}-globulin) (West *et al*, 1966; Engelfriet *et al*, 1970), may bind intact to the cell surface, or it may be split either before or after binding to the cell surface, leaving C$\overline{3d}$ alone on the membrane. The cell surface binding is probably through hydrophobic bonding; some C3b molecules also bind to the antibody (Leddy *et al*, 1965; Petz *et al*, 1968).

The C3d fragment of C$\overline{3b}$ appears to carry the binding site that attaches the molecule to the cell surface. The binding of this site, like that on C$\overline{4b}$, is believed to be very brief, of the order of 0.1 second (see Müller-Eberhard, 1975).

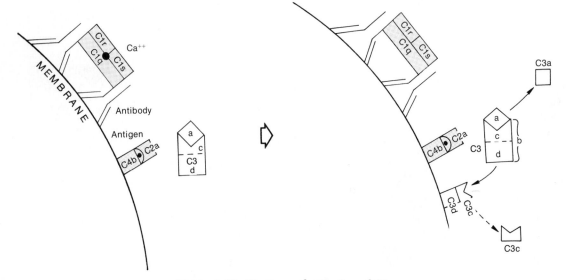

Figure 2–23   Fixation and activation of C3.

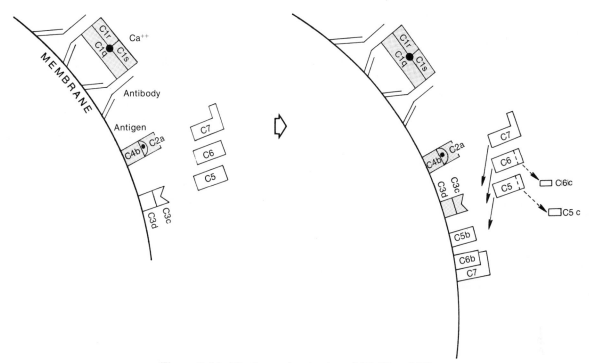

Figure 2-24 Fixation and activation of C5, C6 and C7.

Which component of $\overline{C3}$ reaches the cell surface appears to be of considerable importance with respect to whether the complement-coated cell will or will not be removed from the circulation (Fig. 2–23).

The Terminal Stages: C5 to C9

The $\overline{C4b2a3b}$ ($\overline{C423}$) complex, known as C5 convertase, cleaves C5 into two subcomponents, C5a and C5b. C5a is released into the body fluids where, as anaphylatoxin II, it acts as a mediator of inflammation. C5b attaches to a specific receptor on the cell surface at a site distinct from that of C4b and C3b. C5b then activates both C6 and C7, cleaving C6 into subcomponents C6a and C6b. Subcomponents C5b and C7 become inserted in the phospholipid layer (Fig. 2–24.) C8 is then activated and inserted into the pre-formed channel. It enters into direct contact with the membrane and disrupts it. C9 enhances the activity of C8 (Müller-Eberhard, 1975; Hammer et al, 1975). The presence of C9 is also apparently important in the *formation* of the membrane defect (Green et al, 1959) (Fig. 2–25).

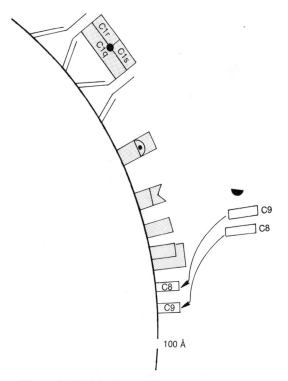

Figure 2-25 Fixation and activation of C8 and C9 with subsequent membrane rupture.

When viewed under the electron micro-scope the defect in the membrane is seen as a very small hole (Humphrey and Dourmashkin, 1965). With respect to human red cells, the diameter of the hole is about 10 nm (100 Å) (Sears *et al*, 1964) and permits the loss of ionic contents, resulting in disequilibrium of water and thus bringing about the lysis of the cell by colloidosmotic lysis (Rosse *et al*, 1966). In the case of red cells, this is caused by swelling and subsequent rupture of the cell.

THE ALTERNATIVE PATHWAY

The alternative pathway of complement activation was originally described as the "properdin" system by Blum *et al* (1959) and is similar in many respects to the classical pathway. Known activators of the alternative pathway are aggregates of IgA and naturally occurring poly-saccharides and lipopolysaccharides. No exam-ples of the activation of the alternative pathway by red cell antibodies have been described. These activator substances convert an "initiat-ing factor" into an activator, which alters C3 proactivator, giving it similar functions with $C\overline{42}$ (C3 convertase). The alternative pathway, therefore, proceeds to the C3 activator stage without the participation or consumption of C1, C4 or C2 (Bitter-Suermann *et al*, 1972) (see also review by Götze and Müller-Eberhard, 1976). Once C3 activator splits C3a from $C\overline{3}$, the ac-tivation sequence proceeds to C9 in the same way as the classical pathway.

DESTRUCTION OF COMPLEMENT *IN VITRO*

The action of complement can be destroyed or inhibited *in vitro* by anticoagulants, heating, normal serum inhibitor or storage.

Anticoagulants. As mentioned, Ca^{++} is needed for the integrity of C1, and Mg^{++} is required for the activation of C42. The addition of *chelating agents*, therefore, prevents comple-ment activity by removing (chelating) the ion-ized calcium (Ca^{++}). In the absence of Ca^{++}, C1 is irreversibly inactivated. For example, the anticoagulant sodium (or potassium) ethylene-diamine tetraacetic acid (EDTA) in the ratio of 2 mg to 1 ml of serum chelates Ca^{++} and com-pletely blocks the activation of complement. *Heparin* is also anti-complementary; Strunk and Colten (1976) reported that 2.5 IU heparin per ml will completely inhibit the cleavage of C4 by $C\overline{1}$. However, Mollison (1979) maintains that much higher concentrations are required. CPD

(citrate phosphate dextrose) and ACD (acid ci-trate dextrose) are anti-complementary insofar as the citrate chelates calcium and thus inter-feres with the binding of C1.

Heating. Heating serum to 56° C for 30 minutes completely inactivates C1 and C2. C4 is damaged to a lesser extent, although after 20 minutes at 56° C, C4 activity may be reduced to 20 per cent of its original strength (Bier *et al*, 1945; Heidelberger and Mayer, 1948).

Normal Serum Inhibitor. Serum normally contains an inhibitor of $C\overline{1}$, which directly af-fects its action (Lepow *et al*, 1965).

Storage. When stored, serum develops anti-complementary activity. The properties causing this are not well understood. Prelimi-nary observations suggest that C4 is principally affected (Margaret J. Polley, unpublished ob-servations, cited by Mollison, 1979).

ANTIBODY ACTIVITY *IN VITRO*

The fundamental reaction between antigen on red cells and its corresponding antibody is simply one of *combination*, which may or may not be followed by *agglutination* of the cells concerned.

There are several types of reaction of antigen-antibody complexes *in vitro*. Each will be considered here in turn, yet first it is neces-sary to study the basic reaction — the simple combination of antigen and antibody, *in vivo* or *in vitro*, known as "sensitization."

Sensitization. An antigen and its specific antibody possess complementary correspond-ing structures that enable the antigenic deter-minants to come into very close apposition with the binding site on the antibody molecule where the two are held together by weak inter-molecular bonds, believed to include opposing charges on ionic groups, hydrogen bonds, hy-drophobic (nonpolar) bonds and Von der Waal's forces. This is not a covalent bond, and in fact is about one tenth as powerful as that of a covalent bond.

The antigen-antibody reaction, which is reversible in accordance with the law of mass action, may be written thus:

$$Ab + Ag \underset{k_2}{\overset{k_1}{\rightleftharpoons}} AbAg$$

where k_1 is the rate constant for the forward reaction and k_2 is the rate constant for the reverse action.

According to the law of mass action (see Hughes Jones, 1963)

$$\frac{(AbAg)}{(Ab) \times (Ag)} = \frac{k_1}{k_2} = K$$

where (Ab), (Ag) and (AbAg), respectively are the concentrations of Ab, Ag and AbAg (the combined product) and K is the equilibrium or association constant, which can be looked upon as a measure of the "goodness of fit" of the antibody to the corresponding antigen. The value of K is ultimately dependent on the strength of the antigen-antibody bonds, and since all antisera contain populations of antibody molecules with a variety of binding strengths, the K value of the serum for any specific reaction is a measure of *average* binding strength of all antibody populations present.

At equilibrium

$$\frac{(AgAb)}{(Ab)} = K(Ag)$$

That is to say, the higher the equilibrium constant, the more will be the amount of antibody combining with antigen at equilibrium. Assuming that a certain minimum number of antibody molecules must be bound to each red cell for agglutination to occur, the ratio of (AgAb) to (Ag) at equilibrium should be as high as possible. In practical terms, this means that a high ratio of serum to cells increases test sensitivity.

Several factors affect the first stage of agglutination (i.e., sensitization) including temperature, pH and ionic strength. These are discussed under the heading Factors Influencing Antigen-Antibody Reactions, p. 58.

Agglutination and Hemagglutination. The phenomenon of "hemagglutination" is a common feature of the antigen-antibody reaction *in vitro*. It occurs when sensitized cells come into contact with one another and are aggregated into clumps, or "agglutinates." When the cells are red cells, this is *hemagglutination*; when they are other than red cells, the phenomenon is called *agglutination*. In most blood bank laboratories, however, the words are used synonymously (i.e., *hemagglutination* is most often referred to simply as *agglutination*).

In hemagglutination, the antigen is referred to as an *agglutinogen*, since it causes the aggregation of cells by direct interaction with the corresponding antibody. The antibody is referred to as an *agglutinin*. Microscopic hemagglutination is shown in Figure 2–26.

In many serologic investigations, it is necessary to "grade" the hemagglutination reaction — that is, to give an indication of its strength. A suggested system, used throughout this text, follows (see also Figs. 2–27 to 2–33). The system given is as recommended by the American Association of Blood Banks.

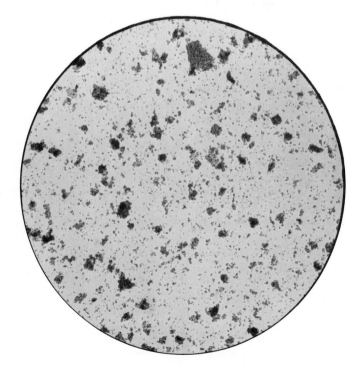

Figure 2–26   Hemagglutination.

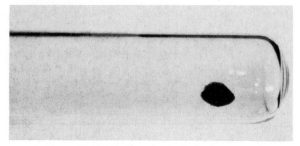

Figure 2-27   4 + Agglutination.

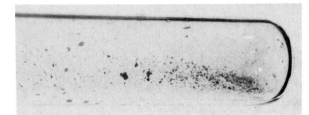

Figure 2-29   2 + Agglutination.

4+   One solid aggregate; no free cells; clear supernatant (macroscopic reading) (Fig. 2-27)

3+   Several large aggregates; few free cells; clear supernatant (macroscopic reading) (Fig. 2-28)

2+   Medium-sized aggregates; some free cells; supernatant clear (macroscopic reading) (Fig. 2-29)

1+   Small aggregates just visible macroscopically; many free cells; turbid reddish supernatant (macroscopic and microscopic reading) (Fig. 2-30)

w+   Tiny aggregates, clumps barely visible macroscopically; many free cells; turbid reddish supernatant (microscopic reading) (Fig. 2-31)

MF   Mixed field; few isolated aggregates; large areas of free cells; red supernatant (Fig. 2-32)

0   Negative; no aggregates; smooth suspension (Fig. 2-33)

Hemolysis. Hemolysis is the breakdown of the red cells, resulting in the release of hemoglobin. Certain blood group antibodies (in this case referred to as *hemolysins*) may be able to damage red cells carrying the corresponding antigen through the activation of *complement*, allowing hemoglobin to be released. The *in vivo* action of complement is basically the same as its action *in vitro*. Hemolysis often obscures agglutination, and its presence is always significant in serological testing. *Note*: Hemolysins act to produce lysis only in the presence of complement (i.e., in fresh serum).

Precipitation. Precipitation involves the interaction of antigen and antibody in optimal proportions, resulting in a visible precipitate. The antigens involved in the precipitin reactions are solutions of molecules that are usually protein or carbohydrate in nature. The simplest form of the precipitin reaction would be the layering of antigen in solution over a small volume of antiserum. Precipitation occurs at the interface of the two reagents, forming a ring (Fig. 2-34).

An explanation for the reaction between antigen and antibody resulting in precipitation was offered by Marrack (1938). This concept, referred to as the "lattice hypothesis," is based on the fact that antibody has more than one valence and therefore may bind with antigen in the form of a coarse "lattice" (Fig. 2-35).

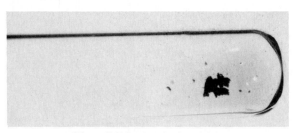

Figure 2-28   3 + Agglutination.

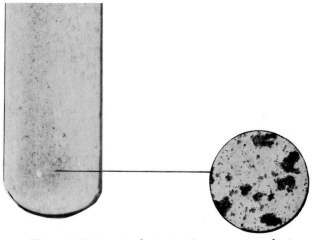

Figure 2-30   1 + Agglutination (macroscopic and microscopic).

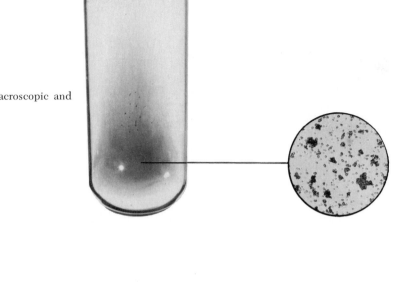

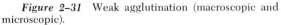

Figure 2-31 Weak agglutination (macroscopic and microscopic).

Figure 2-32 Mixed field agglutination (macroscopic and microscopic). Note dark supernatant.

Figure 2-33 Negative—no agglutination (macroscopic and microscopic).

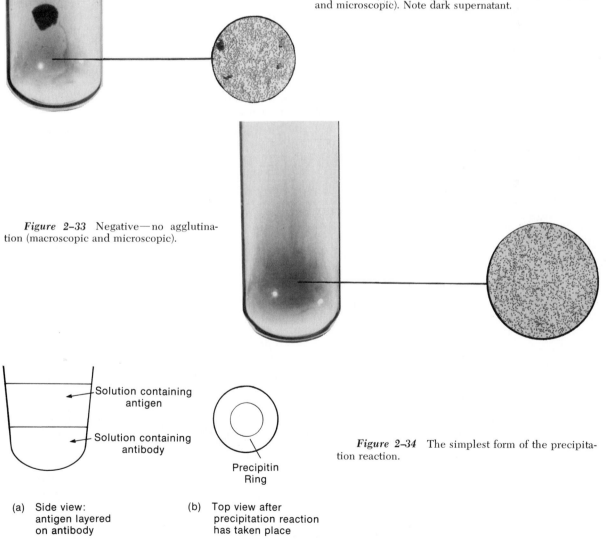

Solution containing antigen

Solution containing antibody

Precipitin Ring

Figure 2-34 The simplest form of the precipitation reaction.

(a) Side view: antigen layered on antibody

(b) Top view after precipitation reaction has taken place

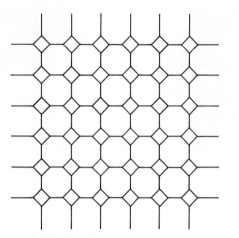

Figure 2–35 The lattice hypothesis: Antigen (◇) bound to antibody (–) to form a "lattice". (From Bryant, N. J.: Laboratory Immunology and Serology. W. B. Saunders Co., Philadelphia, 1979.)

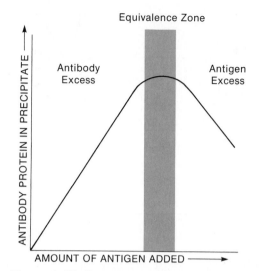

Figure 2–37 Precipitation curve with a constant amount of antibody. (From Bryant, N. J.: Laboratory Immunology and Serology. W. B. Saunders Co., Philadelphia, 1979.)

This reaction is influenced by the quantities of antigen and antibody present. To understand the events that occur, one must assume that antibody molecule has only two reactive sites, whereas antigens have multiple sites that can react with antibody. When a small amount of antigen is added to an excess of antibody, all the valences of the antigen are satisfied, and complexes are formed that are composed of much antibody and little antigen. As increasing amounts of antigen are added to the same amount of antibody, the proportions change until a point of optimal proportion is reached. This point is known as the *equivalence zone*. Further addition of antigen shifts the reaction into the area of antigen excess (Fig. 2–36).

The largest amount of precipitate is found at the equivalence zone, and excess of either reactant may produce false-negative results (Fig. 2–37). This reaction is rarely used now, but it can provide a fairly good quantitative estimate of the amount of antigen or antibody in an unknown if the equivalence zone of the unknown is determined and compared with that of a standard.

The precipitin reaction is of practical use in the laboratory when it takes place in a semisolid media through which soluble molecules can diffuse (e.g., agar gel). In this case, the *location* and *density* of the precipitin bands in the reaction are determined by differences in the concentration and rates of diffusion of the different molecules, which allows for identification of multiple components in mixtures of

◇ = ANTIGEN

—— = ANTIBODY

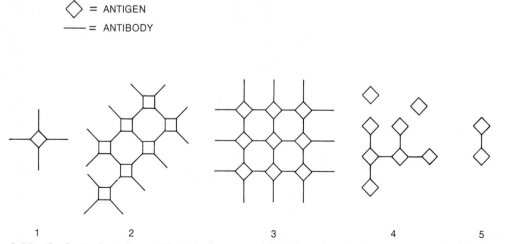

Figure 2–36 The lattice hypothesis. (1) Antibody excess, (2) Moderate antibody excess, (3) Optimal proportions, (4) Antigen excess, (5) Extreme antigen excess. (Modified from Pauling, 1940.)

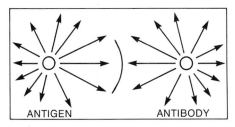

Figure 2-38 A precipitation test showing a single antigen and its corresponding antibody resulting in a single line of precipitation. (From Bryant, N. J.: Laboratory Immunology and Serology. W. B. Saunders Co., Philadelphia, 1979).

antigens and antibodies. Thus a preparation containing only one antigen will give rise to one precipitation line with the corresponding antibody (Fig. 2–38), whereas a preparation containing several antigens will give rise to multiple precipitation lines with the corresponding antibodies (Fig. 2–39). Note that when antigen and antibody are present in optimal proportions the precipitation line formed will generally be concave to the well containing the reactant of higher molecular weight, be it antigen or antibody. This is caused by slower diffusion rates of larger-sized molecules.

A useful procedure for the differentiation of antigens within a mixture is *immunoelectrophoresis*, which combines the principles of gel diffusion and electrophoresis (i.e., molecules are encourgaed to diffuse by the application of an electrical current). This method is especially useful for the study of proteins. In principle, antigen migrates through a gel medium (agar) under the influence of an electrical current, after which the current is stopped and a "trough" is cut in the gel and filled with antibody, resulting in the formation of a precipitin arc. Because antigen (theoretically at a point source) diffuses radically — whereas antibody from a trough diffuses with a plane front — the reactants meet in optimal proportions for precipitation along an arc. The arc is closest to the trough at a point

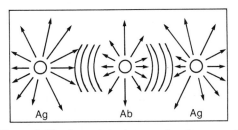

Figure 2-39 A precipitation test showing several antigens with their corresponding antibodies, resulting in several precipitation lines. (From Bryant, N. J.: Laboratory Immunology and Serology. W. B. Saunders Co., Philadelphia, 1979.)

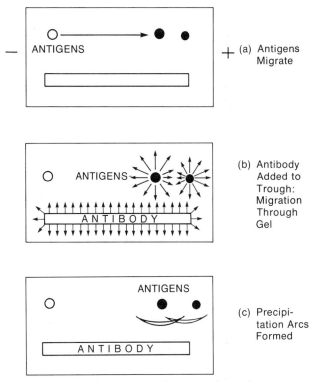

Figure 2-40 The principle of immunoelectrophoresis.

where antigen is in highest concentration. This technique may be used in two-dimensional or multidimensional forms; antigens are then separated on the basis of their electrophoretic mobility (Fig. 2–40). It should be noted that the precipitation reaction by immunoelectrophoresis is fairly insensitive when used for detecting antibody when less than 10 gN/milliliter of serum is present.

Inhibition   (Neutralization). Antibody reactions can be *inhibited (neutralized)* by the addition of soluble forms of blood group antigens or substances having similar terminal structures. The degree of inhibition (i.e., the extent to which the reaction is suppressed) is related to the concentration of soluble antigen and antibody and to the affinity of the antibody molecules for the antigen.

Soluble forms of blood group antigens are found in varying amounts in saliva, serum or plasma, urine and in hydatid cyst fluid.

Inhibition tests are widely used in immunohematology, in particular for the determination of ABH or Lewis secretor status (see Chapter 3), Chido and Rogers phenotypes and antibody specificity (see Chapter 13), Lewis antibody specificity (see Chapter 4) and anti-Sd[a] specificity (see Chapter 23).

Complement Fixation. Complement is widely used as an indicator for immunologic

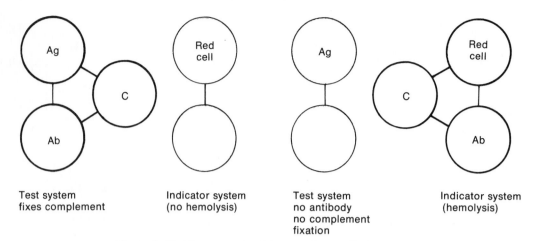

Figure 2–41 The principle of the complement fixation text.

reactions because of its capacity to combine with many antigen-antibody complexes. Immune reactions can therefore be detected even when antigen-antibody reactions such as agglutination or precipitation are absent. Either soluble or insoluble antigens can be employed. The complement fixation test depends on the two basic properties of complement — namely, the binding of complement by antigen-antibody aggregation and the lysis of sensitized red cells.

A suggested method for complement fixation is to introduce into the serum under test a specified dose of complement and an appropriate amount of antigen and to allow them to react at a given temperature. Sensitized sheep cells are then added and the mixture is incubated at 37° C for one hour. If the serum contains antibody to the antigen used, the complement will be *fixed* when combination of antigen with antibody occurs and is therefore no longer available to lyse the sensitized red cells.

A failure to obtain lysis, therefore, denotes a positive result. Complete hemolysis denotes a negative result, indicating that the serum did not contain antibody to the antigen employed. The reaction may also be used to detect antigen, using a serum containing "known" antibody (Fig. 2–41).

It should be noted that the complement-fixation test is of limited usefulness, since it is applicable to IgM antibodies only and the antigen involved must be free of "anti-complementary" activity.

FACTORS INFLUENCING ANTIGEN-ANTIBODY REACTIONS

Antigen-antibody reactions leading to red cell agglutination can occur spontaneously in a saline medium (in the case of IgM molecules —

e.g., anti-A) or, in the case of IgG molecules, by reducing the distance between the cells or the net negative charge exerted by the cells at the slipping plane (see under the heading Electrical Repulsion between Red Cells). In addition, agglutination of IgG-sensitized cells can be achieved by the addition of "antiglobulin" serum that allows the binding of antibody molecules, by providing a sort of "joining piece" (Fig. 2–42). (This phenomenon is further described under the heading "The Antiglobulin Technique," Chapter 21).

"Reduced" IgG.   Romans *et al* (1977) described a method of converting "incomplete" IgG antibodies to direct agglutinins by a process of mild reduction of interchain disulphide bonds with dithioerythritol. This allows for the use of IgG antibodies in a test system without the need for antiglobulin sera or other agents to produce agglutination, and certain sera have been produced commercially in this way.

The Effect of Antibody Size.   It appears that, for agglutination to occur, the distance between red cells can be greater with IgM molecules than with IgG molecules, simply because IgM molecules are bigger and can bridge a wider gap (Pollack *et al*, 1965). According to Green (1969), IgG molecules can bind sites that are up to 140 Å (14 nm) apart, whereas IgM molecules can bind sites up to 350 Å (35 nm) apart (see Fig. 2–43).

Electrical   Repulsion   Between   Red Cells.   Red cells carry negative electric charges on their surfaces when suspended in saline and therefore repel one another and attract positively charged sodium ions (cations), resulting in an ionic cloud around each cell.

Some of these cations travel in a constant configuration around each red cell and become a part of the kinetic unit of the cell. The cloud of positively charged cations around the cell

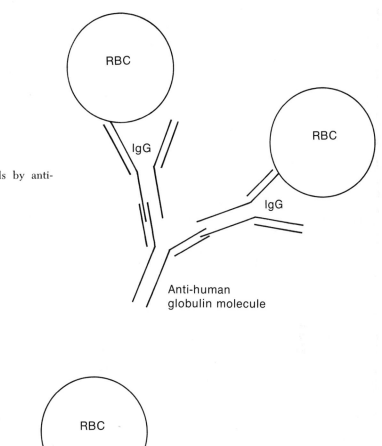

Figure 2–42 Agglutination of red cells by anti-human globulin molecule.

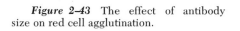

Figure 2–43 The effect of antibody size on red cell agglutination.

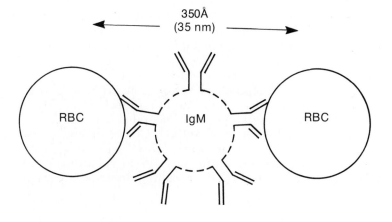

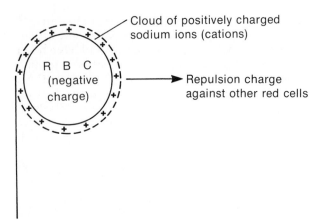

Cloud of positively charged sodium ions (cations)

R B C (negative charge)

Repulsion charge against other red cells

Plane of shear, or "slipping plane"

Figure 2–44 Electromagnetic forces affecting the red cell.

causes a reduction in the net negative charge of the cell. Consequently, the cells repel one another less and are mutually able to approach more closely. The edge of the cloud of cations is known as the *slipping plane* or the *plane (boundary) of shear;* this theoretical boundary separates those cations that move with the cell and those that do not move with the cell (Fig. 2–44). *Zeta potential* is a measurement (in mV) of the net charge exerted by the cell at the boundary of shear (which differs according to the type of media in which the cells are suspended). The zeta potential is therefore directly related to the electrostatic repulsion between cells—for normal red cells suspended in saline, the value is about −15 mV.

Effect of Enzymes. The surface charge exerted by red cells is due to the carboxyl group of sialic acid (sialic = pertaining to saliva), which is contained by certain glycoprotein molecules on the red cell membrane. Treatment of red cells with proteolytic enzymes (e.g., trypsin, ficin, bromelin or papain—see Chapter 19) liberates a sialomucopeptide containing *N*-acetyl-neuraminic acid (a sialic acid), which results in a reduction of the net negative charge of the cells (and thus the zeta potential) and allows the cells to approach one another more closely. It has been postulated that protease treatment may promote cell-to-cell contact, resulting in an ability of IgG blood group antibodies to agglutinate in a saline medium by the simple reduction in the distance between the cells, allowing IgG molecules to bridge the gap between antigen sites. While this cell-to-cell contact was confirmed through electron microscope studies of Voak *et al* (1974), it was shown by Stratton *et al* (1973) that this cannot be the

sole cause of the increased rate of antibody binding subsequent to protease treatment. It has been suggested by these authors that changes in the deformability and plasticity of the cell membrane resulting from enzyme treatment may also result in changes in the *accessibility* and *distribution* of antigenic determinants. It has been shown by Singer (1974) and by Luner *et al* (1975) that protease treatment increases the mobility of the Rh antigen and allows clustering. Enhanced agglutinability may then be due to the formation of multiple bridges between clusters on two adjacent sites.

Effect of Colloids. Antibodies that fail to agglutinate red cells suspended in saline may agglutinate red cells suspended in bovine albumin (Cameron and Diamond, 1945; Diamond and Denton, 1945). Several synthetic colloids (e.g., dextran) have a similar effect (Grubb, 1949).

Pollack (1965) suggested that the enhancing effect of these various colloids may be due to the fact that they *increase* the dielectric constant of the medium and thus reduce zeta potential, though this is probably not the only cause. Chien *et al* (1977) suggest that the effect may be due to reversible adsorption of the polymers onto the red cell surface leading to bridging between adjacent cell structures. Osmotic influences leading either to *deformation* of the cell membrane or to decreases in the chemical potential of intercellular water, or both, may also play a role (van Oss, Mohn and Cunningham, 1978). Bovine albumin is believed to absorb ions from the surrounding medium (see Goldsmith *et al.* 1976).

Effect of Ionic Strength. The rate of association of antibody with antigen is increased by lowering ionic strength (Hughes-Jones *et al*, 1964). These authors found that the titer of most blood group antibodies was enhanced by diluting the serum in a medium of low ionic strength (0.2 per cent NaC1 in 7 per cent glucose) rather than in normal saline. Lincoln and Dodd (1978), however, while conceding that low ionic strength enhances antibody uptake (sensitization), point out that it has a deleterious effect on agglutination unless polycations or proteases are used in conjunction with it.

The practical value of using a low ionic strength medium in the detection of blood group antibodies is discussed in Chapter 22.

Influence of Antigen Characteristics. *The Number of Antigen Sites.* Although many human IgG antibodies fail to agglutinate red cells suspended in saline, there are certain exceptions, notably IgG anti-A and anti-B. This is probably due to the fact that there are many A and B antigen sites on the cell membrane (in fact 100 times more than the number of Rh sites). Further evidence of the influence of the number of antigen sites in determining agglutination has been provided by Leikola and Parsanen (1970) in experiments using a hapten covalently coupled to red cells in different amounts. It was found that when hapten density fell below a certain level, IgG antibodies failed to agglutinate untreated red cells, yet when hapten density was high no treatment of the red cells was required for agglutination to occur.

Projection from the Cell Membrane. The degree to which an antigen site projects beyond the cell membrane may also influence agglutination. It is believed that some antigens protrude from the red cell surface, while others are deeply buried in the cell membrane.

Proximity of Antigen Sites. Agglutination is influenced by the proximity of antigen sites on the cell membrane, though this variable will depend on the number of antigen sites per red cell, on the extent to which the sites occur normally in *clusters* and on the extent to which the antigens are capable of forming clusters after combining with antibody. While there is evidence that antigen mobility may be a prerequisite for antibody-mediated hemagglutination, this does not seem to be an absolute requirement, since IgG anti-Rh will agglutinate Rh-positive red cells in albumin in circumstances in which clustering does not occur (Victoria *et al*, 1975).

Effect of the Number of Antibody Molecules. A minimum number of antibody molecules per red cell are required for agglutination to occur. In comparisons between IgG and IgM molecules, Economidou *et al* (1967) found that IgM anti-A required about 7000 molecules per red cell for agglutination to occur. Different figures were offered by Greenbury *et al* (1963), yet the conclusion is the same.

Enhancing Effect of Serum or Plasma. Weiner *et al* (1947), Pickles (1949) and Stratton and Diamond (1955) reported that a mixture of human plasma (or serum) and concentrated bovine albumin is superior to albumin alone as a medium for the agglutination of Rh-positive red cells with IgG anti-Rh. These observations indicate that plasma (or serum) contains an agglutination-enhancing factor that is different from albumin, yet what this factor (or factors) is has yet to be elucidated. (For further discussion, see Mollison, 1979).

Effect of pH. Most blood group antibodies demonstrate optimal activity between pH 6.5 and 7.5. In a pH out of this range antigen-antibody reactions are depressed and have been known to fail altogether. Exceptions to this generalization include examples of anti-M, which have been reported to be dependent on an acid pH for reactivity (Beattie and Zuelzer, 1965) and antibodies of the Pr (Sp$_1$) group, which are enhanced at a pH below 6.5 (Marsh and Jenkins, 1968).

Effect of Temperature. Certain blood group antibodies react best with their corresponding antigen at warm temperatures (so-called "warm" agglutinins) while others favor a colder temperature for optimal reaction (so-called "cold" agglutinins). Temperature changes in the surrounding media affect either the equilibrium constant or the rate (speed) of the reaction, or both. Since antigen-antibody reactions are accompanied either by absorption or release of heat, a value $\Delta H°$, which represents a measurement of the change in temperature during reaction, can be calculated for various antibody specificities. (This $\Delta H°$ value is normally expressed as a negative parameter.)

If the value of $\Delta H°$ is close to zero (as is the case with warm antibodies), the equilibrium constant is unaffected by temperature changes. The speed of reaction, however, is enhanced with increase in temperature because of an increase in Brownian motion. On the other hand, if the $\Delta H°$ has a significant negative value (as is the case with cold antibodies), decreases in temperature enhance the equilibrium constant yet reduce the speed of the reaction.

Several explanations have been offered to elucidate the reasons for the effect of temperature on antigen-antibody reactions, yet all are subject to exception. For example, Cooper (1977) suggested that the increase in the amount of antigen-antibody complex formed at low temperatures by the I-anti-I reaction may depend on the loss of fluidity of the red cell membrane at low temperatures; however, Lau and Rosse (1975) found that the major sialoglycoprotein of red cells (glycophorin) isolated from human red cells was able to fix complement in the presence of anti-I as well or better at 37° C than at 4° C.

Effect of Centrifugation. Some IgG antibodies that will not agglutinate saline-suspended red cells under normal conditions may do so if the mixtures are centrifuged. In most cases, however, this enhancement is only striking when the cells are suspended in saline and when the centrifugal force is sufficiently high. For example, Solomon (1964) found that agglutination of IgG anti-Rh with Rh-positive red cells suspended in saline began at 4430 g and there was no further enhancement above 17,750 g.

Effect of Time. Incubation time can affect the association of antigen and antibody in saline. If incubation time is too short, reactions will generally be weaker; if incubation time is prolonged, antigen-antibody complexes may disperse (dissociate) and this dissociation rate may overtake the rate of association.

Effect of "Dosage. The number of antigen sites on the red cell membrane may affect the strength of an antigen-antibody reaction by what is known as *dosage effect*, which refers to different reaction strengths depending on the amount of specific antigen on the red cells. In some instances, the amount of antigen present is directly proportional to the genotype of the individual whose red cells are under test; e.g., M-positive red cells from an individual of genotype *MM* possess far more M antigen than those from an individual of genotype *MN*. Antibodies of the Rh system (notably anti-C, anti-c̄ and anti-E) may show marked dosage effect; anti-D, on the other hand, shows little, if any.

Antibodies of the ABO system never show dosage effect.

THE MATUHASI-OGATA PHENOMENON

When red blood cells of, for example, group A $Rh_0(D)$ negative are incubated with a serum containing both anti-A and anti-D, *both* antibodies may bind to the cells despite the absence of D antigen receptor sites. This occurrence was first described by Matuhasi (1959), and was further studied by Matuhasi *et al* (1960) and by Ogata and Matuhasi (1962, 1964). It is known as the *Matuhasi-Ogata phenomenon*. Studies of 45 antibody mixtures by Allen *et al* (1969) demonstrated the phenomenon in 31 of the mixtures tested. It has been shown that the phenomenon does not depend on the occurrence of agglutination and that it occurs with mixtures of sera each containing a single antibody as well as with serum containing two or more antibodies (Ogata and Matuhasi, 1962, 1964). In performing absorption and elution tests, this phenomenon must be borne in mind. (See Chapter 23.)

TYPICAL EXAMINATION QUESTIONS

Choose the phrase, sentence or symbol that correctly answers the question or completes the statement. More than one answer may be acceptable for each question. Answers are given at the back of the book. The heading in parentheses given after each question refers to the section of the chapter in which the subject of the question is discussed.

1. Antibodies produced by an individual in response to antigens contained in the tissues of another of the same species are known as
   (a) alloantibodies
   (b) xenoantibodies
   (c) heterophile antibodies
   (d) autoantibodies
   (Humoral Defense)

2. Placental transfer from mother to fetus of antibodies that provide temporary immunity from disease is an example of
   (a) artificial acquired passive immunity
   (b) natural acquired active immunity
   (c) natural acquired passive immunity
   (d) artificial acquired active immunity
   (Acquired Immunity)

3. The fluid portion of blood, from which fibrinogen has been removed, is called
   (a) plasma
   (b) serum

   (c) fibrinogen-poor plasma
   (d) none of the above
   (The Composition of Blood)

4. The red cell membrane is composed of three layers. The internal and external layers are known as
   (a) hydrophobic layers
   (b) phospholipid layers
   (c) moisture-absorbing layers
   (d) hydrophilic layers
   (The Red Cell Erythrocytes)

5. The antigen precursor substance on the red cell membrane is composed of
   (a) one molecule of D-galactose
   (b) one molecule of N-acetyl-galactosamine
   (c) two molecules of N-acetyl glucosamine
   (d) two molecules of D-galactose
   (e) one molecule of N-acetyl-glucosamine
   (Chemical Characteristics of Blood Group Antigens)

6. Molecules with a molecular weight of 14,000
   (a) are poor antigens
   (b) fail to act as antigens
   (c) are poor antigens unless conjugated with adjuvants
   (d) are good antigens
   (e) are the best antigens
   (Essentials for Antigenic Substances)

7. The two types of light chains on immunoglobulin molecules are
   (a) kappa and lambda
   (b) kappa and delta
   (c) delta and lambda
   (d) kappa and alpha
   (Blood Group Antibodies—
   Structure of the Molecule)

8. Treatment of IgG with the enzyme pepsin results in a split in the molecule producing
   (a) one Fab fragment
   (b) one Fc fragment and two Fab fragments
   (c) two F(ab')₂fragments
   (d) one F(ab')₂ and several small fragments
   (Blood Group Antibodies—
   Structure of the Molecule)

9. The term *extravascular* means
   (a) outside the blood vessels
   (b) outside the body
   (c) within the blood vessels
   (The Function of Immunoglobulin)

10. IgG accounts for
    (a) 20 per cent of the total immunoglobulin in humans
    (b) 98 per cent of the total immunoglobulin in humans
    (c) 85 per cent of the total immunoglobulin in humans
    (d) 5 per cent of the total immunoglobulin in humans
    (IgG)

11. Allelic genes governing the production of blood group antigens are usually
    (a) amorphic
    (b) recessive
    (c) co-dominant
    (d) dominant
    (e) sex-linked
    (Red Cell Antigens—
    Gene Products on the Red Cell)

12. The Fab fragment of an IgG antibody consists of
    (a) kappa chains only
    (b) a portion of an alpha chain
    (c) the constant region of the gamma chains
    (d) a kappa or lambda light chain and a portion of the gamma heavy chain
    (Immunoglobulin)

13. The cellular elements of blood include(s)
    (a) albumin
    (b) erythrocytes
    (c) fibrinogen
    (d) leukocytes
    (The Composition of Blood)

14. Which of the following classes of antibody is found chiefly in secretions?
    (a) IgG
    (b) IgM
    (c) IgA
    (d) IgD
    (Types of Immunoglobulin)

15. The first four components of complement react in which of the following orders?

(a) C1, C2, C3, C4
(b) C2, C1, C4, C3
(c) C1, C3, C4, C2
(d) C1, C4, C2, C3
(Complement)

16. The term *sensitized red cell* usually refers to
    (a) red cells coated with C1
    (b) red cell antigens combined with antibody *in vivo* or *in vitro*
    (c) red cells that are hemolyzed
    (d) red cells coated with antibody, which may or may not be agglutinated
    (Antibody Activity in Vitro)*

17. IgM molecules
    (a) have a molecular weight of 900,000
    (b) have a normal serum concentration in an adult within the range 0.47 - 1.47 g/l
    (c) are unaffected by heating to 56° C for 3 hours
    (d) possess mu (μ) heavy chains
    (IgM)

18. Complement activity in an antigen-antibody reaction is prevented by
    (a) 2 mg EDTA in 1 ml of serum
    (b) Heating to 56° C for 30 minutes
    (c) Storage of serum at room temperature
    (d) All of the above
    (Destruction of Complement in Vitro)*

19. The two types of immunity that may be produced in response to antigenic stimulus are
    (a) passive or cellular
    (b) active or humoral
    (c) natural or passive
    (d) cellular or humoral
    (Types of Immunity Involving Antibody)

20. The treatment of red cells with proteolytic enzymes may increase the uptake of certain blood group antibodies. What substance do the enzymes remove from the surface of the red cell?
    (a) Lipid
    (b) Neuraminidase
    (c) Sialic acid
    (d) Rh antigens
    (e) Lewis antigens
    (Effect of Enzymes)

21. The demonstration of hemolysis due to an antigen-antibody reaction requires the presence of
    (a) albumin
    (b) calcium and magnesium ions
    (c) protein media
    (d) anti-human globulin
    (e) fresh serum
    (Hemolysis — Complement)

22. A secondary response to a foreign antigen usually
    (a) results in a low titer
    (b) disappears very rapidly
    (c) results in rapid production of antibody
    (d) results in antibody occurring at least six months later
    (Primary and Secondary Responses)

23. Antigen-antibody reactions are influenced by
    (a) ionic strength

(b) pH
(c) temperature
(d) (a) and (c)

(Factors Influencing Antigen-Antibody Reactions)

24. IgG
    (a) molecules are made up of one basic structural unit
    (b) molecules are capable of crossing the placenta
    (c) comprises 40 per cent of the total immunoglobulin
    (d) has a sedimentation coefficient of 7S

    (IgG)

25. Factors affecting the first stage of agglutination include
    (a) ionic strength of the medium
    (b) the number of antigen sites
    (c) the location of the antigen sites
    (d) temperature

    (Sensitization—Factors Affecting Antigen-Antibody Reactions)

26. Complement
    (a) is a mixture of alpha, beta and gamma globulins
    (b) consists of at least nine different components
    (c) can be bound to antigen-antibody complexes

(d) can cause hemolysis of red cells

(Complement)

27. The forces that hold antigen-antibody complexes together are believed to include
    (a) ionic bonds
    (b) van den Bergh's forces
    (c) hydrogen bonds
    (d) hydrophilic bonds

    (Antibody Activity in Vitro — sensitization)

28. Which of the following subclasses of IgG is least abundant in normal adult serum
    (a) IgG1
    (b) IgG2
    (c) IgG3
    (d) IgG4

    (Subclasses of IgG)

29. The concentration of IgM in newborns as compared to adult serum is
    (a) 5–10 per cent
    (b) 40–50 per cent
    (c) 60–65 per cent
    (d) 90–95 per cent

    (Production of IgM in Newborns)

30. IgA
    (a) is known to have three subclasses
    (b) is known to have two subclasses
    (c) is known to have four subclasses
    (d) is not known to have subclasses

    (Subclasses of IgA)

GENERAL REFERENCES (SUGGESTED READING)

1. Alexander, J. W. and Good, R. A.: Fundamentals of Clinical Immunology. W. B. Saunders Co., Philadelphia, 1977. *(A well written, easy to understand text. Students of Immunohematology will find the Historical Perspectives [Chapter 1], Development of the Immune Response [Chapter 2], The Immunoglobulins [Chapter 6], and Complement [Chapter 7] particularly useful and informative.)*

2. Bellanti, J. A.: Immunology II. W. B. Saunders Co., Philadelphia, 1978. *(The first section of this book deals with the principles of immunology in a clear, richly illustrated way. The student who wishes to expand his/her knowledge of basic processes will find this book useful and extremely readable.)*

3. Bellanti, J. A.: Immunology: Basic Processes, W. B. Saunders Co., Philadelphia, 1979. *(A "minitext" that concentrates on the principles of immunology*

with little emphasis on the clinical correlations. All sections of the book will be useful to the student of Immunohematology)*

4. Mollison, P. L.: Blood Transfusion in Clinical Medicine. Blackwell Scientific Publications, Oxford, 1979. *(Considered by many to be the "Bible" of Blood Transfusion. Chapter 6, Red Cell Antigens and Antibodies and their Interactions, covers the subjects discussed in this chapter. While coverage may be in too great depth for the average student, the book will serve as an excellent source of reference.*

5. Roitt, I. M.: Essential Immunology, 2nd Ed. Blackwell Scientific Publications, Oxford, 1974. *(An excellent text that will serve the student who wishes a clear, concise explanation of basic processes without unnecessary frills.*

Section Three

SYSTEMS

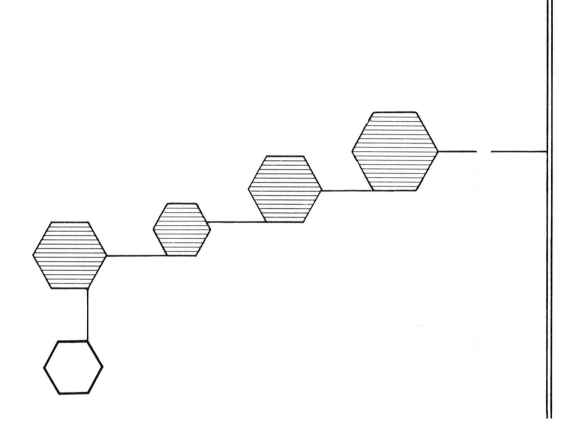

Landsteiner's law states that antibodies are present in plasma only when
the corresponding antigens are not present on the erythrocytes.

3

THE ABO BLOOD GROUP SYSTEM

OBJECTIVES — THE ABO BLOOD GROUP SYSTEM

The student shall know, understand and be prepared to explain:

1. A brief history of the ABO blood group system (Landsteiner's discoveries)
2. The inheritance of the ABO groups, specifically to include:
   (a) Bernstein's original theory
   (b) The four-allele theory
   (c) The cis-AB condition
   (d) Genotypes and phenotypes in the ABO blood group system
3. The distribution of the ABO groups in U.S. whites and blacks
4. The role of the gene H in the expression of A and B genes
5. The antigens of the ABO blood group system, specifically to include:
   (a) The A_1 and A_2 antigens
   (b) Other subgroups of A and B (A_3, A_x (A_4, A_5, A_z, A_o), Am, A_{int}, A_{end}, A_{finn}, A_{el}, B_3, B_x and B_{el})
6. The O_h (Bombay) phenotype, including:
   (a) Genetic theories
   (b) Classification and notations
7. The secretion of blood group substances, including:
   (a) Frequency in U.S. whites and blacks
   (b) Genetic theories
   (c) Water and alcohol forms of ABH substances and body fluids in which they are found
8. Current numbers of A and B antigen sites on red cells
9. ABH on cells other than red cells
10. The acquired B antigen
11. The development of A_1, B and H antigens in newborns
12. The antibodies of the ABO blood group system, specifically to include:
    (a) The development of anti-A and anti-B (environmental and genetic theories)
    (b) Anti-A and anti-B: immunoglobulin class; "natu-

rally occurring" and "immune"; as autoantibodies
    (c) Cross-reacting anti-A_1B
    (d) Anti-A_1 and anti-A, including:
        (1) Sources
        (2) Frequency
        (3) Lectins
    (e) Anti-H: characteristics; from lectins
13. Techniques of ABO grouping, including:
    (a) Sources of cells and sera
    (b) Rules for practical work
    (c) The slide method of ABO grouping (general principles)
    (d) The tube method of ABO grouping (general principles)
14. Other techniques related to the ABO blood group system, specifically:
    (a) Subgrouping with *Dolichos biflorus* (Anti-A_1)
    (b) Grouping with *Ulex europaeus* (Anti-H)
    (c) Secretor saliva tests to determine secretor status
    (d) Hemolysin tests for high titer anti-A and anti-B
    (e) 2-Mercaptoethanol for differentiation of IgG and IgM
    (f) Tests for non-neutralizable anti-A and anti-B
    (g) The preparation of anti-A_1 from *Dolichos biflorus* seeds
    (h) The preparation of anti-H from *Ulex europaeus* seeds
15. Anomalous results in ABO testing caused by:
    (a) Technique
    (b) Serum abnormalities
    (c) Sensitization
    (d) Recent transfusion
    (e) Unusual genotype
    (f) Misgrouping
    (g) Disease
    (h) Polyagglutination
    (i) Chimerism
    (j) Acquired B

(k) Protein abnormalities
(l) Blood group–specific substances
(m) Irregular antibodies
(n) Unwashed cells
(o) Hypogammaglobulinemia
(p) Drugs

(q) Dyes
(r) False reaction
(s) Age
(t) Preservatives

16. The general management of ABO anomalies in the laboratory

History: Landsteiner's Discoveries

Blood groups and the inherent differences in human blood from one individual to another were first discovered by a German scientist, Karl Landsteiner (1900, 1901), who took samples of blood from six of his colleagues, separated the serum and prepared saline suspensions of the red cells. When each serum sample was mixed with each red cell suspension, he noticed that agglutination of the cells had occurred in some mixtures and not in others.

Classification of the blood "groups" was based on the realization that agglutination had occurred because the red cells possessed an *antigen* and the corresponding specific *antibody* was present in the serum. When no agglutination had occurred, either the antigen or the antibody was missing from the mixture. Landsteiner isolated and recognized two separate antigens, now known as "A" and "B." The antibody that reacted with the A antigen was known as "anti-A" and the antibody that reacted with the B antigen as "anti-B."

From these observations, Landsteiner recognized three separate groups, named according to the antigen present on the red cells. Individuals who possessed the A antigen (i.e., their red cells showed agglutination with anti-A) were classified as belonging to group A and individuals who possessed the B antigen (i.e., their red cells showed agglutination with anti-B) were classified as belonging to group B. Red cells from certain individuals showed no agglutination with either anti-A or anti-B, and were classified as belonging to group O — the symbol O denoting zero or the lack of A and B antigens on the red cells. A fourth group was discovered by Landsteiner's pupils von Decastello and Sturli (1902). The red cells of individuals in this group showed agglutination with both anti-A and anti-B, and the group was called AB.

It was further observed that individuals who possessed the A antigen on their red cells also possessed anti-B in their serum; individuals who possessed the B antigen had anti-A in their serum; individuals who possessed neither A nor B antigens (group O) had both anti-A and anti-B in their serum; and individuals with both A and B antigens (group AB) had neither anti-A nor anti-B in their serum (see Table 3–1). (For an explanation of the reasons for the presence of these antibodies, see under the heading Natural Anti-A and Anti-B.)

INHERITANCE OF THE ABO GROUPS

Epstein and Ottenberg (1908) suggested that the ABO groups were inherited characters, and this was proved by von Dungern and Hirszfeld (1910). In 1924, Bernstein postulated three allelic genes — A, B and O — of which each individual inherits two, one from each parent. He also believed that these genes determine which ABO antigens will be present on the red cells (the O gene being amorphic). In 1911, von Dungern and Hirszfeld showed that the A antigen could be divided into subgroups A_1 and A_2 and in 1930, Thompson *et al* proposed a four-allele theory of inheritance to encompass these subgroups. This extended though did not significantly alter the theory of Bernstein, and is still accepted as being substantially correct.

Under the terms of the theory of Thompson *et al*, four allelic genes, A_1, A_2, B and O, give rise to six phenotypes, A_1, A_2, B, O, A_1B and A_2B. Since each individual inherits one chromosome from each parent for each chromosome pair, two genes are inherited for each characteristic, and these four allelic genes give rise to ten possible *genotypes* (Table 3–2).

In group AB, the A gene is normally carried on one chromosome and the B gene on the other, each being co-dominant, although rare

Table 3–1 CLASSIFICATION OF THE ABO BLOOD GROUPS

Antigen on Red Cells	Antibodies in Serum	Blood Group
A	Anti-B	A
B	Anti-A	B
Neither A nor B	Anti-A and anti-B	O
A and B	Neither anti-A nor anti-B	AB

Table 3–2 PHENOTYPES AND GENOTYPES IN THE ABO BLOOD GROUP SYSTEM

Phenotypes	Genotypes
A$_1$	A$_1$A$_1$
	A$_1$A$_2$
	A$_1$O
A$_2$	A$_2$A$_2$
	A$_2$O
B	BB
	BO
A$_1$B	A$_1$B (or A$_1$B/O)
A$_2$B	A$_2$B (or A$_2$B/O)
O	OO

families have been described in which both A and B have been shown to be inherited from one parent (so-called *cis*-AB). (See Seyfried *et al*, 1964; Yamaguchi *et al*, 1965, 1966, 1970; and Reviron *et al* 1967, 1968). In serological testing, individuals of this type have a weaker than normal B antigen (Bouguerra-Jacquet *et al*, 1969) and possess some kind of anti-B in their serum.

Based on this information, it can be seen that if two group A individuals mate, it is possible for the offspring to be group O if both parents are of genotype AO and each passes the O gene. Other possible and impossible groups from the various ABO matings are given in Table 3–3.

With the use of ABO antisera anti-A, anti-B and anti-A$_1$, which are readily available from commercial sources, all six phenotypes can be distinguished, yet only three genotypes, namely A$_1$B, A$_2$B and OO, are apparent (if one ignores the rare *cis*-AB condition). The exact genotypes of A$_1$, A$_2$ and B individuals, however, are sometimes disclosed by blood-grouping other family members. Figure 3–1 gives an example of this. In examining Figure 3–1, it can be seen that since child No. 2 (Generation II) is of phenotype O and therefore of genotype OO, the gene O must have been inherited from both parents. Since the phenotypes of the parents are A and B, respectively, it follows that both must be heterozygous (i.e., AO and BO). Since child 1 and child 3 (Generation II) possess the A and B antigen respectively, the O gene must be present on the opposite chromosome, as shown in Figure 3–2. (See also under the heading Inheritance of Subgroups.)

The Distribution of the ABO Groups

In 1919, Hirszfeld and Hirszfeld discovered that ABO blood group distribution differed among different population groups. Several

studies followed this discovery and results were collected and published by Boyd (1939). A huge review of world blood group distribution was published by Mourant *et al* (1954); the material is much more comprehensive in the second edition of that book, published in 1976 (see Mourant *et al*, 1976). From information provided by Mourant and his colleagues, the distribution of the ABO groups in U.S. whites and blacks is as given in Table 3–4.

The Gene *H*: Its Role in Expression of *A* and *B* Genes

The expression of the A and B genes (i.e., the way in which they produce detectable products on the red cells) appears to depend on the action of another gene, known as H. Most individuals are homozygous for this gene (i.e., HH), though since its allele, h, is an amorphic gene, the heterozygote Hh cannot be recognized. The phenotype h (genotype hh) is extremely rare. (See O$_h$ [The Bombay Phenotype] later in this chapter.)

The genetic sequence leading to the expression of *ABH* genes on the red cell is believed to be as follows:

1. A precursor mucopolysaccharide substance (i.e., the basic precursor substance of all antigens studied so far — see Fig. 2–5) is converted by the H gene to H substance.

2. This "altered" precursor substance (H substance) is partly converted by the A and/or B genes to A and/or B antigen. Some H substance remains unconverted. The O gene, being amorphic, effects no conversion of H substance (Fig. 3–3). Since no conversion of H substance takes place by the action of the O gene, the H antigen is found in greatest concentration in group O individuals.

The chemical analysis of blood group antigens further supports this theory. As discussed, the basic precursor substance of all blood group antigens studied so far consists of four molecules of three different sugars, N-acetyl-galactosamine, D-galactose and N-acetyl-glucosamine (shown in Fig. 2–5). The addition of a sugar known as L-fucose to the terminal D-galactose of this precursor substance (Type 1 or Type 2 chains) gives the resultant molecule "H" specificity (i.e., it will now react with and is capable of stimulating "anti-H" (Fig. 3–4). The fucose molecule is bound in alpha (1→2) linkage.

The presence of an A gene results in the attachment of the sugar N-acetyl-galactosamine to the substrate formed by the H gene. This gives the resultant molecule "A" specificity

Table 3-3 POSSIBLE AND IMPOSSIBLE OFFSPRING GROUPS FROM VARIOUS PHENOTYPE AND GENOTYPE MATINGS (FROM BRYANT, 1980)

Phenotype Mating	Genotype Mating(s)	Possible Offspring Groups (Phenotypes and Genotypes)	Impossible Offspring Groups (Phenotypes)
$O \times O$	$OO \times OO$	$O\ (OO)$	$A_1, A_2, B,$ A_1B, A_2B
$O \times A_1$	$OO \times A_1A_1$ $OO \times A_1A_2$ $OO \times A_1O$	$A_1\ (A_1O)$ $A_2(A_2O)$ $O\ (OO)$	B, A_1B, A_2B
$O \times A_2$	$OO \times A_2A_2$ $OO \times A_2O$	$A_2\ (A_2O)$ $O\ (OO)$	A_1, B, A_1B, A_2B
$O \times B$	$OO \times BB$ $OO \times BO$	$B\ (BO)$ $O\ (OO)$	A_1, A_2, A_1B, A_2B
$O \times A_1B$	$OO \times A_1B$ $OO \times A_1B/O$	$A_1\ (A_1O)$ $B\ (BO)$ $A_1B\ (A_1B/O)°$ $O\ (OO)°$	A_2, A_2B
$O \times A_2B$	$OO \times A_2B$ $OO \times A_2B/O°$	$A_2\ (A_2O)$ $B\ (BO)$ $A_2B\ (A_2B/O)°$ $O\ (OO)°$	A_1, A_1B
$A_1 \times A_1$	$A_1A_1 \times A_1A_1$ $A_1A_1 \times A_1A_2$ $A_1A_1 \times A_1O$ $A_1A_2 \times A_1A_1$ $A_1A_2 \times A_1A_2$ $A_1A_2 \times A_1O$ $A_1O \times A_1A_1$ $A_1O \times A_1A_2$ $A_1O \times A_1O$	$A_1\ (A_1A_1)$ $A_1\ (A_1A_2)$ $A_1(A_1O)$ $A_2\ (A_2A_2)$ $A_2\ (A_2O)$ $O\ (OO)$	B, A_1B, A_2B
$A_1 \times A_2$	$A_1A_1 \times A_2A_2$ $A_1A_1 \times A_2O$ $A_1A_2 \times A_2A_2$ $A_1A_2 \times A_2O$ $A_1O \times A_2A_2$ $A_1O \times A_2O$	$A_1\ (A_1A_2)$ $A_1\ (A_1O)$ $A_2\ (A_2A_2)$ $A_2\ (A_2O)$ $O\ (OO)$	B, A_1B, A_2B
$A_1 \times B$	$A_1A_1 \times BB$ $A_1A_1 \times BO$ $A_1A_2 \times BB$ $A_1A_2 \times BO$ $A_1O \times BB$ $A_1O \times BO$	$A_1\ (A_1O)$ $A_2\ (A_2O)$ $B\ (BO)$ $A_1B\ (A_1B)$ $A_2B\ (A_2B)$ $O\ (OO)$	None
$A_1 \times A_1B$	$A_1A_1 \times A_1B$ $A_1A_1 \times A_1B/O°$ $A_1A_2 \times A_1B$ $A_1A_2 \times A_1B/O°$ $A_1O \times A_1B$ $A_1O \times A_1B/O°$	$A_1\ (A_1A_1)$ $A_1\ (A_1A_2)$ $A_1\ (A_1O)°$ $A_2\ (A_2O)°$ $B\ (BO)$ $A_1B\ (A_1B)$ $A_1B\ (A_1B/O)°$ $A_2B\ (A_2B)$ $O\ (OO)°$	None
$A_1 \times A_2B$	$A_1A_1 \times A_2B$ $A_1A_1 \times A_2B/O°$ $A_1A_2 \times A_2B$ $A_1A_2 \times A_2B/O°$ $A_1O \times A_2B$ $A_1O \times A_2B/O°$	$A_1\ (A_1A_2)$ $A_1\ (A_1O)°$ $A_2\ (A_2A_2)$ $A_2\ (A_2O)°$ $B\ (BO)$ $A_1B\ (A_1B)$ $A_2B\ (A_2B)$ $A_2B\ (A_2B/O)°$ $O\ (OO)°$	None
$A_2B \times B$	$A_2A_2 \times BB$ $A_2A_2 \times BO$ $A_2O \times BB$ $A_2O \times BO$	$A_2\ (A_2O)$ $B\ (BO)$ $A_2B\ (A_2B)$ $O\ (OO)$	A_1, A_1B

°Rare *cis*–AB condition. See text.

Phenotype Mating	Genotype Mating(s)	Possible Offspring Groups (Phenotypes and Genotypes)	Impossible Offspring Groups (Phenotypes)
$A_2 \times A_1B$	$A_2A_2 \times A_1B$ $A_2A_2 \times A_1B/O°$ $A_2O \times A_1B$ $A_2O \times A_1B/O°$	$A_1 (A_1A_2)$ $A_1 (A_1O)$ $A_2 (A_2O)°$ $B (BO)$ $A_1B (A_1B/O)°$ $A_2B (A_2B)$ $O (OO)°$	None
$A_2 \times A_2B$	$A_2A_2 \times A_2B$ $A_2A_2 \times A_2B/O°$ $A_2O \times A_2B$ $A_2O \times A_2B/O°$	$A_2 (A_2A_2)$ $A_2 (A_2O)°$ $B (BO)$ $A_2B (A_2B)$ $A_2B (A_2B/O)°$ $O (OO)$	A_1, A_1B
$B \times B$	$BB \times BB$ $BB \times BO$ $BO \times BO$	$B (BB)$ $B (BO)$	A_1, A_2, A_1B, A_2B
$B \times A_1B$	$BB \times A_1B$ $BB \times A_1B/O°$ $BO \times A_1B$ $BO \times A_1B/O°$	$A_1 (A_1O)$ $B (BB)$ $B (BO)°$ $A_1B (A_1B)$ $A_1B (A_1B/O)$ $O (OO)°$	A_2, A_2B
$B \times A_2B$	$BB \times A_2B$ $BB \times A_2B/O°$ $BO \times A_2B$ $BO \times A_2B/O°$	$A_2 (A_2O)$ $B (BB)$ $B (BO)$ $A_2B (A_2B)$ $A_2B (A_2B/O)°$ $O (OO)°$	A_1, A_1B
$A_1B \times A_1B$	$A_1B \times A_1B$ $A_1B \times A_1B/O$ $A_1B/O \times A_1B$ $A_1B/O° \times A_1B/O°$	$A_1 (A_1A_1)$ $A_1 (A_1O)°$ $B (BB)$ $B (BO)°$ $A_1B (A_1B)$ $A_1B (A_1B/O)°$ $O (OO)°$	A_2, A_2B
$A_2B \times A_2B$	$A_2B \times A_2B$ $A_2B \times A_2B/O°$ $A_2B/O° \times A_2B$ $A_2B/O° \times A_2B/O°$	$A_2 (A_2A_2)$ $A_2 (A_2O)°$ $B (BB)$ $B (BO)°$ $A_2B (A_2B)$ $A_2B (A_2B/O)°$ $O (OO)$	A_1, A_1B

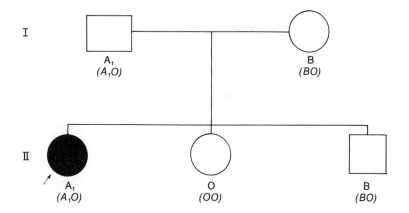

Figure 3–1 A family study that reveals the exact ABO genotypes of all family members.

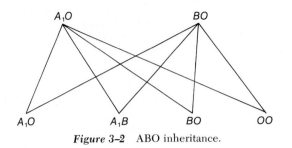

Figure 3–2   ABO inheritance.

Table 3–4   PHENOTYPE AND PERCENTAGES OF GENE FREQUENCIES OF THE ABO BLOOD GROUPS AMONG U.S. WHITES AND BLACKS (FROM BRYANT, 1980)

	Phenotype Frequencies (Percentages)			Gene Frequencies (Percentages)	
Phenotype	Whites	Blacks	Gene	Whites	Blacks
A_1	31.87	19.17	A_1	19.14	13.84
A_2	8.74	8.47	A_2	6.19	3.84
B	10.69	19.23	B	7.51	12.24
O	45.38	48.95	O	67.16	71.05
A_1B	2.54	2.67			
A_2B	0.78	1.49			

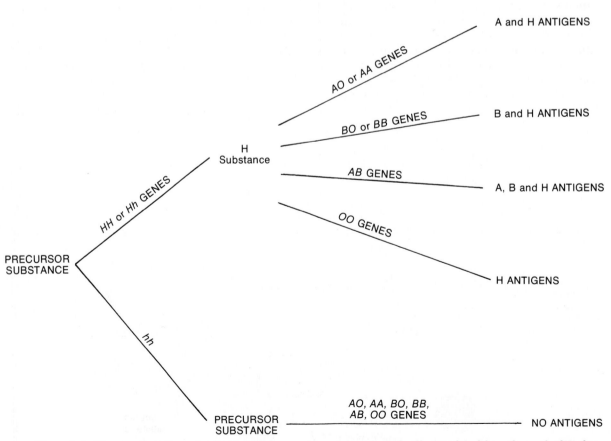

Figure 3–3   The genetic pathway leading to *ABH* gene expression on the red cells. (Modified from the work of Watkins [1959] and Cepellini [1959].)

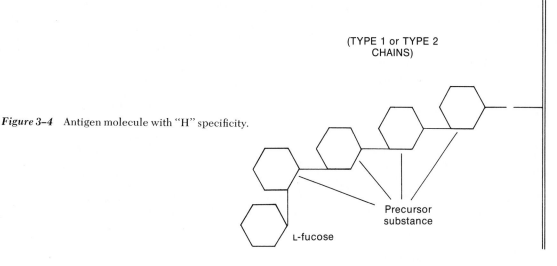

Figure 3–4   Antigen molecule with "H" specificity.

(TYPE 1 or TYPE 2 CHAINS)

Precursor substance

L-fucose

(Fig. 3–5). In much the same way, the presence of the *B* gene results in the attachment of D-galactose to the substrate formed by the *H* gene.

It should be noted that the antigenic determinants so formed are carbohydrates and not proteins and therefore they cannot be direct gene products. It is believed, therefore, that the actual gene products are glycosyltransferases (i.e., enzymes), which effect the transfer of a specific sugar to the precursor substance.

In the absence of the *H* gene, no L-fucose will be added to the *terminal sugar*. The *A* and *B* genes, in this case, will not be expressed. An individual of genotype *hh* will therefore group as "O" even when the *A* or *B* (or both) genes have been inherited (see Fig. 3–3). (See also O_h [The Bombay Phenotype].)

The amount of H substance (antigen) on the red cells varies according to the ABO group of the individual. In group A or group B individuals, much of the H substance on the red cell will have been converted to A or B substance (antigen). Since the *O* gene is amorphic, group O individuals possess only unconverted H substance. For this reason, the order of red cell

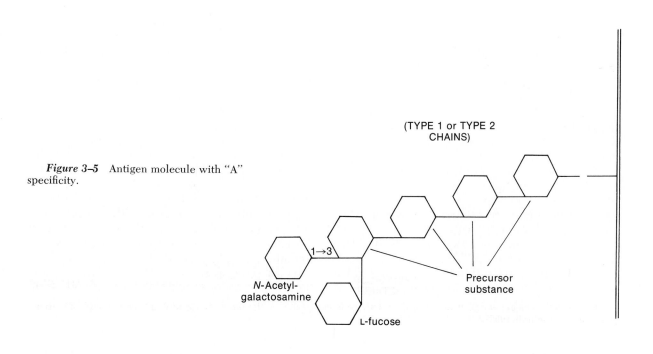

Figure 3–5   Antigen molecule with "A" specificity.

(TYPE 1 or TYPE 2 CHAINS)

1→3

N-Acetyl-galactosamine

Precursor substance

L-fucose

reactivity with anti-H varies considerably, being dependent on the amount of unconverted H substance on the cells. The order of reactivity usually follows the pattern $O > A_2 > A_2B > B > A_1 > A_1B$.

THE ANTIGENS OF THE ABO BLOOD GROUP SYSTEM

The A_1 and A_2 Antigens

Subgroups of A were first described by von Dungern and Hirszfeld (1911), though it was not until the early 1930's that a clear definition of them became available (Thompson *et al,* 1930). It was found that the cells of group A persons did not react equally well with anti-A serum, and it was further discovered that certain weaker-reacting group A individuals were capable of producing an antibody that reacted with the cells of many (but not all) other group A individuals, yet failed to react with the cells of persons of other blood groups. In U.S. whites, 78.48 per cent of group A individuals belong to subgroup A_1 and almost all of the rest are A_2. The distinction between the two groups is most conveniently made with the use of specific anti-A_1 prepared from the seeds of the plant *Dolichos biflorus* (see Lectins, Chapter 19). (See also under the heading Anti-A_1.)

There still appears to be some division of opinion as to whether the A_1, A_2 difference is *qualitative* (related to the quality of the antigen) or *quantitative* (related to the differences in the number of antigen sites on the red cell).

The qualitative difference is supported by the following evidence:

1. A_2 and A_2B individuals are capable of producing a specific anti-A_1 that is occasionally reactive at 37° C and may be capable of causing the destruction of A_1 cells.

2. Potent human anti-A, when subjected to immunodiffusion against sonicated red cell stroma from A_1 and A_2 individuals, reveals two determinants being carried by A_1 cells and only one by A_2 (Milgrom, 1977).

3. A-like rabbits produce potent, specific anti-A_1 when stimulated with red cells (or saliva) from an A_1 secretor, yet produce no anti-A when stimulated with red cells (or saliva) from an A_2 secretor, suggesting that rabbit and human A are alike, but that A_1 is something different (Mohn *et al,* 1975).

The quantitative difference is supported by the work of Greenburg *et al* (1963) and Economidou *et al* (1967), both of whom reported considerable variation in the number of A an-

tigen sites in individuals of group A_1, A_2, A_1B and A_2B (see Table 3–8).

Based on the information given in Table 3–8 and on other evidence, it is believed that A_1 is a composite of two antigens, A and A_1, while A_2 possesses only one antigen, A; also that anti-A sera (from group B donors) contains two antibodies, anti-A and anti-A_1.

Other Subgroups of A and B

Several other subgroups of A have been recognized, though all of them may be classified as extremely rare. These include A_3, A_x (A_4, A_5, A_z, A_0), A_m, A_{int}, A_{end}, A_{finn} and A_{el}.

A_3. First recognized by Friedenreich (1936), this subgroup reveals itself by a characteristic agglutination appearance with anti-A and most anti-A+B (i.e., group O) sera: very small clumps outnumbered by unagglutinated red cells (known as a "mixed field"). About 1 in 1000 group A bloods belong to subgroup A_3 (Gammelgaard, 1942) and the serum of A_3 individuals usually contains anti-A_1 (Dunsford, 1959; Salmon *et al,* 1959). Secretors of subgroup A_3 have A substance in their saliva (see under the heading Secretors and Nonsecretors).

Both Friedenreich (1936) and Gammelgaard (1942) showed A_3 to be an inherited character, representing an allele at the A_1A_2BO locus. Our present way of looking at the genetics of this subgroup is to consider that it is a weaker form belonging to the A_1A_2 series and that it is controlled by an allele, A_3.

In practical work, the assignment of an A_3 phenotype must be preceded by consideration of the possibility of chimera and other blood group mixtures — and from leukemic change (see Weakening of the A Antigen in Leukemia, later in this chapter). The expected reactions with subgroups of A in practical testing are given in Table 3–5.

A_x (A_4, A_5, A_z, A_0). Fischer and Hahn (1935) first described this extremely rare type of blood, which distinguishes itself through red cells that are agglutinated weakly or not at all by the serum of group B donors but are agglutinated by the serum from most group O donors and by anti-H. Eluates reveal that while A_x cells often fail to agglutinate with anti-A, the antigen and antibody do combine (i.e., anti-A can be eluted from the cells, which are therefore sensitized, though not agglutinated). The frequency of A_x, calculated by Salmon (1960) in France, was reported to be one in 40,000. The serum of A_x individuals usually contains anti-A_1 (Dunsford, 1959; André and Salmon, 1957), and A_x secre-

Table 3–5 EXPECTED REACTIONS WHEN DEALING WITH SUBGROUPS OF A AND B

Group	Anti-A	Anti-B	Anti-A, B	Anti-A$_1$	A$_1$ Cells	A$_2$ Cells	B Cells	Secretor Saliva
A$_1$	Pos	Neg	Pos	Pos	Neg	Neg	Pos	A + H
A$_2$	Pos	Neg	Pos	Neg	Neg	Neg	Pos	A + H
A$_3$	Mixed field	Neg	Mixed field	Neg	Pos°	Neg	Pos	A + H
A$_x$	Weak or neg	Neg	Pos	Neg	Pos°	Neg	Pos	H
A$_m$	Weak or neg	Neg	Neg	Neg	Neg	Neg	Pos	A + H
A$_{int}$†	Pos(w)	Neg	Pos	Neg	Neg	Neg	Pos	A + H
A$_{end}$	Mixed field	Neg	Mixed field	Neg	Pos°	Neg	Pos	H
A$_{finn}$‡	Mixed field	Neg	Mixed field	Neg	Pos°	Neg	Pos	H
A$_{el}$	Neg	Neg	Neg	Neg	Pos°	Neg	Pos	H
A$_{bantu}$	Mixed field	Neg	Mixed field	Neg	Pos°	Neg	Pos	H
B$_3$	Neg	Mixed field	Pos	—	Pos	Pos	Neg	B + H
B$_x$	Neg	Weak	Pos	—	Pos	Pos	Weak	B-like + H
B$_{el}$	Neg	Neg	Pos	—	Pos	Pos	Neg	H

°Due to presence of anti-A$_1$.
†Distinguished from A$_1$ and A$_2$ by strong reaction with anti-H.
‡Distinguished from A$_{end}$ by enhancement of reaction with anti-A by enzymes (see text).

tors have H but no A in their saliva, though trace amounts of A have been detected by various workers, including Alter and Rosenfield (1964) and Vox (1964).

Subgroups A$_4$, A$_5$, A$_z$ and A$_o$ are now classified under the heading A$_x$, since they almost certainly represent the same thing. This conclusion is supported by the fact that A$_x$ can vary in expression, even within one family.

The A$_x$ phenotype is probably heterogeneous (i.e., consisting of different elements or ingredients). The inheritance of the subgroup is not clear, appearing straightforward (i.e., due to an allele, A_x, at the ABO locus) in some families and not in others. The expected reactions of A$_x$ with ABO antisera, cells and saliva are given in Table 3–5.

A$_m$. Like A$_x$, A$_m$ red cells are weakly agglutinated or not at all by the serum of group B donors. A$_m$, however, is also not agglutinated by the serum of group O donors (i.e., anti-A + B). Eluates prepared from the cells, however, contain anti-A; the saliva of A$_m$ secretors contains a normal amount of A substance. The serum of individuals of subgroup A$_m$ does not contain anti-A$_1$.

The A_m gene is an allele at the ABO locus, and its inheritance appears to be straightforward (Salmon et al, 1958, 1964; Kindler, 1958; Hrubiška et al, 1966a, 1966b and Serim, 1969). For expected reactions in practical work, see Table 3–5.

A$_{int}$. Landsteiner and Levine (1930) first noted this subgroup, which appeared to be intermediate in its reaction between A$_1$ and A$_2$ (hence the name). Reactions with anti-H, however, are much stronger with A$_{int}$ cells than with A$_2$ cells (Bird, 1958) and therefore A$_{int}$ appears to represent a distinct subgroup, since if it were intermediate between A$_1$ and A$_2$, the anti-H

reactions should also be intermediate. The phenotype is more common in blacks than in whites. For expected reactions in practical work, see Table 3–5.

A$_{end}$. Weiner, Sanger and Race (1959) first described this subgroup, apparently the result of an allele at the ABO locus, later named A$_{end}$ by Sturgeon et al (1964). Reactions give the appearance of an A$_3$, although the saliva of secretors contains H but no A. Anti-A$_1$ is present in the serum of individuals of this subgroup (see Table 3–5).

A$_{finn}$. This subgroup, which is very like A$_{end}$, was described by Mohn et al (1973) and is commoner in Finland than anywhere else. The only distinction between A$_{finn}$ and A$_{end}$ is that the weak reaction with anti-A in the case of A$_{finn}$ can be improved by enzymes, whereas no improvement is seen with A$_{end}$ red cells (see Table 3–5).

A$_{el}$. Red cells of this phenotype are not agglutinated by anti-A or anti-A + B, but eluates prepared from the cells have anti-A specificity. The saliva of secretors contains H but no A substance and the serum of A$_{el}$ individuals may contain anti-A$_1$ (Reed and Moore, 1964). The inheritance of A$_{el}$ appears to be straightforward (see Solomon and Sturgeon, 1964) (see Table 3–5).

Others. A$_{bantu}$ is found in 4 per cent of South African Bantu samples of blood group A. Reactions are similar to those of A$_3$, but the saliva of secretors contains H but no A. Anti-A is regularly present in the serum (Brain, 1966). Still other isolated examples of weaker-reacting group A bloods have been described, which to date have not been fully elucidated or named (see Gold and Dunsford, 1960; Furuhata et al, 1959 and Kitahama, 1959).

Subgroups of B are even rarer than sub-

Table 3–6 OTHER BOMBAY-LIKE PHENOTYPES

Phenotype	Reaction with Anti A	B	A, B	H	Anti-H in Serum	Substances in Saliva of Secretors
A_h	Wk	Neg	Wk	Neg	Yes	None
B_h	Neg	Wk	Wk	Neg	Yes	None
O_{Hm} or O_m^H	Neg	Neg	Neg	Neg (trace)	Some	H
O_{Hm}^A or A_m^H	Wk	Neg	Wk	Neg	Some	A and H
O_{Hm}^B or B_m^h	Neg	Wk	Wk	Neg	Some	B and H
O_{Hm}^{AB} or AB_m^h	Wk	Wk	Wk	Neg	Some	A, B and H

groups of A. While there is no subgroup of B analogous to subgroup A_2, various others have been described that parallel (in terminology) the A subgroups (see Salmon, 1976).

B_3. This subgroup shows a "mixed-field" agglutination pattern with anti-B. The saliva of secretors of this subgroup possesses B substance. *Note:* Moullene *et al* (1955) also used the term "B_3" to describe a very weak B in which no B substance was found in the saliva of secretors (Table 3–5).

B_x. This subgroup shows a weak agglutination pattern with anti-B, and the saliva of secretors contains a type of B substance (B-like), which inhibits the reaction between anti-B and B_x. Weak anti-B is found in the serum of individuals of this phenotype (Table 3–6).

B_{el}. Red cells of this phenotype are not agglutinated by anti-B but will absorb anti-B, which can subsequently be eluted. H substance but not B substance is found in the saliva of secretors (Table 3–5).

Perhaps the most useful test in distinguishing subgroups of A and B that could be mistaken for group O is the preparation of an eluate; in fact, it appears that on the whole, the weaker the antigen, the more potent the eluate (see Celano *et al*, 1957). Elution techniques are given in Chapter 23 of this text.

O_h (THE BOMBAY PHENOTYPE)

The O_h (Bombay) phenotype was first described by Bhende (1952) and is found in individuals who lack the *H* gene (i.e., they are of genotype *hh*). Since the *H* gene is required for the conversion of precursor substance to H substance, an individual of genotype *hh* cannot produce A or B substances (antigens) even when normal *A* or *B* genes or both have been inherited.

In blood grouping tests, therefore, the red cells of an *hh* individual appear to be group O and also fail to react with anti-H. The sera of these individuals contain anti-A, anti-B and

anti-H, whereas sera from normal group O individuals would contain only anti-A and anti-B. The strongly reactive anti-H that is present in O_h (Bombay) individuals causes their serum to agglutinate the red cells of normal group O individuals. The red cells of O_h individuals usually give the reaction Le(a+b−), although O_h Le(a−b−) individuals have been reported (Giles *et al*, 1963; Gandini *et al*, 1968; Petty *et al*, 1969; Moores, 1972). From these investigations it has been shown that the *Hh* genes are not controlled from the *Le* locus (see The Lewis Blood Group System, Chapter 4). An *hh* individual who possesses the secretor gene *(Se)* (see under the heading Secretors and Nonsecretors) does not secrete A, B or H substance, since there is no substance to secrete.

Notations for Bombay bloods are given as O_h^{A1}, O_h^{A2} and O_h^B and so forth, the superscript indicating the antigen that fails to act, demonstrated through family studies — since the "suppressed" gene may be manifested in the offspring of O_h individuals (shown in Fig. 3–6).

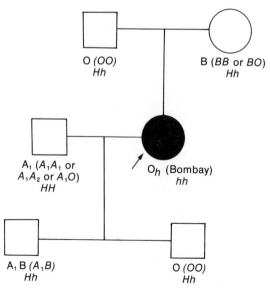

Figure 3–6 Family study demonstrating the suppression of the B antigen. On the basis of this, the proposita can be classified as O_h^B.

When it cannot be shown which ABO gene is suppressed (or is present but prevented from acting), the individual is classified simply as O_h (notation suggested by Levine). The suppressed gene, however can be ascertained without recourse to family studies by fixation-elution studies (Lanset *et al*, 1966; Dzierzkowa-Borody *et al*, 1972). These workers observed that anti-A or anti-B antigens or both of O_h red cells, while failing to agglutinate, must be present in some form.

Several other phenotypes that are similar to O_h have been described. These are shown in Table 3–6 with their normal patterns of reaction. It would appear that all of these phenotypes are similar in genetic background, owing to partial suppression of the expression of the *H* gene, which in turn affects the expression of the *A* or *B* genes or both. The interested reader is referred to *Blood Groups In Man* by R. R. Race and Ruth Sanger for additional information and appropriate references.

Secretors and Nonsecretors

Approximately 77 per cent of U.S. whites and 75 per cent of U.S. blacks secrete water-soluble substances in saliva that have the same specificity as the antigens on their red cells. The term "secretor" refers to individuals who secrete A, B or H substances; substances of the Lewis system, also found in saliva, are not taken into account.

The appearance of ABH antigens in saliva is controlled by a secretor gene inherited independently of *ABO* and *H* genes. The relevant gene is called *Se*, and its allele, which is amorphic, is called *se*. Individuals who are homozygous or heterozygous for the *Se* gene (i.e., *SeSe* or *Sese)* are secretors; individuals who lack the *Se* gene and are therefore homozygous for the amorphic allele *se* (i.e., *sese)*, are nonsecretors.

All secretors secrete H substance, regardless of their ABO group. Thus the saliva of a group O secretor contains H substance, the saliva of a group A secretor contains A and H substances, the saliva of a group B secretor contains B and H substances and the saliva of a group AB secretor contains A, B and H substances. O_h (Bombay) individuals do not secrete A, B or H substances, even when the *Se* gene is present (Table 3–7).

Water-soluble A, B and H antigens (substances) are present in most body fluids (seminal fluid, urine, sweat, tears, digestive juices, bile and milk) of a secretor. A second form of the antigens, which are *alcohol*-soluble, are present in all tissues of the body (except the brain) and on the red cells but are not present in the secretions. These alcohol-soluble antigens are not influenced by the secretor gene (see Hartmann, 1941).

In 1948, Grubb showed that the secretor phenomenon is closely associated with the Lewis blood groups — this is discussed in Chapter 4. Secretor status is determined by the inhibition (neutralization) test, which is detailed under the heading Inhibition Tests for Secretor Status).

The Number of A and B Antigens on Red Cells

Several studies have been performed to determine the number of A and B antigen sites on the red cells (Greenburg *et al*, 1963; Economidou *et al*, 1967a; Cartron *et al*, 1974; Cartron, 1976). While the exact numbers of sites are of academic interest only, differences do serve to explain the quantitative theory of the A sub-

Table 3–7 ABH SUBSTANCES IN THE SALIVA OF SECRETORS AND NONSECRETORS

Blood Group	Secretor Genotype	ABH Substance in Saliva
O	SeSe	H
	Sese	H
	sese	None
A	SeSe	A + H
	Sese	A + H
	sese	None
B	SeSe	B + H
	Sese	B + H
	sese	None
AB	SeSe	A + B + H
	Sese	A + B + H
	sese	None
O_h	SeSe or Sese	None
	sese	None

Table 3–8 ESTIMATES OF THE NUMBER OF A AND B ANTIGEN SITES ON THE RED CELLS OF ADULTS AND NEWBORNS OF VARIOUS PHENOTYPES

Antigen	Number of Sites
A_1 (adults)	810,000–1,170,000 A sites
A_1 (newborn)	250,000–370,000 A sites
A_2 (adults)	240,000–290,000 A sites
A_2 (newborn)	140,000 A sites
A_3 (adults)	35,000 A sites
A_x (adults)	4,800 A sites
A_{end} (adults)	3,500 A sites
A_m (adults)	700 A sites
A_1B (adults)	460,000–850,000 A sites
A_1B (adults)	310,000–560,000 B sites
A_2B (adults)	140,000 A sites
A_1B (newborn)	220,000 A sites
B (adults)	750,000 B sites
B (newborn)	200,000 B sites

groups. Figures, based on the work of the aforementioned authors, are given in Table 3–8.

ABH Antigens on Cells Other Than Red Cells

A, B and H antigens are found in most secretions and tissues of the human body, and are also widely distributed in nature, having been found in animals, plants and bacteria. Among the cellular components of the human body, ABH antigens have been found on normoblasts (Yunis and Yunis, 1963, 1964a, 1964b), platelets (Gurevitch and Nelken, 1954a, 1954b, 1955), white cells (Thomsen, 1930), epidermal and epithelial cells (Coombs *et al*, 1956), cancer cells (Davidsohn *et al*, 1969, 1971a, 1966, 1971b), and spermatozoa (Edwards *et al*, 1964).

In addition to the cells of the body, ABH antigens are also found in serum (see Høstrup, 1962, 1963; Fried *et al*, 1968 and Holburn and Masters, 1974).

Acquired B Antigen

In 1959, Cameron *et al* described seven individuals of blood group A_1 with an acquired B-like antigen. The serum of these individuals contained normal anti-B but the red cells were agglutinated by some anti-B sera, though not as strongly as normal group B red cells. The saliva of those who were secretors contained A and H but no B substance. Of the seven subjects, five had cancer and six were over 60 years of age.

Gerbal *et al* (1976), in investigating nine similar cases, suggested that "acquired B" may result from the action of the bacterial deace-

tylase, which converts N-acetyl-galactosamine to x-galactosamine, which is very similar to galactose, the chief determinant of B. There also appears to be an association between acquired B- and T-activation, in which case the cells are polyagglutinable (see Polyagglutination, Chapter 24).

Bird (1977) described a second type of acquired B caused by the adsorption of B-like bacterial products onto O or A red cells *in vitro* but not *in vivo*.

The A, B and H Antigens in Newborns

A, B and H antigens are detectable long before birth. Kemp (1930) detected the A antigen in a 37-day-old fetus. The strength of the A and B antigens does not increase during fetal life (Constantoulakis and Kay, 1962), being weaker in absorptive power and qualitatively different when compared to adult cells. The H antigen was shown to be the same; though not fully expressed on fetal cells, it is detectable on these cells of all ABO groups (Constantoulakis *et al*, 1963).

In newborns, some difficulty may be experienced in distinguishing between A_1 and A_2 cells (Wiener, 1943). However, after birth the strength of both A and B rises (Bjorum and Kemp, 1929), reaching adult levels at about three years of age, where it remains for life (Grundbacher, 1964).

THE ANTIBODIES OF THE ABO BLOOD GROUP SYSTEM

The Development of Anti-A and Anti-B

An explanation of the fact that anti-A or anti-B antibodies or both occur in all individuals (except those of group AB) has been the subject of debate for some time. The two extreme views are that the antibodies are the result of contact with A and B substances in the environment subsequent to birth or that they are wholly genetically determined. It now appears likely that the truth is midway between the two theories.

The "environment" theory is supported by observations of Springer *et al* (1959), who found that white Leghorn chicks do not produce "natural" antibody if maintained in a germ-free environment. If we apply this observation to humans, an infant of, for example, group A, who comes into contact with A and B substances in the environment will "recognize" the A substance yet will not recognize the B substance and so will produce an antibody — anti-B — to protect itself against this substance. Similarly, a group B infant will produce anti-A to protect itself against A substance. This theory was easier to accept as the *only* explanation when it was believed that newborn infants did not produce anti-A or anti-B or both and that these antibodies, when present in a newborn, were passively acquired from the mother. It is now known through the work of Toivanen and Hirvonen (1969) that this is not true. They found anti-A and/or anti-B that were clearly not of maternal origin in 8 of 44 neonatal sera.

The theory that anti-A and anti-B are genetically determined is supported by the work of Filitti-Wrumser *et al* (1954) on the physiochemical differences between the anti-B produced by persons of different A_1 genotypes (i.e., A_1A_1, A_1A_2 and A_1O) and on the observations of Salmon (1965) with respect to the physical properties of anti-B in persons whose A antigen has been "altered" by leukemia or by massive transfusion of washed O cells (see under the heading Causes of Anomalous Results in ABO Testing). In short, it would appear likely that the presence of anti-A or anti-B or both involves the genetics of the red cells as well as the environment.

Anti-A and Anti-B

As discussed, the anti-A and anti-B antibodies are present in the serum of an individual when the corresponding antigen is absent from the red cells. The strength (titer) of the antibodies varies considerably in different sera, though in general the strength of anti-A in group B and group O subjects tends to be greater than the strength of anti-B in group A and group O subjects. With the exception of group AB subjects, complete absence of anti-A or anti-B or both is very rare in healthy subjects, occurring in approximately 1 in 10,000 donors (Dobson and Ikin, 1946).

Anti-A or anti-B or both are often present in very low concentrations in patients with hypogammaglobulinemia (see under the heading Causes of Anomalous Results in ABO Testing).

Anti-A may be wholly IgM, or partly IgM and partly IgG (Fudenberg *et al*, 1959), partly IgM and partly IgA, or a mixture of all three immunoglobulins (Kunkel and Rockey, 1963). IgG anti-A and anti-B occur more commonly in individuals of group O than in individuals of group A or group B (Rawson and Abelson, 1960). IgM anti-A and anti-B can be inactivated by treatment with 2-mercaptoethanol (2-ME); IgA anti-

A and anti-B are reduced but not completely inactivated by treatment with 2-ME (Rawson and Abelson, 1964; Ishizaka *et al*, 1965; Adinolfi *et al*, 1966) (see under the heading Methods).

Both IgM and IgG anti-A and anti-B are capable of binding complement (Rawson and Abelson, 1960). All examples of IgG anti-A and about 90 per cent of IgM anti-A have been shown by Polley *et al* (1963) to be readily hemolytic. IgA anti-A and anti-B fail to bind complement (Adinolfi *et al*, 1966).

There are two kinds of IgM anti-A and anti-B, so-called "naturally occurring" and "immune." As the name implies, immune anti-A and anti-B are the result of direct stimulus with A or B substance, by pregnancy or by the transfusion of incompatible blood or plasma. Immune anti-A and anti-B may also result from the injection of horse serum, antitetanus toxin or the nondialyzable part of influenza virus vaccine (Springer, 1963). Immune anti-A or anti-B is indicated by a rise in titer, increase of avidity, increased difficulty in neutralizing the antibodies with A or B substance, the appearance of hemolysis, and serological activity which is greater at 37° C than at 4° C (i.e., a reverse of the normal behavior).*

Anti-A and anti-B are sometimes present in neonatal sera. In infants between the ages of 3 and 6 months, the titer of these agglutinins increases, reaching a maximum in the individual at 5 to 10 years of age, after which it gradually decreases (Thomsen and Kettal, 1929). The agglutinins are found in human milk and in ascitic fluid (Weiner, 1943) and also in saliva (see Putkonen, 1930).

Anti-A and anti-B sometimes occur as autoantibodies, though they usually then show cross-reactive specificity with the Ii blood group system (i.e., they shown anti-A_1I anti-BI or anti-Bi specificity). Two cases of autoimmune hemolytic anemia associated with the presence of anti-A in the serum have been described in an A_1 patient (Szymanski *et al*, 1976; Parker *et al*, 1978).

Cross-Reacting Anti-A_1B

Landsteiner and Witt (1926), confirming the earlier observations of Hektoen (1907) and Moss (1910), showed that elution of group A cells mixed with anti-A_1B (group O serum) would produce in the eluate both anti-A and

---

*It may be interesting to note, too, that immune anti-A will react with pig A cells, whereas "naturally occurring" anti-A will not (Polley *et al*, 1963).

anti-B and that group B cells treated in the same way would do so also. These unexpected elution results are not seen when anti-A + anti-B (taken from group A and group B individuals, respectively, and mixed) is used (Dodd, 1952; Bird, 1953).

Several serological explanations have been offered for this phenomenon, yet to date there is no agreement on any of them. (For further discussion see Race and Sanger (1975), page 48.)

Anti-A$_1$

The serum of group O and group B individuals after absorption with an equal volume of group A$_2$ cells will agglutinate A$_1$ cells but will no longer agglutinate A$_2$ cells, whereas if absorption is performed using A$_1$ cells, no agglutination will be seen with A$_1$ or A$_2$ cells. Based on this observation, it is clear that two separate populations of anti-A molecules occur in group O and group B individuals: anti-A, which reacts with both A$_1$ and A$_2$ cells and anti-A$_1$, which reacts only with A$_1$ cells. The anti-A$_1$ isolated from group B individuals is usually IgM; however, anti-A$_1$ from group O individuals was found by Plischka and Schafer (1972) to be wholly IgG.

Anti-A$_1$ also occurs as a separate antibody in 1 to 2 per cent of A$_2$ bloods and 25 per cent of A$_2$B bloods (Taylor et al, 1942; Juel, 1959), although different frequencies have been reported by Speiser et al (1951). The antibody is rare in infants (Speiser, 1956).

Most examples of anti-A$_1$ in A$_2$ or A$_2$B individuals are reactive at temperatures below 25° C and as such are of no clinical significance. Antibodies that are reactive at temperatures above 25° C may bring about the destruction of A$_1$ cells in vivo when therapeutic quantities of blood are given; however, such cases are extremely rare.

Anti-A and Anti-A$_1$ From Other Sources

Anti-A has been found in a number of seed extracts (so-called plant agglutinins, or lectins), the most useful of which is found in *Dolichos biflorus* (Bird, 1951, 1952), which agglutinates A$_1$ and A$_1$B cells strongly and to high dilution and A$_2$ and A$_2$B cells very weakly. An excellent anti-A$_1$ can be prepared from these seeds at suitable dilution and commercial preparations are available (see Lectins, Chapter 19). Lectins that are specific for anti-B and anti-A + B have

also been described but are not generally used.

Prokop et al (1965 a, b, c) showed that the familiar snail *Helix hortensis* contains powerful anti-A that agglutinates A$_1$ and A$_2$ cells at the same strength; the receptor in man was given the name A$_{hel}$ (later called A$_{HP}$, A$_{HH}$, etc.). This opened up a new area of study, which over the years has grown considerably. The interested reader is directed to a review published by Prokop et al (1968), which covers the whole subject of agglutinins in snails and fish roes and also sets down a standard notation.

Anti-H

"Pure" anti-H is found in individuals of the very rare O$_h$ (Bombay) phenotype as a hemolysin and as an agglutinin that is almost as active at 37° C as at O° C (Bhende et al, 1952; Bhatia et al, 1955; Parkin, 1956 and Pettenkover et al, 1960). Anti-H, found in persons who are not of phenotype O$_h$, tends to be weaker and reacts only at low temperatures. The antibody reacts (agglutinates) more strongly with group O red cells and hardly at all with A$_1$ and A$_1$B red cells.

Reagents with anti-H specificity can be obtained from the plant *Ulex europaeus*, which is commonly used by most workers. Other sources of anti-H, from the seeds of the plant *Lotus tetragonolobus* and from the sera of the eel *Anguilla anguilla*, are less satisfactory (see Lectins, Chapter 19).

TECHNIQUES

ABO Grouping

A patient or donor of unknown ABO group is usually tested by *forward grouping* and by *reverse grouping*. This means that the individual's red cells are combined with serum containing known antibody (forward grouping), and his serum is combined with red cells possessing known antigen (reverse grouping).

Sera for Forward Grouping. As has been described, persons of blood group A produce anti-B in their plasma and persons of blood group B produce anti-A in theirs. These antibodies normally build to a titer (strength) of between 1/16 and 1/64 (i.e., the antibody will still show agglutination with its corresponding antigen when diluted 16 to 64 times using one drop of plasma or serum and up to 64 drops of normal saline). The antibodies in certain persons of groups A and B can be stimulated to much greater titers by injection of specific A or B substances, and this provides the source for anti-A and anti-B testing sera used in forward grouping. Anti-A + B (group O), also in common use in most laboratories, is derived from the serum of group O individuals whose anti-A *and* anti-B have been stimulated to high titers. The serum when combined with unknown cells will show agglutination with red cells of group A_1, A_1B (including some A subgroups) and B, yet it will show no agglutination with red cells of group O. The main reason for the use of this serum is to allow distinction between red cells of group O and red cells that belong to a subgroup of A — which might otherwise be indistinguishable.

Cells for Reverse Grouping. For the reverse grouping, red cells from group A and group B individuals are used. The red cells from group A individuals are separated into those belonging to group A_1 and those to subgroup A_2, and both are made available commercially. A_1 cells are used primarily in routine reverse grouping.

RULES FOR PRACTICAL LABORATORY WORK

1. Perform all tests according to the manufacturer's directions. Each manufacturer provides detailed instructions for the use of each antiserum. These instructions differ from one manufacturer to another so that a single set of instructions cannot be used for all reagents of a particular specificity.
2. Always run controls. With respect to ABO grouping most laboratories control the antisera once per day as part of a routine quality assurance program. This eliminates the need to run individual controls each time the reagents are used (see Quality Control, Chapter 20).
3. Always label tubes and slides fully and clearly. Do not rely on colored dyes to identify the antibody.
4. Always add serum *before* adding cells, and

examine each tube after the serum has been added to ensure that none has been missed.
5. Use only high-titered antisera that has been approved for laboratory use.
6. Inspect each tube *individually* against a well-lighted background.
7. Use an optical aid to examine reactions that appear to be negative by the naked eye.

ABO GROUPING (TUBE METHOD)

1. Label each tube to identify the antisera and cells.
2. Mix the antisera with known red cells and the unknown serum with the known cells in ratios as recommended by the manufacturer. *Note:* If "home-made" reverse grouping cells are used, they should be a 2 per cent to 5 per cent suspension of washed cells in saline prepared freshly each day and should be added in the ratio of two drops of serum to one drop of red cells.*
3. Mix all tubes by gently shaking. To enhance agglutination in the reverse grouping, tubes may be incubated for five minutes or more at *room temperature.*
4. Centrifuge at speed and time determined to be optimal (manufacturer's directions).
5. Observe supernatant fluid against a well-lighted white background for presence of hemolysis.
6. Gently disperse cell button and inspect for agglutination, using a well-lighted background and optical aid if necessary.

Interpretation
Table 3–9 gives the results and interpretation of routine ABO grouping.

ABO GROUPING (SLIDE METHOD)

Forward grouping may be performed on a slide because reagent antibodies agglutinate most cell samples without the need for centrifugation.

*AABB recommendation.

Table 3–9 INTERPRETATION OF RESULTS OF ABO GROUPING

Anti-A	Anti-B	Anti-A + B	A_1 Cells	B Cells	Group
−	−	−	+	+	O
+	−	+	−	+	A
−	+	+	+	−	B
+	+	+	−	−	AB

Positive (+) = cells are agglutinated.
Negative (−) = cells are not agglutinated.

Reverse grouping, however, is more reliable performed by the tube method.

Tests are performed according to the manufacturer's directions with respect to cell suspension and diluents. The following instructions, however, apply to all slide tests.*

1. Ensure that slides are clean and dry before use.
2. Label the sections of the slide to identify the antisera (and cells).
3. Mix the red cells and the antisera gently but thoroughly over an area about 1 inch in diameter.
4. Use a separate clean stick to mix red cells with each antiserum.
5. Do not place slide on or over a warmed view box.
6. Keep red cell–serum mixture in continuous, gentle motion and observe for 2 minutes before concluding that agglutination is absent.
7. Do not confuse drying around the edges with agglutination.
8. Avoid touching the red cell–serum mixture with fingers.

Notes on ABO Grouping

Antibodies of the ABO system cause agglutination of saline-suspended red cells at room temperature or below. Heating to 37° C weakens the reaction and a high-protein medium does not interfere with agglutination but does not enhance it. See under the heading Anomalous Results in ABO Grouping.

OTHER TECHNIQUES

Subgrouping with *Dolichos biflorus* Extract (Anti-A₁)

Subgrouping with *Dolichos biflorus* extract (anti-A$_1$) can be performed on a slide or by tube method using commercially prepared reagent. The same general instructions given for ABO slide and tube methods apply. The reagent must be controlled using known A$_1$ and A$_2$ red cells each time the test is performed unless this forms part of the routine quality control performed daily.

Grouping with *Ulex europaeus* Extract (Anti-H)

Methods of testing with *Ulex europaeus* extract (anti-H) are identical to those employed

*AABB recommendations.

when using the anti-A$_1$ lectin, substituting the *Ulex europaeus* extract for the *Dolichos biflorus* extract.

SECRETOR SALIVA TESTS (TO DETERMINE SECRETOR STATUS)

1. Collect about 0.5 ml of saliva into a clean, dry beaker. This can be done in an infant by using a very small cotton wool swab held in Spencer-Wells forceps, which absorbs the saliva and is then squeezed, expressing the drops into a small tube. Alternatively, a plastic pipette can be used by holding the infant's mouth open and recovering saliva from under the tongue. In adults who have difficulty, a wad of wax in the mouth will help to increase salivation.
2. Centrifuge the saliva at about 3400 rpm for 10 minutes, then pour the supernatant into a hard glass test tube.
3. Boil the supernatant saliva in a boiling water bath for 10 minutes; this procedure is most important, because it will destroy the enzymes that would otherwise inactivate the group-specific substances and will also destroy anti-A and anti-B, which are often present in secretions. The saliva can now be stored and will keep well at −20° C. If the saliva is frozen, a clearer supernatant will result.
4. When testing for secretor status, it is normally sufficient to test for H substance alone, by using dilutions of the extract of *Ulex europaeus* against group O cells. If no conclusion can be reached and the subject is group A, B or AB, an additional test, using dilutions of serum containing the appropriate antibody, can be performed for the presence of A or B substance using A$_2$ cells with anti-A and B cells with anti-B.
5. It is important to run controls in parallel with the test, using the saliva of several secretors and several nonsecretors.

Interpretation

If the test for H substance is negative (i.e., no agglutination; antibody activity has been completely neutralized), the individual is a secretor. Partial or no inhibition (i.e., a positive test) reveals a nonsecretor. *Note:* In all neutralization (inhibition) tests, no agglutination or hemolysis is a positive result.

The amount of blood group substance can be estimated by making serial dilutions of the saliva in saline (i.e., performing a *titration* — see Chapter 23) (Table 3–10).

Table 3–10 TITRATIONS OF SECRETOR AND NONSECRETOR SALIVA

| | Dilutions in Saline | | | | | |
	1/1	1/10	1/20	1/40	1/320	Continued
Secretor	–	–	–	–	w	2+
Secretor (Weak)	–	–	–	1+	2+	2+
Nonsecretor	2+	2+	2+	2+	2+	2+

Notes. Despite the difference between the reactivity of A_1 and A_2 red cells with anti-A, saliva from A_1 and A_2 secretors shows virtually no difference in reactivity. Immune anti-A and anti-B are not neutralized by blood group specific substances A and B. If potent substances are used, however, partial neutralization may occur.

HEMOLYSIN TESTS FOR HIGH-TITER ANTI-A AND ANTI-B

Hemolysin tests are used to determine the ability of anti-A and anti-B (in group O subjects) to cause the hemolysis of cells and therefore to determine their "safety" when utilized as unmatched blood or when transfusing group O whole blood to individuals of other blood groups. It should be noted, of course, that in these days of component therapy and minimal use of "unmatched" blood, this test has little application. The common solution nowadays is to remove the plasma from unmatched blood and transfuse the red cells.

Method*

1. Since complement is important to the reaction, use only fresh, complement-containing serum, not plasma or aged or inactivated serum.
2. Place two drops of serum in each of two tubes, labeled A and B.
3. Add two drops of 2 per cent to 5 per cent saline suspension of washed A_1 cells to tube A and two drops of B cells to tube B.

Note. Use of a weaker cell suspension or larger amounts of serum will increase incidence of hemolytic activity (Weiner et al, 1953).

4. Mix gently and incubate at 37° C for 10 to 15 minutes.
5. Centrifuge and examine supernatant against a well-lighted white background to detect hemolysis. Any shade of pink or red indicates hemolysis.

6. Record results as negative or a quantitative estimate on positives.

Note. As a positive control, add two drops of a known hemolytic group O serum to two drops of the suspensions of A_1 and B cells. As a negative control, add two drops of inert AB serum to two drops of the suspensions of A_1 and B cells. Run these in parallel with the test.

2-MERCAPTOETHANOL FOR DIFFERENTIATION OF IgG AND IgM

This test is useful in the serologic investigation of hemolytic disease of the newborn, since only IgG antibodies are capable of crossing the placenta (see Chapter 2). It is also useful in the test for non-neutralizable anti-A and anti-B. Treatment of IgM antibodies with 2-mercaptoethanol results in the breaking of the disulfide bonds of the antibody molecules and hence destroys the serologic activity. Similar treatment of IgG antibodies has no effect.

Method

1. Add 1 ml serum from the individual being tested to 1 ml of freshly prepared 0.1 M 2-mercaptoethanol in pH 7.4 buffer.
2. Add 1 ml of serum plus 1 ml of pH 7.4 buffer to a separate tube. This serves as a control.
3. Incubate the tubes at 37° C for two hours.
4. Dialyze the tubes overnight against 1 liter of pH 7.4 buffered saline at 4° C. Harvest the serum and test for serologic activity (i.e., titrate).

Interpretations

In titrations of serum containing IgG antibodies, little difference or no difference will be noted between untreated serum and 2-mercaptoethanol-treated serum. In titrations of serum containing IgM antibodies, almost complete neutralization of the antibodies may be observed. With mixtures of IgG and IgM antibodies, titers of serum treated with 2-mercaptoethanol will be greatly reduced; however, powerful reactions will still be observed with undiluted serum.

TESTS FOR NON-NEUTRALIZABLE ANTI-A AND ANTI-B*

If both coating and agglutinating antibodies of the same specificity are present in a serum, the

---

*AABB recommended method.

*Reprinted from AABB Technical Manual, 8th edition. Copyright © 1981 American Association of Blood Banks.

existence of coating antibodies will be masked by agglutination. The agglutinins must be removed before coating antibodies can be demonstrated. IgM agglutinins can be inactivated by treatment with 2-mercaptoethanol or dithiothreitol.

Agglutinins are neutralized by soluble blood group substances more readily than are coating antibodies. Elevated levels of non-neutralizable coating antibodies occur in the serum of mothers whose offspring have ABO hemolytic disease of the newborn. It is not clear which level constitutes a threat to the fetus, but activity below 1:10 dilution appears to be insignificant. The following procedure demonstrates activity at 1:10 dilution. To quantitate beyond this level, the neutralized serum can be further diluted.

Method*

1. Add 0.2 ml soluble blood group material (A and B) to 1 ml serum.
2. Mix and leave at room temperature for 5 minutes.
3. Add 0.1 ml of neutralized serum to 0.9 ml saline, for a 1:10 dilution.
4. Add one drop of diluted serum to each of two tubes, labeled A and B.
5. Add one drop of a 2 per cent to 5 per cent saline suspension of A cells to tube A and one drop of B cells to tube B.
6. Centrifuge and examine for agglutination. If there is no agglutination, proceed to step 7. If agglutination occurs, neutralization of agglutinins is incomplete. To the remaining undiluted serum, add another 0.2 ml of soluble blood group substance. Incubate at room temperature for five minutes and repeat steps 3 through 6.
7. Incubate tubes at 37° C for 30 minutes.
8. Wash cells four times in saline, add two drops of antiglobulin serum to each tube, and mix gently.
9. Centrifuge and examine for agglutination. Add sensitized cells as control for negative antiglobulin procedure if desired.

Interpretation

Negative results after antiglobulin testing indicate that the original serum has less than 1:10 level of immunoglobulin capable of sensitizing A or B cells. A positive result indicates that, in addition to the agglutinins readily observed on immediate spin, there is a moderate amount of coating antibody with the same specificity.

---

*Reprinted from AABB Technical Manual, 8th edition. Copyright © 1981 American Association of Blood Banks.

Note that anti-A and anti-B activity may differ widely in strength. On a random basis, anti-A titers are higher than anti-B, but if the immunizing stimulus was group B, a particular individual might have IgG anti-B levels far higher than anti-A.

PREPARATION OF ANTI-A_1 FROM *DOLICHOS BIFLORUS* SEEDS

Method

1. Grind the seeds of *Dolichos biflorus* in a mill.
2. To each gram of meal, add 20 ml of saline.
3. Agitate thoroughly for one hour in a shaking machine.
4. Centrifuge at 3400 rpm for five minutes and recover the supernatant. The supernatant fluid, even though cloudy, can be used immediately, though the appearance can be improved by filtration through a clarifying Seitz filter (pad grade 4).
5. Test the extract with a panel of known cells of subgroups A_1 and A_2. The extract may require dilution so that it gives clear negatives with A_2 cells.
6. Store at 4° C.

PREPARATION OF ANTI-H FROM *ULEX EUROPAEUS* SEEDS

The method of preparation is exactly as for *Dolichos biflorus*. The resulting extract reacts with all human red cells in the following declining order: $O > A_2 > B > A_2B > A_1 > A_1B$. If the extract is to be used for the detection of A_2, dilution should be undertaken to ensure that A_1 and A_1B groups give no reaction.

ANOMALOUS RESULTS IN ABO TESTING

1. *Caused by technique:* Poor technique is one of the major causes of anomalous results in routine ABO testing. This includes:
   - (a) Dirty glassware — false positive results.
   - (b) Improper cell-to-serum concentration — false positive or false negative results.
   - (c) Contamination or inactivation of reagents — false negative or occasionally false positive results.
   - (d) Overcentrifugation — false positive results.
   - (e) Undercentrifugation — false negative results.

(f) Failure to identify hemolysis as a positive result — false negative results.

(g) Careless reading — false negative results.

(h) Failure to use an optical aid — false negative results.

(i) Incorrect identification of specimen or materials — false positive or false negative results.

(j) Incorrect recording of results or interpretation — false positive or false negative results.

All of these can be controlled if rigid policies and procedures are enforced in the laboratory. An anomalous result due to poor technique can result in fatal consequences for the recipient and is always the most difficult type of error to defend.

2. *Caused by serum abnormalities:* Reverse grouping may be affected by Wharton's jelly or serum proteins causing rouleaux. These factors may be present in the patient's serum and remain in the cell suspension tested.

3. *Caused by sensitization:* Antibody-coated (sensitized) red cells in the patient may agglutinate in a high protein medium.

4. *Caused by recent transfusion:* A transfusion of blood of another ABO group prior to testing may provide a sample that is a mixture of cell types, giving a "mixed field" appearance on testing.

5. *Caused by unusual genotype:* The A or B antigens may be weakly expressed because of an unusual genotype (i.e., subgroups of A and B).

6. *Caused by misgrouping:* A_2B and A_3B samples may react weakly with anti-A. If anti-A_1 is present, the sample may be misgrouped as group B. Sera from samples thought to be group B should therefore be tested against A_2 cells as well as A_1 cells to distinguish those with anti-A_1 but no anti-A in the serum.

7. *Caused by disease:* In some subjects with acute leukemia or other nonhematologic malignant disorders, the red cell antigens in the ABO system may be greatly depressed. Diminishing of A_1 and H antigens can also occur in refractory anemia.

8. *Caused by polyagglutination:* Red cells may possess genetic or acquired surface abnormalities that render them polyagglutinable (see Chapter 24).

9. *Caused by chimerism:* A chimera possesses a dual population of red cells resulting in a classic "mixed field" appearance on testing.

10. *Caused by acquired B:* Acquired "B-like" activity can result from the action of gram-negative organisms (Gerbal *et al*, 1975) (see p. 78).

11. *Caused by abnormal proteins:* Abnormal proteins, altered proportions of globulins and high concentrations of fibrinogen may cause rouleaux formation, which could be mistaken for agglutination.

12. *Caused by blood group – specific substances:* In certain conditions (e.g., patients with ovarian cysts) blood group–specific substances may be of such high concentration that anti-A and anti-B are neutralized when unwashed cells are used. At least three washes may be necessary before accurate results can be obtained.

13. *Caused by irregular antibodies:* Besides unexpected antibodies reacting with A_1, B or H antigens, irregular antibodies in some other blood group system may be present that react with antigens on the A or B cells used in reverse grouping.

14. *Caused by unwashed cells:* The use of unwashed cells can cause false positive results due to rouleaux-promoting properties in the subject's serum (e.g., in multiple myeloma).

15. *Caused by hypogammaglobulinemia:* The first indication of hypogammaglobulinemia (diminished amounts of gamma globulin) may be missing or weak reactions in serum (reverse) grouping owing to low over-all immunoglobulin levels.

16. *Caused by drugs, etc.:* Drugs, dextran, and intravenously injected contrast materials may cause cellular aggregation that resembles agglutination.

17. *Caused by dyes:* Antibody to coloring dyes (e.g., acriflavine, used in some countries as a yellow dye in anti-B) can cause false positive results with anti-B. Such a discrepancy would be recognized, however, by the presence of anti-B in the serum.

18. *Caused by false reaction:* In testing with *Dolichos biflorus* extract, it should be noted that the lectin will agglutinate strongly positive Sd(a+) red cells irrespective of ABO group as well as Cad Sd(a++) and Tn cells (see Lectins, Chapter 19).

19. *Caused by age:* Anomalous results may occur when testing infants who have not begun to produce their own antibodies or who possess antibodies that have been passively acquired from the mother or when testing elderly persons whose antibody levels have declined.

20. *Caused by preservatives:* A patient may possess antibodies to elements of the preservatives, suspending mediums or reagent solutions used in testing, resulting in errors in ABO group classification.

Notes on Anomalies in ABO Testing

Many of the anomalies in ABO testing can be resolved by obtaining a new sample of blood from the individual, carefully washing the cells and repeating the tests. If problems are encountered, the results of antibody-screening and antiglobulin tests, serum protein findings and autocontrol result and such information as age of the patient, diagnosis and history of previous medications or transfusions may all help in establishing the cause. Rouleaux factors can often be diminished by adding additional saline to the cell-serum mixture. If anti-I is the cause, it is usually possible to autoabsorb the antibody — though this should *not* be attempted if the patient has been transfused with red blood cells in the preceding four weeks, since the antigens on the *transfused* cells may absorb a developing alloantibody of clinical significance.

Weak examples of A or B can be diagnosed in many cases by testing the cells with many different samples of anti-A and anti-B, by incubation at 18° C or 4° C before testing, by testing the cells for the ability to absorb antibody, by testing the eluate from absorbed cells for agglutinating activity against cells of other unusual activities, by testing the saliva and by studying the blood and saliva from blood relatives, to determine heritability of the abnormality. If polyagglutinability is suspected, various lectins can be employed to establish the different types (See Polyagglutination, Chapter 24).

TYPICAL EXAMINATION QUESTIONS

Choose the phrase, sentence or symbol that correctly answers the question or completes the statement. More than one answer may be acceptable for each question. Answers are given at the back of the book.

1. The antibodies one would expect to find in the serum of an individual who has the O_h (Bombay) phenotype are
   (a) anti-A, anti-D, anti-H
   (b) anti-A, anti-B, anti-H
   (c) anti-A, anti-B, anti-A_1B
   (d) anti-A, anti-B, anti-h
   (e) anti-A, anti-B, anti-A_1
   (O_h [The Bombay Phenotype])
2. The terminal sugars of the antigenic determinants of A and B blood groups are
   (a) D-galactose and N-acetyl-D-glucosamine
   (b) N-acetyl-galactosamine and N-acetyl glucosamine
   (c) N-acetyl-galactosamine and D-galactose
   (d) N-acetyl-glucosamine and L-fucose
   (e) N-acetyl-glucosamine and glucose
   (The Gene H: Its Role in the Expression of A and B Genes)
3. When testing blood samples from individuals with weak subgroups of A, the following may be observed
   (a) The red cells may react with anti-A,B
   (b) The red cells may type as O
   (c) The serum may possess anti-A_1
   (d) The incidence of immune antibodies may be increased
   (Other Subgroups of A and B)
4. Whether or not an individual secretes A, B or H substance in saliva is controlled by
   (a) the ABO blood group
   (b) the presence of the A_1 gene
   (c) the presence of the *Rh* gene
   (d) the presence or absence of the *Se* gene
   (Secretors and Nonsecretors)
5. Parents whose children show all of the phenotypes (excluding subgroups and excluding *cis* AB) in the ABO blood group systems are
   (a) group O and AB
   (b) group A and B
   (c) group B and AB
   (d) group A and AB
   (e) group O and B
   (Table 3–3)
6. The following results are obtained when performing blood grouping on an individual

Anti-A	Anti-A_1	Anti-B	Anti-A,B	A_1 cells	A_2 cells
Pos	Neg	Pos	Pos	Pos	Neg

B cells	O cells
Neg	Neg

   The most probable interpretation would be
   (a) A_1B
   (b) A_2B with anti-A_1 in the serum
   (c) A_2B
   (d) A_2B with anti-A_2 in the serum
   (Anomalous Results in ABO Testing)
7. A_1 and B cells used in ABO reverse (serum) grouping
   (a) will detect subgroups of A and B
   (b) may indicate that a patient has hypogammaglobulinemia
   (c) may detect anti-A_1
   (d) will always be correct and the cell grouping incorrect
   (Anomalous Results in ABO Testing)
8. Leukemia has been reported to weaken the
   (a) A antigen
   (b) B antigen
   (c) A and B antibodies
   (d) antibodies to A_1
   (Anomalous Results in ABO Testing)

9. ABO serum (reverse) grouping is
   (a) unnecessary if anti-A and anti-B are used
   (b) unreliable in newborns
   (c) ignored if it does not agree with the forward group
   (d) the test that may give the first clue that a patient is suffering from a protein abnormality

   (Anomalous Results in ABO Testing–ABO Grouping)

10. A lectin prepared from the seeds of *Dolichos biflorus* will react with
    (a) O$_h$ cells
    (b) A$_1$ cells
    (c) A$_1$ and A$_2$ cells if not suitably diluted
    (d) adult O cells
    (e) A$_3$ cells

    (Anti-A and Anti-A$_1$ From Other Sources)

11. Mixed-field agglutination may occur between commercially prepared anti-A and red blood cells that are group
    (a) A$_m$
    (b) A$_h$
    (c) A$_3$ or B$_3$
    (d) A$_2$
    (e) A$_x$

    (Table 3–5)

Study the diagram and answer the following questions:

(Fig. 3–3)

12. The substance labeled I is
    (a) h
    (b) H
    (c) unidentified
    (d) O
    (e) precursor substance

    (Fig. 3–3)

13. The substance labeled II is
    (a) H
    (b) h
    (c) O
    (d) precursor substance
    (e) A

    (Fig. 3–3)

14. The ABH substance(s) labeled IV in the saliva of a nonsecretor would
    (a) have B and H specificities and be present in small amounts
    (b) have B and H specificities and be present in large amounts
    (c) be absent
    (d) have H specificity only

    (Fig. 3–3)

15. The ABH substance(s) labeled VI in the saliva of a secretor would
    (a) be absent
    (b) neutralize anti-H
    (c) neutralize anti-A,B
    (d) none of the above

    (Fig. 3–3)

16. The red cell antigen(s) labeled VII would be
    (a) A, B and H
    (b) A and B
    (c) neither A, B nor H
    (d) B and H
    (e) A and H

    (Fig. 3–3)

17. The products of *A, B* and *H* genes are
    (a) glycolipids
    (b) transferases
    (c) glycoproteins
    (d) antigens on the red cell surface
    (e) oligosaccharide chains

    (Inheritance of the ABO Groups — See Also Chapter 2)

18. The *h* and *O* genes are thought to be
    (a) alleles
    (b) inherited as mendelian codominants
    (c) amorphs
    (d) detectable in the homozygous state only
    (e) identified by family study only

    (General)

19. Which of the following statements regarding the ABO system is (are) not true?
    (a) Group O blood is found in an individual with two amorphic genes at the ABO locus
    (b) The O$_h$ phenotype is found in individuals who lack the A or B genes or both at the ABO locus
    (c) Red cells of O$_h$ individuals are negative with anti-A, anti-B and anti-H
    (d) Red cells from group O secretors are negative with *Ulex europaeus* extract
    (e) The serum of an O$_h$ individual contains anti-A, anti-B and anti-H

    (General—O$_h$—The Bombay Phenotype)

20. Which of the following red cells will react weak-
    est with anti-H?
    (a) A₂ adult red cells
    (b) O adult red cells

(c) A₂B adult red cells
(d) A₁ adult red cells

*(The Gene H: Its Role in the
Expression of A and B Genes)*

GENERAL REFERENCES

1. AABB Technical Manual, American Association of Blood
   Banks, 7th Ed. 1977. (*Excellent coverage of the
   system in clear language. Discrepancies between
   cell and serum results will prove useful.*)
2. Mollison, P. L.: Blood Transfusion in Clinical Medicine,
   6th Ed. Blackwell Scientific Publications, Oxford,
   1979. (*Section on immune responses to A and B
   antigens (p. 260) is probably the most comprehen-*
   sive available. Coverage of the system will be useful
   to the student wishing to expand basic knowledge.)*
3. Race, R. R. and Sanger, R.: Blood Groups in Man, 6th Ed.
   Blackwell Scientific Publications, Oxford, 1975.
   (*Complete coverage, fully referenced. This book will
   provide a source of reference for the student requiring detailed information on the system.*)

4

THE LEWIS BLOOD GROUP SYSTEM

OBJECTIVES — THE LEWIS BLOOD GROUP SYSTEM

The student shall know, understand and be prepared to explain:

1. A brief history of the discovery of the Lewis blood group system
2. The basic principles of the inheritance of Lewis substance, specifically to include:
   (a) Gene names (original and current)
   (b) The interaction of Lewis genes with ABO, H, secretor genes
   (c) The structure of molecules with Lewis specificity on red cells
3. The effects of the interaction of Lewis genes with ABO, H and secretor genes on the Lewis types of offspring
4. The development of Lewis antigens
5. The antibodies of the Lewis system, specifically to include:
   (a) The types of immunoglobulin
   (b) Anti-Le^a in human sera (frequency and characteristics)
   (c) Anti-Le^a in animal sera
   (d) Anti-Le^b (characteristics, types [Le^{bL} and Le^{bH}])
   (e) Anti-Le^x (characteristics)
   (f) Anti-Le^c (characteristics)
   (g) Anti-Le^d (characteristics)
   (h) Anti-A$_1$Le^b and anti-BLe^b
   (i) Anti-Magard (characteristics)
   (j) Anti-ILe^{bH} (characteristics)
6. The Lewis system at the level of the routine blood bank, specifically:
   (a) Laboratory characteristics
   (b) Transfusion difficulties and requirements
7. The changes in Lewis phenotypes during pregnancy
8. The saliva types — Wiener's classification
9. General detection of Lewis substance in saliva

Introduction

The Lewis blood group system was originally described by Mourant (1946) when he reported the discovery of the antibody anti-Le^a. Two years later, the antithetical antibody anti-Le^b was described by Andresen (1948). Since that time, the Lewis system has been studied in depth and has, in many respects, been found to be unique among blood groups.

Grubb (1948) observed that individuals whose red cells were Le(a+) were nonsecretors of ABH substances; that the saliva of Le(a+) individuals inhibited anti-Le^a and that the majority of Le(a−) subjects also inhibited anti-Le^a but did so less strongly (Grubb, 1948, 1951; Brendemoen, 1949). Brendemoen (1951) also detected Le^a substance in the serum of Le(a+) subjects.

A general theory with respect to the Lewis groups was proposed by Grubb (1951) and sup-ported by the work of Ceppellini (1955a, 1955b) and by Ceppellini and Siniscalco (1955). The theories of Grubb and Ceppellini form the basis of our present view of the Lewis system.

The Genetics of the Lewis System

Lewis is a system of *soluble* antigens present in saliva and plasma; the determinants are not indigenous to the red cells. The red cells, however, acquire their Lewis phenotype by adsorption of Lewis substances from the plasma (Sneath and Sneath, 1955) (Fig. 4–1).

Ceppellini (1955) showed that the presence of Le^a in the saliva was controlled by a dominant gene, which he called *L*. The allele was originally called *l*, but the appellations of both genes were later changed by Ceppellini and other workers to *Le* and *le*.

The red cells of adults have the possible

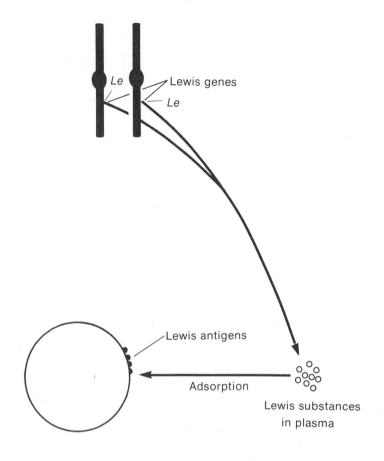

Figure 4–1   The expression of Lewis genes.

Lewis phenotypes Le(a+b−), Le(a−b+) and Le(a−b−). The Le(a+b+) phenotype is possessed by subjects of group O and A_2 who also possess the *H, Se* and *Le* genes, though the reaction with anti-Le[a] is usually weak and not consistent with all anti-Le[a] sera. The phenotype Le(a−b−) has not been found in adults of group A_1, probably because they make less Le[a] substance as a result of competition between the A_1 and *Le* gene products for substrate (see later discussion). The Lewis phenotype is determined genetically and is controlled by the interaction of three sets of independently inherited genes, *Lele, Hh* and *Sese*. Because Lewis substances (antigens) are formed only in secretions and serum and *not* directly on red cells, the interaction of the three sets of genes actually determines which Lewis antigens will be in the serum and will thus be adsorbed onto the red cells.

Individuals who inherit the *Le* gene can produce Le[a] substance; thus their red cells will have the phenotype Le(a+b−). In order for Le[b] substance to be produced, *Le, H* and *Se* genes must all be inherited, and the simultaneous presence of these three genes will produce the Le(a−b+) phenotype.

The *H* gene is very common and ABH antigens are nearly always present on *red cells*. In secretions, however, the presence of ABH substances is genetically controlled by the "regulator" genes, *Sese*. Individuals who are genetically *SeSe* or *Sese* are called secretors of ABH substances. Nonsecretors of ABH substances are genetically *sese*. *Note: Sese* genes control the secretion of ABH substances only; they have no control over the secretion of Lewis substances.

In each of the three systems, the alleles *le, h* and *se* are amorphic, and therefore produce no product. The red cells of *lele* individuals are Le(a−b−), since no Lewis substance can be made. Since *Sese* genes are inherited independently and control only the secretion of ABH substances, Le(a−b−) individuals may either inherit the *Se* gene and be secretors of ABH substances or be homozygous for the amorphic *se* gene and be nonsecretors of ABH substances (Table 4–1).

In addition, the Lewis phenotype may be modified by the ABO phenotype; e.g., the A_1 gene may interfere with the expression of the Le[a] antigen in Le(b+) subjects (Cutbush *et al*, 1956). Some of the interactions of the *Hh, Sese, ABO* and *Lele* genes are shown in Table 4–2.

The Lewis genes, like the *ABH* genes,

Table 4–1 GENETIC INFLUENCES ON THE LEWIS PHENOTYPE OF RED CELLS

Genes Inherited*	Secretor Status	Lewis Phenotypes of Red Cells
Le, H, se	Nonsecretor	Le (a+b−)
Le, H, Se	Secretor	Le (a−b+)
le, H, Se	Secretor	Le (a−b−)
le, H, se	Nonsecretor	Le (a−b−)

*The rare *hh* (Bombay) phenotype has been omitted.

control the production of specific transferase enzymes that cause the addition of a single sugar residue to a preformed precursor substance (Watkins and Morgan, 1959). The basic precursor substance is the same for both *ABH* and *Le* genes (see Figure 2–5, Chapter 2). As discussed in Chapter 2, two types of precursor substance exist, known as Type 1 and Type 2 chains. The *Le* gene controls the conversion of Type 1 chains to Le^a substance through the addition of a fucose molecule to the subterminal N-acetyl-glucosamine sugar of the precursor substance in alpha (1–4) linkage (Lloyd *et al*, 1968; Rege *et al*, 1964) (Fig. 4–2).

Le^b specificity results when both fucose residues are present on the Type 1 precursor chain (Marr *et al*, 1967). The fucose residue on the terminal galactose residue is controlled by the H gene. The *simultaneous* presence of both fucose units results in almost complete loss of Le^a activity (Fig. 4–3). This demonstrates how, in individuals who have inherited the *Le* and *H* genes, the substance is converted to Le^b substance. Some Le^a substance, although little, remains unconverted and can be demonstrated in the saliva of Le(a−b+) individuals by hemagglutination inhibition techniques. The *Se* gene is also necessary for the conversion of Le^a to Le^b because it controls the function of the *H* gene in secretory cells.

A basic summary of this information is given under the heading The Lewis System (Study Aid).

Table 4–2 EXAMPLES OF INTERACTIONS OF *Hh, Sese, ABO,* AND *Lele* GENES*

Genes	Blood Group Substances	
	In Secretions	On Red Cells
H, Se, A, Le	H, A, Le^a, Le^b	H, A, Le^b
H, se, A, Le	Le^a	H, A, Le^a
H, Se, A, le	H, A	H, A
H, Se, O, Le	H, Le^a, Le^b	H, (Le^a), Le^b
h, Se, A, Le	Le^a	Le^a

*Based on Watkins (1966). Modified from Mollison (1979).

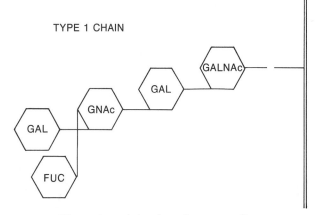

Figure 4–2 Molecule with Le^a specificity.

LEWIS MATINGS

Andresen (1948) showed that the genes responsible for the Le^a antigen are not straightforward in their action. It was discovered that parents of Le(a+) individuals could both be Le(a−). Subsequently, based on Ceppellini's theory, it was also discovered that Le(b−)

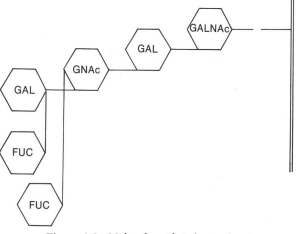
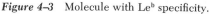

Figure 4–3 Molecule with Le^b specificity.

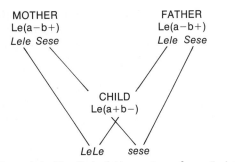

Figure 4–4 Two Le(a−b+) parents produce a Le(a+b−) child.

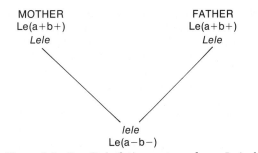

Figure 4–6 Two Le(a+b+) parents produce a Le(a−b−) child.

parents can produce Le(b+) offspring. This can be explained in the light of the theories of Grubb (1951) and Ceppellini (1955) (Fig. 4–4). Both parents in the example shown in Figure 4–4 have passed the *Le* gene to their offspring. Both, however, are heterozygous for the secretor genes. The child has inherited the *se* gene from both parents, and is therefore a nonsecretor of ABH substances. As explained, nonsecretors who inherit the *Le* gene are of phenotype Le(a+b−).

In Figure 4–5, both parents are Le(b−), yet the child has inherited the *Se* gene from one parent and the *Le* gene from the other parent, thereby acquiring the red cell phenotype Le(a−b+).

Similarly, parents of phenotype Le(a+b+) who are heterozygous for the *Le* gene could pass the *le* gene to their offspring, resulting in an Le(a−b−) individual (Fig. 4–6).

THE DEVELOPMENT OF LEWIS ANTIGENS

Almost all newborn infants type as Le(a−b−) (Rosenfield and Ohno, 1953; Jordal, 1956). Lewis antigens, however, are present in saliva and serum at birth, though they are absent from the red cells (Lawler and Marshall, 1961a, 1961b). Soon after birth, the antigens appear on the cells, and by age three months over 80 per cent of children give the reaction Le(a+b−). By the age of 2, this has fallen to the

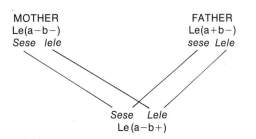

Figure 4–5 Parents lacking the Le[b] antigen produce a Le(a−b+) child.

adult level of 20 per cent. Le[b] only reaches adult frequency (70 per cent) by the age of 6 (see Andresen, 1948; Jordal and Lyndrup, 1952; Jordal, 1956; Brendemoen, 1961). Le[x] is well developed at birth.

THE ANTIBODIES OF THE LEWIS SYSTEM

Type of Immunoglobulin. Almost all Lewis antibodies tested by the indirect antiglobulin test behave as if they were solely IgM. Only one example of anti Le[a] that appeared to be solely IgG has been reported (Mollison, 1967) and one example of IgG anti-Le[b] was found by G. Garratty (unpublished, cited by Mollison, 1979). Holburn (1974) revealed a mixture of IgG and IgM in *potent* anti-Le[a] sera, a finding which is confirmed by Mollison (1979) who suggests that if potent anti-Le[a] sera are tested after 2-ME treatment, it might be possible to demonstrate IgG antibody in some of them.

Anti-Le[a] in Human Sera. Anti-Le[a] is relatively common in human sera when compared with other red cell antibodies (excluding anti-A and anti-B). The antibody is found only in persons who secrete ABH substances and who are genetically Lewis negative (i.e., *lele*) and who therefore have the Lewis phenotype Le(a−b−). With rare exceptions, all examples of Lewis antibodies have the ability to bind complement and cause hemolysis *in vitro*. Approximately 20 per cent of the adult white population react with anti-Le[a] sera.

The majority of anti-Le[a] sera also contain some weak anti-Le[b]. Both antibodies are usually too weak to be useful — most are non-red cell–immune and react best at temperatures below 37° C, though some are enhanced by the indirect antiglobulin test or by the use of the enzyme papain. The antibody occasionally appears to be immune in origin, and as such has been implicated in hemolytic transfusion reactions (see deVries and Smitskamp, 1951; Matson *et al*, 1952; Merrild-Hansen and Munk-Andersen, 1957; Peterson and Chisholm, 1958).

Anti-Le^a in Animal Sera. Anti-Le^a sera have been produced in chickens, rabbits and goats by the injection of nonsecretor saliva, of substances isolated from ovarian cysts of nonsecretors and of tanned rabbit red cells coated with Le^a substance (Brown *et al*, 1959; Baer *et al*, 1959; Toyama, 1956; Glynn *et al*, 1956; Iseki *et al*, 1957; Levine and Celano, 1960; Tsuganezawa, 1956; Kerde *et al*, 1960; Marcus and Grollman, 1966; Marcus *et al*, 1967). These antibodies are either of the precipitating or agglutinating type.

Anti-Le^b. Anti-Le^b is most often found as a weak antibody in serum that contains a relatively potent anti-Le^a. Like anti-Le^a, the antibody is produced (without anti-Le^a) in nonsecretors of ABH who are always of phenotype Le(a−b−) (Miller *et al*, 1954). However, rare examples of anti-Le^b in A_1 or A_1B, Le(a+b−) nonsecretors have been reported (Brendemoen, 1950; Garratty and Kleinschmidt, 1965; Komstad, 1969) that are of the anti-Le^{bH} type.

Potent anti-Le^b sera often contain some anti-H and possess three properties in common with anti-H: (1) they react more strongly with O and A_2 cells; (2) salivas that inhibit anti-H also inhibit anti-Le^b; and (3) most anti-Le^b are produced by A_1 or A_1B individuals.

There are some anti-Le^b sera (see Brendemoen, 1950) that react specifically with A_1, A_2 and O cells — most, however, like the original example of Andresen (1948) react specifically *only* with A_2 and O cells. Based on these observations it is now generally agreed that there are two kinds of anti-Le^b sera: anti-Le^{bH} and anti-Le^{bL}.

Anti-Le^{bH}. This antibody is neutralized (inhibited) by the salivas of all ABH secretors (including Le(a−b−) secretors) and reacts *only* with A_2 and O red cells.

Anti-Le^{bL}. This antibody is not neutralized (inhibited) by the saliva of Le(a−b−) secretors of ABH but is neutralized by the saliva of Le(a−b+) individuals and reacts with A_1 red cells and with those of other groups.

Anti-Le^{bL} can be thought of as "true" anti-Le^b (i.e., the antibody that reacts with the Le^b antigen). It has been suggested (Bird, 1958, 1959) that anti-H may be thought of as anti-H + H_1 (comparable with anti-A + A_1) and that anti-Le^{bH} may in fact be anti-H_1.

Both anti-Le^{bL} and anti-Le^{bH} are mostly IgM and are efficient at binding complement, though only a few examples have the ability to cause hemolysis *in vitro*. It is rare for the antibodies to cause a hemolytic transfusion reaction, and they have never been implicated in hemolytic disease of the newborn. Approximately 70 per cent of the adult white population react with anti-Le^{bL}.

Anti-Le^x. Anti-Le^x, originally called anti-X, was described by Andresen and Jordal (1949). It was considered by many workers to be anti-Le^a plus anti-Le^b, not necessarily in a separate state. Jordal (1956), however, showed that anti-Le^x, unlike anti-Le^a and anti-Le^b, reacts with almost the same proportion of cord samples as adult samples. The antibody reacts equally well with O, A_2 and A_1 red cells. It was concluded by Andresen (1961) that anti-Le^x must be detecting on the red cells a product of the *Le* gene (then called *Le^a*).

Anti-Le^x, according to Andresen (1961), must be considered as a specific agglutinin with a corresponding specific receptor (X) that is closely related to Le^a substance, since when the X receptor is present on the red cells, Le^a substance is always present in the secretions. Le^x is, in fact, present in the saliva of all individuals with the *Le* gene (Arcilla and Sturgeon, 1974). The Le^x receptor is not affected by the *Sese* or *Hh* genes (Sturgeon and Arcilla, 1970).

Anti-Le^c. Anti-Le^c was described by Iseki *et al* (1957), produced by injecting a rabbit with Le(a−b−) secretor saliva and absorbing the immune serum with enzyme treated Le(a+b−) and Le(a−b+) red cells. The antibody reacts well with Le(a−b−) red cells from individuals of genotype *lele, sese* (i.e., nonsecretors) and also with those of genotype *lele, hh*, and is inhibited by saliva from individuals of the same genotypes. The first example of anti-Le^c in a patient (of group O, Le(a−b+)) was reported by Gunson and Latham (1972).

Anti-Le^c reacts with red cells that have taken up Le^c from the plasma. Since Le^c is not determined by the Lewis genes, Mollison (1979) suggests that a new name be found for this antibody that would dissociate it from the Lewis system.

Anti-Le^d. Anti-Le^d reacts with Le(a−b−) red cells from individuals of genotype *lele, H, Se* (i.e., secretors) (Potapov, 1970). It is now known that the antibody reacts with red cells that have taken up Type IH and that Le^d, like Le^c, is not part of the Lewis system.

Anti-A_1Le^b and Anti-BLe^b. Anti-A_1Le^b was discovered by Seaman *et al* (1968) in a patient whose serum reacted with red cells possessing both A_1 and Le^b antigens but not with red cells possessing only one or neither of these two antigens. The antibody was inhibited *only* by saliva from A_1Le(b+) individuals. A second example was found in a chimeric twin by Crookston *et al* (1970). A third example was described in an A_1 donor who secreted some A but no H. The antibody was inhibited by A alone or by Le^b without A (Gundolf, 1973).

Anti-BLe^b has been detected in lymphocytotoxicity tests (as has anti-ALe^b) (Jeannet *et al*, 1972, 1974). This antibody reacts with red cells possessing both B and Le^b antigens but not with red cells possessing only one or neither of these two antigens.

Anti-Magard. The antibody "Magard" was detected by Andersen (1958) in an A_2 Le(a−b+) individual who reacted only with the red cells of A_1, Le(a−b−) secretors and, rather less strongly, with those of A_2Le(a−b−) secretors. The antibody was inhibited by A substance but not by B, H, Le^a or Le^b substances. Mollison (1979) suggests that it may be an antibody directed against Type I glycolipid with A specificity (i.e., anti-A_1Le^d).

Anti-ILe^{bH}. Tegoli (1971) described an antibody that reacted with O or A_2, Le(a−b+), I positive red cells in an A_1Le(a−b−) individual. The antibody was inhibited by saliva from O or A_1, Le(a−b+), I positive individuals and A_1, i adult, Le(a−b+) individuals but not by saliva from O or O_h Le(a+b−), I positive individuals.

LEWIS AT THE LEVEL OF THE ROUTINE BLOOD BANK

Lewis antibodies are both common and confusing in routine serologic tests. They are frequently found in individuals who have not been exposed to red cell antigenic stimulus and can therefore be considered to be non-red cell–immune (or "naturally occurring"). It is not known if individuals whose serum lacks anti-Le^a may form the antibody as a result of antigenic stimulus, although it is known that the titer of an *existing* Lewis antibody may increase dramatically after antigenic stimulus.

There is no doubt that Lewis antibodies, when potent, can cause rapid destruction of transfused red cells, although reactions of this type are comparatively rare.

The transfusion of Le(a−b−) blood to subjects with potent Lewis antibodies is desirable when available. Among whites, the incidence of Le(a−b−) is about 3 to 6 per cent, although it is much higher in blacks.

Lewis antibodies are predominantly IgM and seem almost always to bind complement. This results in the kind of red cell destruction that is most often serious, namely intravascular hemolysis. The reason why hemolytic transfusion reactions due to Lewis incompatibility are rare is because plasma contains Lewis substances that may wholly or partially *neutralize* the circulating antibody so that red cells that are theoretically incompatible would survive normally in the circulation for a limited time. Therefore, the injection of plasma in small amounts can act to neutralize all detectable antibody and allow the subsequent normal survival of Le(a+b−) or Le(a−b+) blood. In addition to this, after transfusion of blood to a Le(a−b−) individual, Le(a+) and/or Le(b+) red cells lose their Lewis antigens and become Le(a−b−). Since this transformation occurs within a few days of transfusion, the transfused red cells are likely to have become Le(a−b−) by the time that Lewis antibodies have reached a high concentration in the recipient's plasma.

In practice, weak Lewis antibodies in the recipient do not cause problems for the reasons just given, but potent antibodies that cause *in vitro* hemolysis certainly could, and the infusion of Le(a−b−) red cells, in the latter case, should be considered essential. If anti-Le^a is principally present, Le(a−b+) blood may be safe, since it would still partially neutralize anti-Le^a; when only anti-Le^b is present, Le(a+b−) blood may be used because Le(a+) individuals do not usually produce any Le^b antigen.

Lewis Antigens in Pregnancy

Lewis antigens become weaker during pregnancy to a point at which women of phenotype Le(a−b+) may type as Le(a−b−) (Brendemoen, 1952). Mollison (1972) suggested that this may be due to steroid hormones produced during pregnancy. Lewis antibodies are frequently encountered in the sera of pregnant women (Kissmeyer-Nielsen, 1965) and are generally more commonly found in women in the reproductive period (Andersen and Munk-Andersen, 1957). These antibodies do not cause hemolytic disease of the newborn, however, since they are predominantly IgM and since the red cells of newborn infants are usually Le(a−b−).

Saliva Types

Wiener *et al* (1964), adopting the notations of previous workers, have presented the following classification of the Lewis types:

1. Les = presence of Lewis substance in the saliva

2. nL = absence of Lewis substance from the saliva
3. Sec = secretors of H substance
4. nS = nonsecretors of H substance

Since the Lewis and the H substances are genetically *independent* of one another, in combination they determine four *saliva* types:

1. Les Sec = saliva contains Lewis and H substance
2. Les nS = saliva contains Lewis substance but no H substance
3. nL Sec = saliva contains H substance but no Lewis substance
4. nLnS = saliva contains neither Lewis nor H substance

SUMMARY: THE LEWIS SYSTEM (STUDY AID)

1. The phenotype Le(a+b−) is found in nonsecretors of ABH.
2. The phenotype Le(a−b+) is found in secretors of ABH.
3. The phenotype Le(a−b−) is found in individuals of genotype *lele*. These individuals are *usually* secretors (80 per cent).
4. Le(a+b−) individuals (nonsecretors of ABH) secrete Le[a] substance.
5. Le(a−b+) individuals secrete ABH, Le[a] and Le[b] substances.

TECHNIQUES

In testing for Lewis substances in saliva or on red cells, it has been found that red cell reactions may vary even in the same individual, the reactions being dependent to some extent on the subject's age and the techniques employed. Tests on saliva, however, are usually more reliable, since they yield fairly consistent results. This situation is not as true now as it was a few years ago, however, since the advent of anti-Le[a] and anti-Le[b] produced in goats has provided a reagent that gives powerful reactions when testing red cells. In many laboratories, this has now become the technique of choice.

Method of Detection of Lewis Substances in Saliva

1. Centrifuge saliva and recover supernatant into a separate test tube.
2. Immerse the supernatant in a boiling water bath for ten minutes to inactivate enzymes that would otherwise inactivate the blood group substances.
3. Dilutions of saliva to be tested are then added to equal volumes of anti-Le[a]. Allow 15 minutes for inhibition to occur, then add Le(a+) red cells and examine macroscopically for agglutination.

Note. Controls are of major importance. The negative control (saliva from a Le(a−b−) *(lele)* subject) must be carefully selected, since a small proportion of subjects whose red cells group as Le(a−b−) secrete Le[a] substance in their saliva. Saliva from a subject of phenotype Le(a+b−) or Le(a−b+) may be used as a positive control.

4. Results are interpreted as shown in Table 4–3.

Method of Detection of Lewis Substances on Red Cells

1. Mix one drop of anti-Le[a] reagent with one drop of a washed 5 per cent suspension of red cells from the individual under test.
2. Incubate at the temperature recommended by the manufacturer, or at the temperature at which the serum is known to give its best reaction.
3. Shake gently and examine microscopically for agglutination, macroscopically for hemolysis.

Note. Since Lewis antibodies almost always bring about the binding of complement components to red cells at 37° C, antiglobulin techniques for the detection of Lewis substances on red cells should be performed using the freshest possible antisera and should be adequately and strictly controlled. In the selection of controls, Le(a+b−), Le(a−b+) and Le(a−b−) red cells should be used. When the cells to be typed are group A_1 or A_1B, select A_1 controls with anti-Le[b].

Table 4–3 INTERPRETATION OF SALIVA TESTS FOR DETECTION OF LEWIS SUBSTANCES

Tests with Anti-Le[a] Plus Le(a+) Red Cells°				
Dilutions of Saliva				
1/1	*1/80*	*1/320*	*1/1280*	*Interpretation*
2+	2+	2+	2+	Le (a−b−)
−	−	−	1+	Le (a+b−)
−	−	1+	2+	Le (a−b+)

°It is unnecessary to test for Le[b] substance because when Le[a] and H are present, its presence is inferred.

TYPICAL EXAMINATION QUESTIONS

Select the phrase, sentence or symbol that com-
pletes the statement or best answers the question.
More than one answer may be correct in each case.
Answers are at the back of the book.

1. An individual is group B, Le(a+b−). The blood
   group substance(s) detectable in the patient's
   saliva should be
   (a) B substance
   (b) B substance and Le^a substance
   (c) Le^a substance
   (d) B substance and H substance
   (e) B substance, H substance and Le^a substance
                        (Summary: The Lewis System)
2. What is the most probable genotype of cells with
   the phenotype Le(a−b−)?
   (a) *lele*
   (b) *Le^{a}le*
   (c) *Lele*
   (d) *leLe^b*
   (e) *LeLe*
                        (Summary: The Lewis System)
3. A mother is known to be Le(a−b+). The father is
   known to be Le(a+b−). Which of the following
   genotypes is possible in their children?
   (a) *Sese*
   (b) *Le(a−b+)*
   (c) *Le(a+b−)*
   (d) *SeSe*
   (e) *sese*
                                        (General)
4. An individual who is genotype *AO, Lele, Sese*
   will be
   (a) a nonsecretor
   (b) Le(a−b+)
   (c) Le(a+b−)
   (d) Le(a−b−)
   (e) a secretor of H substance only
                        (Table 4–1, Table 4–2)
5. The term *secretor* usually refers to
   (a) an individual whose red blood cells possess
   no detectable A, B or H antigens
   (b) an individual whose red cells are Le(a−b−)
   and whose saliva does not contain H substance
   (c) an individual whose secretions contain ABH
   substances
   (d) red blood cells that are agglutinated by anti-
   Le^a
                        (The Genetics of the Lewis System)
6. The Le(a+b+) phenotype
   (a) does not exist
   (b) is possessed by subjects who are group A$_1$
   (c) is possessed by subjects who are group A$_2$
   and O and who also possess the *H, Se* and *Le*
   genes
   (d) usually gives weak reactions with anti-Le^a
                        (The Genetics of the Lewis System)
7. If an individual possesses the genes *H, Se, A* and

Le, which of the following blood group substances will be found in his secretions?
(a) H and A only
(b) Le^a only
(c) Le^b only
(d) H, A, Le^a, Le^b
(e) Le^a and Le^b only
                                        (Table 4–2)
8. The *Le* gene
   (a) controls the conversion of Type I chains to
   Le^a substance
   (b) controls the conversion of Le^a substance to
   Le^b substance
   (c) controls the addition of a fucose molecule to
   the terminal sugar of Type I chain of the
   precursor substance
   (d) controls the addition of a fucose molecule to
   the subterminal sugar of Type I chain of the
   precursor substance
   (e) controls the conversion of H substance to Le
   substance
                        (The Genetics of the Lewis System)
9. Almost all newborn infants type as
   (a) Le(a+b−)
   (b) Le(a−b+)
   (c) Le(a+b+)
   (d) Le(a−b−)
                        (The Development of Lewis Antigens)
10. Almost all Lewis antibodies are
    (a) IgG
    (b) IgM
    (c) IgA
    (d) a mixture of IgG and IgM
                        (Type of Immunoglobulins)
11. Anti-Le^b, if neutralized by the saliva of all ABH
    secretors and reactive *only* with A$_2$ and O red
    cells, is known as
    (a) anti-Le$_1$
    (b) anti-Le^{bH}
    (c) anti-Le^{bL}
    (d) anti-Le^a
                                        (Anti-Le^b)
12. *Anti-Le^x*
    (a) was originally called anti-X
    (b) is anti-Le^a plus anti-Le^b
    (c) reacts equally well with cord samples as
    adult samples
    (d) is present in all individuals with the *Le*
    gene
                                        (Anti-Le^x)
13. Lewis antibodies
    (a) are frequently found in individuals who have
    not been exposed to red cell antigenic stimu-
    lus
    (b) are always clinically significant
    (c) may cause intravascular hemolysis
    (d) become weaker through pregnancy
    (e) are more commonly found during the re-
    productive period
*(Lewis at the Level of the Routine Blood Bank —
                Lewis Antigens in Pregnancy)*

14. The classification of saliva that contains Lewis substance but no H substance is
    (a) Les Sec
    (b) nL
    (c) Les
    (d) Les nS
    (e) nL nS

    (Saliva Types)

15. In the detection of Lewis substances in saliva, the saliva must be immersed in a boiling water bath for ten minutes
    (a) to inactivate enzymes
    (b) to clarify the saliva
    (c) to ensure that the controls will work
    (d) to activate the blood group substances

    (The Detection of Blood Group Substances in Saliva)

Answer True or False

16. Individuals who are Le(a+) are nonsecretors of ABH substances.

    (Introduction)

17. Red cells acquire their Lewis phenotype by adsorption of Lewis substances from the plasma.

    (The Genetics of the Lewis System)

18. Lewis genes are called Le^a and Le^b.

    (The Genetics of the Lewis System)

19. A Le(a−) × Le(a−) mating cannot produce Le(a+) offspring.

    (Lewis Matings)

20. Potent anti-Le^a sera may be a mixture of IgM and IgG.

    (Type of Immunoglobulin)

GENERAL REFERENCES

1. Mollison, P. L.: Blood Transfusion in Clinical Medicine. 6th Ed. Blackwell Scientific Publications, Oxford, 1979. *(Excellent, concise review of the Lewis system. The section on the chemistry of Lewis antigenic determinants (page 285) will be useful to the student interested in this aspect.)*

2. Race, R. R., and Sanger, R.: Blood Groups in Man. 6th Ed. Blackwell Scientific Publications, Oxford, 1975.

   (Comprehensive coverage of the Lewis system — especially useful with respect to various theories of antigens, and genetic inheritance.

3. Erskine, A. G.: The Principles and Practice of Blood Grouping. C. V. Mosby Co., St. Louis, 1973. *(Interesting and useful approach to the Lewis system with special emphasis on the saliva types.)*

5

THE Rh/Hr BLOOD GROUP SYSTEM

OBJECTIVES — THE Rh/Hr BLOOD GROUP SYSTEM

The student shall know, understand and be prepared to explain:

1. A brief history of the Rh/Hr blood group system
2. The principles of Fisher-Race nomenclature, including the genetic theory of three closely linked loci
3. Wiener nomenclature, including the genetic theory of a single complex locus and multiple alleles
4. Rosenfield nomenclature and numerical equivalents between this and the nomenclatures of Wiener and Fisher-Race
5. The method of determination of Rh phenotypes and probable genotypes, specifically to include:
   (a) Assignment of genotype based on frequencies of antigens and gene complexes
   (b) Percentage of error in each case
6. The antigens of the Rh/Hr blood group system, specifically to include:
   (a) Chemical nature of the antigens
   (b) Characteristics of the antigens C, D, E, c and e
   (c) Alleles at the D locus, including D^u (practical and theoretical aspects, genetics and clinical significance); the theory of the D antigen mosaic, the categories of D antigen, D^w, Go^a (brief description)
   (d) Alleles at the Cc locus, including C^w, C^x, c^v, C^u, c-like, C^G (with the exception of C^w, these antigens are briefly described as to characteristics)
   (e) Alleles at the Ee locus, including E^w, E^u, hr^s, hr^B, e^s, e^i, E^T (brief description of characteristics only)
   (f) Compound antigens, general description, specifically to include: f, Ce, CE, cE, G and V
   (g) Depressed antigens, including R^N, Rh33 and Be^a (brief description only)
   (h) Suppressions, including Rh_{null} (genetic theories, types, disease association and characteristics), Rh_{mod} (brief description) and other suppressions ($-D-$ and C^wD-).
   (i) A brief description of recently discovered antigens of the Rh system
   (j) The LW antigen (characteristics, discovery and relationship to Rh)
   (k) The number of antigen sites on the red cells
   (l) Clustering of D antigen sites
   (m) Tissues that carry Rh antigens other than red cells
   (n) Development of Rh antigens in the fetus and newborn
7. The antibodies of the Rh/Hr blood group system, specifically to include:
   (a) Immunoglobulin classes and subclasses
   (b) "Naturally occurring" antibodies
   (c) Immune antibodies
   (d) The ability to bind complement
   (e) Mixtures of Rh antibodies commonly found
   (f) Clinical significance of Rh antibodies
8. A general understanding of the theories of techniques used in Rh antigen detection in the routine laboratory
9. The specifics of the techniques so described, specifically to include:
   (a) $Rh_o(D)$ typing (technique and controls) (slide and tube methods)
   (b) The causes of false positive and false negative reactions in $Rh_o(D)$ typing
   (c) D^u typing using the indirect antiglobulin test
   (d) Tests for other Rh antigens (C, E, c and e)
   (e) Causes of false positive and false negative reactions in Rh typing

Introduction

The Rh/Hr blood group system is probably the most complex of all red cell blood group systems. The account provided here is written for the student; it emphasizes the information required at that level and provides only a basic overview of the more obscure material. Extensive sources from the literature are available on the subject, some of which have been listed at the end of this chapter.

History

Levine and Stetson (1939) reported an antibody in the mother of a stillborn fetus who suffered a hemolytic reaction to the transfusion of her husband's blood. Upon testing, the mother's serum was found to agglutinate approximately 80 per cent of randomly selected ABO-compatible donors. The corresponding antigen was found to be independent of all other blood groups discovered before that time.

In 1940, Landsteiner and Wiener, injecting blood from the monkey *Maccacus rhesus* into rabbits and guinea pigs, discovered that the resulting antibody agglutinated both the monkey's red cells and about 85 per cent of human donors. Those donors whose red cells were agglutinated by the antibody were called Rh-positive and the remaining 15 per cent were called Rh-negative.

Wiener and Peters (1940) showed that the antibody anti-Rh could be found in the serum of certain individuals who had had transfusion reactions following ABO group–compatible transfusions. The antibody was reported to be indistinguishable from the antibody discovered by Levine and Stetson in 1939.

Levine *et al* (1941a, 1941b, 1941c) showed that erythroblastosis fetalis (hemolytic disease of the newborn) was the result of Rh group incompatibility between mother and child.

In fact, rabbit anti-rhesus and human anti-Rh are not the same, as came to be realized later, yet the vast literature that had accumulated made it impossible to change the name of the human antibody from anti-Rh. At Levine's suggestion, therefore, the rabbit antibody was renamed anti-LW in honor of Landsteiner and Wiener, who had discovered it, and the human antibody retained the title anti-Rh.

NOMENCLATURES AND GENETIC THEORIES

Since 1940, a vast body of knowledge about the Rh system has been accumulated, and three terminology systems have been devised, two of which are based on different genetic theories.

The Fisher-Race Nomenclature

By 1943, four antibodies known to be part of the Rh system had been described by Race *et al* (1943), and studies by Fisher (1944) showed that the reactions of two of them were "antithetical" (i.e., at least one of the corresponding antigens was always present). Fisher therefore postulated that the genes controlling these antigens were alleles, and he called them *C* and *c*. The other two antibodies did not show antithetical relationship and the corresponding an-

tigens were called *D* and *E*. The *D* and *E* genes were assumed to have allelic forms *d* and *e* producing d and e antigens that would be capable of stimulating the production of anti-d and anti-e.

From this information, the Rh gene complex was assumed to possess closely linked genes, which could be assembled in eight different ways: *CDe, cDE, cde, cDe, cdE, Cde, CDE* and *CdE*. Note that some workers assemble the complex as DCE, because of the order of discovery and also because it was stated that this is the order in which the genes appear on the chromosomes. Since there is no way to examine the genes on a chromosome with respect to order, the latter reason is considered to be invalid, and this text will follow the CDE order in keeping with the majority of authoritative texts on the subject (see Mollison, 1979; Race and Sanger, 1975; Issitt and Issitt, 1976).

In summary, the Fisher-Race theory states that there are three closely linked loci, each with a primary set of allelic genes (*D* and *d*, *C* and *c*, *E* and *e*). These three loci are thought to be so closely linked that crossing over occurs only very rarely, and the three Rh genes are inherited as a complex. (Thus a *CDe/cDE* individual will pass only *CDe* or *cDE* to offspring and no other combination.)

In terms of nomenclature, the Rh antigens are therefore named C, D, E, c, d, e. The antigen d (and its corresponding antibody, anti-d) has never been discovered and is thought not to exist. The symbol "d" is used, however, to denote the *absence* of D. All individuals who lack the D antigen are said to be Rh-negative, regardless of whether the C or E antigen or both are present. The most frequent genotype among D-negative individuals, however, is *cde/cde*.

The theory of Fisher-Race was confirmed when the two unknown reactions of *CDE* were shown to be as predicted (Murray *et al*, 1945) and when anti-e was discovered (Mourant, 1945). The only weakness in the theory, therefore, was the failure to find the expected antigen d. (The Fisher-Race theory is shown diagrammatically in Figure 5–1). Other antigens since found to be part of the Rh system have been classified using the same basic principles.

The Wiener Nomenclature

Wiener (1943) proposed his own genetic theory of the Rh blood types; it differed from the Fisher-Race theory and has remained the subject of considerable controversy since that time. Wiener visualized multiple alleles — an

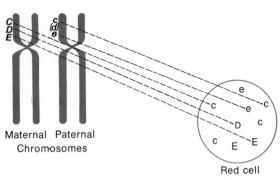

Figure 5–1 The Fisher-Race theory of Rh inheritance.

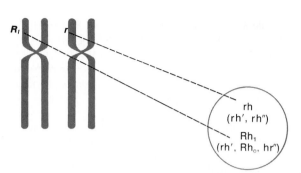

Figure 5–2 The Wiener theory of Rh inheritance.

infinite number of them — at a *single complex locus*, each allele determining its own particular agglutinogen (antigen). The agglutinogens comprise multiple factors (depending on which genes are present) and are recognized by whichever factors are detectable. The two genes (i.e., one paternal and one maternal) may be alike (homozygous) or different (heterozygous). Therefore, multiple alleles may exist at this locus. The eight major alleles are called R^1, R^2, r, R^0, r', r'', R^z and r^y.

In simple terms, for example, the R^1 gene produces a complex antigen, Rh_1, on the red cell that is made up of at least three factors, **rh′**, **Rh₀** and **hr″**. The **rh′** factor is the C factor of the Fisher-Race nomenclature; the **Rh₀** factor is the D antigen and the **hr″** factor is the e antigen. Wiener uses boldface type to indicate factors (i.e., each separately reacting part of the genetic structure), roman type to indicate agglutinogens, and in keeping with general practice, italics to convey the concept of gene symbols. Thus R_0 determines **Rh₀**, which comprises **hr′**, **Rh₀**, **hr″** (i.e., **Rh₀** = cDe, whereas **Rh₀** = D).

The eight different ways in which the Rh antigens can be assembled now compare with the Fisher-Race system as shown in Table 5–1.

In comparing the two theories, it becomes obvious that the only practical difference be-

tween the two is that Fisher and Race envision a complex gene, whereas Wiener envisions a complex antigen. The factors, although possessing different names, refer to the same cell substances identifiable with specific antisera. It can, of course, be said that the Fisher-Race theory is based on a faulty genetic premise, since the d antigen (and the d gene) has not been shown to exist. This does not invalidate the nomenclature, however, which remains easier to understand and to explain than Wiener's theory. The CDE nomenclature can, in effect, be used to simplify the reactions obtained with particular cells. For example, C^wCDe, which is plainly seen as C^w + C + D + e, is given in Wiener's nomenclature as $Rh_2{}^wRh_1$, which does not allow for easy recognition. The Wiener theory, for comparison with Figure 5–1, is shown diagrammatically in Figure 5–2.

The Rosenfield Nomenclature

Rosenfield *et al* (1962) developed a numerical terminology for the Rh groups based on a proposal of Murray (1944a and b) to eliminate certain difficulties in classification using the Fisher-Race and Wiener nomenclatures and to pave the way for the storage of such information in computers. The nomenclature proposes a system that describes reactions with particular antisera, is free of any genetic implication and gives equal importance to positive and negative reactions.

The antigens are numbered in chronological order of discovery, and the system has certain obvious advantages. In practice, however, it is difficult to apply; e.g., Rh_1rh (CDe/cde) would be given as Rh:1,2, −3, 4, 5, 6, 7, −8, 9, −10, −11, 12 and so on, depending on how many further antigens had been tested for.

The antigens of the Rh system are given in Table 5–2, with their equivalents in the Rosenfield, Fisher-Race and Wiener nomenclatures.

Table 5–1 COMPARISON OF FISHER-RACE AND WIENER NOMENCLATURES

Fisher-Race	Wiener
CDe	Rh_1 (**rh′**, **Rh₀**, **hr″**)
cDE	Rh_2 (**hr′**, **Rh₀**, **rh″**)
cde	rh (**hr′**, **hr″**)
Cde	rh′ (**rh′**, **hr″**)
cdE	rh″ (**hr′**, **rh″**)
CdE	rh^y (**rh′**, **rh″**)
CDE	Rh_z (**rh′**, **Rh₀**, **rh″**)
cDe	Rh_0 (**hr′**, **Rh₀**, **hr″**)

Table 5-2 COMPARISON OF NOMENCLATURES OF ANTIGENS OF THE Rh SYSTEM*

Wiener	Fisher-Race	Rosenfield
Rh_0	D	Rh1
rh'	C	Rh2
rh''	E	Rh3
hr'	c	Rh4
hr''	e	Rh5
hr	ce or f	Rh6
	CE	Rh22
rh_i	Ce	Rh7
rh_{ii}	cE	Rh27
rh^{w1}	C^w	Rh8
rh^x	C^x	Rh9
rh^{w2}	E^w	Rh11
	E^T	Rh24
rh^G	G	Rh12
	C^G	Rh21
hr^v	V or ce^s	Rh10
	VS or e^s	Rh20
Hr_0		Rh17
Hr		Rh18
hr^s		Rh19
hr^H		Rh28
Rh^A		Rh13
Rh^B		Rh14
Rh^C		Rh15
Rh^D		Rh16
	D^w	Rh23
	L^W	Rh25
	c-like ("Deal")	Rh26
	RH ("Total Rh")	Rh29
	D^{cor} (Go^a)	Rh30
hr^B		Rh31
	(R^N)	Rh32
	(R^{oHar})	Rh33
Hr^B	(Bas)	Rh34
	(1114)	Rh35
	(Be^a)	Rh36*
	(Evans)	Rh37*
	(Duclos)	Rh38*
		Rh39
		Rh40
		Rh41
Ce^s		Rh42

*Classification suggested by Issitt *et al* (1979).

Rh INHERITANCE

In terms of the basic antigens, C, D, E, c and e, the genetics of the Rh blood group system can be considered straightforward. The gene complex is inherited and families may be analyzed in terms of separate antigens: D or its absence (d), C or c and E or e. (Rh inheritance is shown diagrammatically in Figures 5–3 and 5–4.)

Chalmers and Lawler (1953), Goodall *et al* (1953; 1954) and Lawler and Sandler (1954) demonstrated genetic linkage between the genes for Rh and for oval red cells (elliptocytosis). This and later linkages involving Rh finally

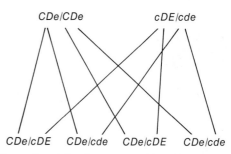

Figure 5-3 Rh inheritance with Fisher-Race nomenclature.

assigned the *Rh* locus to chromosome No. 1; see Race and Sanger (1975) for more details.

The Determination of Rh Phenotypes and Probable Genotypes

In reporting the phenotype of an individual, only those factors that are detected by direct testing are listed (e.g., CcDEe or CDEe and so forth). The determination of the Rh *genotype* of an individual is complicated by two facts: (1) The d antigen has not been found to exist, and therefore its presence or absence cannot be determined. (2) It is not possible to determine the *arrangement* of the genes on the two chromosomes. Consider the following example.

"Unknown" red cells are tested against these antisera:

1. Anti-C: Red cells agglutinate (positive reaction), indicating the presence of the C antigen.
2. Anti-D: Red cells agglutinate (positive reaction), indicating the presence of the D antigen.
3. Anti-E: Red cells fail to agglutinate (negative reaction), indicating the absence of the E antigen.
4. Anti-c: Red cells agglutinate (positive reaction), indicating the presence of c antigen.
5. Anti-e: Red cells agglutinate (positive reaction), indicating the presence of the e antigen.

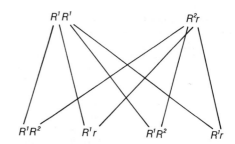

Figure 5-4 Rh inheritance with Wiener nomenclature.

Table 5–3 THE 18 DIFFERENT REACTION COMBINATIONS IN TESTING RED CELLS WITH THE FIVE MOST COMMON Rh ANTISERA AND ALL THEIR POSSIBLE GENOTYPES*

	Reactions with					
Anti-C	Anti-D	Anti-E	Anti-c	Anti-e	Phenotype	Possible Genotypes
+	+	+	+	+	CcDEe	CDe/cDE (R^1R^2) or CDe/cdE (R^1r'') or cDE/Cde (R^2r') or CDE/cde (R^zr) or CDE/cDe (R^zR^0) or cDe/CdE (R^0r^y)
−	+	+	+	+	cDEe	cDE/cde (R^2r) or cDE/cDe (R^2R^0) or cDe/cdE (R^0r'')
−	+	−	+	+	cDe	cDe/cde (R^0r) or cDe/cDe (R^0R^0)
+	+	−	+	+	CcDe	CDe/cde $(R'r)$ or CDe/cDe (R^1R^0) or cDe/Cde (R^0r')
+	+	−	−	+	CDe	CDe/CDe (R^1R^1) or CDe/Cde (R^1r')
+	+	+	−	+	CDEe	CDE/CDe (R^zR^1) or CDE/Cde (R^zr') or CDe/CdE (R^1r^y)
+	+	+	−	−	CDE	CDE/CDE (R^zR^z) or CDE/CdE (R^zr^y)
+	+	+	+	−	CcDE	CDE/cDE (R^zR^2) or CDE/cdE (R^zr'') or cDE/CdE (R^2r^y)
−	+	+	+	−	cDE	cDE/cDE (R^2R^2) or cDE/cdE (R^2r'')
−	−	−	+	+	ce	cde/cde (rr)
+	−	+	+	+	CcEe	Cde/cdE $(r'r'')$ or CdE/cde (r^yr)
−	−	+	+	+	cEe	cdE/cde $(r''r)$
+	−	−	+	+	Cce	Cde/cde $(r'r)$
+	−	−	−	+	Ce	Cde/Cde $(r'r')$
+	−	+	−	+	CEe	CdE/Cde (r^yr')
+	−	+	−	−	CE	CdE/CdE (r^yr^y)
+	−	+	+	−	CcE	CdE/cdE (r^yr'')
−	−	+	+	−	cE	cdE/cdE $(r''r'')$

*Modified from Bryant (1980).

Table 5–4 ESTIMATIONS OF PROBABILITIES IN Rh GENOTYPING AND THE PERCENTAGE OF ERROR

	Reactions with Anti-				Possibilities		Percentage of Error With First Choice
C	D	E	c	e	Probable	Second Choice	
+	+	−	+	+	CDe/cde (R^1r)	CDe/cDe (R^1R^0)	7
+	+	−	−	+	CDe/CDe (R^1R^1)	CDe/Cde (R^1r')	5
+	+	+	+	+	CDe/cDE (R^1R^2)	CDe/cdE (R^1r'') or CDE/cde (R^2r) or cDE/Cde (R^2r')	13
−	+	+	+	+	cDE/cde (R^2r)	cDE/cDe (R^2R^0)	6
−	+	+	+	−	cDE/cDE (R^2R^2)	cDE/cdE (R^2r'')	16
−	+	−	+	+	cDe/cde (R^0r)	cDe/cDe (R^0R^0)	4
−	−	−	+	+	cde/cde (rr)	−	−

Table 5–5 COMMON Rh GENE COMPLEXES (IN ORDER OF FREQUENCY FOR WHITES: NOTE DIFFERENT FREQUENCIES FOR BLACKS)

| Gene Complex | Percentage Frequency | |
	Whites	Blacks
CDe (R¹)	40.79	8.18
cde (r)	37.13	24.88
cDE (R²)	16.97	7.20
cDe (Rᵒ)	2.69	48.80
cdE (r″)	0.86	0.99
Cde (r′)	0.71	2.23
CDE (Rᶻ)	0.40	0.51
CdE (rʸ)	0.001	–

Table 5–7 THE 36 POSSIBLE Rh GENOTYPES IN ORDER OF FREQUENCY AMONG WHITES

Genotype	Frequency (Percentage)
CDe/cde (R¹r)	32.6808
CDe/CDe (R¹R¹)	17.6803
cde/cde (rr)	15.1020
CDe/cDE (R¹R²)	11.8648
cDE/cde (R²r)	10.9657
CDe/cDe (R¹Rᵒ)	2.1586
cDe/cde (Rᵒr)	1.9950
cDE/cDE (R²R²)	1.9906
CDe/cdE (R¹r″)	0.9992
cdE/cde (r″r)	0.9235
CDe/Cde (R¹r′)	0.8270
Cde/cde (r′r)	0.7644
cDE/cDe (R²Rᵒ)	0.7243
cDE/cdE (R²r″)	0.3353
cDE/Cde (R²r′)	0.2775
CDE/CDe (RᶻR¹)	0.2048
CDE/cde (Rᶻr)	0.1893
CDE/cDE (RᶻR²)	0.0687
cDe/cDe (RᵒRᵒ)	0.0659
cDe/cdE (Rᵒr″)	0.0610
cDe/Cde (Rᵒr′)	0.0505
Cde/cdE (r′r″)	0.0234
cdE/cdE (r″r″)	0.0141
CDE/cDe (RᶻRᵒ)	0.0125
Cde/Cde (r′r′)	0.0097
CDE/cdE (Rᶻr″)	0.0058
CDE/Cde (Rᶻr′)	0.0048
CDe/CdE (R¹rʸ)	0.0042
CdE/cde (rʸr)	0.0039
cDE/CdE (R²rʸ)	0.0014
CDE/CDE (RᶻRᶻ)	0.0006
cDe/CdE (Rᵒrʸ)	0.0003
CdE/cde (rʸr)	0.0001
CdE/cdE (rʸr″)	0.0001
CdE/CdE (rʸrʸ)	0.0000
CDE/CdE (Rᶻrʸ)	0.0000

From the results of the tests it has been determined that the red cells carry the antigens C, D, c and e but not E. It is assumed that since *E* and *e* are alleles, the e gene is present on both chromosomes at the *Ee* locus — that is, the individual is homozygous for *e (ee)*. In addition, it has been determined by direct testing that the individual is heterozygous for *C (Cc)*. Therefore, the known genotype at this point is *Ce/ce*. In the case of the *D* gene, however, it cannot be determined if the individual is homozygous *(DD)* or heterozygous *(Dd)*. The presence or absence of the *(d)* gene must be postulated using information gained from tests for the antigens C, D, E, c and e based on probabilities as defined by large numbers of family studies. In the example described, the genotype could be either *CDe/cde (R¹r)* or *CDe/cDe (R¹Rᵒ)*. It has been discovered (through family studies) that 32.7 per cent of individuals with these results are *CDe/cde (R¹r)* whereas only 2.2 per cent are *CDe/cDe (R¹Rᵒ)*. So it follows that the genotype *CDe/cde* is more probable.

Based on the reactions with the five antisera — anti-C, anti-D, anti-E, anti-c and anti-e — 18 different reaction combinations are possible. These are listed in Table 5–3, along with all of the possible genotypes. The "most probable" genotypes and the percentage of error in each case are given in Table 5–4.

The genotyping of individuals with respect to Rh is largely based on frequencies of antigens and gene complexes and individual genes. These frequencies are given in Tables 5–5, 5–6 and 5–7.

THE ANTIGENS OF THE Rh/Hr BLOOD GROUP SYSTEM

Chemical Nature

Although several attempts have been made to define the chemical nature of Rh antigens, very little progress has been made. There is, however, considerable evidence that the Rh antigen is protein (Green, 1967; Kaufman and Masouredis, 1963), the structure of which is maintained by surrounding lipid. If this is so, Rh antigen cannot be extracted from red cells in a soluble form — and this, of course, hinders chemical analysis. Rh activity is not lost when lipid is extracted from red cell membranes, suggesting that the lipids do not carry the antigenic determinants but may be essential for

Table 5–6 COMMON Rh ANTIGENS IN ORDER OF FREQUENCY AMONG WHITES

Antigen	Frequency (Percentage)
e (hr″)	98
D (Rhₒ)	85
G (Rhᴳ)	85
c (hr′)	80
C (rh′)	70
f (ce) (hr)	64
E (rh″)	30

the conformation of the determinants (Green, 1968).

The Rh$_0$(D) antigen has been estimated to have a molecular weight of 174,000 (Folkerd *et al*, 1977).

The Antigens C, D, E, c and e

Rh$_0$(D) can be considered the most clinically significant of all the red cell antigens after the A and B antigens of the ABO blood group system. The antigen is highly antigenic; it has been shown that 50 per cent of Rh-negative individuals form anti-Rh$_0$(D) following a single transfusion of Rh-positive blood (Diamond, 1947; Pickles, 1956), although the immunizing dose can be considerably less — in fact, as little as 10 ml (Freda *et al*, 1966).

The antigens C, c and E, e for most practical purposes behave as pairs of antithetical antigens, although alternative alleles occur at the *Cc*, *D* and *Ee* loci (discussed later). Individuals who lack any of these antigens may be stimulated to produce the corresponding antibodies by transfusion or pregnancy. Of these antibodies, anti-c, anti-E and anti-e occur fairly frequently either as single antibodies or in combination with one another or with antibodies outside the Rh system. Anti-C is rare as a single antibody, although it occurs more commonly in Rh-negative subjects in combination with anti-D.

Alleles at the *D* Locus

D^u

A new allele at the *D* locus, called *D*^{u}, was first described by Stratton (1946). Race *et al* (1948) defined D^u as red cells that give some but not all of the reactions expected of D—specifically that D^u red cells were agglutinated by some anti-D sera and not by others. Masouredis (1960) showed that D^u cells, when compared with normal D cells, take up only 7 to 25 per cent as much anti-D. Stratton (1946), Race *et al* (1948) and Stratton and Renton (1948) showed the antigen to be genetically inherited (discussed later).

From a laboratory standpoint, D^u may simply be regarded as a weak form of the D antigen (i.e., possessing relatively few D sites). In practical terms, however, D^u cannot simply be categorized in terms of standard or usual reactions because there are many *grades* of D^u; it appears, in fact, that no two are exactly alike. Red cells of the "higher" grade of D^u are agglutinated by certain anti-D sera while red cells of the

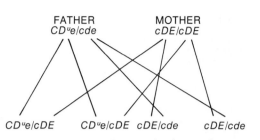

Figure 5–5   Diagram showing the direct inheritance of *D*^{u}.

"lower" grade are detectable only by the indirect antiglobulin test. Certain lower grade D^u's may only be detectable by absorption and elution of anti-D from the red cells; examples of these were recognized by Yvart *et al* (1974) and Garretty *et al* (1974).

The Genetics of D^u — Direct Inheritance and "Position" Effect

D^u was originally shown to be an inherited character due to an abnormal *D* gene that was passed in the normal way to successive generations (Stratton, 1946; Race *et al*, 1948; Stratton and Renton, 1948) (Fig. 5–5). It has further been shown that if parents have high-grade D^u, any children who inherit D^u also have high-grade D^u. Similarly, if parents have low-grade D^u, the children will also have low-grade D^u.

It is now known that certain high-grade D^u's are *not* the result of an abnormal allele, *D*^{u}, but of a position effect exerted by *Cde* on a normal *D* gene in the opposite gene complex (i.e., in *trans* position); for example, blood from a person of genotype *CDe/Cde* may behave as D^u (Ceppellini *et al*, 1955). When this "weakened" D is passed to a successive generation, if it is not paired again with *Cde* it will behave as a normal D antigen (Fig. 5–6). It has also been reported that the *C* gene in *cis* position (i.e., on the same chromosome) may also weaken the expression of *D* (Bush *et al*, 1974).

A third type of D^u has also been described that represents individuals who, through genetic control or influence, lack part of the Rh antigen mosaic (discussed later).

The Clinical Significance of D^u

D^u is a much less effective antigen than D with respect to the stimulation of anti-D; however, D^u red cells may be destroyed at an increased rate by anti-D, and a D^u infant can suffer from hemolytic disease of the newborn if the mother possesses anti-D (Mollison and Cutbush, 1949). In addition, a severe hemolytic transfusion reaction may result from the transfu-

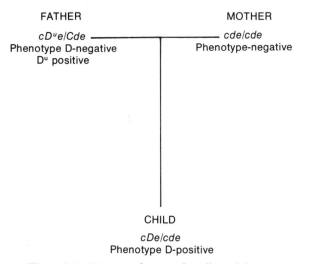

Figure 5–6 Diagram showing the effect of the *C* gene in the "trans" position.

sion of D^u-positive red cells to a recipient whose serum contains anti-D (Diamond and Allen, 1949).

D^u As It Affects the Laboratory

1. In practical testing, since it is not usual to use more than one anti-$Rh_o(D)$ antiserum, a sample is classified as D^u if it reacts with anti-D by the indirect antiglobulin test *only*. It should be noted, however, that this distinction is nowadays complicated by the fact that many "slide and rapid tube" anti-D reagents will react even with so-called "low-grade" D^u cells *without* the use of the indirect antiglobulin test, the reaction strength being influenced by the strength of the red cell suspension, temperature, duration of incubation and so forth. While this may complicate accurate classification, it is well to note that D^u cells will not react with genuine saline anti-D, which may be used in doubtful cases or when accurate classification is essential (see later discussion).

2. D^u subjects who are blood donors must be classified as $Rh_o(D)$-positive, since the infusion of D^u cells to an individual who possesses preformed anti-D (i.e., an **$Rh_o(D)$-negative** individual) may result in a hemolytic transfusion reaction in the recipient.

3. D^u subjects who are recipients of blood transfusion are most safely classified as $Rh_o(D)$-negative. Theoretically, of course, they can be classified as $Rh_o(D)$-positive if they are the type of D^u that differs only quantitatively from normal D. If they are the type of D^u resulting from missing portions of the mosaic (D variants, see later discussion) they should be classified as

$Rh_o(D)$-negative. In practical terms, of course, the argument regarding accurate classification wears thin in light of the fact that the actual risk of provoking the formation of anti-D in a D^u subject through the transfusion of D-positive blood is extremely small (Mollison, 1979). (*Note well:* There is no specific anti-D^u antibody.)

Subgroups (Subdivisions) of D (D Variants); The D Antigen Mosaic

$Rh_o(D)$-positive and D^u-positive individuals have been reported to have formed anti-D that is *not* an autoantibody (see Argall *et al*, 1953; Geiger and Wiener, 1958; Anderson *et al*, 1958). Based on this observation, it was suggested that the D-antigen is not a single entity but rather a mosaic structure of several different component parts. In other words, the antigen known as "D" is a name commonly used to describe a group of antigens that may all be present on red cells, as $Rh_o(D)$-positive or may all be absent, as $Rh_o(D)$-negative. Unger and Wiener (1959a, b, c) and Unger *et al* (1959) named the component parts A, B, C and D. Individuals possessing all of the portion are classified as Rh^{ABCD}. Individuals who are so-called "D variants" lack one or more of the A, B, C and D determinants and may produce a corresponding antibody. Whenever a portion of the mosaic is missing, the capital letter is replaced by a small letter. Thus an individual lacking Rh^D but possessing all other portions of the mosaic is classified as Rh^{ABCd}. This individual if transfused with Rh^{ABCD} blood could produce anti-Rh^D (Fig. 5–7).

$Rh_o(D)$-positive blood samples very rarely lack any of the mosaic components; however,

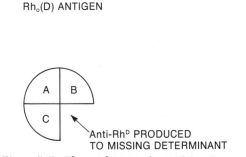

$Rh_o(D)$ ANTIGEN

Anti-Rh^D PRODUCED
TO MISSING DETERMINANT

Figure 5–7 The production of anti-Rh^D to the missing determinant of the D antigen mosaic.

about 50 per cent of D^u samples lack one or more of these antigens (Unger et al, 1959).

A different system of classifying D-positive individuals who produced anti-D was devised by Tippett and Sanger (1962). Six categories of the D antigen were described as follows:

Category I. The anti-D in these individuals is always very weak. Red cells from these individuals react with all anti-D sera (whether from D+ or D− individuals) except their own. So far, all individuals in this category have been white.

Category II. Only three unrelated propositi in this group.

Category III. The serum used to define this category is the original anti-Rh^D, and individuals in this category are classified as Rh_0^d (Sacks et al, 1959; Wiener and Ungar, 1962). Most subjects are black and many are cDe, VS+, V−.

Category IV. Black category IV members are Go(a+); white category IV members are Go(a−). Selected anti-D sera show Go(a+) category IV members to have elevated D.

Category V. The original member of this category formed anti-Rh^C. The category has both black and white members. The red cells of all members react with anti-D^W, and the D^W gene segregates with the unusual D gene.

Category VI. All of the many members of this category are white. Only a very small proportion of anti-D antisera react with the red cells of individuals belonging to category VI. These cells are often called Rh^B (or D^B); however, the classification is incorrect because Rh^B has been shown to be a normal component of the D antigen (Unger et al, 1959).

D^W (Rh23)

This allele at the D locus was first described by Chown et al (1962) who discovered the "new" antigen, at first called Wiel and later D^w. The D^w gene was originally found in the alignment cD^we in three families (two black, one white) and subsequently in the alignment CD^we in a white family (Chown et al, 1962; Chown et al, 1964; Lewis et al, 1956). The antigen is more frequent in blacks than in whites — 9 in 235 vs. 0 in 13,000 (Chown et al, 1964).

Go^a (D^{cor}, Rh30)

A "new" antibody, called anti-Go^a, was reported by Alter et al (1962) to be the cause of mild hemolytic disease of the newborn. In

1967, Lewis et al showed Go^a to be part of the Rh system, a finding supported by subsequent work of Alter et al (1967) and Chown et al (1968). Anti-Go^a is believed to react with the facet of D missing from D^{IV} (i.e., Category IV).

ALLELES AT THE Cc LOCUS

C^W (Rh8; rh^{w1})

The antigen C^W was first described by Callender and Race (1946). The corresponding antibody, anti-C^W, was found in the serum of a CDe/CDe (R^1R^1) individual who had been transfused with blood of genotype C^wDe/CDe ($R^{1w}R^1$). Anti-C^W has been shown to give marked dosage effect. The antigen frequency is low (approximately 1 per cent of U.S. whites), and several examples of the antibody have been found, some for which there was no known antigenic stimulus (Chown and Lewis, 1954; Kornstadt et al, 1960). In a few cases, anti-C^W, which is an IgG antibody, has been shown to be the cause of a hemolytic transfusion reaction and of hemolytic disease of the newborn.

C^x (Rh9; rh^x)

Stratton and Renton (1954) reported an antibody for a rare antigen called C^x, which was responsible for a case of hemolytic disease of the newborn. The antibody is very rare and is not normally found in anti-C sera (unlike anti-C^w); though it does occur fairly frequently in patients with acquired hemolytic anemia (Cleghorn, 1961). About one person in a thousand is C^x positive.

c^v and C^u

The antigens c^v and C^u, originally described by Race et al (1948), were later shown to be weakened forms of c and C, respectively (Race et al, 1960). It is possible that C^u is an allele of C similar to D^u, but it is also possible that it is merely a "depressed" C, written (C). It has now been established that c^v is not an allele at the Cc locus, but is the expression of C in the alignment CDE (see under the heading Compound Antigens).

c-like (Rh26)

Huestis et al (1964) discovered a sample of blood that reacted with all available anti-c sera but one. Two further samples were subsequently found in testing 1900 randomly selected C-positive individuals. The odd c antigen was found to be directly inherited and was called Rh26. No further examples of the antibody have been found.

C^G (Rh21)

Levine et al (1961) gave the name C^G to the antigenic component of r^Gr^G or r^Gr red cells (see later discussion) that reacts with some anti-C sera. There is no specific anti-C^G serum.

ALLELES AT THE *Ee* LOCUS

E^w (rh^{w2}; Rh11)

The antigen E^w was discovered by the finding of an antibody implicated as the cause in a case of hemolytic disease of the newborn (Greenwalt and Sanger, 1955). E^w-positive red cells are agglutinated by some anti-E sera and a specific anti-E^w exists. The allele is very rare.

E^u

The antigen E^u was found in the complex cDE^u by Ceppellini *et al* (1950); it distinguished itself by giving some but not all of the reactions expected of E (i.e., similar to D^u). No anti-E^u has been found.

hr^s (Rh19)

An antibody called anti-hr^s was found in the blood of a Bantu woman by Shapiro (1960). The cells of the proposita were found to lack a component of the **hr"** (e) antigen, and that component was given the name **hr^s**. The antibody is contained in most if not all anti-**hr"** (e) sera and seems to be the major or even the only component of some sera.

hr^B (Rh34)

Anti-hr^B, which, like anti-**hr^s**, defines another antigen associated with **hr"** (e), was described by Shapiro *et al* (1972). The antibody was detected in a South African black woman (Mrs. Bas) who was found to be of genotype r$^{/nH}$ R^{odH} (Cde^s/cD^{III}e). The antibody is directed against another "negro variant" of which there appear to be an infinite number.

e^s (VS) (Rh20)

Sanger *et al* (1960) gave the name e^s (or VS) to this, another allele of e found mostly in the blood of blacks. The antibody, anti-e^s, agglutinated the red cells of black people of phenotype V (**ce^s**) and Cde^s. (*NOTE:* The superscript s was used for both e^s and **hr^s** in papers that were published around the same time; this is unfortunate because e^s and **hr^s** are not the same antigen.)

e^i

This allele at the *Ee* locus was found by Layrisse *et al* (1961) who reported that about 20 per cent of Chibcha Indians possessed the gene complex cDe^i. Homozygotes are similar to the suppressed genotype cD−/cD− (discussed later), but they give weak reactions with some anti-e sera.

E^T (Rh24)

Vos and Kirk (1962) discovered the antibody (which they called anti-E^T) in the serum of an Australian aboriginal of phenotype CDe/cDE. The antibody appeared to be "naturally occurring." In tests so far, all white people who have E have been found to possess the antigenic component E^T, whereas about one third of Australian aboriginals with E lack the E^T component.

COMPOUND ANTIGENS

Rosenfield *et al* (1953a, 1953b) proposed the idea of a *combined* antigen in an attempt to explain the reactions of anti-f, which they had discovered. Since that time, the idea that f and certain other antigens are the combined effect of the *c* and *e* alleles in the *cis* position has gained general acceptance, in spite of the fact that it may not be the final answer.

1. *The antigen f (ce) (Rh6):* The antibody defining the f antigen was discovered in the serum of a white man of genotype CDe/cDE who had received multiple blood transfusions (Rosenfield *et al*, 1953). The antibody was found to react with a product of the gene complexes cde, cDe and cD^{u}e, but not with, for example, red cells of genotype CDe/cDE, in which c and e are in *trans*. The antigen was therefore considered to be a compound formed by the genes ce when they are in the *cis* position. It should be noted that there are several facts that dispute the likelihood that anti-f is simply anti-ce. For example, the gene complex cD− reacts with anti-ce (f) when a negative is expected; and the gene complex r^L, which has depressed c and e activity, gives a normal reaction with anti-ce (f). It has therefore been postulated by Boorman and Lincoln (1962) that f may in fact be a compound antigen of only part of the ce complex. An opposing viewpoint has also been offered by Perrault (1972). Anti-f is useful in making a distinction between CDe/cDE (f negative) and CDE/cde (f positive) red cells.

2. *The antigens Ce(rh$_i$) (Rh7); CE (Rh22); cE (rh$_{ii}$); Rh27):* Rosenfield and Haber (1958) proposed that when C and e are in *cis* they produce a compound antigen which they called **rh$_i$** (Ce). Therefore, the corresponding antibody (anti-**rh$_i$**) will react with red cells possessing the product of C and e in *cis* — which is not produced when these genes are in *trans* position. Similarly, when C and E are in *cis*, the compound CE (Rh22) is produced; and when c and E are in *cis*, the compound cE (**rh$_{ii}$**; Rh27) is produced. Examples of antibodies to each of these compounds have been reported (Dunford, 1962; Keith *et al*, 1965; Gold *et al*, 1961). These

compounds, like anti-f, are useful in distinguishing certain genotypes.

3. *The antigen G (rh^G; Rh12):* Allen and Tippett (1958) investigated the red cells of a white blood donor, Mrs. Crosby, which, though apparently Rh-negative, reacted with most "anti-CD" sera. This was explained by postulating an antigen "G" present on Mrs. Crosby's red cells but normally present only on red cells possessing the D or C antigens. The genotype proposed for Mrs. Crosby was *r^Gr* and anti-CD sera were assumed to have an anti-G component. Anti-G was isolated from anti-CD sera by elution using Mrs. Crosby's red cells, and subsequent tests showed that all common gene complexes except *cde* and *cdE* contained G.

The existence of G explained several puzzles — including that cde/cde women who are never transfused but are immunized by a fetus can make apparent anti-CD although their husbands lack C. The antibody is in fact anti-D + anti-G and does not contain anti-C.

The rare genotype r^Gr^G was discovered by Levine *et al* (1961), and a sample possessing D yet lacking G was reported by Stout *et al* (1963), thus confirming that G is a distinct Rh antigen.

4. *The antigen V, or ce^s (Rh10):* Anti-V was discovered by DeNatale *et al* (1955) in the serum of a *cde/cde (rr)* individual who had received many blood transfusions. The antigen V is only found in individuals possessing the gene complexes *CDe, cde* or *cD^ue* and is found predominantly in blacks. It was originally thought that V was an allele of *f* and therefore that V was a combined antigen, ce^s, "allelic" to f (ce). This view is not supported by all investigators (e.g., see Shapiro, 1964; Rosenfield *et al*, 1973).

DEPRESSED ANTIGENS

1. $\overline{\overline{\mathbf{R}}}^N$ (Rh32) and *(C) D (e) (Rh35):* Gene complexes producing weak C and e antigens (with a normal D) were found in a black family by Rosenfield *et al* (1960), who named the complex $\overline{\overline{\mathbf{R}}}^N$. Distinct from this negroid $\overline{\overline{\mathbf{R}}}^N$ is the complex (C) D (e) found in whites, which displays a different pattern of reactions with anti-C and anti-e and is nonreactive with specific anti-$\overline{\overline{\mathbf{R}}}^N$ antibodies. About 1 per cent of American blacks have the $\overline{\overline{\mathbf{R}}}^N$ complex, which has shown to be inherited in a straightforward fashion.

The (C) D (e) complex was discovered by Broman *et al* (1963) and was shown to be of two kinds — one producing normal and the other an elevated D antigen. Giles and Skov (1971)

found an antibody specific for the product of (C) D (e) without enhanced D, which was given the number anti-Rh35.

2. Rh33 or R_o^{Har}: This antigen was described by Giles *et al* (1971). It appeared to be associated with a variant of D and depression of e, and is defined by a specific antibody, anti-Rh33.

3. Be^a(Berrens) (Rh36): Anti-Be^a was described by Davidsohn *et al* (1953), but it was not until 1974 that Ducos *et al* described a family (Koz) which demonstrated that Be^a is part of the Rh system. The antigen is extremely rare; no random Be(a+) person was found in testing more than 25,000 donors of various races. Yet the antibody has been implicated as the cause of hemolytic disease of the newborn. In three generations of the Koz family, the Be(a+) members were found to have an unusual *cde* complex, resulting in weak c, e and ce antigens.

SUPPRESSIONS

Suppressions refer to the rare conditions in which some or all of the expected Rh antigens are missing. Many of these are of minor interest to the student, and as such have been treated briefly with some emphasis placed on the Rh_null condition. Further information can be obtained from Race and Sanger (1975).

Rh_null. Vos *et al* (1961) described a sample of blood that completely failed to react with all Rh antibodies. The phenomenon was given the name Rh_null by Ceppellini (cited by Levine *et al*, 1964). Further examples of Rh_null by Levine *et al* (1964, 1965a, 1965b) and by Ishimori and Hasekura (1966, 1967) revealed two distinct genetic backgrounds for the Rh_null condition.

The first kind of Rh_null appears to be the result of an amorphic gene at the Rh locus in double dose (Fig. 5–8). As can be seen from the figure, an apparent *cDe/cDe × CDe/CDe* mating has produced a *CDe/CDe* offspring. This would appear to be impossible, since the *CDe/CDe* child would then have inherited no gene at all from the *cDe/cDe* (or *cDe/cde*) parent. The propositus being Rh_null provides the genetic explanation, since it is then obvious that both parents must be heterozygous for the rare --- gene (called $\overline{\overline{r}}$ in the Wiener terminology) and this gene has been inherited paternally by the second son and both maternally and paternally by the propositus.

The second type of Rh_null, of which there are more examples, appears to be caused by a regulator gene that is not part of the Rh complex locus. The Rh_null propositus of this type carries

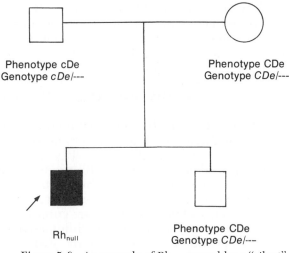

Phenotype cDe
Genotype *cDe/---*

Phenotype CDe
Genotype *CDe/---*

Rh$_{null}$

Phenotype CDe
Genotype *CDe/---*

Figure 5–8 An example of Rh$_{null}$ caused by a "silent" or amorphic allele at the *Rh* locus.

two normal genes at the *Rh* locus that are prevented from expressing themselves in terms of Rh antigens because of the operation of a suppressor (regulator) gene in double dose. Levine *et al* (1964, 1965a, 1965b), in interpreting the results of the original family study, proposed that in "normal" individuals a gene that they called *X'r* prepares a substrate on which *CDE* genes can act; whereas the Rh$_{null}$ individuals inherit two rare recessive *X°r* genes that are unable to prepare this substrate so that normal *CDE* genes are unable to act to produce

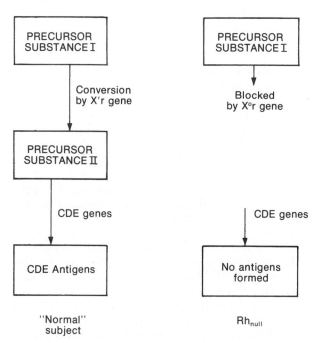

PRECURSOR SUBSTANCE I		PRECURSOR SUBSTANCE I
Conversion by X'r gene		Blocked by X°r gene
PRECURSOR SUBSTANCE II		No antigens formed
CDE genes		CDE genes
CDE Antigens		
"Normal" subject		Rh$_{null}$

Figure 5–9 Genetic pathway of regulator type Rh$_{null}$.

CDE antigens (Fig. 5–9). The regular type of Rh$_{null}$ therefore reveals itself when either parent or child of the propositus has normal Rh genes.

In Rh$_{null}$ individuals, the antibody formed in response to transfusion or pregnancy reacts with all cells except Rh$_{null}$ cells and is called anti-Rh29, although Rh$_{null}$ subjects may produce Rh antibodies of other specificities (Race and Sanger, 1975).

The red blood cells of Rh$_{null}$ individuals appear as "stomatocytes" (red cells with a light-staining, oblong-shaped center area). This suggests that they lack some membrane component, although no particular abnormality of membrane lipids or electrophoretic mobility has been demonstrated (Sturgeon, 1970). The majority of Rh$_{null}$ individuals have a compensated anemia, which is usually mild and may require sophisticated tests to detect. They often have increased reticulocyte counts and increased fetal hemoglobin or bilirubin or both. In addition, they usually have reduced hemoglobin, hematocrit and haptoglobin levels. Their red cells do not survive for the normal lengths of time either in normal individuals (when injected) or in Rh$_{null}$ individuals. It has been shown that the Rh antigens are an integral part of the red cell wall (Nicholson *et al*, 1971), and it is therefore assumed (Levine, 1972) that the Rh$_{null}$ condition is responsible for a defect in the structure of the wall.

The condition described, originally known as Rh$_{null}$ disease, is now more commonly referred to as Rh$_{null}$ syndrome.

Rh$_{null}$ red cells give weak or negative reactions with anti-U, anti-S and anti-s when the indirect antiglobulin test is used, though not when an agglutination test in saline or albumin is used (Race and Sanger, 1975).

Rh$_{mod}$. Chown *et al* (1972) described a case of *incomplete* suppression of Rh antigen development by a variant of the regulator gene responsible for one type of Rh$_{null}$. The condition was called Rh$_{mod}$. The red cells of these individuals were found to be abnormal, like Rh$_{null}$ red cells, in that they had a reduced survival and that they revealed some depression of Ss and U antigens.

Other Suppressions. Rare genes exist within the Rh system that fail to produce the "expected" Rh antigens (i.e., samples fail to react with anti-C and anti-c and/or with anti-E and anti-e). One such complex is known as −D−, which produces D but no Cc and Ee antigens. Red cells possessing the −D− complex appear to have large amounts of D antigen and are capable of agglutination in saline with most sera containing "incomplete" anti-D (Race *et al*, 1951).

Samples that fail to react with either anti-E or anti-e (cD−/cD−) were described by Tate *et al* (1960). C^{w}D− was described by Gunson and Donohue (1957) and *(C)* D^{IV}− was described by Salmon *et al* (1969).

In general, suppressions appear to be inherited as if they are "deleted" alleles at the *CDE* locus. In some families, however, inheritance appears straightforward. There is a high consanguinity rate among parents of individuals with suppressed antigens (Race and Sanger, 1968).

Other Recently Discovered Antigens of the Rh System. In the 40 years since the Rh blood group system was first described, such extensive work has been performed to explain its curiosities that one would think that the end had been reached in terms of new antigens — yet each year, almost without exception, they continue to be discovered. Those not described in the preceding pages include the Rh antigen Evans, described in 1978 by Contreras *et al* and given the number Rh37 by Issitt *et al*, 1979, who also suggest that the antigen Duclos, which bears at least as much relationship to Rh as does LW, be called Rh38 (see Habibi *et al*, 1978).

Anti-Rh39 (Issitt *et al*, 1979), is an autoantibody that resembles anti-C in specificity, yet the corresponding antigen is present in −D−/−D− *and cD−/cD−* red cells.

The Rh antibody most recently identified (at the time of writing) is anti-Ce^s (Moulds *et al*, 1980), which was found to react with r′^{s}r (Ccde^s) red cells. The new antigen has been called Rh42 in the numerical system of nomenclature.

THE LW ANTIGEN

As mentioned, the antibody produced in guinea pigs after injection of rhesus monkey red cells (Landsteiner and Wiener, 1940) was at first considered identical with anti-Rh produced in humans after challenge with Rh-positive red cells either by transfusion or pregnancy.

The first evidence that the guinea pig (Rhesus monkey) antibody was different from human anti-Rh was produced by Fisk and Foord (1942) when they found that the guinea pig antibody reacted equally strongly with Rh-negative and Rh-positive cord blood red cells. Further evidence of differences soon followed (Murray and Clark, 1952; Levine *et al*, 1961a, 1961b) and in 1963 Levine *et al*, in reporting a D-positive woman with the anti-*rhesus* antibody in her serum, suggested that the guinea pig antibody be referred to as "anti-LW" in honor of Landsteiner and Wiener.

The similarity between anti-Rh$_0$ (D) and anti-LW is due to the inter-relationship of their corresponding antigenic pathways. Swanson and Matson (1964) were able to show that the gene responsible for LW is inherited independently of the Rh genes, the relationship being between the LW and Rh gene products. Tippett

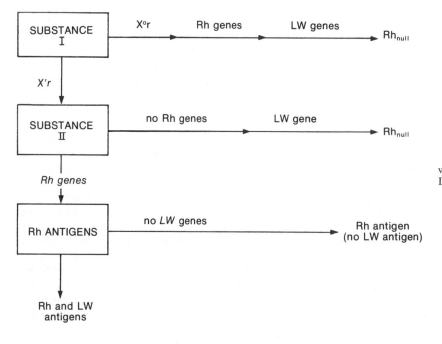

Figure 5–10 Possible pathways for the synthesis of Rh and LW antigens.

(1972) suggested that LW is formed by the action of an *LW* gene on Rh antigen. (The genetic pathways suggested are shown in Figure 5–10.)

Further distinctions in the LW system have now been recognized. Swanson *et al* (1974) described two kinds of LW antibody and two kinds of LW-positive antigens. One antibody is anti-LW + LW_1 (analogous to anti-A + A_1) and the other is anti-LW_1 (analogous to anti-A_1). Anti-LW_1 distinguishes two different LW antigens, LW_1 and LW_2 — with most individuals possessing the LW_1 antigen. Further subdivisions were subsequently described by White *et al* (1975), called LW_2 and LW_4. LW_3 individuals can produce anti-LW that reacts with LW_1 (Rh-positive) and LW_2 (Rh-negative) red cells, but not with LW_3 or LW_4 (LW-negative) red cells. LW_4 individuals can produce anti-LW, which reacts with LW_1, LW_2 and LW_3 red cells.

THE NUMBER OF Rh ANTIGEN SITES

The number of D antigen sites on red cells of different phenotypes was estimated by Rochna and Hughes-Jones (1965) using purified ^{125}I-labeled anti-IgG. Results of this study are given in Table 5–8.

In addition, four examples of $-D-/-D-$ red cells were examined by Hughes-Jones *et al* (1971) and found to have between 110,000 and 202,000 D sites per red cell. In the same study, Hughes-Jones and his colleagues estimated the numbers of c, e and E antigen sites per red cell, with the following results:

c sites (cc red cells): 70,000 to 85,000
(cC red cells): 37,000 to 53,000
e sites (ee red cells): 18,200 to 24,000
(eE red cells): 13,400 to 14,500

A great variation in the number of E antigen sites was found according to the source of anti-E and the phenotype of the red cells. Results varied from 450 to 25,600 sites per cell.

Table 5–8 THE NUMBER OF D ANTIGEN SITES ON RED CELLS OF DIFFERENT PHENOTYPES

Phenotype	Probable Genotype	D Antigen Sites
CcDe	*CDe/cde* (*R¹r*)	9900–14,600
cDe	*cDe/cde* (*R⁰r*)	12,000–20,000
cDEe	*cDE/cde* (*R²r*)	14,000–16,600
CDe	*CDe/CDe* (*R¹R¹*)	14,500–19,300
CcDEe	*CDe/cDE* (*R¹R²*)	23,000–31,000
cDE	*cDE/cDE* (*R²R²*)	15,800–33,300

°From Rochna and Hughes-Jones (1965).

The results given are substantially different from those reported by Masouredis *et al* (1976).

Clustering of D Antigen Sites. The distribution of the Rh antigen sites on the red cell membrane, particularly $Rh_0(D)$, has been studied by a number of workers (see Nicholson *et al*, 1971; Romano *et al*, 1975; Voak *et al*, 1974). The results of the study by Nicholson *et al* (1971) suggested that the D sites are present as single molecular entities distributed in "a periodic and random two dimensional array," a finding confirmed by Romano *et al* (1975). The latter workers also provided evidence that treatment of the cells with the enzyme papain produced clustering of the antigen sites — and that $-D-$ red cells showed a clustering of D sites without enzyme treatment, which may in part explain why IgG anti-D is capable of agglutinating untreated $-D-$ red cells in saline. Voak *et al* (1974) also observed clustering of D sites after enzyme treatment of red cells.

Rh Antigens on Tissues Other Than Red Cells. Rh antigens (substances) have not been detected on leukocytes, platelets (Gurner and Coombs, 1958; Barnes *et al*, 1963; Ashhurst *et al*, 1956), or in saliva (Wiener and Forer, 1941; Levine and Katzin, 1941; Mohn and Witebsky, 1948) or in amniotic fluid (Walker and Bailey, 1956; Lawler and Shatwell, 1962).

Development of Rh Antigens. Rh antigens are well developed at birth (Bornstein and Israel, 1942; Stratton, 1943). In fact the $Rh_0(D)$ antigen has been demonstrated on fetal red cells as early as 38 days after conception in a 10 mm embryo (Bergstrom *et al*, 1967). Race and Sanger (1975) report that they have found the antigens V (ce^s), f (ce), VS (e^s), and rh$_i$ (Ce) to be well developed in cord cells.

THE ANTIBODIES OF THE Rh/Hr BLOOD GROUP SYSTEM

Immunoglobulin Classes and Subclasses. The majority of Rh antibodies are IgG (7S) and do not agglutinate saline-suspended Rh-positive red cells (with the exception of $-D-$ cells) but can be detected using a colloid medium (e.g., bovine albumin) or by the indirect antiglobulin test. A few anti-D sera contain some IgM antibody (which is almost always accompanied by IgG antibody) and these sera will agglutinate saline-suspended red cells if the IgM component is present in sufficient concentration. Rare anti-D sera contain some IgA antibody but this is (in all examples detected so far) present as a minor component in a serum containing predominantly IgG antibody.

In the early stages of the immune response it appears that IgG and IgA antibodies are formed, followed by IgM antibody (Davey *et al*, 1969; Gunson *et al*, 1970). Jakobowicz *et al* (1972), however, reported that the earliest antibody to appear was IgM, followed by IgG with the property of agglutinating saline-suspended cells (an activity of more potent IgM anti-Rh) developing last. This final IgM, upon subsequent stimulation, was found to be the first to disappear.

IgG antibody molecules are predominantly of the IgG_1 and IgG_3 subclasses (Natvig and Kunkel, 1968), although some may be partly IgG_2 (Abramson and Schur, 1972) or IgG_4 (Frame *et al*, 1970).

Non-red cell–immune Rh Antibodies ("Naturally Occurring"). Anti-D that is not the direct result of antigenic stimulus is extremely rare, although several examples of anti-E of this type have been described (Harrison, 1970; Kissmeyer-Nielsen, 1965; Dybkjaer, 1967). Some examples of non-red cell–immune anti-E agglutinate red cells suspended in saline and react stronger at 20° C than at 37° C; others are detected only by the agglutination of enzyme-treated red cells. The frequency of non-red cell–immune anti-E was reported to be 0.1 per cent in studies performed by Kissmeyer-Nielsen (1965) on over 200,000 individuals.

A few examples of "naturally occurring" anti-C, anti-C^w and anti-C^x have been described (Beck *et al*, 1968; Chown and Lewis, 1954; Plaut *et al*, 1958).

Immune Rh Antibodies. Rh antibodies are most commonly stimulated by transfusion or pregnancy (i.e., as a result of immunization by red cells) and generally develop from two to six months after the initial challenge. Studies by Diamond (1947) revealed that following transfusion of one or more units of Rh positive blood, anti-Rh_0(D) appears in the serum of about 50 per cent of Rh-negative individuals. In spite of repeated stimulation with Rh-positive blood, about 33 per cent of Rh-negative individuals fail to form anti-Rh_0(D) (Mollison, 1967; Davey, 1976) and are termed "nonresponders." Secondary immunization in subjects who are primarily immunized to Rh_0(D) may result in maximal increase in antibody concentration within three weeks.

Following a single pregnancy with an Rh-positive (ABO-compatible) infant, anti-Rh_0(D) becomes serologically detectable within 6 months in about 7 per cent of Rh-negative women (see Chapter 16).

The formation of anti-Rh_0(D) as a consequence of transfusion or pregnancy is now uncommon, since Rh-negative subjects are routinely transfused with Rh-negative blood and since Rh-immune globulin is used to suppress Rh immunization during or following pregnancy. After anti-Rh_0(D), anti-G is now probably the most common Rh antibody formed, followed by anti-c and anti-E.

Complement Binding. The majority of Rh antibodies do not bind complement, because the triggering of the complement cascade calls for at least two IgG molecules to be bound to the cell in close proximity. Rh antigens are too far apart on the red cell membrane to allow IgG molecules to collaborate with one another, and therefore the condition is not fulfilled. Rare examples of complement-binding Rh antibodies, however, have been described (Waller and Lawler, 1962; Ayland *et al*, 1978).

Rh Antibodies and Antibody Mixtures Commonly Found. As mentioned, after anti-Rh_0(D), anti-G is probably the most common Rh antibody formed, followed by anti-c and anti-E. Anti-f (ce) is present in most sera containing anti-c and in most sera containing anti-e (Rosenfield *et al*, 1953; Jones *et al*, 1954).

Anti-CE is sometimes formed with anti-D (Race and Sanger, 1968) or with anti-C (Dunsford, 1962). Anti-C is commonly a mixture of anti-C and anti-Ce and is rarely formed without anti-D. Anti-V (Ce^s) and anti-VS (e^s) are most commonly found in blacks.

The Clinical Significance of Rh Antibodies. Rh antibodies in the plasma of a recipient of blood transfusion are capable of causing severe hemolytic transfusion reactions if the patient is transfused with blood possessing the offending antigen, and these antibodies must be considered to be very important clinically. In addition, Rh antibodies, being IgG, are capable of crossing the placenta and are a cause of hemolytic disease of the newborn (see Chapter 16).

In cases in which Rh-negative blood is unavailable, Rh-positive blood is often transfused to individuals who do not possess Rh antibodies rather than withhold blood from a patient whose need for blood is critical. Since up to 70 per cent of Rh-negative recipients will form anti-Rh_0(D) after transfusion with Rh-positive blood, this practice should not be encouraged and should be specifically avoided (when possible) in women of childbearing age.

In certain cases it is possible to prevent immunization with large doses of Rh_0(D) Immune Globulin (Human) when only one unit of

Rh-positive blood has been given to an Rh-negative recipient. Pollack *et al* (1971) reported that 15 to 20 ml of Rh Immune Globulin is required to prevent immunization by 1 unit of blood. In general, the number of vials of Rh Immune Globulin needed (each vial containing 300 μg) can be calculated by dividing the volume of transfused red blood cells by 15.

It should be noted that giving excess Rh Immune Globulin does not harm the Rh-negative patient; therefore, it is better to err by overestimating the volume required than by underestimating. (See Rh Immune Globulin, Chapter 16.)

$Rh_o(D)$ Typing. $Rh_o(D)$ typing may be performed on a slide (tile) or in tubes using either anti-$Rh_o(D)$ serum (for slide or rapid tube) or saline-reactive serum. In general, the "slide or rapid tube" serum is used in routine situations, with the saline-reactive serum reserved for special circumstances, as when cells agglutinate spontaneously or form rouleaux when suspended in a high-protein medium, or when cells are coated (sensitized) with anti-$Rh_o(D)$ (in hemolytic disease of the newborn) or other antibodies (in autoimmune hemolytic anemia) and when antiserum for slide and rapid tube tests gives equivocal results.

TECHNIQUES

In most routine situations, cell typing involves only $Rh_o(D)$ with full phenotyping being performed only when there are specific reasons for doing so (e.g., family studies, paternity testing, transfusion when Rh antibodies are present, prenatal testing when attempts are being made to determine homozygosity or heterozygosity).

Controls When Typing With Slide and Rapid Tube Reagent

The macromolecular nature of the suspending medium and specific substances in the reagents may cause cellular aggregation that resembles antibody-mediated agglutination in slide and rapid tube tests for $Rh_o(D)$ typing. Therefore, a control using immunologically inert reagents must accompany the test.

The most satisfactory control medium to detect these false reactions is the material used as a suspending medium for the specific antibody. Many commercial houses offer these immunologically inert high-protein mediums, which lack the specific antibody yet resemble the reagent in all other ways. This material should be used as a control, run in parallel with all tests for the $Rh_o(D)$ antigen. If the material is not available, 22 per cent or 30 per cent bovine albumin may be used.

Controls When Typing With Saline-Reactive Reagent

Saline-reactive anti-$Rh_o(D)$ agglutinates saline-suspended cells; therefore, the use of high-protein medium or the aforementioned control is not indicated. The American Association of Blood Banks (AABB) recommends that if the reagent is used occasionally, the test should be accompanied by known positive and negative controls. If the test is done frequently, however, the reagent should be tested as part of the routine quality control program (see Chapter 20).

METHODS*

$Rh_o(D)$ Typing (Slide Technique)

1. **Place 1 drop of reagent anti-$Rh_o(D)$ on a labeled slide.**
2. **Place 1 drop of albumin or other control medium on another labeled slide.**
3. **To each slide add 2 drops of well-mixed 40 per cent to 50 per cent suspension of cells in plasma or serum.**
4. **Thoroughly mix the cell suspension and reagent, using a clean stick for each slide, and spread the mixture evenly over most of the slide.**
5. **Place both slides on a viewing surface (lighted) and tilt gently and continuously. Observe for agglutination. Do not allow cell mixture to come in contact with hands. (*Note:* the viewing surface should be kept lighted at all times to preserve a temperature of 45° to 50° C. Reagents placed on a glass slide in contact with the surface should then reach 37° C, the optimum temperature for reaction, within two minutes.)**

Interpretation. **A positive test has agglutination with anti-$Rh_o(D)$ and a smooth suspension of cells in the control. A negative test has a smooth suspension of cells in both the test and the control. If there is agglutination or irregularity in the control, the test results must be considered invalid, and a saline test performed.**

---

*All methods given are those recommended by the American Association of Blood Banks (AABB). Variables may exist in manufacturer's directions, of course, and these should always be followed.

Causes of False Reaction in Slide Tests

1. False positives may be caused by the following:
   (a) Drying on the slide, which may be confused with agglutination
   (b) Small fibrin clots may give the appearance of agglutination
   (c) Blood incompletely anticoagulated, which may clot on the heated slide
2. False negatives may be caused by the following:
   (a) Saline-suspended cells reacting poorly or not at all
   (b) If the cell suspension is too weak (as in a severely anemic patient), cells may agglutinate poorly
   (c) Weakly active cells may take the full 2 minutes to agglutinate and may therefore be misinterpreted if read too soon
   (d) Failure to properly identify reagents at the time of use may result in the wrong reagent used in place of anti-Rh_o(D).

Rh_o(D) Typing (Tube Technique)

1. Place 1 drop of antiserum in a tube labeled "test."
2. Place 1 drop of albumin or control medium in a tube labeled "control."
3. Add 1 or 2 drops (depending on manufacturer's directions) of a recommended cell suspension (usually 2 to 5 per cent) in serum or saline to each tube *or* use clean, separate applicator stick to dislodge enough cells from the clot to approximate cell volume of 1 drop of 5 per cent suspension in each tube.
4. Mix well and centrifuge according to manufacturer's directions.
5. Gently resuspend the cell button and observe for agglutination.
   (*Note:* If an applicator stick was used to transfer the cells, the addition of 1 drop of saline to the tube before resuspending the cell button will provide more fluid and make resuspension and reading easier.)

Interpretation. A positive test has agglutination with anti-Rh_o(D) and a smooth suspension of cells in the control. A negative test has a smooth suspension of cells in both the test and the control. If there is agglutination or irregularity in the control, the test results must be considered invalid and a saline test performed.

Causes of False Reaction in Tube Tests

1. False positives may be caused by the following:
   (a) The anti-Rh_o(D) used may contain (in addition to anti-Rh_o(D), antibodies of another specificity (e.g., anti-Bg).
   (b) If an antibody complex (e.g., anti-G) is used instead of pure anti-Rh_o(D), red cells that lack the Rh_o(D) antigen but possess the C antigen will be agglutinated.
   (c) If cells and serum remain together too long before the test is read, the high protein medium may produce rouleaux, which resembles agglutinates.
2. False negatives may be caused by the following:
   (a) Inadvertent failure to add the reagent.
   (b) Failure to properly identify reagents, resulting in the wrong reagent being used in place of anti-Rh_o(D).
   (c) If cells and serum remain together too long before the test is read, antibody may elute from weakly-reactive cells and small agglutinates may disperse.

D^u Typing Using the Indirect Antiglobulin Technique

1. Place 1 drop of anti-Rh_o(D) serum in a labeled test tube.
2. Add 1 or 2 drops of a 2 to 5 per cent suspension of red cells (according to the manufacturer's directions). (*Note:* If the initial Rh_o(D) typing was performed in a tube, this tube can be used directly for D^u testing.)
3. A control is required, which may either consist of one or two drops of the original cell suspension in a labeled control tube (which need not be incubated), or the albumin or reagent control tube from Rh_o(D) typing may be used.
4. Mix gently and incubate at 37° C. (The time of incubation will be specified by the manufacturer.)
5. Wash cells in both "test" and "control" tubes 3 or 4 times in large volumes of saline.
6. Decant thoroughly after *each* wash and blot the rim of the tubes until they are quite dry.
7. Add 1 or 2 drops of antiglobulin reagent to each tube (according to manufacturer's directions).
8. Mix gently and centrifuge (time and speed of centrifugation according to manufacturer's directions).
9. Gently resuspend the cell button and observe for agglutination.
10. Add known sensitized cells as a control of the antiglobulin procedure, if desired.

Interpretation. Agglutination in the tube containing anti-Rh_o(D) indicates a Rh variant, and blood may be classified as Rh_o(D) positive, D^u-positive provided that the control is negative. A negative result is absence of agglutination in both the test and the control; blood is then classified as $Rh_o(D)$ negative. If the control is positive, the test result must not be considered valid. If the blood is from a donor, it should not be used for transfusion; if the blood is from a patient requiring transfusion, Rh-negative blood should be used.

It should be noted that when the albumin or reagent tube is used for antiglobulin testing, globulins in the medium may coat the cells during incubation, resulting in a false positive reaction. To distinguish this from a truly positive direct antiglobulin test, repeat the antiglobulin test on well-washed unincubated red cells. If this is negative, the reagents used for incubation should be investigated for the possible presence of immunologically active protein.

For further discussion of the antiglobulin test and the causes of false reactions, see Chapter 21.

$Rh_o(D)$ Typing (Saline Tube Test)

1. Place 1 drop of saline-reactive anti-$Rh_o(D)$ in a properly labeled test tube.
2. Add 1 drop of a 2 to 5 per cent saline suspension of well-washed red cells.
3. Mix gently and incubate at 37° C. (Time of incubation according to the manufacturer's directions.)
4. Centrifuge. (Time and speed according to manufacturer's directions.)
5. Gently resuspend the cell button and observe for agglutination.

Note. A saline suspension of known $Rh_o(D)$-positive and $Rh_o(D)$ negative cells should be run in parallel with the test as a control. Ensure that the concentration of cells in the control is comparable to that of the test cells.

Interpretation. Agglutination in the test substance indicates that the red cells are $Rh_o(D)$-positive. D^u cells will not normally be agglutinated. This test is performed only on recipients of transfusion; any seemingly negative recipient should be given Rh-negative blood. Saline-reactive anti-$Rh_o(D)$ cannot be used for D^u testing (i.e., in the antiglobulin test).

Tests for Other Rh Antigens

Both saline-reactive and slide or rapid tube test reagents are commercially available for the Rh antigens rh' (C), rh'' (E), hr' (c) and hr'' (e), and should be used according to the manufacturer's directions. Red cells that are known to be positive and negative should be used as controls, and these should be run in parallel with the test unless they are frequently used, in which case they should be controlled as part of a daily program (see Chapter 20). A high-protein control should be used with slide or rapid tube test reagents as for anti-$Rh_o(D)$. It should be noted that these reagents may contain antiglobulin-reactive antibodies other than those specified on the label and therefore, unless the instructions clearly indicate their suitability, these reagents should not be used in the antiglobulin test.

Other Causes of False Positive and False Negative Results in Rh Testing

1. False positives in routine Rh typing may also be caused by:
   (a) Contaminating antibody. A contaminating antibody with specificity other than that indicated by the label could cause "false" positive results. While this is not a common problem, it must be kept in mind and tested for when using any reagent.
   (b) Polyagglutination. Polyagglutinable red cells may be agglutinated by any human protein reagent, because the causative antibodies are present in all human sera. This situation will reveal itself through discrepant ABO cell and serum tests — except in the case of group AB red cells.
   (c) Serum-suspended cells from a patient with abnormal serum proteins. This situation may cause rouleaux formation, which could be mistaken for agglutination. The situation will reveal itself in a positive albumin or reagent medium control, and can be resolved by using well-washed saline-suspended red cells with saline-reactive reagents.
2. False negatives in routine Rh typing can also be caused by:
   (a) A reagent antibody that recognizes only a compound antigen, which will not react with red cells carrying the individual's specificities as separate gene products. (For example, anti-hr (f), or ce would give negative results with R^1R^2 *(CDe/cDE)* red cells or any other cells on which the hr'' (e) antigen was part of a gene product that did not include the compound antigen.) A well-defined quality control program should obviate the problem.
   (b) Red cells with variant antigens (e.g., C^w, ce^s) may fail to react with standard reagents. There is no easy way to detect this problem, which may reveal itself only in family studies or in the investigation of antibody that is directed against the variant.

TYPICAL EXAMINATION QUESTIONS

Choose the phrase, sentence or symbol that correctly answers the question or completes the statement. More than one answer may be acceptable for each question. Answers are at the back of the book.

1. A patient's red cells are tested with Rh antisera and the following results were obtained: positive with anti-D, anti-C, anti-e; negative with anti-E and anti-c and anti-f. The Rh phenotype in the Rosenfield terminology is
   (a) Rh 1, 2, 3, −4, −5, −6
   (b) Rh 1, 2, −3, −4, 5, 6,
   (c) Rh 1, Rh2, Rh−3, Rh−4, Rh5, Rh−6
   (d) Rh1, 2, 5
   (e) Rh1, 2, −3, −4, 5, −6
   (The Rosenfield Nomenclature)

2. A person of genotype $r''r''$ could produce which of the following alloantibodies?
   (a) Anti-E
   (b) Anti-G
   (c) Anti-f
   (d) Anti-e
   (General)

3. The most common Rh genotype is
   (a) rr
   (b) R^1R^2
   (c) R^2r
   (d) R^1r
   (e) R^1R^0
   (Table 5–7)

4. The Rh genotype R^2r is the same as
   (a) cDE/cde
   (b) cdE/cDe
   (c) $rh'Rh_0rh''/hr'hr''$
   (d) $hr'\ Rh_0\ hr''/hr'hr''$
   (e) $hr'Rh_0rh''/hr'hr''$
   (Table 5–1)

5. Which of the following statements is/are correct?
   (a) D^u is a variant of the D antigen
   (b) C^u is a variant of the C antigen
   (c) G^u is a variant of the G antigen
   (d) E^u is a variant of the E antigen
   (General)

6. Which antibody could be produced if an R^1r individual received R^2R^2 blood?
   (a) Anti-c
   (b) Anti-G
   (c) Anti-E
   (d) Anti-ce
   (e) Anti-Ce
   (General)

7. Which of the following is not an allele at the Ee locus?
   (a) E^w
   (b) hr^s
   (c) hr^B
   (d) rh^x
   (e) VS
   (Alleles at the Ee Locus)

8. Anti-f will react with the products of which of the following genotypes?
   (a) R^0r^y
   (b) R^1r
   (c) R^ZR^0
   (d) $r'r'$
   (e) $r''r''$
   (Compound Antigens)

9. Which of the following antigens is not part of the Rh blood group system?
   (a) V
   (b) G
   (c) Be^a
   (d) Jk^a
   (General)

10. The majority of Rh antibodies
    (a) bind complement
    (b) do not bind complement
    (c) are non-red cell immune
    (d) are clinically significant
    (The Antibodies of the Rh/Hr
    Blood Group System)

11. IgG Rh antibodies are predominantly of the
    (a) IgG_1 and IgG_3 subclasses
    (b) IgG_4 subclass
    (c) IgG_2 subclass
    (d) IgG_2, and IgG_4 subclasses
    (Immunoglobulin Classes and Subclasses)

12. When a blood transfusion is needed for a patient who has anti-C, the percentage of compatible blood is appproximately
    (a) 98
    (b) 31
    (c) 70
    (d) 3
    (e) 12
    (Table 5–6)

13. Rh antibodies
    (a) are a cause of hemolytic disease of the newborn
    (b) are most commonly stimulated by pregnancy but are generally not stimulated by transfusion
    (c) are capable of crossing the placenta
    (d) usually react better at 37° C than at 22°C
    (The Antibodies of the Rh/Hr
    Blood Group System)

14. Select the correct equivalents for the following
    (a) R^1r: CDe/cde
    (b) rr: hr' hr''/rh' rh''
    (c) R^0R^0: rh'Rh₀hr''/rh' Rh₀hr''
    (d) $r'r$: rh' hr''/hr' hr''
    (The Wiener Nomenclature)

15. Enter the Wiener nomenclature for the following genotypes
    (a) CDe/cde _____
    (b) cDE/CdE _____
    (c) CDE/cDe _____
    (d) CDe/CdE _____
    (e) CDe/cDE _____

(f) *Cde/Cde* _____
(g) *cdE/cdE* _____
(h) *CDe/cDe* _____
(i) *cdE/cde* _____
(j) *CDe/CDe* _____
(k) *Cde/cdE* _____

(l) *cDE/cDE* _____
(m) *cde/cde* _____
(n) *CdE/cdE* _____
(o) *cDE/Cde* _____
(p) *Cde/cde* _____

(General–Nomenclatures)

16. **Fill in the blanks as indicated:**

	C	D	E	c	e	Phenotype (Fisher-Race Nomenclature)	Probable Genotype (Fisher-Race and Wiener Nomenclatures)
		*Red Cell Reactions With Anti-*					
(a)	−	+	−	+	+	_____	_____
(b)	−	−	−	+	+	_____	_____
(c)	+	+	−	+	+	_____	_____
(d)	+	+	−	−	+	_____	_____
(e)	−	+	+	+	+	_____	_____
(f)	+	+	+	+	+	_____	_____
(g)	+	−	−	−	+	_____	_____
(h)	−	+	+	+	−	_____	_____

(General – Nomenclature)

17. The *Rh* locus has been assigned to chromosome number _____.

(Rh Inheritance)

18. D^u subjects who are blood donors must be classified as Rh _____.

(D^u As It Affects the Laboratory)

19. An individual lacking Rh^D but possessing all other portions of the mosaic is classified as _____.

(Subgroups of D: The D Antigen Mosaic)

20. Rh antibodies are most commonly stimulated by _____ or _____.

(Immune Rh Antibodies)

21. The most common antibody in the Rh system is _____.

(Rh Antibodies and Antibody Mixtures Commonly Found)

22. In slide tests for Rh antigens, saline-suspended red cells may produce a false-_____ reaction.

(Causes of False Reactions in Slide Tests)

23. The antigen Rh12 is given as _____ in the Fisher-Race nomenclature.

(Table 5–2)

24. The complex antigen Rh_2 is made up of factors _____.

(Table 5–11)

25. The phenotype of red cells which are Rh_1Rh_0 is _____.

(General)

GENERAL REFERENCES

The references provided in Chapter 4 will also prove useful in the study of the Rh blood group system. In addition, A. G. Erskine's The Principles and Practice of Blood Grouping discusses Wiener's approach to the Rh system and will prove useful to students who are experiencing difficulty with that theory. Students may also find the following useful:

1. Boorman, K. E., Dodd, B. E., and Lincoln, P. L.: Blood Group Serology. Churchill-Livingstone, New York, 1977. (*Clearly written with emphasis on the Fisher-Race theory. Methods of Rh typing will prove interesting as a comparison of used methods.*)

2. Issitt, P. D., and Issitt, C. H.: Applied Blood Group Serology. Spectra Biologicals, 1976. (*Excellent description of the Rh system. Useful as a reference text.*)

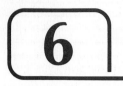

THE KELL BLOOD GROUP SYSTEM

OBJECTIVES — THE KELL BLOOD GROUP SYSTEM

The student shall know, understand and be prepared to explain:

1. A short history of the discovery of the antigens and antibodies in the Kell system
2. The nomenclatures in the Kell blood group system, specifically to include:
   (a) Original names (Kell, Cellano, etc.)
   (b) Original symbols (K, k, Kp[a], etc.)
   (c) Numerical symbols (K1, K2, etc.)
3. The basic principles of the inheritance of Kell genes
4. The antigens of the Kell system, specifically to include:
   (a) Antigens K and k (general characteristics, frequency, antigenicity)
   (b) Antigens Kp[a] and Kp[b] (general characteristics, frequency)
   (c) Antigen Kp[c] (characteristics)

(d) Antigens Js[a] and Js[b] (characteristics)
(e) A brief outline of the characteristics of other antigens in the Kell blood group system (K8–K19)
(f) A general summary of the K[o] phenotype, the McLeod phenotype and depressed Kell antigens in hemolytic anemia and as a result of depression effects by other Kell genes
(g) The number of K and k antigen sites on the red cells
(h) The development of the Kell antigens at birth
5. The antibodies of the Kell system, to include characteristics, stimulus, immunoglobulin class, frequency and clinical significance
6. The technique used in the detection of antigens in the Kell system, and the controls commonly used in such detection

Introduction

The Kell blood group system was discovered within a few weeks of trials with the newly described antiglobulin test (Coombs, Mourant and Race, 1946). In the serum of a mother, Mrs. Kellacher, who had given birth to an infant affected by hemolytic disease of the newborn, there was an antibody that sensitized the blood of her husband and her elder child and about 7 to 9 per cent of random blood samples. The definitive antigen was shown to be independent of all other blood group systems known at the time, and the newly recognized blood group was given the name Kell, after the patient.

A second example of anti-K was found by Wiener and Sonn-Gordon (1947), although it was not at first recognized as such and was named Si. Other examples of anti-K soon followed.

The antithetical antibody anti-k was discovered by Levine et al (1949). The proposita in this case did not wish her name to be used for the new antigen, and so a partial anagram of her name, Cellano, was used.

For eight years, Kell remained a simple two-antigen system; this simple arrangement abruptly ended with the discovery of anti-Kp[a] and anti-Kp[b], which were shown to be related to the Kell system (Allen and Lewis, 1957). In the same year, rare individuals were discovered who apparently lacked all Kell antigens — referred to as K[o] (Chown et al, 1957).

Then, in 1965, Stroup et al discovered that the Sutter groups originally described by Giblett (1958) belonged to the Kell system. These antigens, which have retained the names Js[a] and Js[b], represent the third set of antithetical antigens. The antigens K11 (Côté) (Guévin et al, 1971 and K17 (Weeks) (Strange et al, 1974)

Table 6–1 ANTIGENS OF THE KELL BLOOD GROUP SYSTEM: COMPARISON OF NOMENCLATURES

Original Name	Numerical Term	Year of Original Report
K (Kell)	K1	1946
k (Cellano)	K2	1949
Kp^a (Penney)	K3	1957
Kp^b (Rautenberg)	K4	1958
K$_o$ (Peltz)	K5	1957
Js^a (Sutter)	K6	1958
Js^b (Matthews)	K7	1963
K^w	K8	1965
KL (Claas)	K9	1965
Ul^a	K10	1968
Côté	K11	1971
Bøc	K12	1973
Sgro	K13	1974
San	K14	1976
Kx	K15	1975
K-like	K16	1975
Wk^a (Weeks)	K17	1974
—	K18	1975
—	K19	1979
Kp^c (Levay)		1979

represent the fourth and to date final set of antithetical antigens.

At the present time there are in total 20 Kell-related antigens, many of which are associated in some way with the "null" phenotype (K$_o$). The genetic relationship of these K$_o$-associated antigens to the Kell system is not yet understood, and they are often referred to as "para-Kell" (Race and Sanger, 1975).

Nomenclatures

The antigens of the Kell blood group system were originally named after the individuals in whom the antibodies were first found. Allen and Rosenfield (1961) proposed a numerical nomenclature after the model of the Rosenfield Rh nomenclature in an attempt to ease the difficulties of communication. The antigens of the Kell system are given in Table 6–1 together with their numerical equivalents.

The Genetics of the Kell System

Several theories of Kell inheritance have been suggested, yet all involve a certain amount of guesswork in light of newer discoveries that appear not to fit into the pattern (see Zmijewski and Fletcher, 1972; Race and Sanger, 1975; Issitt and Issitt, 1975).

At a basic yet convenient level, the Kell locus can be considered to be a complex of four series of allelic genes, *K* and *k*, *Kp*^{a} and *Kp*^{b}, *Js*^{a} and *Js*^{b} and *K11* and *K17*. If we ignore for the moment the allelic pair *K11* and *K17* and the K$_o$ phenotype, genetic control of the antigens K, k, Kp^a, Kp^b, Js^a and Js^b can be seen to be similar to that of the Rh system — namely, that the three allelic genes occupy three closely linked loci or three subloci within a single complex genetic locus. Under this scheme, there are eight theoretically possible gene complexes in the

Table 6–2 THE 8 GENE COMPLEXES, 36 "PAIRINGS" AND 27 PHENOTYPES THEORETICALLY POSSIBLE IN THE KELL SYSTEM USING 6 KELL ANTISERA (FROM BRYANT, 1980)

Gene Complexes	Pairing	Phenotypes
K Kp^a, Js^a*	K Kp^a Js^a × K Kp^a Js^a	K Kp^a Js^a
	K Kp^a Js^a × K Kp^a Js^b	K Kp^a Js^a Js^b
	K Kp^a Js^a × K Kp^b Js^a	K Kp^a Kp^b Js^a
	K Kp^a Js^a × K Kp^b Js^b	K Kp^a Kp^b Js^a Js^b
	K Kp^a Js^a × k Kp^a Js^a	Kk Kp^a Js^a
	K Kp^a Js^a × k Kp^a Js^b	Kk Kp^a Js^a Js^b
	K Kp^a Js^a × k Kp^b Js^a	Kk Kp^a Kp^b Js^a
	K Kp^a Js^a × k Kp^b Js^b	Kk Kp^a Kp^b Js^a Js^b
K Kp^a Js^b	K Kp^a Js^b × K Kp^a Js^b	K Kp^a Js^b
	K Kp^a Js^b × K Kp^b Js^a	K Kp^a Kp^b Js^a Js^b†
	K Kp^a Js^b × K Kp^b Js^b	K Kp^a Kp^b Js^b
	K Kp^a Js^b × k Kp^a Js^a	Kk Kp^a Js^a Js^b†
	K Kp^a Js^b × k Kp^a Js^b	Kk Kp^a Js^b
	K Kp^a Js^b × k Kp^b Js^a	Kk Kp^a Kp^b Js^a Js^b†
	K Kp^a Js^b × k Kp^b Js^b	Kk Kp^a Kp^b Js^b†
K Kp^b Js^a*	K Kp^b Js^a × K Kp^b Js^a	K Kp^b Js^a
	K Kp^b Js^a × K Kp^b Js^b	K Kp^b Js^a Js^b
	K Kp^b Js^a × k Kp^a Js^a	Kk Kp^a Kp^b Js^a†
	K Kp^b Js^a × k Kp^a Js^b	Kk Kp^a Kp^b Js^a Js^b†
	K Kp^b Js^a × k Kp^b Js^a	Kk Kp^a Kp^b Js^a†
	K Kp^b Js^a × k Kp^b Js^b	Kk Kp^b Js^a Js^b
K Kp^b Js^b	K Kp^b Js^b × K Kp^b Js^b	K Kp^b Js^b
	K Kp^b Js^b × k Kp^a Js^a	Kk Kp^a Kp^b Js^a Js^b†
	K Kp^b Js^b × k Kp^a Js^b	Kk Kp^a Kp^b Js^b†
	K Kp^b Js^b × k Kp^b Js^a	Kk Kp^b Js^a Js^b†
	K Kp^b Js^b × k Kp^b Js^b	Kk Kp^b Js^b
k Kp^a Js^a*	k Kp^a Js^a × k Kp^a Js^a	k Kp^a Js^a
	k Kp^a Js^a × k Kp^a Js^b	k Kp^a Js^a Js^b
	k Kp^a Js^a × k Kp^b Js^a	k Kp^a Kp^b Js^a
	k Kp^a Js^a × k Kp^b Js^b	k Kp^a Kp^b Js^a Js^b
k Kp^a Js^b*	k Kp^a Js^b × k Kp^a Js^b	k Kp^a Js^b
	k Kp^a Js^b × k Kp^b Js^a	k Kp^a Kp^b Js^a Js^b†
	k Kp^a Js^b × k Kp^b Js^b	k Kp^a Kp^b Js^b
k Kp^b Js^a	k Kp^b Js^a × k Kp^b Js^a	k Kp^b Js^a
	k Kp^b Js^a × k Kp^b Js^b	k Kp^b Js^a Js^b
k Kp^b Js^b	k Kp^b Js^b × k Kp^b Js^b	k Kp^b Js^b

*Gene complex has never been found.
†Phenotype occurs more than once in table.

Table 6–3   ANTIGEN AND PHENOTYPE FREQUENCIES IN THE KELL SYSTEM*

Antigen	Percentage of Positives		Phenotype	Percentage Frequency	
	Whites	Blacks		Whites	Blacks
K	9.0	3.5	K+ k−	0.2	<0.1
k	99.8	>99.9	K+ k+	8.8	3.5
Kp^a	2.0	<0.1	K− k+	91.0	96.5
Kp^b	>99.9	>99.9	Kp(a+b−)	<0.1	<0.1
Js^a	<0.1	19.5	Kp(a+b+)	2.0	< 0.1
Js^b	>99.9	98.9	Kp(a−b+)	98.0	>99.9
			Js(a+b−)	<0.1	1.1
			Js(a+b+)	<0.1	18.4
			Js(a−b+)	>99.9	80.5

*From Bryant, 1980.

system, which can be paired in 36 different ways. These 36 possible genotypes make 27 phenotypes that would be distinguishable with the six antisera, anti-K, anti-k, anti-Kp^a, anti-Kp^b, anti-Js^a and anti-Js^b (Table 6–2).

Unlike the Rh system, however, in which all possible combinations of C, D, E, c and e have been found, only four of the eight possible gene complexes and only nine of the 27 possible phenotypes have actually been found (see Table 6–2). Several explanations have been offered for this (see Race and Sanger, 1975; Chown, 1964) yet the most likely appears to be that the antigens K (and Kp^a) and Js^a are most mutually exclusive in whites and blacks (respectively), whose interbreeding presumably has been confined to recent centuries. This would give little time for recombination to produce the "missing" alignments. The finding of such alignments would prove the accuracy of this theory. The frequencies of Kell system antigens and phenotypes are given in Table 6–3.

With respect to other genes in the Kell system, K11 and K17, as mentioned, represent a fourth series of alleles (Strange *et al*, 1974). The gene UI^a (K10) must also be considered an allele at the Kell complex, since no evidence has been found to tie it to the *K, Kp* or *Js* series (Furuhjelm *et al*, 1968).

The gene *K^o* may be considered as an allele at the *Kell* structural locus that produces no Kell antigens or as a rare allele at the Kell operator site that depresses all activity of its neighboring *K, Kp* and *Js* sites. Studies by Nunn *et al* (1966) and Lombardo *et al* (1972) showed the phenotype K$_o$ to be due to homozygosity at the *Kell* complex. Families revealing an unattached regulator locus (the background of most Rh$_{null}$ phenotypes) have not yet been reported.

The genetic pathways of the Kell antigens are still largely a matter of conjecture, yet most involve a precursor substance and interacting genes. Interesting suppositions have been offered by Race and Sanger (1975) and Issitt and Issitt (1975).

THE ANTIGENS OF THE KELL SYSTEM

Antigens K (K1) and k (K2). The antigen K (K1) is found in 7 to 9 per cent of randomly selected whites, who would possess the genotype *KK* (0.2 per cent) or *Kk* (99.8 per cent). The gene *K*, which has a frequency in North American whites of 0.0438, is directly inherited as a mendelian characteristic, co-dominant with its allele *k*, which has a frequency of 0.9562 in white North Americans. K-positive and k-positive individuals, therefore, must have at least one parent who is K-positive or k-positive, respectively. Both the K(K1) and k (K2) antigens are highly antigenic. Outside of the ABO and Rh systems, anti-K is the most common immune red cell antibody (see under the heading Antibodies of the Kell System).

Antigens Kp^a (K3) and Kp^b (K4). The antigen Kp^a (K3) occurs in approximately 2.4 per cent of random North American white blood. The gene *Kp^a* is inherited as a dominant mendelian character (Race and Sanger, 1975) codominant with its allele *Kp^b*. The incidence of the Kp^a antigen in K+ individuals is only about half that in the general population; this suggests that a gene complex capable of producing both the K and Kp^a antigens might not exist, and that K and Kp^a, when they do exist together, are due to K and Kp^a genes in *trans* position. Studies by Lewis *et al* (1960); Allen and Lewis (1957), Cleghorn (1961), Wright *et al* (1965) and Dichupa *et al* (1969) have supported this theory.

In persons who are K+, Kp(a+), the antigen k is weaker than usual when it is produced by the gene complex that also produces Kp^a (Allen and Lewis, 1957). This is important in practical testing since it is a common pitfall for the unwary when screening for k-negative units.

The antigen Kp[a] has not been reported in blacks.

The antithetical antigen Kp[b] (K4) is extremely common; only two Kp(b−) samples were found by Allen *et al* (1958) in tests on 5500 whites.

Antigen Kp[c]. A "new" allele, *Kp[c]*, at the *Kell* complex locus was described by Yamaguchi *et al* (1979). The proposita produced an antibody, anti-Kp[c], which was directed against the *Kp* part of the *Kell* locus. Later tests on the original serum by Gavin *et al* (1979) have revealed that a low-frequency antigen, "Levay," which was discovered in England 33 years ago (and not assigned to any system), is the antigen Kp[c] of the Kell system. The Kp[c] antigen was not given a numerical designation in the original paper, and it is therefore suggested that K20 be used in keeping with the present sequence.

Antigens Js[a] (K6) and Js[b] (K7). The antigen Js[a] was discovered by Giblett (1958). The antibody, anti-Js[a], was found to sensitize about 20 per cent of black donors but failed to sensitize any of the 240 white donors originally tested. Subsequent tests have confirmed Js[a] to be an important black antigen, rarely encountered in whites (see Giblett and Chase, 1959).

The antigen Js[b] was reported by Walter et al (1963, 1964). The gene was found to be an allele of *Js[a]*. Both *Js[a]* and *Js[b]* belong to the Kell system.

OTHER ANTIGENS OF THE KELL SYSTEM

The known complexity of the Kell system has increased rapidly since 1965. The following is a brief summary of the "newer" antigens. Readers requiring more information are referred to the list of general references at the end of this chapter.

Antigen K[w] (K8). The antibody anti-K[w] was first described by Bove *et al* (1965) and was found to be present in approximately 8 per cent of anti-K (−K1) sera. In studies of K-negative blood, K[w] (K8) was found in 5.2 per cent of whites and 18 per cent of blacks. It should be noted that the antigen K[w] (K8) has not been proved to belong to the Kell system.

Antigen KL (Claas) (K9). Van der Hart *et al* (1968) recorded the investigation of a boy, Claas, who possessed an antibody that reacted with all cells tested (including K_o) except his own. Later studies revealed that the antibody did not react with cells of the McLeod phenotype (described later) — which represents its only association with Kell. The corresponding antigen, usually referred to as KL, could therefore be classed as a "Kell-related" or "para-Kell" antigen.

Antigen UI[a] (K10). Furuhjelm *et al* (1968) described an antibody, anti-UI[a], which defined an antigen of low frequency (approximately 3 per cent in Finnish blood donors). Furuhjelm *et al* (1969), in studies of three informative families, showed that the gene UI[a] belongs to the *Kell* complex locus. The allelic gene *UI[b]* has not been found; however, when and if it is, then *UI* would add another series of alleles to those already known.

Antigen K11 (Côté). Anti-K11 was discovered by Guévin *et al* (1971). The antibody anti-K11 was found to react with all red cells tested except K_o, the maker's own cells and those of two of her eight sibs. Strange *et al* (1974) showed that *K11* and *Wk[a] (K17)* are alleles, and this was later confirmed (see Stroup, 1974). The alleles, in accordance with other nomenclatures, could be regarded as Wk[a] (K17) and Wk[b] (K11).

Antigen K12 (Bøc). The antigen K12, discovered through its corresponding antibody (Heisto *et al*, 1973), is a high-frequency antigen that is classed as Kell-related or para-Kell. The antibody, anti-K12, reacts with all cells except K_o and with the maker's own cells. There is as yet no evidence that K12 is an inherited character.

Antigen K13 (Sgro). Anti-K13 was discovered by Marsh *et al* (1974). The corresponding antigen, K13, is another high-frequency Kell-related or para-Kell antigen. The individual in whom the antibody was first discovered (and one of his five sibs) was found to have weaker than normal Kell antigens — though not as weak as red cells of the McLeod phenotype.

Antigen K14 (San). The antibody defining the K14 antigen was reported at the same time as K11 (Heisto *et al*, 1973). The antigen is another high-frequency Kell-related or para-Kell antigen. Only one example of the antibody has been found and no family members were tested. Therefore, we have no evidence that K14 is an inherited character.

Antigen K15 (Kx). In investigations of anti-KL (K9), van der Hart *et al* (1968) prepared, by absorption and elution, one fraction that reacted more strongly with K−k+ red cells than with K_o red cells and another fraction that gave the opposite reaction. The fraction that reacted more strongly with K_o red cells gave trace reactions with red cells of common Kell type and reacted with intermediate strength against known heterozygous K^o samples. It was given the name anti-K_x by Marsh *et al* (1974, 1974). The K_x antigen is absent in individuals of the McLeod phenotype and from the white cells of patients with chronic granulomatous disease (CGD) (discussed later). Marsh *et al* (1973) suggested that the K_x antigen is necessary for the Kell system genes to express themselves in terms of antigenic determinants.

Antigen K16. The antigen K16 is a Kell-related or para-Kell high frequency character reported by Marsh and Allen in 1974 (unpublished). The antigen, which appears to be related in some way to k (K2) and K11, is still under investigation.

Antigen K17 (Weeks, Wk^a). This low-frequency antigen, discovered by Strange *et al* (1974), is the product of an allele of K11.

Antigen K18. This is another high-frequency Kell-related or para-Kell antigen discovered by Marsh *et al* (1975). The antibody, anti-K18, like others of this type, reacts with all samples of blood tested except those of the K_o phenotype and with the red cells of the maker.

Antigen K19. A new Kell-related or para-Kell antigen of high frequency, this was reported by Sabo *et al* (1979). The antibody reacted with all random cells tested but failed to react with red cells of the K_o phenotype. Studies of the proposita's family have provided evidence that the K19 antigen is a genetically determined inherited characteristic.

The K_o Phenotype

The K_o phenotype was discovered by Chown *et al* (1957) and was the name given to individuals who lacked all Kell antigens. The proposita (Peltz) was found through the investigation of an antibody, called anti-Ku, in her serum that reacted with all K+ or k+ red cells. A second example of K_o was reported by Kaita *et al* (1959), found as a result of a deliberate search in which 10,838 samples were tested with the anti-Ku of the original proposita. In these original investigations, both individuals were found to be K–k– Kp(a–b–). The observation that both propositi were also Js(a–b–) was an important step in placing the Js groups in the Kell system.

The gene responsible for the K_o phenotype is believed to be an allele at the *Kell* complex locus. Several families have been investigated, which confirms this (Nunn *et al*, 1966; Lombardo *et al*, 1972). Race and Sanger (1975) think of K^o as a rare allele at an operator site that "switches off" all activity at the *Kell* structural loci.

The majority of K^o propositi have anti-Ku in their serum (this being the name given to the antibody that reacts with all cells except those of the K_o phenotype).

Depressed Kell Antigens

The McLeod Phenotype: Chronic Granulomatous Disease. The McLeod phenotype was first encountered by Allen *et al* (1961): the red cells of the propositus, McLeod, were found to react extremely weakly with anti-k, anti-Kp^b and anti-Js^b (the latter realized later — Stroup *et al*, 1965). The cells also failed to react with anti-K or anti-Kp^a — that is, K–kwKp(a–bw) Js(a–bw).

The antibody Claas (anti-K9, anti-KL) was later found to be compatible with McLeod cells (von der Hart *et al*, 1968), yet all other cells, including K_o, were incompatible. Then in 1971, Giblett *et al* made the observation that the phenotypes K_o or McLeod are commonly found among sufferers of chronic granulomatous disease (CGD), a condition in which repeated bacterial infections occur that are often impossible to control even with antibiotics. The sufferers are children, and usually male. Whether these patients are *genetically* K_o or McLeod or whether their Kell antigens are oppressed by the process of the disease is not fully known. Evidence to support the genetic theory has been provided by Swanson *et al* (1972) and by Marsh *et al* (1973, 1975).

Hemolytic Anemia. Depressed Kell antigens have been noted in a patient with autoimmune hemolytic anemia (Seyfried *et al*, 1972). During the disease, the red cells gave the McLeod picture and anti-Kp^b was found in the patient's serum. After recovery, the Kell antigens were found to be normal.

Other Depressed Kell Antigens. The *Kp^a* and *K13* genes appear to have a *cis*-modifying effect on other *Kell* genes (Allen and Lewis, 1957; Marsh *et al*, 1974).

Some individuals who are Gerbich negative have markedly weakened k, Kp^b, Js^b, K11, K12 and K18 antigens. This suggests a relationship between the two blood groups, although the genes are known to segregate independently (Rosenfield *et al*, 1960). The exact nature of the relationship, if any, awaits explanation.

OTHER NOTES ON THE KELL ANTIGENS

The Numbers of K and k Antigen Sites. Hughes-Jones and Gardner (1971), using ^{125}I-labeled anti-K, found that the average number of K-antigen sites was 6100 on *KK* red cells and 3500 on *Kk* red cells. Masouredis (1976) estimated that there are 3800 k antigen sites on of the K_o phenotype).

The Development of Kell Antigens. The antigens K, k, Kp^a, Kp^b, Js^a and Js^b are all well developed at birth (see Toivanen and Hirvonen, 1973; Giblett and Chase, 1959; Huestis *et al*, 1963).

THE ANTIBODIES OF THE KELL SYSTEM

"Naturally occurring" antibodies in the Kell system are rare, although occasional examples of anti-K and anti-Kp^a have been identified in persons who have no history of exposure to the reactive antigen (see Marsh *et al*, 1976; Allen and Lewis, 1957). An example of naturally-occurring anti-Js^a (K6) was also recently reported in a Japanese female (Ito *et al*, 1979). Anti-K (and anti-k) are usually IgG, reacting best in the indirect antiglobulin test. Some examples of IgG anti-K bind complement. Anti-k is immune in nature (no "naturally occurring" example has yet been reported). Both anti-K and anti-k can cause hemolytic disease of the newborn — though it is unusual with anti-k since the causative antigen is so rare in the general population (2 in 1000).

All other antibodies of the Kell system are extremely rare.

Table 6–4 CONTROLS FOR USE WHEN TESTING FOR THE PRESENCE OF KELL ANTIGENS

Antigen	Positive Control	Negative Control
K (K1)	Kk	kk
k (K2)	Kk	KK
Kp^a (K3)	Kp(a+b+)	Kp(a−b+)
Kp^b (K4)	Kp(a+b+)	Kp(a+b−)
Js^a (K6)	Js(a+b+)	Js(a−b+)
Js^b (K7)	Js(a+b+)	Js(a+b−)

Clinical Significance

Anti-K has caused many severe hemolytic transfusion reactions, sometimes with hemoglobinuria (see Young, 1954; Ottensooner *et al*, 1954; Mollison, 1975). As mentioned, both anti-K and anti-k can cause hemolytic disease of the newborn (see van Loghem *et al*, 1953; Levine *et al*, 1949).

All other Kell antibodies, when encountered, must be considered to be clinically significant.

TECHNIQUES

Kell antigens are usually detected using the indirect antiglobulin test (see Chapter 21). In testing for Kell antigens, known heterozygous cells should be used as a positive control. The recommended controls are given in Table 6–4.

TYPICAL EXAMINATION QUESTIONS

Select the phrase, sentence or symbol which completes or answers the question. More than one answer may be acceptable in each case. Answers are given in the back of the book.

1. The K (K1) antibody sensitizes
   (a) 20–25 per cent of random bloods
   (b) 7–9 per cent of random bloods
   (c) 91 per cent of random bloods
   (d) 50 per cent of random bloods
   (Introduction)

2. The K4 antigen is also known as
   (a) k (Cellano)
   (b) Rautenberg
   (c) Js^a
   (d) Kp^b
   (e) Kp^a (Penney)
   (Table 6–1)

3. In the numerical nomenclature, K_o is known as:
   (a) K2
   (b) K9
   (c) K18

   (d) K4
   (e) K5
   (Table 6–1)

4. Which of the following are alleles?
   (a) K11 and K15
   (b) K11 and K17
   (c) K3 and K4
   (d) K5 and K9
   (The Genetics of the Kell System)

5. The K1 antigen
   (a) is highly antigenic
   (b) is a dominant mendelian character
   (c) occurs commonly in whites
   (d) occurs in less than 10 per cent of randomly selected whites
   (The Antigens K(K1) and k(K2))

6. The incidence of the Kp^a antigen is
   (a) 95 per cent
   (b) less in K+ individuals than in the general population
   (c) 50 per cent
   (d) 2.4 per cent
   (The Antigens Kp^a (K3) and Kp^b (K4))

7. The antigen k
   (a) occurs as a mendelian-recessive character
   (b) is extremely rare
   (c) is weaker than usual in K+Kp(a+) individuals
   (d) is extremely common
   (The Antigens K (K1) and k (K2))
   (The Antigens Kpᵃ (K3) and Kpᵇ (Ku))

8. Select the most common phenotype in the Kell system
   (a) K+k− Kp(a−b+) Js(a−b+)
   (b) K−k+ Kp(a+b−) Js(a+b−)
   (c) K−k+ Kp(a−b+) Js(a−b+)
   (d) K−k+ Kp(a−b+) Js(a+b+)
   (General)

9. Which of the following is not a Kell system antigen:
   (a) Côté
   (b) Gerbich
   (c) Claas
   (d) K_x
   (General)

10. Which of the following antibodies is commonly found in persons of the K_o phenotype
    (a) anti-Ku
    (b) anti-KL
    (c) anti-K_x
    (d) anti-K7
    (The K_o phenotype)

11. The antibody Claas (K9) is
    (a) compatible with K_o cells
    (b) compatible with McLeod cells
    (c) incompatible with K_o cells
    (d) incompatible with McLeod cells
    (The McLeod Phenotype: Chronic Granulomatous Disease)

12. Kell antibodies are
    (a) usually non-red cell immune
    (b) usually immune in nature
    (c) clinically insignificant
    (d) with the exception of anti-K1, extremely rare
    (The Antibodies of the Kell System)

13. Fill in the blanks:

(a) _____	(_____)	K2		(original name and alternative)
(b) Kpᵃ	(_____) _____			(alternative name and numerical equivalent)
(c) _____	(Matthews) _____			(original name and numerical equivalent)
(d) K_o	(_____) _____			(alternative name and numerical equivalent)
(e) _____	(Sutter)	K6		(original name)

(Table 6–1)

Answer true or false

14. Not all of the possible gene complexes in the Kell system have been found.
    (The Genetics of the Kell System)

15. The genes *K11* and *K17* are alleles.
    (The Genetics of the Kell System)

16. The antigen Kpᵃ is common in blacks.
    (The Antigens Kpᵃ (K3) and Kpᵇ(Ku))

17. The antigen Jsᵃ is common in whites.
    (The Antigens JSᵃ (K6) and Jsᵇ (K7))

18. The antigen Kʷ (K8) has not been proved to belong to the Kell system.
    (The Antigen Kw (K8))

19. Persons of the McLeod phenotype have weak reactions with anti-k, anti-Kpᵇ and anti-Jsᵇ.
    (The McLeod Phenotype)

20. The K (K1) antigen is well developed at birth.
    (The Development of Kell Antigens)

21. Some examples of anti-K bind complement.
    (The Antibodies of the Kell System)

GENERAL REFERENCES

1. Issitt, P. D. and Issitt, C. H.: Applied Blood Group Serology. Spectra Biologicals, 1975. *(Excellent general review of the Kell system; especially useful in terms of genetic theories.)*

2. Race, R. R., and Sanger, R.: Blood Groups in Man. Blackwell Scientific Publications, Oxford, 1975. *(Useful coverage of antigens up to K18).*

3. Marsh, W. L.: The Kell Blood Group. A two-part review of Recent Developments. Spectra Biologicals (undated). *(A useful general review of the Kell system.)*

THE DUFFY BLOOD GROUP SYSTEM

OBJECTIVES — THE DUFFY BLOOD GROUP SYSTEM

The student shall know, understand and be prepared to explain:

1. A brief history of the discovery of the Duffy groups
2. The nomenclature commonly used in the Duffy system (including the numerical nomenclature)
3. The inheritance of the Duffy genes in whites and blacks
4. The assignment of the Duffy locus to chromosome No. 1
5. The characteristics of antigens of the Duffy system
6. The effects of enzymes on Duffy antigen receptors
7. The number of Fy^a sites on red cells
8. The development of the Duffy antigens
9. The serological characteristics of the Duffy antibodies
10. The influence of ionic strength on the activity of anti-Fy^a and anti-Fy^b sera
11. The clinical significance of Duffy antigens
12. The techniques used in the detection of Duffy antigens

Introduction

Cutbush, Mollison and Parkin (1950) and Cutbush and Mollison (1950) described an antibody in the serum of a hemophiliac patient (Mr. Duffy) who had been transfused several times during the preceding 20 years. The patient's name was used as the systemic name; the antibody was termed anti-Fy^a and the corresponding antigen, which was found on the red cells of 66 per cent of randomly selected blood samples of whites, was termed Fy^a. A second example of the antibody (at first named anti-Pluym) was described by van Loghem and van der Hart (1950), and several further examples were soon reported (Ikin *et al*, 1950; James and Plaut, 1951; Rosenfield *et al*, 1950). The gene, Fy^a, was found to be inherited as a dominant character.

The antithetical antibody, anti-Fy^b, was discovered by Ikin *et al* (1951). The corresponding antigen, Fy^b, was found to occur in about 80 per cent of randomly selected blood samples of whites and the gene Fy^b was found to be co-dominant with the gene Fy^a. In whites, therefore, possible genotypes were Fy(a+b−), Fy(a+b+) and Fy(a−b+) and possible genotypes, Fy^aFy^a, Fy^aFy^b and Fy^bFy^b, respectively.

In 1955, Sanger *et al* discovered that the majority of blacks were of the phenotype Fy(a−b−), a phenotype not found in whites. The gene symbol Fy was used to describe the gene or genes responsible for the condition. The gene Fy was thought to exist in the heterozygous state in whites (Race and Sanger, 1962); however, Chown *et al* (1965, 1972) established that the majority of these white heterozygotes were in fact heterozygous for a gene called Fy^x, which makes a small amount of Fy^b antigen.

In 1971, Albrey *et al* reported an antibody that failed to react with Fy(a−b−) cells from blacks yet reacted with Fy(a−b±); that is, Fy^xFy^x cells. The antibody was called anti-Fy3 and the corresponding antigen Fy3.

Two other antigens defined by specific antibodies, Fy4 and Fy5, have also been reported (Behzad *et al*, 1973; Colledge *et al*, 1973).

In 1963, the *Duffy* locus was assigned to chromosome No. 1 (see below).

Nomenclature

Following the example of other blood group systems, a numerical notation is used to describe the antigens and antibodies of the

125

Table 7–1 THE ANTIGENS, ANTIBODIES AND GENES OF THE DUFFY BLOOD GROUP SYSTEM

Antigen			
Original Term	Numerical Notation	Antibody	Gene
Fy^a	Fy1	Anti-Fy^a (−Fy1)	Fy^a (Fy^1)
Fy^b	Fy2	Anti-Fy^b (−Fy2)	Fy^b (Fy^2)
−	Fy3	Anti-Fy3	Fy^3
−	Fy4	Anti-Fy4	Fy^4
−	Fy5	Anti-Fy5	Fy^5

Duffy blood group system. Under this notation, the Fy^a and Fy^b antigens become Fy1 and Fy2, respectively. The antigens, antibodies and genes of the system are given in Table 7–1. A phenotype in which the Fy^a, Fy3 and Fy5 antigens, for example, were detectable and the Fy^b and Fy4 were not would be written as Fy:1, −2, 3, −4, 5.

INHERITANCE IN WHITES

The Genes Fy^a and Fy^b. Fy^a and Fy^b are co-dominant genes with an allelic relationship. In tests with both anti-Fy^a and anti-Fy^b phenotype frequencies have been calculated in North American whites (see Mourant, 1976) and these are given in Table 7–2. Six different matings are possible in the Duffy system if only genes Fy^a and Fy^b are considered, though the inclusion of the genes Fy and Fy^x (discussed later) increases this number to 55.

The Fy^x Gene. The variant Duffy allele Fy^x was described by Lewis *et al* (1965, 1972) and was found to occur not infrequently in whites. The gene determines the production of a red cell antigen that reacts weakly with anti-Fy^b sera but not at all with anti-Fy^a. The difference between Fy^b and Fy^x appears to be *quantitative* rather than *qualitative*, and because of this, cells that are of phenotype Fy^{a}Fy^x or Fy^{b}Fy^x cannot be recognized as such. The Fy^x and the Fy genes are independent (i.e., Fy^x is not the equivalent in whites of Fy.)

Family studies have not revealed if the Fy^x phenotype results from the activity of independent modifying genes affecting the expression of a normal Fy^b gene; the gene does not appear to be a graded or heterogenous character.

Red cells that result from the genotype Fy^{x}Fy^x react more strongly with anti-Fy^b than cells resulting from the genotype Fy^{a}Fy^x (Lewis et al, 1965). In persons of genotype Fy^{x}Fy^x, red cells also have weak Fy3 and Fy5 antigens (Marsh, 1973).

The gene Fy occurs as an extreme rarity in whites.

INHERITANCE IN BLACKS

Sanger *et al* (1955) applied the second example of anti-Fy^b serum to a series of blood samples of American blacks in conjunction with anti-Fy^a and found that almost 70 per cent were Fy(a−b−). This was subsequently confirmed in further tests (Race and Sanger, 1968). These results were interpreted as being caused by a third allele, Fy, for which blacks were assumed to be homozygous. It has also been considered that the inheritance of an independent modifying gene may be inhibiting the expression of the Fy^a and Fy^b genes (Sanger et al, 1955).

All family studies performed so far have supported the "silent allele" theory in that the matings Fy(a−b−) with Fy(a−b−) always produced Fy(a−b−) children. No evidence has been found to support the "independent modifying gene" theory. However, if such genes do exist, they must be very closely linked to the *Duffy* locus, and this, for all practical purposes, would be the same thing as a silent Fy allele. A pedigree giving the typical inheritance patterns in black families is given in Figure 7–1.

Assignment to Chromosome No. 1

Renwick and Lawler (1963), in studying a large family in which a type of congenital nuclear cataract was present, found that the determining gene, *Cae*, was closely linked to the *Duffy* locus. Five years later, an inherited visible abnormality of chromosome No. 1 (called

Table 7–2 PHENOTYPE FREQUENCIES IN NORTH AMERICAN WHITES AND BLACKS

Phenotype	Percentage Frequencies	
	Whites	Blacks
Fy (a−b−)	38.29	19.87
Fy (a+b−)	15.45	9.82
Fy (a+b+)	46.26	2.68
Fy (a−b−)	−	67.63

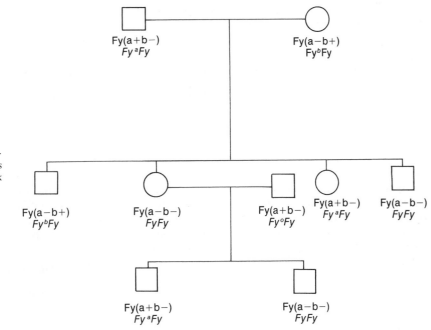

Figure 7–1 A pedigree showing the typical inheritance patterns of Duffy blood groups in a black family.

Uncoiler 1 [Un–1]) was also found to be closely linked to the *Duffy* locus, thus placing all three genes *(Un–1, Cae* and *Duffy)* on that chromosome (Donahue *et al,* 1968). Supportive data was obtained in a family in which a structural rearrangement of chromosome No. 1 was found to correlate with distribution of the Duffy groups (Lee et al, 1974).

Duffy has the distinction of being the first locus in man to be assigned to a particular autosome.

THE ANTIGENS OF THE DUFFY SYSTEM

Characteristics. Duffy antigens do not exist naturally in a soluble form. The Fy^a antigen was not detected in the aqueous phase of a chloroform-methanol extraction of red cell stroma (Hamaguchi and Cleve, 1972).

The Fy^a, Fy^b and Fy3 antigenic determinants are thermolabile, being inactivated by heating red cells to 56° C for 10 minutes. The antigens are also denatured by treatment with formaldehyde (Marsh *et al,* 1974). Both of these observations indicate that the Duffy receptors are protein in nature.

Antigens Fy^a (Fy1) and Fy^b (Fy2). The Fy^a and Fy^b antigens constitute the main antithetical pair in the system. Because they do not occur in a natural, soluble form, little is known of their chemical nature. Both antigens have low antigenicity, and so, while the risk of immunization is 34 per cent (with respect to

Fy^a), in practice alloimmunization to Fy^a is an uncommon event. Immunogenicity of Fy^a appears to be about 40 times less than K1 (Kell) (Marsh, 1975).

Enzymes markedly reduce or eliminate activity of the red cell Fy^a and Fy^b receptors (discussed later).

The Fy^a and Fy^b receptors on the erythrocyte membrane are thought to be associated with susceptibility to malaria. Studies by Miller *et al* (1975, 1976) showed that Fy(a–b–) red cells are resistant to invasion *in vitro* with *Plasmodium knowlesi.* Of 17 volunteers exposed to the bites of *Plasmodium vivax*–infected mosquitoes, only those with the red cell phenotype Fy(a–b–) were resistant to erythrocyte infection. It was concluded therefore that the Fy^a or Fy^b receptors or both on the red cell membrane are required for invasion by *vivax* merozoites.

The Antigen Fy3. The antibody which defines the Fy3 antigen was detected in the serum of a white woman of phenotype Fy(a–b–) who had been previously transfused and was pregnant for the third time (Albrey *et al,* 1971). The antibody, anti-Fy3, was found to react with all Fy(a+) or Fy(b+) red cells and also with red cells of phenotype Fy(a–b±) (i.e., *Fy^{x}Fy^x*), and therefore appeared to contain anti-Fy^a plus anti-Fy^b. Absorption experiments, however, failed to separate these antibody components, and so it was concluded that anti-Fy3 was detecting another antigen that was a product of an allele at the *Duffy* locus. In addition to this, enzyme treatment was found not to affect the Fy3 receptor.

Although thousands of blacks of Fy(a−b−) phenotype must have received transfusions of blood from Fy(a+) or Fy(b+) donors, only one example of anti-Fy3 has been reported in a black individual (Oberdorfer et al, 1974), suggesting that the genetic backgrounds of "white" Fy(a−b−) and "black" Fy(a−b−) are subtly different. There is as yet, however, no scientific evidence to support this.

The Antigen Fy4. The antibody that defines the Fy4 antigen, anti-Fy4, was discovered by Behzad et al (1973). It was found to react with all Fy(a−b−) samples and with the majority of black Fy(a+b−) and Fy(a−b+) samples. To date no other example of this antibody has been found. Like Fy3, the Fy4 receptor was found to be unaffected by treatment with enzymes.

The Antigen Fy5. The antibody anti-Fy5 was found in a black male child of phenotype Fy(a−b−) (Colledge et al, 1973) and was originally thought to be another example of anti-Fy3. It was distinguished by the fact that it gave positive reactions with the red cells of the original patient with anti-Fy3 and that it reacted negatively with Rh$_{null}$ red cells of normal Duffy phenotypes and weakly with −D−/−D− red cells, suggesting some interaction between Rh and Duffy. No further example of anti-Fy5 has been reported, and so the nature of that interaction, if any, remains unknown.

The Effects of Enzymes on Duffy Antigen Receptors. Both anti-Fy^a and anti-Fy^b are inactive against enzyme-treated red cells (Morton and Pickles, 1951; Morton, 1957). Of the four proteolytic enzymes commonly used, ficin has the most pronounced effect (Haber and Rosenfield, 1957), bromelin and papain slightly less and trypsin the least (Unger and Katz, 1951). Enzyme treatment denatures the Fy^a and Fy^b antigens to a point where they lose their ability to absorb the corresponding antibodies (Marsh, 1973).

The denaturing effect on Fy^a and Fy^b receptors appears to be an effect of protease activity against membrane proteins, and not the effect of sialic acid removal (as is the case with M and N receptors — see Chapter 10) from the red cell membrane. This is known because neuraminidase (an enzyme that specifically removes sialic acid) destroys M and N antigenicity (Springer and Ansell, 1958), yet has no effect on the Fy^a and Fy^b receptors. The denaturing effect on the Fy^a and Fy^b receptors is often useful in the laboratory when dealing with mixtures of antibodies.

Enzymes have no effect on the Fy3, Fy4 and Fy5 receptors.

Number of Antigen Sites. Masouredis (1976) performed studies using ferritin-conjugated anti-IgG and electron microscopy, and estimated the number of Fy^a sites on Fy^a Fy^a red cells to be 12,000.

Development of Duffy Antigens. The Fy^a and Fy^b antigens appear to be well developed on the red cells of infants at birth (Cleghorn, 1968; Toivanen and Hirvonen, 1969; Toivanen and Hirvonen, 1973). The Fy3 antigen does not appear to be fully developed at birth (Oberdorfer et al, 1974), but Fy5 does (Colledge et al, 1973). No studies on the development of Fy4 have been reported.

THE ANTIBODIES OF THE DUFFY SYSTEM

Serological Characteristics

Anti-Fy^a. Only one example of non-red cell-immune anti-Fy^a has been reported (Rosenfield et al, 1950). Most examples of the antibody are IgG, detectable only by the indirect antiglobulin test. About 50 per cent of anti-Fy^a antibodies bind complement.

Occasional examples of anti-Fy^a agglutinate Fy(a+) red cells suspended in saline (Race et al, 1953). In these cases, dosage is almost always observed (i. e., the antibody reacts with Fy(a+b−) red cells more strongly than with Fy(a+b+) red cells).

Anti-Fy^b. Anti-Fy^b occurs much more rarely than anti-Fy^a. The antibody is most often IgG, and usually reacts best by the indirect antiglobulin test, though a few examples agglutinate red cells suspended in saline. Some examples of anti-Fy^b show dosage. Non-red cell-immune anti-Fy^b has not been reported.

Anti-Fy3, Anti-Fy4, Anti-Fy5. The characteristics of these antibodies are described under the headings The Antigen Fy3; The Antigen Fy4 and The Antigen Fy5).

Influence of Ionic Strength

The activity of some anti-Fy^a and anti-Fy^b sera is enhanced by reducing the ionic strength and pH of the suspending media (see Elliot et al, 1964; Hughes-Jones et al, 1964).

Clinical Significance

Incompatibility involving anti-Fy^a may cause severe hemolytic transfusion reactions, and has been implicated in hemolytic disease of the newborn (see Greenwalt et al, 1959).

Table 7–3 CONTROLS FOR USE WHEN TESTING FOR THE PRESENCE OF DUFFY ANTIGENS

Antigen	Positive Control	Negative Control
Fy^a	Fy (a+b+)	Fy (a−b+)
Fy^b	Fy (a+b+)	Fy (a+b−)

Anti-Fy^b has been implicated as the cause of a fatal transfusion reaction (Badehere *et al*, 1970), yet has not been found to be the cause of hemolytic disease of the newborn. Most examples of anti-Fy^b do not persist for long periods of time in the sera of immunized subjects and may disappear within a few months of its detection (Levine *et al*, 1955; Blumenthal and Pettenkover, 1952).

TECHNIQUES

The majority of anti-Duffy sera react best by the indirect antiglobulin test (see Chapter 21). In testing for the presence of the Fy^a and Fy^b antigens, cells known to be heterozygous should be used as a positive control (Table 7–3).

TYPICAL EXAMINATION QUESTIONS

Choose the phrase, sentence or symbol that completes or answers the question. More than one answer may be correct in each case. Answers are given in the back of the book.

1. A phenotype in which Fy^a, Fy3 and Fy4 are present and Fy^b and Fy5 are absent would be given in the numerical nomenclature as
   (a) Fy:−1, 2, −3, 4, 5
   (b) Fy: 1, 3, 4
   (c) Fy: 1, −2, 3, −4, 5
   (d) Fy: 1, −2, 3, 4, −5
   (Nomenclature)

2. The most common Duffy phenotype in whites is
   (a) Fy(a−b+)
   (b) Fy(a+b+)
   (c) Fy(a+b−)
   (d) Fy(a−b±)
   (e) Fy(a−b−)
   (Inheritance in Whites: Table 7–2)

3. The *Fy^x* gene
   (a) occurs not infrequently in whites
   (b) is independent of the *Fy* gene
   (c) is the equivalent in whites of the *Fy* gene
   (d) produces a red cell antigen that reacts weakly with anti-Fy^b
   (The Fy^x Gene)

4. The percentage of bloods of blacks that are Fy(a−b−) is approximately
   (a) 10 per cent
   (b) 95 per cent
   (c) 70 per cent
   (d) 100 per cent
   (Inheritance in Blacks)

5. The *Duffy* locus has been assigned to
   (a) Chromosome No. 1
   (b) Chromosome No. 2
   (c) Chromosome No. 6
   (d) Autosome No. 1
   (Introduction)

6. The *Duffy* locus is closely linked to the loci for
   (a) *Un–1*
   (b) *Cae*
   (c) *Rh*
   (d) *Kell*
   (Assignment to Chromosome No. 1)

7. The Fy^a, Fy^b and Fy3 antigens are
   (a) thermostable
   (b) thermolabile
   (c) inactivated by heating red cells to 56° C for 30 seconds
   (d) denatured by treatment with formaldehyde
   (e) probably protein in nature
   (The Antigens of the Duffy Blood Group System: Characteristics)

8. There appears to be an association between the Fy^a and Fy^b antigenic receptors and susceptibility to
   (a) malaria
   (b) syphilis
   (c) hepatitis
   (d) none of the above
   (The Antigens Fy^a (Fy1) and Fy^b(Fy2))

9. Anti-Fy3
   (a) reacts with all Fy(a+) and Fy(b+) red cells
   (b) reacts with cells of phenotype Fy(a−b±)
   (c) is a mixture of anti-Fy^a and anti-Fy^b, separable by absorption
   (d) is commonly found in blacks
   (The Antigen Fy3)

10. The antigen Fy4
    (a) reacts with all Fy(a−b−) samples
    (b) reacts with the majority of black Fy(a+b−) and Fy(a−b+) samples
    (c) is unaffected by enzymes
    (d) is denatured by enzymes
    (The Antigen Fy4)

11. Anti-Fy5 fails to react with
    (a) cells of phenotype Fy(a−b±)
    (b) Rh$_{null}$ red cells
    (c) −D−/−D− red cells (reacts weakly)
    (d) none of the above
    (The Antigen Fy5)

12. Enzymes denature which of the following antigens?

(a) Fy^a, Fy^b, Fy4
(b) Fy^a, Fy^b
(c) Fy3, Fy5
(d) Fy^a, Fy^b, Fy3, Fy4 and Fy5
*(The Effects of Enzymes
on Duffy Antigen Receptors)*

13. Which of the following antigens does not appear to be fully developed at birth?
(a) Fy^a
(b) Fy^b
(c) Fy3
(d) Fy5
(Development of Duffy Antigens)

14. Anti-Fy^a
(a) always binds complement
(b) is usually IgG
(c) is commonly non-red cell immune
(d) is usually detected in the indirect antiglobulin test
(e) is enhanced by reducing the ionic strength and pH of the suspending media
*(Serological Characteristics:
Influence of Ionic Strength)*

Answer true or false

15. The gene symbol *Fy* is used to describe the genes responsible for the Fy(a−b−) phenotype.
(Introduction) (Inheritance in Blacks)

16. The *Fy*^{a} gene is dominant; the *Fy*^{b} gene is recessive.
(Inheritance in Whites)

17. The difference between Fy^x and Fy^b appears to be qualitative.
(The Fy^x gene)

18. The most common Duffy phenotype in blacks is Fy(a−b−).
(Inheritance in Blacks)

19. Duffy antigens do not exist naturally in a soluble form.
*(The Antigens of the Duffy
System: Characteristics)*

20. The denaturing effect of enzymes on Fy^a and Fy^b receptors is due to sialic acid removal from the red cell membrane.
*(The Effects of Enzymes
on Duffy Antigen Receptors)*

GENERAL REFERENCES

1. Issitt, P. D. and Issitt, C. H.: Applied Blood Group Serology. Spectra Biologicals, 1975. *(Excellent general coverage of the Duffy system. Particularly interesting with respect to proposed genetic pathways.)*
2. Marsh, W. L.: Present status of the Duffy blood group system. Critical reviews in Clin. Lab. Sci. March, 1975. *(Probably the best review article to appear on the Duffy system.)*
3. Race, R. R. and Sanger, R.: Blood Groups in Man. Blackwell Scientific Publications, Oxford, 1975. *(Excellent, useful coverage of the Duffy system.)*

8

THE KIDD (Jk) BLOOD GROUP SYSTEM

OBJECTIVES — THE KIDD BLOOD GROUP SYSTEM

The student shall know, understand and be prepared to explain:
1. A brief history of the discovery of the Kidd antigens and antibodies
2. The inheritance of Kidd genes
3. The serologic characteristics of the antibodies of the Kidd system

4. The clinical significance of Kidd antibodies
5. The development of Kidd antigens
6. The anthropologic uses of the Kidd system
7. The techniques used in the detection of Kidd antigens

Introduction

The Kidd blood group system was discovered by Allen *et al* (1951) through a "new" antibody in the serum of a mother, Mrs. Kidd, whose child suffered from hemolytic disease of the newborn as a result of the antibody. The corresponding antigen, Jk^a, was found to be present in about 77 per cent of white donors, inherited as a mendelian-dominant character.

Plaut *et al* (1953) were the first to discover the antithetical antibody, anti-Jk^b. Further reports of examples of both anti-Jk^a and anti-Jk^b quickly followed.

In 1959, Pinkerton *et al* discovered the phenotype Jk(a−b−), presumed to be due to a third, silent allele, *Jk*. Again, further examples were soon found, mainly among people of the Pacific area. Some Jk(a−b−) individuals were found to possess an antibody giving the reactions of anti-Jk^a plus anti-Jk^b (anti-Jk^{a}Jk^b). This antibody is known as anti-Jk3.

Individuals who are heterozygous for the *Jk* allele were first reported by Crawford *et al* (1961) among Europeans. The genetic background of this phenomenon, or whether it is the same as the "eastern" *Jk*, is not known.

Inheritance

Jk^a and Jk^b inheritance is straightforward. The genes *Jk*^{a} and *Jk*^{b} are inherited as mendelian co-dominants, and the phenotype Jk(a−b−) is presumed to be due to a silent allele, *Jk*. The most common phenotype among whites is Jk(a+b+); among blacks Jk(a+b−) is more common (Table 8–1). Homozygous (*JkJk*) individuals are extremely rare and are practically confined to Filipino-Spanish, Hawaiian-Chinese, Chinese, Polynesians, Thais and Mato Grosso Indians — though heterozygotes are known to exist in whites. This can cause problems in paternity testing, as illustrated in Fig-

Table 8–1 PHENOTYPE FREQUENCIES IN THE KIDD SYSTEM*

Phenotype	*Percentage Frequencies*	
	Whites	*Blacks*
Jk (a−b+)	20.42	6.27
Jk (a+b−)	27.63	54.79
Jk (a+b+)	51.95	38.94
Jk (a−b−)	—	—

*Based on information from Mourant.

131

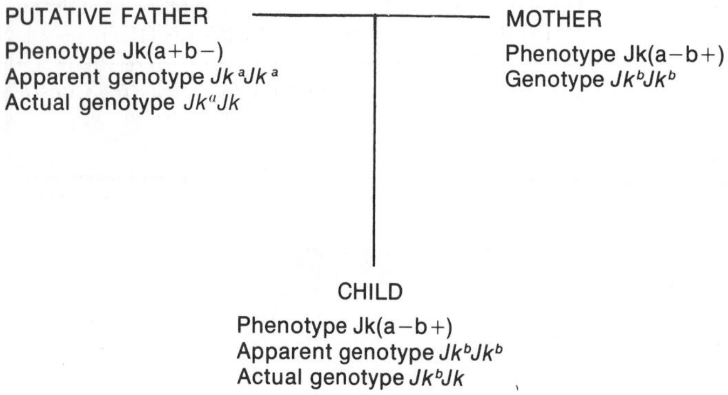

PUTATIVE FATHER ————————┐   ┌——→ MOTHER
Phenotype Jk(a+b−)   Phenotype Jk(a−b+)
Apparent genotype *Jk*ᵃ*Jk*ᵃ   Genotype *Jk*ᵇ*Jk*ᵇ
Actual genotype *Jk*ᵃ*Jk*

CHILD
Phenotype Jk(a−b+)
Apparent genotype *Jk*ᵇ*Jk*ᵇ
Actual genotype *Jk*ᵇ*Jk*

Figure 8–1 Apparent exclusion of paternity explained by the existence of the gene *Jk* in the heterozygous state.

ure 8–1. The gene *Jk* is estimated to have a frequency of 0.66 per cent among whites and 0.82 per cent among blacks. Other antigen frequencies among North American whites and blacks are given in Table 8–2.

THE ANTIBODIES OF THE KIDD SYSTEM

Anti-Jkᵃ and Anti-Jkᵇ

Both anti-Jkᵃ and anti-Jkᵇ are usually IgG (but may be IgM); they are best detected by the indirect antiglobulin technique. The antibodies commonly (probably always) bind complement — to a point at which reactions with anticomplement may be the only ones observed in indirect antiglobulin testing (see Stratton *et al*, 1965). Both antibodies occur rarely and then most often in serum that also contains other immune blood group antibodies. Upon storage, both antibodies deteriorate rapidly. Characteristically, patients producing these antibodies frequently cease production soon after exposure to the antigen has ceased, leading to rapid deterioration *in vivo*. For this reason, Kidd antibodies have frequently been the cause of delayed hemolytic transfusion reactions (see under the heading Clinical Significance).

In the detection of very weak Kidd antibodies, enzyme treatment with ficin or trypsin may be helpful. Anti-Jkᵃ commonly shows dosage so

that positive results may only be obtained with Jk(a+b−) (*Jk*ᵃ*Jk*ᵃ) red cells (von der Hart and von Loghem, 1953). In using ficin-treated red cells, anti-Jkᵃ may lyse Jk(a+b−) (*Jk*ᵃ*Jk*ᵃ) red cells completely while only lysing 25 per cent of Jk(a+b+) (*Jk*ᵃ*Jk*ᵇ) red cells (Haber and Rosenfield, 1957).

Anti-Jkᵃ sera occasionally agglutinate red cells suspended in saline (Mollison, 1975).

Anti-JkᵃJkᵇ (Anti-Jk3)

The antibody anti-JkᵃJkᵇ(Jk3), first described by Pinkerton *et al* (1959), was found to behave as "inseparable" anti-Jkᵃ plus anti-Jkᵇ. Evidence that the antibody is not crossreacting anti-Jkᵃ-anti-Jkᵇ was provided by Marsh *et al* (1974), who found that the neutrophil leukocytes of Jk(a+) and Jk(b+) individuals do not absorb anti-Jkᵃ or anti-Jkᵇ, though both types of neutrophil absorb anti-Jk3. Further supportive evidence was provided by Humphrey and Morel (1976).

An example of non-red cell–immune anti-Jk3 was described by Arcara *et al* (1969).

Clinical Significance

Antibodies in the Kidd system have been implicated in both hemolytic transfusion reactions and in hemolytic disease of the newborn. Because Kidd antibodies rapidly deteriorate *in vivo*, they are a common cause of delayed hemolytic transfusion reaction (e. g., see Degnan and Rosenfield, 1965). These antibodies may be undetectable at the time of crossmatching yet may attain considerable levels soon after transfusion of red cells possessing the offending antigen.

A case of hemolytic disease of the newborn

Table 8–2 THE FREQUENCIES OF GENES IN THE KIDD BLOOD GROUP SYSTEM

| *Gene* | *Percentage Frequencies* | |
	Whites	*Blacks*
*Jk*ᵃ	53.60	73.88
*Jk*ᵇ	46.40	26.12
Jk	0.66	0.82

due to anti-Jk3 has recently been reported (Pierce *et al*, 1980).

OTHER NOTES ON THE KIDD GROUPS

Development of Kidd Antigens

The Jk^a and Jk^b antigens are well developed at birth. They have been detected in fetuses between 7 and 20 weeks' gestation (Toivanen and Hirvonen, 1973).

ANTHROPOLOGIC USES

The Kidd groups make useful anthropologic markers because of their striking differences in distribution among various races (see Mourant, 1974). For example, the phenotype Jk(a+) occurs in 93 per cent of American blacks (Rosenfield *et al*, 1953), about 77 per cent of Europeans and about 50 per cent of Chinese. There is also a remarkable association of the phenotype Jk(a−b−) with Polynesians.

Table 8–3 CONTROLS FOR USE WHEN TESTING FOR THE PRESENCE OF KIDD ANTIGENS

Antigen	Positive Control	Negative Control
Jk^a	Jk (a+b+)	Jk (a−b+)
Jk^b	Jk (a+b+)	Jk (a+b−)

TECHNIQUES AND CONTROLS

As mentioned, antigens and antibodies of the Kidd blood group system are best detected by the indirect antiglobulin test. Very weak Kidd antibodies are generally enhanced when the test cells are enzyme treated with ficin or papain. In some instances, the addition of complement can also prove helpful (Stratton, 1956; Crawford *et al*, 1961). Race and Sanger (1975) state that they prefer an antiglobulin test on papainized cells. In all tests with Kidd antibodies, dosage effect should be borne in mind.

In testing for Kidd antigens, known heterozygotes should always be used as a positive control (Table 8–3).

TYPICAL EXAMINATION QUESTIONS

Choose the phrase, sentence or symbol that completes or answers the question. More than one answer may be acceptable in each case. Answers are given in the back of the book.

1. The percentage frequency of the Jk^a antigen in whites is approximately
   (a) 10
   (b) 97
   (c) 77
   (d) less than 1
   (e) 50
   (Introduction)
2. The gene Jk^a is
   (a) inherited as a mendelian dominant
   (b) due to a silent allele at the *Kidd* locus
   (c) an allele of Jk^b
   (d) more common in blacks than in whites
   (Inheritance: Table 8–2)
3. Homozygous *JkJk*
   (a) is extremely rare among whites
   (b) has not been found
   (c) is found in Polynesians
   (d) is extremely common
   (Inheritance)
4. The frequency of the gene *Jk* is
   (a) 0.66 per cent in whites
   (b) 0.2 per cent in whites

   (c) 0.82 per cent in blacks
   (d) the same in all races
   (Inheritance)
5. Anti-Jk^b
   (a) is usually IgG
   (b) may be IgM
   (c) commonly binds complement
   (d) occurs frequently in whites
   (Anti-Jk^a and Anti-Jk^b)
6. Anti-Jk^a and anti-Jk^b
   (a) deteriorate very slowly *in vitro*
   (b) deteriorate rapidly *in vivo*
   (c) are frequently associated with delayed hemolytic transfusion reactions
   (d) may be enhanced by enzyme treatment
   (Anti-Jk^a and Anti-Jk^b)
7. Anti-Jk^a
   (a) has never been implicated in hemolytic disease of the newborn
   (b) has never been implicated in hemolytic transfusion reactions
   (c) may occasionally agglutinate red cells suspended in saline
   (d) is best detected by the indirect antiglobulin test
   (e) commonly shows dosage effect
   (Anti-Jk^a and Anti-Jk^b: Clinical Significance)

8. Anti-Jk3
   (a) is anti-Jk^a plus anti-Jk^b in a separable form
   (b) is anti-Jk^{a}Jk^b in an inseparable form
   (c) is usually non-red cell immune
   (d) has not been found
   (Anti-Jk^{a}Jk^b (Anti-Jk3))

9. When testing for the presence of the Jk^a antigen, which of the following should be chosen as a positive control?
   (a) Jk(a+b+) red cells
   (b) Jk(a+b−) red cells
   (c) Jk(a−b−) red cells
   (d) None of the above
   (Techniques and Controls)

10. The percentage frequency of the Jk^a antigen in blacks is reported to be
    (a) 10
    (b) 93
    (c) 1
    (d) 100
    (Anthropologic Uses)

Answer true or false

11. The phenotype Jk(a−b−) is presumed to be due to the presence of a rare, silent allele, *Jk*.
    (Introduction: Inheritance)

12. The most common Kidd phenotype among blacks is Jk(a+b+).
    (Inheritance)

13. Heterozygotes for the gene *Jk* are known to exist in whites.
    (Inheritance)

14. The estimated frequency of the *Jk* allele is less than 1 per cent among whites and blacks.
    (Inheritance)

15. Occasionally, anti-complement may be the only reactant in indirect antiglobulin testing for anti-Jk^a and anti-Jk^b.
    (Anti-Jk^a and Anti-Jk^b)

16. Neutrophil leukocytes of Jk(a+) individuals readily absorb anti-Jk^a.
    (Anti-Jk^{a}Jk^b (Anti-Jk3))

17. Hemolytic disease of the newborn due to anti-Jk3 has not yet been reported.
    (Clinical Significance)

18. The Jk^a and Jk^b antigens are well developed at birth.
    (Development of the Kidd Antigen)

19. Jk(a+) occurs less frequently in Chinese than in whites.
    (Anthropologic Uses)

20. Enzyme treatment of red cells fails to enhance weak Kidd antibodies.
    (Techniques and Controls)

GENERAL REFERENCES

1. Issitt, P. D. and Issitt, C. H.: Applied Blood Group Serology. Spectra Biologicals, 1975. *(General coverage of the Kidd system.)*
2. Mollison, P. L.: Blood Transfusion in Clinical Medicine. Blackwell Scientific Publications, Oxford, 1979. *(Emphasis on characteristics of Kidd antibodies.)*
3. Race, R. R. and Sanger, R.: Blood Groups in Man. Blackwell Scientific Publications, Oxford, 1975. *(Excellent general coverage of the Kidd system.)*

9

THE LUTHERAN (Lu) BLOOD GROUP SYSTEM

OBJECTIVES — THE LUTHERAN BLOOD GROUP SYSTEM

The student shall know, understand and be prepared to explain:
1. A brief history of the discovery of the Lutheran antigens and antibodies.
2. The inheritance of *Lutheran* genes (including the linkage between *Lutheran* and *secretor* genes, recessive and dominant Lu(a−b−) inheritance.
3. The antigens of the Lutheran blood group system, characteristic of:
   (a) Lu^a
   (b) Lu^b
   (c) Lu6 and Lu9
   (d) Other Lutheran-related antigens
4. The development of the Lutheran antigens (Lu^a and Lu^b)
5. The characteristics of the antibodies of the Lutheran blood group system:
   (a) Anti-Lu^a
   (b) Anti-Lu^b
   (c) Anti-Lu3
   (d) Other Lutheran antibodies and para-Lutheran antibodies
6. The clinical significance of anti-Lu^a and anti-Lu^b
7. The techniques used in the detection of Lutheran antigens

Introduction

The Lutheran blood group system was first discovered by Callender *et al* (1945) and more fully described by Callender and Race (1946). The antibody appeared after a transfusion of blood from a donor by the name of Lutheran; this blood was subsequently found to contain the provocative antigen. The antithetical antibody was discovered by Cutbush and Chanarin (1956). The original antigen was named Lu^a and the antithetical antigen, Lu^b.

In 1961, Crawford *et al* discovered the phenotype Lu(a−b−) and in 1963, Dornborough *et al* found an antibody that reacted with all red cells except those of phenotype Lu(a−b−) (i.e., anti-Lu^{a}Lu^b).

A second set of alleles, *Lu^9* and *Lu^6*, recognized by Molthan *et al* (1973), were found to be related to the Lutheran locus in the same way as *C* and *c* are related to *E* and *e* at the *Rh* complex locus.

Many other antibodies have been described that fail to react with Lu(a−b−) red cells but react with the red cells of other rare Lutheran phenotypes; the nature of the relationship of most of these antibodies to Lutheran is not yet clear.

Inheritance

Callender and Race (1946), after testing the blood of relatives of Lu(a+) propositi, concluded that the Lu^a antigen was inherited as a dominant character.

In 1961, however, the rare phenotype Lu(a−b−) was discovered by Crawford *et al*, and with it a complication arose to dispute the straightforward appearance of Lutheran inheritance. By "normal" rules (i.e., those that hold for most other blood group systems) it would be expected that the Lu(a−b−) phenotype would be due to homozygosity for a rare allele *Lu*, (i.e., genotype *LuLu*) that is either amorphic or producing some antigen yet undetected. Indeed, in some families, the Lu(a−b−) phenotype behaves as though reflecting recessive inheritance. In other families, however, the very rare Lu(a−b−) type appears to be transmitted as a dominant character. It has been postulated (Race and Sanger, 1968) that another locus, spatially independent of the *Lu* locus, exists where a rare dominant allele converts the Lu precursor substance into a form by which it is unable to effect the production of normal Lu antigens. This postulation was later proved by Tippett (1971) and by Taliano *et al* (1973), who suggested the symbol *In(Lu)* to describe the independent locus and also the rare allele responsible for the inhibition, and *In(lu)* for the very common "normal" allele. Later, *In(Lu)* was found to inhibit (in addition to the Lu antigens) the Au^a antigen, the P$_1$ antigen and the i antigen (Crawford *et al*, 1974), although *In(Lu)* has been shown not to be a part of the *P* locus (Contreras and Tippett, 1934). No information is yet available about its genetic relationship to the *Au(Auberger)* or *Ii* loci.

In 1951, evidence of linkage between the *Lutheran* and the *secretor* loci was presented by Jan Mohr in Copenhagen; in fact, this was the first convincing evidence of autosomal linkage in man. The subsequent relationship postulated between the Auberger and the Lutheran groups (Tippett, 1963), in which seven Lu(a−b−) individuals were found to be Au(a−) whereas six other individuals (i.e., of other phenotypes) were all Au(a+), can be explained in terms of the *In(Lu)* gene, which inhibits Au^a expression.

THE ANTIGENS OF THE LUTHERAN BLOOD GROUP SYSTEM

Lu^a and Lu^b (Lu1, Lu2). The majority of white and black individuals are of phenotype Lu(a−b+) (93.47 and 95.14 per cent respectively). The phenotype Lu(a+b−) occurs in 0.17 per cent of whites and as an extreme rarity in blacks, and the phenotype Lu(a+b+) occurs in 6.37 per cent of whites and 4.86 per cent of blacks, based on U.S. population studies (information from Bryant, 1980). With the use of the antisera anti-Lu^a and anti-Lu^b, four phenotypes can be distinguished, giving rise to six possible genotypes (Table 9–1).

The Lu^a antigen varies in strength in different heterozygous individuals (Mainwaring and Pickles, 1948; Race and Sanger, 1962) and shows dosage difference in strength between homozygotes and heterozygotes (Greenwalt *et al*, 1967). A similar pattern of reaction strength is seen with the antigen Lu^b (Cutbush and Chanarin, 1956; Greenwalt and Sasaki, 1957; Metaxas *et al*, 1959; Kissmeyer-Nielsen, 1960; Greenwalt *et al*, 1967).

The Antigens Lu6 and Lu9. The antigen Lu9 was described by Molthan *et al* (1973), who showed it to be a dominant character linked to the *Lutheran* locus. The relationship of Lu9 to Lutheran is believed to be like that of C to D or E in the Rh system.

Anti-Lu6 was described by Marsh (1972). In later studies, two unrelated individuals of phenotype Lu−6 and two Lu−6 relatives of one of them were all found to be Lu9, providing evidence that *Lu6* belongs to the *Lutheran* complex locus. In addition, the red cells of these four Lu−6 individuals reacted more strongly with anti-Lu9 than did the red cells of heterozygous Lu9 individuals, suggesting that *Lu6* is an allele of *Lu9* (Molthan *et al*, 1973). However, the story may not be as simple as this, for similar reactions were not found in a family studied by Dybkjear *et al* (1974).

Other Antigens Related to the Lutheran System. Recent studies have documented an increase in the number of antigens that appear to be related to the Lutheran blood group system, yet in a way that is not yet understood. In 1971, the first antibody showing such relationship was reported and called anti-Lu4 (Bove *et al*, 1971). This antibody defined a common red cell antigen and agglutinated all red cell types except those of the Lu(a−b−) phenotype. The discovery of anti-Lu4 sparked off a sudden and rapid investigation of the Lutheran-related antibodies, defining both high- and low-frequency antigens. In the case of high-frequency antigens, these were all recognized by antibodies that define antigens which are different from Lu^b, but are absent on red cells of the Lu(a−b−)

Table 9–1 PHENOTYPES AND POSSIBLE GENOTYPES IN THE LUTHERAN BLOOD GROUP SYSTEM

Reactions With Anti-		Phenotypes	Possible Genotypes
Lu^a	*Lu^b*		
+	−	Lu (a+b−)	Lu^a Lu^a or Lu^a Lu
+	+	Lu (a+b+)	Lu^a Lu^b
−	+	Lu (a−b+)	Lu^b Lu^b or Lu^b Lu
−	−	Lu (a−b−)	Lu Lu or (In (Lu))

Table 9–2 ANTIGENS THAT ARE PART OF
(OR ARE BELIEVED TO BE PART OF)
THE LUTHERAN BLOOD GROUP SYSTEM

High Frequency	Low Frequency
Lu^b (Lu2)	Lu^a (Lu1)
Lu3	Lu9
Lu4	Lu10
Lu5	Lu14
Lu6	
Lu7	
Lu8	
Lu11	
Lu12	
Lu13	
Lu15	
Lu16	

phenotype. That different antigenic determinants are involved in each case is supported by the fact that these blood samples are all incompatible with one another.

The number of Lutheran-related antigens has now reached Lu16. Of these, mention should be made of the antigen Lu12 (Much) since there is indirect evidence that this antigen is not controlled by the *Lutheran* locus. The *Lutheran* genes of the Much family were found not to be segregating, but the *secretor* genes were. Since it is therefore clear that the locus responsible for the Much antigen is not close to the *secretor* locus, it must also not be close to the *Lutheran* locus (Sinclair *et al*, 1973).

The latest Lutheran-related antigen, Lu16, was described by Sabo *et al* (1980). Only one of the three propositae had a family that was available for testing, and no information was provided in these tests as to the linkage of the corresponding antigen to other systems or its genetic relationship to Lutheran. Table 9–2 gives a list of antigens that are part of, or believed to be related to, the Lutheran blood group system.

The Development of Lutheran Antigens. Greenwalt *et al* (1967) reported that in the heterozygote the Lu^a antigen is only weakly expressed at birth and that its strength increases until about age 15. The Lu^b antigen of Lu(a−b+) cord cells is weaker than that of adults (Kissmeyer-Nielsen, 1960; Greenwalt *et al*, 1967) and weaker still in Lu(a+b+) infants (Greenwalt *et al*, 1967).

The Swann Antigen. This low-frequency antigen has in several publications been associated with Lutheran, yet the suggestive evidence of linkage between the *Lutheran* and *Swann* genes was shattered by one family reported by Metaxas-Bühler *et al* (cited by Race and Sanger, 1975, page 440).

THE ANTIBODIES OF THE LUTHERAN BLOOD GROUP SYSTEM

Anti-Lu^a (Anti-Lu1). The frequency of anti-Lu^a is low, probably because of the rarity of the provocative antigen rather than its immunizing capacity. The antibody usually occurs as a cold agglutinin that reacts best at 12° C and that shows some dosage effect. The antibody appears to be mainly IgG (Mollison, 1979) and may be "naturally occurring" (Greenwalt and Sasaki, 1957; Gonzenbach *et al*, 1955; Shaw *et al*, 1954) or immune (Callender and Race, 1946; Mainwaring and Pickles, 1948; Holländer, 1955). Some examples of anti-Lu^a have the ability to bind complement but not to cause *in vitro* lysis.

The appearance of the agglutination of Lu(a+) red cells by anti-Lu^a is seen as large agglutinates surrounded by many "free" cells (Callender and Race, 1946).

Anti-Lu^b (Anti-Lu2). Anti-Lu^b is found not uncommonly in Lu(a−b−) individuals following transfusion or pregnancy. Most examples fail to react with red cells suspended in saline but give more reliable results in the antiglobulin test. Three examples of anti-Lu^b studied by Greenwalt *et al* (1967) were mainly IgA and partly IgG. This finding was disputed by Mollison (1979), who tested several examples of anti-Lu^b (and anti-Lu^a) and found that they appeared to be mainly IgG with no definite evidence of an IgA component. Some examples of the antibody show the ability to bind complement but not to cause *in vitro* lysis. Most anti-Lu^b examples are immune, but "naturally occurring" examples have been noted. The antibody causes great crossmatching difficulties because of the frequency of the corresponding antigen and therefore the problem of finding compatible blood.

Anti-Lu^{a}Lu^b (Anti-Lu3). The antibody with this specificity, in which anti-Lu^a and anti-Lu^b are inseparable, was reported by Darnborough *et al* (1963) in the serum of an individual of the rare phenotype Lu(a−b−). The antibody appeared to be immune, and reacted, like all subsequently described examples, more strongly by indirect antiglobulin than by saline tests. The antibody appears to be made by individuals of the recessive type and not by those of the dominant type of Lu(a−b−).

Other Lutheran Antibodies and Para-Lutheran Antibodies. Anti-Lu6 and anti-Lu9 are extremely rare. One example of anti-Lu9 has been reported (Molthan *et al*, 1973), which appeared to be immune and reacted best by the antiglobulin test. Anti-Lu6 has been reported by Marsh (1972), Wrobel *et al* (1972) and Dybkjaer *et al* (1974) — all three examples appeared to be immune.

The majority of Lutheran-related antibodies (e.g., anti-Lu4, anti-Lu5, anti-Lu6, etc.) react with high-frequency antigens; negative reactions are rare. Only anti-Lu9, anti-Lu10 and anti-Lu14 are of the "private" type (i.e., they react with low-frequency antigens).

The Clinical Significance of Anti-Lu^a and Anti-Lu^b

Anti-Lu^a has not been clearly incriminated as the cause of hemolytic transfusion reaction or of hemolytic disease of the newborn. Greendyke and Chorpenning (1962) reported the normal survival of Lu(a+) red cells in a patient with fairly potent anti-Lu^a in her serum.

Anti-Lu^b, however, has caused the destruction of transfused Lu(b+) red cells (Mollison, 1956; Metaxas *et al*, 1959; Tilley *et al*, 1977), has caused hemolytic transfusion reaction (Molthan and Crawford, 1966), has caused delayed transfusion reaction (Greenwalt and Sasaki, 1957; Metaxas [cited by Mollison, 1979]) and has been blamed for hemolytic disease of the newborn (Kissmeyer-Nielsen, 1960; Scheffer and Tamaki, 1966).

TECHNIQUES

Depending on the antisera used, most tests for the presence of the Lu^a antigen are performed at 12 to 15° C using equal quantities of antisera and a 2 to 5 per cent suspension of red cells. The mixture is incubated, centrifuged and read macroscopically or microscopically. Known Lu(a+b+) red cells and known Lu(a−b+) are always run with the test as positive and negative controls respectively.

Lu^b typing is usually performed using the indirect antiglobulin test (see Chapter 21). Again Lu(a+b+) red cells serve as a positive control and Lu(a+b−) red cells serve as a negative control, run with each set of tests.

TYPICAL EXAMINATION QUESTIONS

Choose the phrase, sentence or symbol that completes the statement or answers the question. More than one answer may be correct in each case. Answers are given in the back of this book.

1. The Lu^a antigen is inherited as
   (a) a recessive character
   (b) a dominant character
   (c) an amorphic character
   (d) none of the above
   (Inheritance)
2. The Lu(a−b−) type is transmitted as
   (a) a dominant character
   (b) a recessive character
   (c) an independent antigen which produces some Lu^a
   (d) none of the above
   (Inheritance)
3. The *In(Lu)* refers to an allele responsible for the inhibition of
   (a) the Lu^a antigen
   (b) the Lu^b antigen
   (c) the Au^a antigen
   (d) the Rh antigens
   (Inheritance)
4. The *In(Lu)* is a part of the
   (a) *Lutheran* locus
   (b) *P* locus
   (c) *Secretor* locus
   (d) none of the above
   (Inheritance)
5. There is evidence of genetic linkage between
   (a) the *Lewis* and *Lutheran* loci

(b) the *ABO* and *Lutheran* loci
(c) the *secretor* and *Lutheran* loci
(d) the *Kell* and *Lutheran* loci
(Inheritance)
6. The Lu^a antigen
   (a) is extremely common in whites
   (b) varies in strength in different heterozygous individuals
   (c) shows dosage effect
   (d) none of the above
   (Lu^a and Lu^b (Lu1, Lu2))
7. The antigens Lu6 and Lu9 are believed to be
   (a) alleles
   (b) not related to the Lutheran system
   (c) antithetical
   (d) none of the above
   (Lu6 and Lu9)
8. The high-frequency antigens (Lu4, Lu5, etc), which are related to the Lutheran system in a way not clearly understood,
   (a) are the same as Lu^b
   (b) are absent from red cells of phenotype Lu(a−b−)
   (c) are present on red cells of phenotype Lu(a+b−)
   (d) are probably alleles of *Lutheran* at the Lu^a-Lu^b complex locus
   (Other Antigens Related to the Lutheran System)
9. The Lu^9 antigen
   (a) is fully developed at birth
   (b) is only weakly expressed at birth in the heterozygote (Lu(a+b+))

(c) increases in strength until about age 15 in the heterozygote

(d) is weakly expressed in individuals of phenotype Lu(a−b+)

(The Development of Lutheran Antigens)

10. Anti-Lu^a (Anti-Lu1)
    (a) usually reacts best at 12° C
    (b) usually shows dosage effect
    (c) is always immune
    (d) frequently causes *in vitro* lysis

    (Anti-Lu^a (Anti-Lu1))

11. Anti-Lu^b (Anti-Lu2)
    (a) usually reacts best in the antiglobulin test at 37° C
    (b) is not uncommonly found as an immune antibody in Lu(a−b−) individuals
    (c) always binds complement
    (d) does not cause *in vitro* lysis

    (Anti-Lu^b (Anti-Lu2))

12. Anti-Lu^b
    (a) has not been implicated as the cause of hemolytic disease of the newborn
    (b) has not caused hemolytic transfusion reaction
    (c) has caused the destruction of transfused Lu(a+b−) red cells
    (d) has been implicated as the cause of delayed hemolytic transfusion reaction

    (The Clinical Significance of Anti-Lu^a and Anti-Lu^b)

Answer true or false

13. The Lu^a antigen is inherited as a dominant character.

    (Inheritance)

14. The *In(Lu)* allele inhibits Au^a antigen expression.

    (Inheritance)

15. The most common Lutheran phenotype is Lu(a+b+).

    (Lu^a and Lu^b (Lu1, Lu2))

16. The Lu^a antigen varies in strength in various heterozygous individuals.

    (Lu^a and Lu^b (Lu1, Lu2))

17. The antigen Lu12 (Much) is believed not to be controlled by the *Lutheran* locus.

    (Other Antigens Related to the Lutheran System)

18. The *Swann* gene is linked to the *Lutheran* genes.

    (The Swann Antigen)

19. The antibody anti-Lu^{a}Lu^b (anti-Lu3) appears to be made by individuals of the dominant type and not those of the recessive type of Lu(a−b−).

    (Anti-Lu^{a}Lu^b (Anti-Lu3))

20. A normal survival of Lu(a+) red cells in a patient with a fairly potent anti-Lu^a has been reported.

    (The Clinical Significance of Anti-Lu^a and Anti-Lu^b)

GENERAL REFERENCES

1. Mollison, P. L.: Blood Transfusion in Clinical Medicine, 6th Ed. Blackwell Scientific Publications, Oxford, 1979. *(Good discussion of "major" antigens. No coverage of Lutheran-related antigens.)*
2. Race, R. R. and Sanger, R.: Blood Groups in Man, 6th Ed. Blackwell Scientific Publications, Oxford, 1975. *(Useful, well-referenced chapter on Lutheran with general discussion of Lutheran-related antigens. Particularly useful with respect to genetics of the system.)*

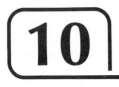

THE MNSs BLOOD GROUP SYSTEM

OBJECTIVES — THE MNSs BLOOD GROUP SYSTEM

The student shall know, understand and be prepared to explain:

1. A brief history of the discovery of the MNSs blood groups
2. The inheritance of the MNSs antigens (current theories)
3. The antigens of the MNSs blood group system (characteristics), including:
   (a) Antigens controlled by alleles at the MN locus (M^g, M_1, M^c, M^r, M^z, M^v, M^a, N^a, Tm and Sj)
   (b) Antigens controlled by alleles at the Ss locus ($U(S^u)$, S_2, Z)
   (c) Antigens associated with the MNSs system (Hu, He, Vr, Ri^a, St^a, Mt^a, Cl^a, Ny^a, Sul and Far)
   (d) The Miltenburger series of antigens
   (e) Biochemistry of the M and N antigens
   (f) Development of antigens in the MNSs system
4. The antibodies of the MNSs blood group system (characteristics), including:
   (a) Anti-M
   (b) Anti-N
   (c) Anti-S
   (d) Anti-s
   (e) Anti-M_1
   (f) Anti-M'
   (g) Anti-U
   (h) Anti-Mg
   (i) Anti-M^k
   (j) Anti-Tm
   (k) Anti-Sj
   (l) Anti-Hu
   (m) Anti-He
   (n) Anti-M^v
   (o) Anti-Vr
   (p) Anti-Mt^a
   (q) Anti-Cl^a
   (r) Anti-Ny^a
   (s) Anti-Sul
   (t) Anti-Far
   (u) Antibodies to the Miltenburger series of antigens
5. The techniques commonly used in detection of MNSs antigens

Introduction

The MNSs blood group system was discovered through the injection of human red cells into rabbits and subsequent absorption of the resulting rabbit serum, which was then tested against other human red cells. As a result of this work, the antigen M was described (Landsteiner and Levine, 1927), and later in the same year the antigens N and P (see Chapter 11) (Landsteiner and Levine, 1927).

During the subsequent 30 years, several rare antigens were identified — some of which were shown to be alleles of M and N. Others, though not alleles, obviously belonged to the MN system. In 1947, Walsh and Montgomery discovered a "new" antibody that was shown to recognize an antigen associated with M and N (Sanger and Race, 1947; Sanger et al, 1948). The new antigen was called S; while the gene S could be shown to be not an allele of M and N, it was believed to be related to M and N in the same way as C, D and E are related in the Rh system. The anticipated allele s was discovered through the identification of the antibody anti-s by Levine et al (1951).

Greenwalt et al (1954) made the discovery that less than 1 per cent of blood samples of blacks lack both S and s; this is presumed to be the result of inheritance of a pair of allelic genes U and u (described later).

Several other antigens have since been described that are related to the MNSs system. These will be discussed briefly.

Inheritance

The original theory of *M* and *N* inheritance was proposed by Landsteiner and Levine (1927). According to this theory, two allelic genes *M* and *N* determine the presence of the M and N antigens, allowing for three possible genotypes (*MM, MN* and *NN*) and three phenotypes (M, MN and N).

The recognition of *S* and *s* enlarges the theory to encompass two sets of allelic genes, yet the basic concept is the same.

The genes *M, N, S* and *s* are inherited as dominant genes.

Several observations suggest that the relation of N to M may be similar to that of H to A and B in the ABO system (i.e., that N is a precursor of M) (see Figur and Rosenfield, 1965). This theory is based on the fact that anti-N can be absorbed from serum by any sample of human red cells except those of the rare type *MS*ᵘ*MS*ᵘ, suggesting that *MM* red cells normally contain some "unconverted" N substance. Supportive evidence was presented by Uhlenbruck (1960) (see Prokop and Uhlenbruck, 1969), who found that M cells treated with pronase are converted to N cells, and by Springer *et al* (1971), workers who found that mild acid treatment, which removes some sialic acid from the MN glycoprotein, destroys M activity and results in a large transient increase in N activity. Yet despite this suggestive evidence, N is not *known* to be a precursor of M and opposing viewpoints have been offered by Lisowska and Duk (1975), Dahr *et al*, (1975) and Wasniowska *et al* (1977). All these investigators suggest rather that *M* and *N* determine different amino acid sequences of a polypeptide chain onto which glycosyl transferases, determined by genes unrelated to the *MN* locus, attach sialic acid residues.

Antigen, phenotype and gene frequencies with respect to M, N, S and s are given in Table 10–1.

Theoretical pathways of MN characters were proposed by Uhlenbruck (1960) (see Prokop and Uhlenbruck, 1969), based on the theory that N is the precursor of M. Until this last statement is proved, they lack the substance for general acceptance.

THE ANTIGENS OF THE MNSs BLOOD GROUP SYSTEM

Besides the M, N, S and s antigens, there are several other antigens that are associated with the system. For the purpose of this discussion these will be split into those antigens that are controlled by alleles at the *MN* or *Ss* loci, and those associated with the MNSs system, though not controlled by alleles at the *MN* or *Ss* loci.

ANTIGENS CONTROLLED BY ALLELES AT THE *MN* LOCUS

The Antigen Mᵍ. The Mᵍ antigen was discovered by Allen *et al* (1958). Its frequency appears to be one of the lowest (outside Switzerland and Sicily) of all known blood group antigens. Neither anti-M nor anti-N react with the Mᵍ antigen.

Being an allele at the *MN* locus, Mᵍ occupies the locus normally occupied by an *M* or *N* gene. Blood representing the genotype *M*ᵍ*M* gives only a single dose reaction against titrations of anti-M sera — yet in routine testing gives the reaction of M (i.e., *MM*). Similarly, blood representing the genotype *M*ᵍ*N* gives only a single dose reaction against titrations of anti-N sera, yet in routine testing gives the reaction of N (i.e., *NN*). This can cause serious

Table 10–1 PERCENTAGE FREQUENCIES OF ANTIGENS, PHENOTYPES AND GENES IN THE MNSs BLOOD GROUP SYSTEM

| Antigens | | Phenotypes | | | Genes | | |
Ag	Whites	Phenotype	Whites	Blacks	Gene	Whites	Blacks
M	78	MS	6.42	1.81	MS	24.73	9.44
N	72	Ms	9.52	15.32	NS	6.91	5.88
S	57	NS	0.46	1.05	Ms	30.63	38.82
s	88	Ns	14.48	19.53	Ns	37.73	45.86
		MSs	14.81	6.39			
		MNS	3.69	3.12			
		MNSs	22.23	11.09			
		MNs	23.30	35.95			
		NSs	5.10	3.3			

errors in paternity testing. For example, a child born to an M^gM father (typing as M) and an NN mother might be M^gN (typing as N) and therefore appear illegitimate.

The antigen M^g had not been found in tests on approximately 105,000 randomly selected people tested in Boston and England up to 1964 (studies by the Boston grouping Laboratory and Cleghorn, cited by Race and Sanger, 1975), yet in Switzerland the frequency of the antigen was found to be approximately 0.153 per cent (Metaxas *et al*, 1966).

Nordling *et al* (1969) found the M^g condition to be associated with certain physiochemical changes to the red cell surface, namely, reduced electrophoretic mobility and sialic acid content. This has increased general interest in M^g.

M^k. The allele M^k, first discovered by Metaxas and Metaxas-Buhler (1964), produces no M, N, S, s or M^g antigen. At first the allele was thought to produce an M^k antigen; investigators now think that what appeared to be an antigen is much more likely to be a reflection of the marked shortage of sialic acid on the surface of the red cells of M^k heterozygotes (Nordling *et al*, 1969). Metaxas *et al* (1970) give the frequency of the gene M^k as 0.00064 among Swiss blood donors.

The Antigen M_1. The antigen M_1 is a "subdivision" of the M antigen, recognized by anti-M_1, which appears to be a component of some human anti-M sera. Anti-M_1 divides the M antigen into two groups in a *qualitative* way (Jack *et al*, 1960). The antigen M_1 is a somewhat graded character, and is more common in blacks than in whites.

The Antigen M^c. The antigen M^c, described by Dunsford *et al* (1953), was found to react with the majority of anti-M and the minority of anti-N rabbit sera. It is considered, therefore, to be intermediate between M and N. There is no specific anti-M^c antibody; the antigen, like others (M^r, M^z, N_z, M^a and N^a), is distinguished by unusual reactions with anti-M or anti-N sera or both. All M^cN propositi tested have been found to be M_1 positive, yet M^c is different from M_1 because M_1N red cells can react with anti-M sera that fail to react with M^c red cells.

The Antigens M^r and M^z. Both M^r and M^z were discovered through unexpected dosage reactions (Metaxas *et al*, 1968). M^r, like M^c, reacts with the majority of anti-M and a minority of anti-N sera, but the reactions do not coincide. However, M^z, unlike M^c, fails to react with anti-M_1 yet reacts with anti-M'; M^r also reacts with most anti-M and some anti-N sera, but it reacts with neither anti-M_1 nor anti-M'. Both M^z

and M^r red cells are St(+) and both, like M^g, etc., have some alteration of the cell surface. M^c, M^z and M^r cells are distinguished as follows:

M^c red cells are M_1+, M' − St(a−)
M^z red cells are M_1-, M' + St(a+)
M^r red cells are M_1-, M' − St(a+)

The Antigen M^v. This antigen was discovered by the finding of an anti-N sera that reacted with 1 in about 400 M samples from white individuals. In 1970, anti-M^v (without the anti-N component) was discovered by Crossman *et al*. The gene M^v therefore produces an antigen that *behaves* like M in being agglutinated by anti-M but not by anti-N sera. It is an interesting contradiction, therefore, that the original anti-M^v — the result of stimulation of an MM mother by an M^vM fetus — behaved like anti-N except that it also reacted with the rare M^vM cells.

The Antigen M^a. The variant M^a appears to lack a part of the normal M antigen. In this respect it is similar to the variants of the $Rh_o(D)$ antigen. The original discoverers (Konugres *et al*, 1966) called the antigen M^a and the antibody, which failed to react with the maker's own MN red cells, anti-M^A.

The Antigen N^a. Booth (1971) found in two Melanesian blood donors an anti-N that failed to agglutinate between 10 and 30 per cent of NN Melanesians of different ethnic groups. The antiserum was called anti-N^A; the positive N cells were called N^A, and those that were negative were called N^a.

The Antigens Tm and Sj. Anti-Tm, which was found to react with the red cells of about 20 per cent of white people and 30 per cent of New York black people, was first discovered by Issitt *et al* (1965). Most of the positive reactors possessed the antigen N. The Tm antigen was found to be very variable in strength. Another antibody called anti-Sj was later separated from the same serum by Issitt *et al* (1968). About 2 per cent of whites and 4 per cent of blacks were found to possess the Sj antigen — and all were found to be Tm+.

The Antigen N_2. Weak N antigens in two propositi were first discovered by Metaxas *et al* (1968). The gene symbol N_2 was used, though this should be distinguished from the weak N associated with a positive direct antiglobulin reaction that is also sometimes called N_2 (discussed later).

ANTIGENS CONTROLLED BY ALLELES AT THE *Ss* LOCUS

The Antigen U(S^u). Wiener *et al* (1953, 1953) described an antibody, anti-U, which was found to react with the red cells of all of 1100 white people tested but which failed to react with 12 out of 989 New York black people. Greenwalt *et al* (1954) showed that the blood samples found to be negative with anti-U were also negative with anti-S and anti-s. Anti-U was therefore considered to be anti-Ss (anti-S + anti-s) with inseparable components.

Francis and Hatcher (1966) showed that not all black people who are S−s− are also U−. In random testing, 84 per cent of blacks were found to be U− and 16 per cent, U+.

Several genetic backgrounds have been offered to explain the S−s− phenotype; probably the most likely being that it is the homozygous expression of a rare allele at the *Ss* locus, and for this reason it is now designated S^u — although with the proviso that it is heterogenous. From family studies, it is clear that the S−s− phenotype is not caused by a suppressor gene, since S−s− individuals do not have S+s+ parents or offspring (Sanger *et al*, 1955; Allen *et al*, 1963; Morton *et al*, 1966; Goldstein, 1966).

The phenotype S−s- has not so far been found in white people. The antibody, anti-S^u, is clinically significant, however, since it has been implicated in a transfusion death, in hemolytic disease of the newborn and as an autoantibody in cases of acquired hemolytic anemia.

The Antigen S_2. The gene S_2 appears to be a straightforward allele at the *Ss* locus that produces a weak S antigen. There is no evidence that the difference is qualitative. Only one family of this type has been reported (Hurd *et al*, 1964).

The Antigen Z. The antigen Z, which appears to be associated with S and s, was described by Booth (1972). The antigen was found to be less common in Melanesians than in Europeans, and the phenotype S+Z− is most common in Melanesians. Only one example of anti-Z, which was non-red cell–immune, has been described so far.

ANTIGENS ASSOCIATED WITH THE MNSs SYSTEM

Many antigens have been reported that, while not alleles at the *MN* or *Ss* loci, have been found to be associated with the MNSs system. At the present time the majority of these are of academic interest only, and therefore will not be described in any detail here. Readers are referred to Race and Sanger's *Blood Groups in Man* for further details.

The Antigens Hu and He. Anti-Hu and anti-He were produced by rabbits in response to injections of red cells of blacks (Landsteiner *et al*, 1934); all blood samples giving positive reactions with anti-Hu belonged to group N or MN, suggesting an association with N. Anti-He has been found to be variously associated with NS, Ns, MS and Ms according to ethnic origin.

The Antigens Vr, Ri^a, St^a, Mt^a, Cl^a, Ny^a, Sul and Far. All of these antigens were brought to light by specific antibodies. All are dominant characters and have no influence on the MNSs antigens with which they segregate. The exception is St^a, which may affect the M antigen (see foregoing discussions of M^z and M^r). St^a is also associated with changes in the red cell surface (see foregoing discussions of M^g and M^k).

The Miltenburger Series of Antigens. The so-called Miltenburger subsystem was proposed by Cleghorn (1966), named because the serum of a Mrs. Miltenburger contained the first example of the antibody now known to be the most comprehensive in its reactions. Four classes were proposed originally and a fifth class has been added following the discovery of an English Miltenburger type (Crossland *et al*, 1970). Each class gives a different pattern of reactions with the types of sera, and all but class V are positive with anti-Mi^a (Miltenburger). This pattern of reactions is given in Table 10–2.

OTHER NOTES ON ANTIGENS OF THE MNSs SYSTEM

Weak M and N Antigens Associated with a Positive Direct Antiglobulin Test. Jakobowicz *et al* (1949, 1950) first made the observation that a positive direct antiglobulin reaction could be an inherited character. The phenomenon has

Table 10–2   THE PATTERNS OF REACTION WITH THE MILTENBERGER SERIES OF ANTIGENS

Red Cells Class	*Types of Antisera*				
	Verweyst (−Vw)	Miltenberger (−Mi^a)	Murell (−Mur)	Hill (−Hil)	Hut (−Hut)
I	+	+	−	−	−
II	−	+	−	−	+
III	−	+	+	+	+
IV	−	+	+	−	+
V	−	−	−	+	−

been found to be segregating with a weak N (Jensen and Freiesleben, 1962; Jeannet *et al*, 1964) and a weak M (Jakobowicz *et al*, 1949).

The globulin involved appeared in these cases to be IgM, and no signs of anemia were seen. Treatment of the red cells with papain abolished the reaction, whereas treatment with neuraminidase had no effect on some examples. The basic abnormality is therefore thought to be caused by an alteration in red cell sialic acid metabolism.

The Biochemistry of M and N. Springer and Ansel (1958) and Mäkelä and Cantell (1958) independently reported that the MN activity of human red cells was inactivated by neuraminidases from influenza viruses and from *Vibrio cholerae*, resulting in the release of sialic acid (*N*-acetylneuraminic acid, NANA) from the cells, Mäkelä and Cantell (1958) therefore concluded that sialic acid is an essential part of the M and N receptors.

The M and N antigens are glycoproteins and appear to be dependent on the presence of sialic acid in appropriate linkages. Springer and Huprikar (1972) reported that there is more β-D-galactopyranosyl in N than in M, but otherwise there is no information on the structures differentiating M and N specificity. Therefore the structures on the glycoprotein molecules that carry M and N specificities have not yet been isolated or characterized.

The Development of Antigens in the MNSs System. The M and N antigens are well developed at birth and are constant throughout life (Schiff and Boyd, 1942), as are the antigens S (see Race and Sanger, 1975), s (Speiser, 1959), U (Burki *et al*, 1968), M^g (Metaxas-Bühler *et al*, 1966), Mt^a, Cl^a, Ny^a, Far and the antigens of the Miltenberger series (see Race and Sanger, 1975). The antigen Tm, however, is not well developed at birth (Issitt *et al*, 1966).

THE ANTIBODIES OF THE MNSs BLOOD GROUP SYSTEM

Anti-M. Anti-M is a rare antibody occurring more commonly in infants than in adults (Strahl *et al*, 1955). When the antibody does occur it is usually a cold agglutinin reacting best at 4° C and weakly or not at all at 37° C (Dahr, 1941; Paterson *et al*, 1942; Unger *et al*, 1946). Auto-anti-M has been described (Fletcher and Zmijewski, 1970), in one case occurring without apparent antigenic stimulus (Vale and Harris, 1980). Anti-M is usually IgG, though IgM anti-M is also frequently found. Studies by Smith and Beck (1979) revealed that 78 per cent of

anti-M sera are composed of IgG, and there appeared to be no correlation between immunoglobulin composition and history of transfusion and pregnancy.

Anti-M of the IgG type may react more strongly in albumin or serum than in saline and may react as well at 37° C as at 4° C (Stone and Marsh, 1959).

Strong dosage effect can occur with anti-M (and anti-N), and the antibody may only react with red cells that are homozygous for the M antigen. Certain rare examples may bind complement, though they do not cause *in vitro* lysis.

Papain, ficin, trypsin and bromelin inhibit MNSs reactions, though the cross reaction of anti-N with M red cells is enhanced by trypsin.

Anti-M may cause fairly rapid red cell destruction in patients who have not previously been transfused, though hemolytic disease of the newborn caused by anti-M is extremely rare, even when the antibody is known to be present in the mother (see Bowley and Dunsford, 1949).

Besides the human antibody, anti-M is found as a weak, "naturally occurring" agglutinin in horse serum. Potent antisera can be produced by the injection of human group O, M-positive red cells (Levine *et al*, 1957), though the resulting antibody shows marked dosage effect. A more satisfactory anti-M sera can be produced in rabbits (see Menolasino *et al*, 1954).

Anti-M is also found in the seeds of *Iberis amara* (see Chapter 19).

Anti-N. Anti-N is found almost exclusively in S-negative, s-negative individuals, since these are the only red cells that are completely N-negative (Telischi *et al*, 1976). The antibody is exceedingly rare — even rarer than anti-M.

At temperatures of 23° C or lower, anti-N will agglutinate M cells, although anti-M will not agglutinate N cells (Hirsch *et al*, 1957). Anti-N will also agglutinate trypsin-treated M cells.

Anti-N fails to react with red cells of phenotype MS^u (genotype $MS^u MS^u$) (Allen *et al*, 1960; Figur and Rosenfield, 1965) and the reaction strength between anti-N and M-positive red cells is influenced by the Ss group of the red cells (Race and Sanger, 1962).

Anti-N produced by S-positive or s-positive individuals reacts only in the cold and is usually poor in strength.

Most examples of anti-N are non-red cell–immune (i.e, "naturally occurring") and are typically IgM cold agglutinins inactive above

20 to 25° C, although one naturally occurring IgG anti-N has been reported (Giblett, cited by Mollison, 1979). Immune anti-N is extremely rare.

In a few cases, anti-N has been found as an auto-antibody (see Moores *et al*, 1970; Perrault, 1973; Hinz and Boyer, 1963). Autoimmune hemolytic anemia has been reported to be associated with IgM auto-anti-N (Bowman *et al*, 1974) and with IgG auto-anti-N (Dube *et al*, 1979).

In 1972, Howell and Perkins reported that 12 out of 416 patients on renal dialysis had developed anti-N, usually active at 4° C and 20° C but never active at 37° C. It was suggested that the stimulus for these antibodies might come from small amounts of red cells left in the dialysis equipment that were denatured by formol treatment. This suggestion has since gained support with the observation that M-positive red cells (i.e., *MM*) treated *in vitro* with formaldehyde acquired reactivity to anti-N (White *et al*, 1975). The antigen formed by formaldehyde treatment is known as formaldehyde-N.

The anti-N–like antibody formed by patients on renal dialysis does not usually affect the survival of transfused N-positive red cells unless the antibody is active at or near 37° C.

Anti-N, like anti-M, often shows dosage and may react only with "*NN*" cells. Most examples do not bind complement or cause *in vitro* lysis. The reactions of anti-N are inhibited by enzymes, though trypsin enhances the crossreaction of anti-N with "*MM*" cells.

Mild hemolytic disease of the newborn caused by anti-N (see Mollison, 1979), has been reported, though this is extremely unusual. While the antibody has not been implicated as a cause of hemolytic transfusion reaction, it must be considered clinically significant when reactive at 37° C.

Several lectins have been described that have anti-N activity, the most notable of which is *Vicia graminea* (see Chapter 19).

Anti-S. Anti-S is most commonly found as an immune antibody in patients having many transfusions, though "naturally occurring" examples have been reported (e.g., see Constantoulis *et al*, 1955). Most examples of immune anti-S are IgG, though two examples have been described that behaved as saline agglutinins and were found to be IgM (Adinolfi *et al*, 1962). Some examples of anti-S have the ability to bind complement, though they do not appear to have the ability to cause *in vitro* lysis. Anti-S has been implicated as a cause of hemolytic transfusion reaction (one of them fatal — see Coombs

et al, 1951) and is also known to have caused hemolytic disease of the newborn (e.g., see Levine *et al*, 1952).

Anti-s. Anti-s is an extremely rare antibody. Most examples have been found to be IgG, yet react more strongly at low temperatures (Lalezari *et al*, 1973). A few examples appear to bind complement, but most do not. The first example of the antibody was the cause of severe hemolytic disease of the newborn (Levine *et al*, 1951), and it has been implicated as a cause of the disease in other subsequent cases (Giblett *et al*, 1958, Lusher *et al*, 1966; Drachman and Brogaard, 1969). Anti-s was successfully induced in two out of 22 rabbits following injections of red cells in 5 weeks (Puno and Allen, 1969).

Anti-M₁. About one third of human anti-M sera also contain anti-M_1 (Jack *et al*, 1960), the antibody detecting a qualitative difference in the M antigen. An example of anti-M_1 without anti-M has been described by Giles and Howell (1974).

Anti-M'. Like anti-M_1, anti-M' lacks clear-cut reactions with some samples. The only difference between the two antibodies is that anti-M fails to react with M^c red cells and does react with M^z red cells, the reverse of the reactions with anti-M_1.

Anti-U. Anti-U is a rare antibody that is now known *not* to be anti-Ss (Francis and Hatcher, 1966). The antibody has been implicated as the cause of hemolytic disease of the newborn, in one instance resulting in stillbirth (Burki *et al*, 1964), and is sometimes the cause of hemolytic transfusion reactions. In rare examples, acquired hemolytic anemia has been attributed to anti-U (Blajchman *et al*, 1971; Nugent *et al*, 1971; Marsh *et al*, 1972). Auto-anti-U has also been described (Beck *et al*, 1972).

OTHER ANTIBODIES OF THE MNSs BLOOD GROUP SYSTEM

Anti-M^g. This is probably the commonest antibody belonging to the MNSs blood group system, having a frequency of 1 to 2 per cent. The antibody reacts more strongly at room temperature than at 37° C (Darnborough, 1957; Zeitlin *et al*, 1958; Allen *et al*, 1958). The antibody has been made in rabbits (Ikin, 1966).

Anti-M^k. Specific anti-M^k does not exist; the reaction observed represents the interaction of immune antisera in general with the changed surface properties of M^k red cells.

Anti-Tm and Anti-Sj. Anti-Tm is not uncommon, but tends to "go off" both *in vivo* and *in vitro* (Issitt *et al*, 1968; Race and Sanger, 1962). Anti-Sj, however, appears to be more stable (Issitt *et al*, 1968). No immune example of anti-Tm has been reported.

Anti-Hu and Anti-He. These antibodies have been produced in rabbits. Only one example of anti-He in human serum has been reported, and was thought to be "naturally occurring" (Macdonald *et al*, 1967).

Anti-M^v is almost certainly immune (Gershowitz and Fried, 1966). The positive reactions with this antibody descend in order of strength from M^{v}N, N, M^{v}M, MN to negative with M red cells (Gershowitz, 1967).

Anti-Vr is extremely rare, with only three examples so far described, two of which were found in anti-S sera. The original example was found to be immune.

Only one example of *anti-Ri^a* has been described (Hart *et al*, 1958) found together with *anti-St^a*. Further examples of anti-St^a have subsequently been described (Madden *et al*, 1964).

Anti-Mt^a was first described as a "naturally occurring antibody (Swanson and Matson, 1962). However, it has caused hemolytic disease of the newborn and was successfully produced in rabbits (Konugres *et al*, 1963).

Anti-Cl^a was first discovered in anti-B serum and was subsequently found to be present in the serum of 0.45 per cent of randomly selected donors in Glasgow and London (Wallace and Izatt, 1963).

Anti-Ny^a has been produced in rabbits. Four examples of the antibody have been found in tests of over 3000 Norwegian donors (Ørjasaeter *et al*, 1964a; Ørjasaeter *et al*, 1964b). The original example was found in a "normal" donor.

Anti-Sul is relatively common — four examples were found in testing only 119 sera of normal donors in Boston (Konugres and Winter, 1967).

The single example of *anti-Far* so far described was the result of feto-maternal immunization (Cregut *et al*, 1968).

ANTIBODIES TO THE MILTENBERGER SERIES OF ANTIGENS

Anti-Mi^a, anti-Vw, anti-Mur, anti-Hil and anti-Hut have only been found in human sera and all have been implicated as the cause of hemolytic disease of the newborn, though anti-Vw is more often "naturally occurring." When it develops immune characteristics, its specificity broadens to become anti-Mi^a (Cleghorn, cited by Mollison 1979). Anti-Vw can also be considered of negligible significance (with respect to hemolytic disease of the newborn) because of the rarity of the corresponding antigen. One example of anti-Mi^a was shown to cause the destruction of red cells *in vivo* by Cutbush and Mollison (1958).

Of the other antibodies to the Miltenberger series of antigens, several examples of anti-Mur have been found (Cleghorn, 1966; Cornwall *et al*, 1968; Smerling, 1971), but only one example of anti-Hil is known (Cleghorn, 1966). Several examples of anti-Hut have been described (Mohn *et al*, 1958; Cleghorn, 1966; Mohn and Macvie, 1967), all of which were the cause of hemolytic disease of the newborn.

TECHNIQUES

The worker should ensure that the method recommended by the manufacturer is carefully followed, since the method of testing will depend on the nature of the antibody. In general, tests for anti-M and anti-N are performed at room temperature in a test tube or on a tile using equal volumes of antibody and an appropriate red cell suspension. The tubes are incubated at room temperature and *not* centri-

Table 10–3   THE USUAL SEROLOGIC BEHAVIOR OF MNSs ANTIBODIES*

		Anti-M	*Anti-N*	*Anti-S*	*Anti-s*
Saline or	4° C	Most	Most	Few	None
Albumin	22° C	Most	Most	Some	Few
	37° C	Few	Few	Some	Few
	IAGT	Few	Few	Some	Most
Enzyme	37° C	None	None	None	Some
	IAGT	None	None	None	Most

*Modified from the Technical Manual of the American Association of Blood Banks, 7th Ed., 1977.

fuged. Reading is macroscopic. Heterozygous (*MN*) red cells are run as a positive control in parallel with the test, as are *NN* or *MM* red cells as a negative control. Negative controls often show weak positive reactions. If the reaction is classified as more than weak (w), the tests should be considered invalid.

Some commercial anti-S sera are the "complete" variety and react best at room temperature. Most anti-s sera, however, react best by the indirect antiglobulin test. Known S-positive and s-positive red cells (Ss) should be run in parallel with the test as a positive control and SS or ss red cells run as a negative control.

The usual serologic behavior of MNSs antibodies is given in Table 10–3.

TYPICAL EXAMINATION QUESTIONS

Choose the phrase, sentence or symbol that correctly answers the question or completes the statement. More than one answer may be acceptable for each question. Answers are given in the back of the book.

1. The M and N antigens were originally discovered
   (a) to be the result of immunization by transfusion
   (b) to be the result of immunization by pregnancy
   (c) through the injection of human red cells into rabbits, then testing the absorbed rabbit serum against other red cells
   (d) by Landsteiner and Levine
   (Introduction)

2. The genes *M, N, S* and *s* are
   (a) co-dominant
   (b) dominant
   (c) recessive
   (d) allelic
   (Inheritance)

3. Antigens controlled by alleles at the *MN* locus include
   (a) M^g
   (b) N^a
   (c) Z
   (d) Hu
   (Antigens Controlled by Alleles at the MN Locus)

4. Which of the following antigens does not belong to the MN^{Ss} blood group system
   (a) Ri^a
   (b) Vw
   (c) Far
   (d) Ge
   (e) none of the above
   (Antigens Associated with the MNSs System – General)

5. An essential part of the M and N receptors is
   (a) neuraminidase
   (b) sialic acid
   (c) *N*-acetylneuraminic acid
   (d) none of the above
   (The Biochemistry of M and N)

6. Which of the following antigens is/are not well developed at birth?

   (a) M
   (b) M^g
   (c) Tm
   (d) Mt^a
   (e) s
   (The Development of Antigens in the MNSs System)

7. Anti-M
   (a) is more common in infants than in adults
   (b) is IgM in all cases
   (c) may show dosage effect
   (d) cross-reacts with N red cells
   (Anti-M)

8. Anti-N
   (a) will agglutinate M red cells at temperatures below 23° C
   (b) will agglutinate trypsin-treated M red cells
   (c) is found almost exclusively in S-negative, s-negative individuals
   (d) reaction strength is influenced by the Ss group of the red cells under test
   (e) is usually IgG
   (Anti-N)

9. Most examples of immune anti-S
   (a) are IgG
   (b) are IgM
   (c) are IgA
   (d) behave as saline agglutinins
   (Anti-S)

10. Anti-s
    (a) has been successfully induced in rabbits
    (b) is usually IgG
    (c) usually reacts more strongly at low temperatures
    (d) has never been implicated as the cause of hemolytic disease of the newborn
    (Anti-s)

11. Anti-U
    (a) is anti-Ss
    (b) has been implicated as the cause of hemolytic disease of the newborn
    (c) has been described as an autoantibody
    (d) is sometimes the cause of hemolytic transfusion reactions
    (Anti-U)

12. Which of the following antibodies have been produced in rabbits?

(a) Anti-M^g
(b) Anti-Hu
(c) Anti-He
(d) Anti-Mt^a

*(Other Antibodies of the MNSs
Blood Group System)*

13. Which of the following antibodies is directed against the Miltenberger series of antigens?
    (a) Anti-Cl^a
    (b) Anti-Far
    (c) Anti-Ny^a
    (d) Anti-Mur

*(Antibodies to the Miltenberger
Series of Antigens)*

Answer true or false

14. Less than 1 per cent of black blood samples lack S and s.

(Introduction)

15. It has been suggested that M may be a precursor to N.

(Inheritance)

16. Anti-M and anti-N fail to react with the M^g antigen.

(The Antigen M^g)

17. A positive direct antiglobulin reaction could be an inherited character segregating with a weak N or a weak M.

*(Other Notes on Antigens
of the MNSs System)*

18. Papain, ficin, trypsin and bromelin inhibit MNSs reactions.

(Anti-M)

19. The M-like antigen formed by patients on renal dialysis is known as formaldehyde-M.

(Anti-N)

20. About one third of human anti-M sera also contain anti-M$_1$.

(Anti-M$_1$)

GENERAL REFERENCES (SUGGESTED READING)

1. Boorman, K. E., Dodd, B. E. and Lincoln, P. J.: Blood Group Serology, 5th Ed. Churchill-Livingstone, Edinburgh, New York, 1977. *(General coverage of the MNSs blood group system – also includes suggested techniques.)*
2. Mollison, P. L.: Blood Transfusion in Clinical Medicine, 6th Ed. Blackwell Scientific Publications, Oxford, 1979. *(General coverage of the MNSs blood group system. Emphasis on "major" antigens.)*
3. Race, R. R., and Sanger, R.: Blood Groups in Man, 6th Ed. Blackwell Scientific Publications, Oxford, 1975. *(Full comprehensive coverage of the MNSs blood group system. Particularly useful to the student requiring further information on the rarer antigens, and references.)*

11

THE P BLOOD GROUP SYSTEM

OBJECTIVES — THE P BLOOD GROUP SYSTEM

The student shall know, understand and be prepared to explain:

1. A brief history of the P blood group system, specifically to include:
   (a) Original discovery and notation
   (b) Changes in notation
   (c) Discovery of other antigens in system
2. The basic genetic inheritance of the P_1 and P_2 antigens
3. The characteristics of the P_1 antigen
4. General aspects of:
   (a) The phenotype p
   (b) The phenotype P^k
   (c) The Luke phenotype
5. The existence of anti-P_1 in hydatid cyst fluid
6. The biochemistry of P system antigens

7. The general characteristics when known (temperature of reaction, immunoglobulin class, ability to bind complement and usual stimulus) of the following antibodies:
   (a) Anti-P_1
   (b) Anti-PP,P^k
   (c) Anti-P
   (d) Anti-Luke
   (e) Anti-p
   (f) Anti-IP$_1$, anti-I^{T}P$_1$ and anti-IP
8. The general characteristics of the Donath-Landsteiner antibody
9. The clinical significance of P antibodies
10. The general principles of the technique for detection of the P_1 antigen

Introduction

The P blood group system was discovered by Landsteiner and Levine in 1927 while testing immune sera prepared by the injection of human red cells into rabbits and subsequent recovery of the rabbit serum. This was an unexpected byproduct of the experiments wherein the MN groups were discovered. (Note that these two systems, P and MNSs, were the only major blood group systems discovered through the injection of human red cells into animals.) The immune rabbit sera were found, after absorption of the species agglutinins, to agglutinate some samples of human red cells and not others, and the two types of blood were called P+ and P−.

The antibody (called anti-P) was found in human serum soon afterward (Landsteiner and Levine, 1930) as well as in normal, non-immune sera from cattle, pigs, horses and rabbits (Landsteiner and Levine, 1931).

In 1951, Levine *et al* discovered the antigen Tj^a (now called PP$_1$P^k), which was shown to be part of the P system by Sanger (1955). The

antigen P later came to be called P_1 when it was discovered that individuals who produced anti-PP$_1$P^k (anti-Tj^a) were P-negative (Sanger, 1955). It was then realized that P-negative individuals share a powerful antigen with P-positive individuals and do not lack an antigen of the system as was originally supposed. The notation was therefore modified in accordance with this discovery; the P-positive phenotype became P_1; the P-negative phenotype became P_2; and anti-P became anti-P_1.

Almost all individuals are either P_1 or P_2. The P_1 phenotype, representing 72.94 per cent of the U.S. white population and 93.1 per cent of the U.S. black population, is by far the most common. P_2 individuals frequently have anti-P_1 in their serum as a cold agglutinin, which is only occasionally active at 20° C or higher.

In 1959, the P system grew in complexity with the discovery of the antigen P^k by Matson *et al*. This rare antigen is almost unique among blood groups in the manner of its inheritance (discussed later). The extremely rare phenotype p was described by Levine *et al* (1951), yet only three examples of the antibody reacting pre-

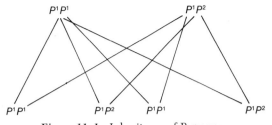

Figure 11-1   Inheritance of P groups.

ferentially with p cells have been described (see later discussion).

Inheritance

Landsteiner and Levine (1930, 1931) showed that the P_1 antigen is probably inherited as a mendelian dominant character, and all subsequent work has supported this. Genotype matings, therefore, result in (among others) the offspring groups shown in Figure 11-1.

There is some evidence that the gene P is linked to ADA (adenosine deaminase) (Edwards *et al*, 1973). The gene is generally believed to be on chromosome No. 20.

A rare inhibitor of P_1 (and other antigens) was found by Crawford *et al* (1974). The inhibitor locus, called *In(Lu)*, is not linked to the P locus (or the *Lutheran locus*) and the antigens Lu^a, Lu^b and Au^a are all affected by it. If this rare dominant inhibitor is present, therefore, individuals who type as P_2 may in fact be genetically P^1 (see Chapter 9).

THE ANTIGENS AND PHENOTYPES OF THE P BLOOD GROUP SYSTEM

The Antigen P_1.   Landsteiner and Levine (1927) defined two grades of P_1 blood samples, one reacting strongly and the other weakly with anti-P_1 sera. In 1929, the same workers recorded four categories that they called an "arbitrary arrangement." Henningsen (1949) realized that it was not possible to subdivide P_1 strength into separate categories, the results showing a normal distribution curve using a modification of Jonsson's titration method. The same worker was also unable to demonstrate any qualitative differences between weak and strong P_1 antigens. Moharram (1942) and Henningsen (1949) (1952) suggested that the strength of the antigen was inherited, and this theory has not as yet been disputed.

The Phenotype p.   The phenotype p, originally classified as Tj(a−), was described by Levine *et al* (1951). All individuals of this phenotype possess anti-PP$_1$P^k (anti-Tj^a) in their serum. The frequency of this phenotype is 5.8 in a million in most parts of the world and slightly higher in parts of North Sweden (Race and Sanger, 1975). The inheritance of the phenotype is unclear, though two possibilities have been suggested: p individuals may be homozygous for a third allele (p) at the P^1P^2 locus (or a suppressor gene at the P^1 or P^2 gene complex) or they may be homozygous for a "regulator" allele at some other locus with the ability to prevent the P^1 and P^2 genes from expressing as antigens.

The possible existence of an antigen p has been suggested (see Engelfriet *et al*, 1971).

The Phenotype P^k.   The phenotype P^k was found to be part of the P blood group system by Matson *et al* (1959), who investigated a sample of blood that possessed an anti-Tj^a–like antibody, though the red cells did not give the expected negative reaction with antibodies from p individuals. The P^k phenotype is even rarer than the p phenotype and is of particular interest because, unlike practically all other blood group antigens, it is not inherited as a straightforward dominant character. In addition, the P^k antigen, while extremely rare on red cells, has been demonstrated on the cultured fibroblasts of practically all P_1 and P_2 individuals, but not on the fibroblasts of p individuals (Fellous *et al*, 1972), suggesting that P^k is an almost universal "public" gene that is somehow prevented from expressing itself on red cells.

The antibody in the serum of p individuals — originally thought to possess only anti-P and anti-P_1 — is now known to possess a third antibody component, anti-P^k. P^k individuals regularly possess anti-P, one of the antibodies in p individuals. The red cells of P^k individuals possess the P^k antigen but lack the P antigen. The majority have the antigen P_1 (phenotype P^k_1) but some lack the P_1 antigen (phenotype P^k_2).

Genetically, the P^k antigen is believed to reflect a recessive homozygous inheritance background (Race and Sanger, 1975) though does not appear to be due to an allele (recessive in effect) at the P_1P_2 locus, since P^k individuals have normal P_1 or P_2 genes. Several schemes for the possible biosynthesis of the P system antigens have been proposed, yet all are, for the moment at least, only speculative (see Fellous *et al*, 1974; Race and Sanger, 1975).

The Luke Phenotype.   Tippett *et al* (1965) discovered an agglutinin in the serum of a male patient, Mr. Luke P., which was like anti-P (in that it failed to react with the red cells of p and P^k individuals) yet which also failed to react with about 2 per cent of P_1 and P_2 individuals. The antibody also reacted very weakly with P_2

red cells and with A_1 and A_1B red cells (whether P_1 or P_2), suggesting a possible relationship between the P and ABO blood group systems.

Family studies have suggested that the Luke-positive property is a dominant character and Luke-negative a recessive, and that the character, while undoubtedly associated with the P blood group system, segregated independently of the P_1P_2 genes (Race and Sanger, 1975).

P_1 Substance in Hydatid Cyst Fluid. Cameron and Staveley (1957) found that two patients suffering from hydatid disease possessed a strong anti-P_1, and this led to the discovery that fluid from hydatid cysts, provided that it contained scolices, inhibited anti-P_1. The fluid was also found to inhibit in part anti-$P+P_1$ sera (Staveley and Cameron, 1958) and anti-P^k strongly, though anti-P was inhibited only weakly or not at all (Matson *et al*, 1959; Kortekangas *et al*, 1959).

Hydatid cyst fluid may therefore be used to establish the specificity of a suspected anti-P_1 antibody; the fluid may be lyophilized and stored without notable loss of reactivity.

The Development of Antigens in the P Blood Group System. The P_1 antigen is usually not fully developed at birth (Henningsen, 1949), though younger fetuses are more frequently and more strongly P_1 than are older fetuses (Race and Sanger, 1954; Ikin *et al*, 1961). The P antigen does appear to be well developed at birth (see Race and Sanger, 1975), as is the Luke antigen (Tippett *et al*, 1965). No P^k individual has yet been tested at birth.

Complete development of the P_1 antigen may not occur until age 7 or higher (Heiken, 1977).

The Biochemistry of P System Antigens. Morgan and Watkins (1962, 1964) demonstrated by chemical analysis of hydatid cyst fluid that the immunodominant sugar of the P_1 antigen is a D-galactose. The substance in hydatid cyst fluid that inhibits anti-P_1 is a glycoprotein. The terminal trisaccharide (Gal (α, $1 \rightarrow 4$) Gal (β, $1 \rightarrow 4$) GlcNAc) has the same structure in hydatid cyst fluid as the terminal trisaccharide of the P_1 glycolipid isolated from red cells (Naiki *et al*, 1975). The P^k antigen has been found to possess the same terminal disaccharide (α-D-galactose) (Voak *et al*, 1973). Anti-P is inhibited by globoside (Naiki and Marcus, 1975; Watkins and Morgan, 1976; Marcus *et al*, 1976), and the antibody called anti-p is inhibited by sialosylparagloboside (Schwarting *et al*, 1977). The P, P^k and P_1 antigens on red cells are glycoshingolipids, as are the P and P^k antigens in plasma.

THE ANTIBODIES OF THE P BLOOD GROUP SYSTEM

Anti-P_1. Anti-P_1 is present in the serum of two thirds of randomly selected P_2 individuals — mostly as a weak, cold-reacting (20° C or lower) agglutinin (Henningsen, 1949). In pregnant women who are P_2, the incidence of anti-P_1 was found to be almost 90 per cent, though this could not be connected with alloimmunization in pregnancy. The antibody can occur "naturally" in human serum and occurs in non-immune sera of animals of several different species. Potent anti-P_1 has been produced in goats and rabbits (Levine *et al*, 1958, 1959; Prokop and Oesterle, 1958; Kerde *et al*, 1960).

Few examples of anti-P_1 will agglutinate red cells at 25° C and fewer still are active at 37° C; those that do agglutinate red cells at or near 37° C may fix complement (Cutbush and Mollison, 1955).

Anti-P_1 is usually a cold-reacting IgM agglutinin. Polley *et al* (1962) showed that potent anti-P_1 would sensitize red cells to agglutination by anti-IgM and anti-complement — but not by anti-IgG. The antibody is usually non–red-cell-immune, though on rare occasions it can be stimulated by transfusion (see Wiener and Peters, 1940; Wiener, 1942) (see later discussion on clinical significance of P antibodies).

Anti-PP_1P^k (anti-Tj^a). This antibody (or mixture of antibodies) is found only in individuals of the rare phenotype p. Absorption of anti-PP_1P^k sometimes leaves the other antibodies when selected cells are used — and sometimes does not — though a satisfactory explanation for this has not yet emerged (see Kortekangas *et al*, 1965). An association between anti-PP_1P^k and habitual abortion has been suggested (Levine and Koch, 1954); however, it is not clear whether the association is a casual one (see Race and Sanger, 1975).

Anti-PP_1P^k is usually IgM in nature, though IgG examples have been reported (see Wurzel *et al*, 1971; Levine *et al*, 1977).

Anti-P. Anti-P, in a pure form, has been found in the serum of all known P^k individuals. The antibody behaves as an agglutinin and hemolysin at room temperature and at 37° C, and reacts equally strongly with P_1 and P_2 red cells. The reaction is not inhibited by hydatid cyst fluid.

Anti-Luke. This antibody, like anti-P, fails to react with p and P^k samples, yet, unlike anti-P, it also fails to react with about 2 per cent of P_1 and P_2 samples. The antibody has been found to react very weakly with P_2 red cells and with A_1 and A_1B red cells (whether P_1 or P_2), suggesting a possible relationship between the P and ABO blood group systems.

Anti-p. Only one example of this antibody has been reported (Engelfriet *et al,* 1971), though the discoverers were not certain about the specificity, and therefore the antibody can only be believed to exist.

Anti-IP₁, Anti-I^T P₁ and Anti-IP. The I antigen is believed to be related to both the ABH antigens and the P_1 antigen, though the mechanics of the relationship are not yet understood. Four antibodies have been described by Issitt *et al* (1968) that had apparent anti-P_1 specificity yet that failed to react with P_1 i red cells. Booth (1970) described an anti-P_1 whose reaction with P_1 cells was related to the I^T strength of the red cells, and Allen *et al* (1974) reported an antibody of specificity anti-IP.

Auto-anti-Tj^a (Anti-Tj^a-Like). Vos *et al* (1964) reported a transient anti-Tj^a–like antibody in the serum of habitual aborters in Australia, described as a "hemolytic activity" found only during pregnancy (Vos, 1965, 1966, 1967). The hemolytic factor is not complement related, nor does it appear to be an immunoglobulin. This strange activity has not been found in habitual aborters in the United States or in Canada (Vos *et al,* 1964).

The Donath-Landsteiner (DL) Antibody. In paroxysmal cold hemoglobinuria (PCH), the patient's serum contains an antibody that is reactive in the cold and classically has the specificity anti-P (Levine *et al,* 1963; Worlledge and Rousso, 1965). The antibody, which is frequently called the Donath-Landsteiner (DL) antibody after its discoverers, produces hemolysis both *in vivo* and *in vitro* when the blood is first cooled and then warmed (known as a biphasic hemolysin). The DL antibody has also been found in such disease states as syphilis and following measles and mumps, chicken pox and so forth, and does not always have anti-P specificity (Wienter et al, 1964). The DL antibody (i.e., of anti-P specificity) is always IgG.

The Clinical Significance of P Antibodies

There is no doubt that anti-P_1 can cause severe adverse transfusion reactions, and yet many patients with cold-reacting anti-P_1 have received P_1-positive blood without adverse effect. Mollison (1979) describes the destruction of P_1 red cells by anti-P_1 as "occasional," although examples that sensitize red cells to anticomplement serum (even if only weekly reactive as agglutinins at 37° C) should be regarded as clinically significant. A fatal transfusion reaction due to anti-P_1 was described by Moureau (1954). Anti-P_1 has not been implicated as the cause of hemolytic disease of the newborn.

Anti-PP₁P^k has been implicated as the cause of hemolytic transfusion reaction (Levine *et al,* 1951) and of hemolytic disease of the newborn (Hayashida and Watanabe, 1968; Levine *et al,* 1977).

TECHNIQUES

The standard tube technique is generally used for typing of red cells with anti-P_1 at the recommended temperature (i.e., according to the manufacturer's direction). Known P_1-positive and P_1-negative red cells should be included with each batch as controls. (*Note*: some laboratories used P_1-strong *and* P_1-weak red cells as a positive control.) Antisera that react at 15° C or higher are preferable to those reactive at 4° C, where other cold agglutinins may interfere with the results. Tests should be read carefully because the agglutinates are often fragile.

The test for the detection of the Donath-Landsteiner antibody is given in Chapter 23.

TYPICAL EXAMINATION QUESTIONS

Choose the phrase, sentence or symbol that completes or best answers the question. More than one answer may be acceptable in each case. Answers are given in the back of the book.

1. In accordance with the discovery that P-negative individuals do not lack an antigen of the P system but share a powerful one with P-positive individuals, the original notation (P+ and P−) was changed as follows
   (a) P-positive became P_1
   (b) P-negative became PP₁P^k
   (c) Anti-P became anti-PP₁P^k
   (d) P-negative became P_2

   (Introduction)

2. The P_2 phenotype
   (a) results from a mendelian-dominant gene, P^2
   (b) was originally referred to as P−
   (c) occurs in individuals possessing the genotype P^2P^2
   (d) none of the above

   (Inheritance)

3. The differences in P_1 antigen strength are believed to reflect
   (a) a qualitative difference in P_1 antigens
   (b) an inherited characteristic
   (c) dosage effect
   (d) none of the above
   (The Antigen P_1)

4. Individuals of phenotype p
   (a) possess anti-PP_1P^k in their serum
   (b) may be homozygous for the allele *p* at the P^1P^2 locus
   (c) may be homozygous for a suppressor gene at the P^1 or P^2 gene complex
   (d) are extremely common
   (The Phenotype p)

5. The P^k phenotype
   (a) is inherited as a straightforward dominant character
   (b) is rarer than the p phenotype
   (c) is not inherited as a straightforward dominant character
   (d) is due to an allele, P^k, at the P_1P_2 locus
   (The P^k Phenotype)

6. Fluid from hydatid cyst fluid containing scolices
   (a) inhibits anti-P_1
   (b) inhibits (in part) anti-$P+P_1$
   (c) strongly inhibits anti-P
   (d) strongly inhibits anti-P^k
   (P_1 Substance in Hydatid Cyst Fluid)

7. The P_1 antigen
   (a) is fully developed at birth
   (b) is not fully developed at birth
   (c) may be more strongly developed in younger fetuses than in older fetuses
   (d) may not be fully developed until age 7 or higher
   (The Development of Antigens in the P Blood Group System)

8. The immunodominant sugar of the P_1 antigen is
   (a) α-D-galactose
   (b) N-acetyl-glucosamine
   (c) the same as that possessed by the P^k antigen
   (d) not yet known
   (The Biochemistry of P System Antigens)

9. Anti-P_1
   (a) occurs in two out of three randomly selected P_2 individuals
   (b) has been produced in goats and rabbits
   (c) is usually a cold-reacting IgM agglutinin
   (d) is usually non–red-cell-immune
   (Anti-P_1)

10. Anti-Luke
    (a) fails to react with p and P^k samples
    (b) reacts with all P_1 and P_2 red cells
    (c) reacts weakly with A_1 and A_1B red cells (whether P_1 or P_2)
    (d) is also known as anti-P
    (Anti-Luke)

11. The Donath-Landsteiner antibody
    (a) classically has the specificity anti-P_1
    (b) is a biphasic hemolysin
    (c) is only found in paroxysmal cold hemoglobinuria
    (d) is always IgG when it is of anti-P specificity
    (The Donath-Landsteiner (DL) Antibody)

12. Anti-P_1
    (a) has been implicated as the cause of hemolytic disease of the newborn
    (b) has never been the cause of adverse transfusion reaction
    (c) has caused a fatal transfusion reaction
    (d) is considered clinically insignificant
    (The Clinical Significance of P Antibodies)

ANSWER TRUE OR FALSE

13. The P blood group system was discovered through the injection of human red cells into animals.
    (Introduction)

14. The rare inhibitor of P_1 is believed to be linked to the *P* locus.
    (Inheritance)

15. The P^k antigen has been demonstrated on the cultured fibroblasts of practically all P_1 and P_2 individuals.
    (The Phenotype P^k)

16. The *Luke* gene is believed to segregate independently of the P^1P^2 genes.
    (The Luke Phenotype)

17. Hydatid cyst fluid cannot be stored.
    (P_1 Substance in Hydatid Cyst Fluid)

18. Anti-P_1 is usually stimulated by transfusion.
    (Anti-P_1)

19. It has been suggested that anti-PP_1P^k may be associated with habitual abortion.
    (Anti-PP_1P^k)

20. Anti-P_1 antisera reactive at 15° C or higher is preferable to those reactive at 4° C, where other cold agglutinins may interfere with the results.
    (Techniques)

GENERAL REFERENCES

1. Boorman, K. E., Dodd, B. E., and Lincoln, P. J.: Blood Group Serology, 5th Ed. Churchill Livingstone, New York, 1977. *(General coverage including techniques for typing with anti-P_1. Writing is clear and easy to follow.)*

2. Issitt, P. D., and Issitt, C. H.: Applied Blood Group Serology. 2nd Ed. Spectra Biologicals, 1975. *(Good general coverage of the P blood group system.)*

3. Mollison, P. L.: Blood Transfusion in Clinical Medicine. 6th Ed. Blackwell Scientific Publications, Oxford, 1979. *(Good general coverage – particularly useful with respect to clinical aspects.)*

4. Race, R. R., and Sanger, R.: Blood Groups in Man. 6th Ed. Blackwell Scientific Publications, Oxford, 1975. *(Detailed coverage of antigens and antibodies in system; laboratory viewpoint.)*

12

THE Ii BLOOD GROUP SYSTEM

OBJECTIVES — THE Ii BLOOD GROUP SYSTEM

The student shall know, understand and be prepared to explain:

1. A brief history of the discovery of the Ii blood group system
2. The inheritance of Ii blood group characters
3. The antigens of the Ii blood group system, specifically to include characteristics of:
   (a) I-adult
   (b) I-cord
   (c) i-adult
   (d) i-cord
   (e) I^T
4. The number of I and i antigen sites on the red cells
5. The I antigen in other species
6. The I antigen on leukocytes and in body fluids, specifically to include:
   (a) Leukocytes
   (b) Saliva
   (c) Milk
   (d) Amniotic fluid
   (e) Urine
   (f) Ovarian cyst fluid and hydatid cyst fluid
   (g) Plasma
7. The I antigen in disease states
8. The antibodies of the Ii blood group system (characteristics), specifically to include:
   (a) Anti-I
   (b) Anti-i
   (c) Anti-I^T
   (d) Anti-HI, −AI, −BI, −Hi and −Bi
   (e) Anti-P$_1$I and −P$_1$I^T
   (f) Anti-HILe^b
9. The clinical significance of Ii antibodies
10. The chemistry of Ii antigenic determinants
11. The heterogenicity of anti-I
12. The techniques used in the detection and identification of anti-I and anti-i

Introduction

For many years an agglutinin, apparently reactive with all human red cells, had been recognized in the serum of persons suffering from acquired hemolytic anemia. The antibody was of the cold type (i.e., reactive at or below room temperature).

In 1956, Wiener *et al* recognized the specificity of this cold agglutinin in an individual with hemolytic anemia whose red cells were found to be compatible with 5 out of 22,000 donor samples. The antibody was called anti-I and the corresponding antigen, I. Wiener *et al* (1956) recognized that a few individuals existed who appeared to lack or who had very little I, and this very rare phenotype was denoted i. The I antigen of "normal" individuals was found to be of varying strength.

Four years later, in 1960, two examples of anti-I were discovered in individuals who pos-

sessed very little I. This precipitated an investigation in which 50 sera thought to contain "nonspecific cold agglutinins" were found to have anti-I specificity (Jenkins *et al*, 1960; Tippett *et al*, 1960). These studies led to the discovery of anti-i by March and Jenkins (1960, 1961).

Most normal sera contain some anti-I. The majority of these antibodies are only clinically significant when they are reactive at a temperature of around 30° C or higher. It should be noted, however, that the presence of anti-I may mask the presence of other clinically important antibodies.

Inheritance

Tippett *et al* (1960) produced a family study providing the first evidence that the I groups are inherited characters, though in this system the manner of inheritance is not straightforward.

Infants, it was found, rarely possess the I antigen; most appear to be of the phenotype i. During the first 18 months of life, however, the red cells gradually come to react strongly with anti-I and weakly with anti-i. The I reactivity then appears to be retained by healthy persons throughout life.

Marsh *et al* (1970) subsequently found that the I antigen has a mosaic structure. I^F (fetal) is the name given to that part of the antigen present in fetal cells and in the cells of i adults, and I^D (developed) to that part which is developed after the first 18 months of life.

The genes that control the Ii specificity, therefore, are thought not to be concerned with the placement of specificity on a preformed substrate but with assistance or nonassistance in the development of i into I. A very common gene (say Z) has been postulated to be necessary for the development of fetal i antigen into I (Jenkins and Marsh, 1961, cited by Race and Sanger, 1975). If this is so, then i-adult is not homozygous *ii* but homozygous *zz*, and is therefore unable to convert i to I.

It should be noted that the I groups are not controlled from the *AB, H* or *P* loci, yet they are in some way entangled with these systems (see later discussion).

THE ANTIGENS OF THE Ii BLOOD GROUP SYSTEM

I-Adult. The I antigen in randomly selected adults shows a great range of strength that fits a normal distribution curve in titration tests (Race and Sanger, 1958) yet I strength in one individual appears to be a constant property of the cells.

The red cells of almost all healthy adults have the I antigen (Wiener *et al*, 1956; Jenkins *et al*, 1960; Tippett *et al*, 1960).

I-Cord. Jenkins *et al* (1960) and Tippett *et al* (1960) found that very weak reactions could be obtained with a powerful anti-I with cord red cells. Marsh *et al* (1971) reported qualitative and quantitative differences in the I antigen of cord and adult red cells.

i-Adult and i-Cord. A very few "normal" adults have little or no I antigen and are classified as belonging to the rare phenotype i. Red cells that fail completely to react with anti-I are classed as i_1. The phenotype is usually found in white persons. Red cells of phenotype i_2 have a small amount of I antigen, are usually from

black persons, and are slightly less rare. While both of these phenotypes and that on cord cells were originally designated i, the following notation has been suggested (see Marsh and Jenkins, 1960, 1961):
1. i_1: fail to react with anti-I, found as a rarity in whites
2. i_2: react weakly with anti-I, found as a rarity in blacks
3. i-cord: found in all cord samples
4. $I_{(Int)}$: found in individuals thought to be heterozygous for I
5. I: found in adults

The phenotypes i_1 and i_2 can be distinguished by the amount of I antigen on the red cells and by absorption tests; i_1 have less I antigen than i_2 and i_2 red cells will absorb some anti-I from the serum of an i_1 individual.

Cord red cells react weakly with anti-I and strongly with anti-i (Marsh and Jenkins, 1960).

I^T. Booth *et al* (1966) detected a cold agglutinin in 76 per cent of the coastal populations of Papua and New Guinea. The antigen was found to be powerful on cord cells, weaker on normal adult cells and weaker still on adult i cells. The name I^T was chosen because the antigen appeared to be best expressed during the "transition" from i to I. However, the description may not be entirely appropriate, since fetal red cells have been found to react more strongly than cord red cells with anti-I^T (Garratty *et al*, 1972).

The Number of I and i Antigen Sites on Red Cells

Evans *et al* (1965) estimated the number of I antigen sites on adult red cells to be 5×10^5, a number confirmed by Rosse *et al* (1966) using PNH red cells. Doinel *et al* (1976) reported the number to be only 1×10^5, suggesting that the higher figure of Evans and associates might have been due to the presence of aggregates in the preparation of ^{125}I-labeled anti-I.

Doinel *et al* (1976) also found the number of i sites on cord red cells to be between 0.2 and 0.65×10^5.

The I Antigen in Other Species

The I antigen has been found on the red cells of many species of animals — rabbits, sheep, cattle and kangaroos (Curtain, 1969). Anti-I can therefore be classified as a heterophile antibody.

The I Antigen on Leukocytes and in Body Fluids

Leukocytes. The I and i antigens can be demonstrated on leukocytes in agglutination tests (Lalezari and Murphy, 1967) or in cytotoxicity tests (Lalezari, 1970). Shumak *et al* (1971), studying three examples of potent anti-i and one of anti-I, showed that the Ii antigens are present on both adult and cord lymphocytes, that they had the same specificity as those present on red blood cells, and that the antibodies were lymphocytotoxic at 25° C. Prozanski *et al* (1975) showed that anti-I and anti-i kill both T and B peripheral lymphocytes and about one third of monocytes and granulocytes.

Saliva. Saliva has been found to inhibit rare examples of anti-I (Dzierzkowa-Borodej *et al*, 1971) and anti-i (Burnie, 1973). The amount of I substance is relatively high in infants at birth and in adult-i individuals, and is not related to the amount of ABH, Lewis or Sd^a substances present. The I antigens of the red cell and secretions are therefore known to develop independently.

Milk. Human milk has been found to contain more I substance than does saliva (Marsh *et al*, 1970), using inhibition tests with allo- or auto-anti-I sera. I substance has also been found in the milk of an i woman (in amounts comparable to I milk) whose allo-anti-I was inhibited by her own milk (Marsh *et al*, 1972).

Amniotic Fluid. Amniotic fluid was shown to contain I inhibiting substance with the same properties as that in milk (Cooper, 1970). Abbal (1971) also found i-inhibiting substance in amniotic fluid.

Urine. Urine has been found to contain small amounts of I substance (Cooper, 1970) and i substance (Abbal, 1971).

Ovarian Cyst Fluid and Hydatid Cyst Fluid. Both of these fluids have been found to inhibit some anti-I sera (Burnie, 1973; Tegoli *et al*, 1967) and some anti-i sera (Burnie, 1973; Marsh, 1961).

Plasma. The i antigen is known to be present in plasma (DeBoissezon *et al*, 1970; Burnie, 1973) at a concentration of 100 to 1300 ng/ml (Slayter *et al*, 1974). Studies by Rouger *et al* (1979) revealed the I antigen in plasma. There appeared to be no reciprocal relationship between the levels of I and i antigens in plasma as there is on the red cell membrane.

THE I AND i ANTIGENS IN DISEASE

The I Antigen. The strength of the I antigen of red cells has been found to be decreased in certain cases of leukemia (Jenkins and Marsh, 1961; McGinniss *et al*, 1964). In one reported case, it was found that the I antigen was depressed and the i antigen increased so that the normal reciprocal relationship of Ii strength was maintained (Jenkins *et al*, 1965).

Red cells treated with extracts of mycoplasma (PPLO) are less well agglutinated by anti-I (Schmidt *et al*, 1965). The relationship of mycoplasma to I specificity is discussed under the heading Anti-I.

The i Antigen. In certain hematologic disorders (e.g., thalassemia major) the strength of the i antigen is increased beyond the normal without any complementary decrease in I antigen (Giblett and Crookston, 1964). Increased agglutinability with anti-i has been found in patients with hypoplastic anemia, sideroblastic anemia, megaloblastic anemia, chronic hemolytic states and acute leukemia (Giblett and Crookston, 1964; Cooper *et al*, 1968). The phenotype i has also been associated with congenital cataract in Japanese people (Ogata *et al*, 1979). A high agglutination score with anti-i was also noted in patients with hereditary erythroblastic multinuclearity with a positive acidified-serum test (HEMPAS) by Crookston *et al*, 1969. The red cells of these patients were found in most cases to be susceptible to lysis both by anti-i and anti-I; this was thought to be due in the case of anti-I to increased uptake of antibody by the red cells (Lewis *et al*, 1970) and to an increased sensitivity to complement (Crookston *et al*, 1969b).

The i antigen reactivity with anti-i in "normal" individuals can be increased by repeated phlebotomy — a fact that led Hillman and Giblett (1965) to suggest that there was an inverse relationship between i reactivity and marrow transit time. It is notable, however, that there is no change in the strength of I or H antigens as the marrow transit time shortens (see Race and Sanger, 1975).

THE ANTIBODIES OF THE Ii BLOOD GROUP SYSTEM

Anti-I. Anti-I is a common autoantibody — particularly in patients suffering from acquired hemolytic anemia of the cold antibody type (see Chapter 15). It is also found as a weak cold agglutinin in the serum of "normal" individuals (Tippett *et al*, 1960). Allo-anti-I is rare, owing to the rarity of i individuals, but it is found in the serum of most i subjects (Jenkins *et al*, 1960; Tippett *et al*, 1960), though enzyme tests may be necessary to demonstrate it. The

THE Ii BLOOD GROUP SYSTEM

antibody varies a little according to the i pheno-type of the subject: in i_1 individuals, the an-tibody fails to react with i_1 and i_2 red cells, whereas in i_2 individuals the antibody does react (though weakly) with i_2 red cells and these cells can absorb some anti-I from these sera. Allo-anti-I does not reveal the gradation of an-tigen strength in I people so clearly revealed by auto-anti-I.

Virtually all anti-I antibodies are IgM and have the ability to bind complement. In sero-logic tests, the antibody usually reacts best at cold temperatures and weakly or not at all with cord red cells.

Anti-I cold autoagglutinins commonly show a transient increase in titer following infection with *Mycoplasma pneumoniae*, re-sulting in an episode of hemolytic anemia in occasional patients.

Anti-i. Anti-i was first described as a cold autoagglutinin in the serum of a patient with reticulosis (Marsh and Jenkins, 1960). The same authors later found two more examples of the antibody, also in patients suffering from some kind of reticulosis, one of whom died from hemolytic anemia. A fourth example was found in a patient suffering from myeloid leukemia (van Loghem *et al*, 1962).

In 1965, transient auto-anti-i was found in the serum of individuals suffering from infec-tious mononucleosis (Jenkins *et al*, 1965; Ro-senfield *et al*, 1965), and in 1967 an antibody presumed to be anti-i was found to be not uncommon in the serum of patients suffering from alcoholic cirrhosis (Rubin and Solomon, 1967).

Anti-i is usually IgM but can be IgG (see Capra *et al*, 1969). Like anti-I, the antibody reacts best with saline-suspended red cells at cold temperatures. No example of allo-anti-i has been described.

Anti-I^T. Anti-I^T antibodies are found in a high proportion of Melanesians (Curtain *et al*, 1965; Booth and MacGregor, 1966), in the coast-al populations of Papua and New Guinea (Booth *et al*, 1966) and in the Yanomama Indians in the Upper Orinoco River of Venezuela (Layrisse and Layrisse, 1968). Garratty *et al* (1972) found the antibody in a white patient with Hodgkin's disease, occurring as a warm IgG alloantibody.

Some of the reactions of anti-I^T are de-scribed in the preceding section on the antigen I^T.

Anti-HI, Anti-AI, Anti-BI, Anti-Hi and Anti-Bi. These compound antibodies react only when both antigens are present on the red cells. Of those listed, anti-HI is the most com-mon. Like anti-H, anti-HI reacts most strongly

with group O red cells and most weakly with A_1B red cells. Of the others, anti-AI was de-scribed by Tippett *et al* (1960); anti-BI by Tegoli *et al* (1967); anti Hi by Bird and Wing-ham (1977) and anti-Bi by Pinkerton *et al* (1977).

Anti-P_1I, Anti-P_1I^T. Tippett *et al* (1960) observed that certain anti-I sera were inhibited or partly inhibited by hydatid cyst fluid. This suggested a link between the I and the P blood group system. Issitt *et al* (1968) recorded anoth-er link when he reported four anti-P_1 sera that reacted with P_1 red cells only when the cells also contained I. The antibody was called anti-P_1I. Anti-P_1I^T, which reacts only with red cells containing the I^T and P_1 antigens, was de-scribed by Booth (1970).

Anti-HILe^b. Described by Tegoli *et al* (1971), this antibody was found to agglutinate red cells that were O, I, Le(a−b+) or A_2, I, Le(a−b+). The antibody was inhibited by sali-va containing I, H and Le^b.

The Clinical Significance of Ii Antibodies

Anti-I has never been implicated as the cause of hemolytic disease of the newborn, being almost invariably IgM. Most examples of anti-I do not cause hemolytic transfusion reactions. However, occasional examples that react at 30 to 37° C *in vitro* produce variable degrees of destruction of red cells *in vivo* that are well correlated with their thermal range *in vitro*. After transfusion of I-positive blood to patients with cold agglutinin disease there may be a substantial destruction of the transfused red cells in the first few hours, presumably until the cells have become resistant to complement-mediated lysis by anti-I.

Anti-i was once implicated as the cause of hemolytic disease of the newborn (Gerbal *et al*, 1971), but has not been known to be the cause of hemolytic transfusion reaction.

OTHER NOTES ABOUT I AND i

An I−i− Phenotype. Joshi and Bhatia (1979) found seven examples of bloods in In-dian donors that failed to react with both anti-I and anti-i, suggesting that these samples had the phenotype I−i−. These samples were found to react weakly with anti-I^T.

Chemistry of the Ii Antigenic Determi-nants. Little is known about the structure of the I and i antigens, probably because the corresponding antibodies are very heterogeneous. It has been suggested, however, that the I antigen may be a branched carbohydrate chain attached at an early stage in the biosynthetic pathway of the ABH antigens (Feizi *et al*, 1971; Gardas, 1976). The Ii antigens occur in secretions as glycoproteins, as does the i antigen in plasma (Cooper and Brown, 1973).

Heterogenicity of Anti-I. It has been suggested that the I antigen is a mosaic and that two main types of anti-I are directed at different parts of the mosaic (Jenkins and Marsh, 1961).

Some anti-I sera react fairly strongly with i_1 and i-cord cells — others scarcely react at all with cord red cells.

TECHNIQUES

For discussion on the detection and identification of anti-I and anti-i, refer to Antibody Identification and Titration, Chapter 22.

TYPICAL EXAMINATION QUESTIONS

Choose the phrase, sentence or symbol that correctly answers the question or completes the statement. More than one answer may be correct in each case. Answers are given in the back of the book.

1. During the first 18 months of life
   (a) the red cells come to react strongly with anti-I and weakly with anti-i
   (b) the red cells come to react strongly with anti-i and weakly with anti-I
   (c) there is no change in the Ii antigens
   (d) the i antigen reactivity decreases
   (Inheritance)

2. The I antigen has a mosaic structure. The component parts are called
   (a) I^D and I^C
   (b) I^F and I^C
   (c) I^D and I^F
   (d) I^A and I^B
   (Inheritance)

3. The I groups are controlled from
   (a) the *AB* locus
   (b) the *H* locus
   (c) the *P* locus
   (d) none of the above
   (Inheritance)

4. The I antigen in randomly selected adults
   (a) shows a great range of strength
   (b) shows weak reactions with anti-I
   (c) shows qualitative and quantitative differences on red cells
   (d) shows constant strength on the red cells of any one individual
   (I-Adult, I-Cord)

5. The antigen of the I system that reacts weakly with anti-I and is found as a rarity in blacks is designated
   (a) i_1
   (b) i_2
   (c) $I_{(Int)}$
   (d) I
   (i-Adult and i-Cord)

6. The antigen I^T
   (a) is usually powerful on cord red cells

   (b) is usually weak on adult i red cells
   (c) refers to "Transitional" I
   (d) none of the above
   (I^T)

7. The I antigen has been found in the red cells of:
   (a) rabbits
   (b) sheep
   (c) kangaroos
   (d) cattle
   (The I Antigen in Other Species)

8. The I antigen has been found:
   (a) in amniotic fluid
   (b) in urine
   (c) in plasma
   (d) all of the above
   (The I Antigen in Leukocytes and in Body Fluids)

9. The i antigen strength
   (a) is increased in thalassemia major
   (b) is increased in patients with HEMPAS
   (c) can be increased by repeated phlebotomy
   (d) is not affected by disease states, although the I antigen strength is
   (The I and i Antigens in Disease)

10. Anti-I
    (a) is a common autoantibody
    (b) is a common alloantibody
    (c) is usually IgM
    (d) commonly shows a transient increase in titer following infection with *Mycoplasma pneumoniae*
    (Anti-I)

11. Anti-i
    (a) has never been implicated as the cause of hemolytic disease of the newborn
    (b) is not uncommon in the serum of individuals suffering from infectious mononucleosis
    (c) is usually IgG
    (d) reacts best with saline-suspended red cells at cold temperatures
    (Anti-i; Clinical Significance of Ii Antibodies)

12. Anti-I
    (a) is clinically insignificant when reactive at 37° C

(b) may be the cause of hemolytic disease of the newborn

(c) may be clinically significant when it reacts at 30 to 37° C *in vitro*

(d) commonly causes hemolytic transfusion reactions

(The Clinical Significance of Ii Antibodies)

ANSWER TRUE OR FALSE

13. Most normal sera contain some anti-I.

(Introduction)

14. The genes that control Ii specificity are known to be directly concerned with the placement of specificity on a preformed substrate.

(Inheritance)

15. Red cells that completely fail to react with anti-I are denoted i_1.

(i-Adult and i-Cord)

16. Fetal red cells have been found to react more strongly than cord red cells with anti-I^T

(I^T)

17. Anti-I cannot be classified as a heterophile antibody.

(The I Antigen in Other Species)

18. The I antigen strength has been found to be increased in certain cases of leukemia.

(The I and i Antigens in Disease)

19. Anti-I antibodies usually bind complement.

(Anti-I)

20. The anti-P_1I^T antibody will fail to react with P_1-negative, I^T-positive red cells.

(Anti-P_1I, Anti-P_1I^T)

GENERAL REFERENCES

1. Burnie, K.: The Ii antigens and antibodies. Can J Med Tech 35:5–26, 1973. *(This paper, which won the Ortho Diagnostics 1972 award in blood bank technique, will provide a clear view of the system to the interested student.)*
2. Mollison, P. L.: Blood Transfusion in Clinical Medicine, 6th Ed. Blackwell Scientific Publications, Oxford, 1979. *(General coverage — particularly useful in terms of clinical aspects.)*
3. Race, R. R. and Sanger, R.: Blood Groups in Man, 6th Ed. Blackwell Scientific Publications, Oxford, 1979. *(General coverage of serological aspects.)*

13

OTHER BLOOD GROUP SYSTEMS: OTHER ANTIGENS ON THE RED CELL SURFACE

OBJECTIVES — OTHER BLOOD GROUP SYSTEMS: OTHER ANTIGENS ON THE RED CELL SURFACE

The student shall know, understand and be prepared to explain:

1. The significant characteristics of antigens in the following blood group systems:
   (a) Diego (Di) blood group system
   (b) Cartwright (Yt) blood group system
   (c) Auberger (Au) blood group system
   (d) Dombrock (Do) blood group system
   (e) Colton (Co) blood group system
   (f) Sid (Sd) blood group system
   (g) Scianna (Sc) blood group system
   (h) Xg blood group system
   (i) Wright (Wr) blood group system

2. The significant characteristics of the following "unrelated" red cell antigens:
   (a) Bg antigens
   (b) The antigen Chido (Chª)
   (c) The antigen Rogers (Rgª)
   (d) Antigens Cost (Csª), York (Ykª), Knops (Knª) and McCoy (McCª)

3. A general understanding of the terms "antigens of high frequency" and "antigens of low frequency" and some examples of these antigens on the red cells.

The following is a short account of blood group antigens that represent independent blood group systems and of other antigens that are as yet unrelated to any existing system. The reader requiring more information on these antigens is referred to Race and Sanger, *Blood Groups in Man*, 6th Edition, 1975.

The Diego (Di) Blood Group System

The antibody anti-Diª was found in a woman whose family was of mixed native Venezuelan and white race and whose infant was affected with hemolytic disease of the newborn (Layrisse *et al*, 1955). The antigen, which appears to be inherited as a dominant character, is extremely rare in whites, but is found in 5 to 15 per cent of Japanese and Chinese people (Layrisse and Arends, 1956) and in 11 per cent of Chippewa Indians (Lewis *et al*, 1956).

Thompson *et al* (1967) discovered the antithetical anti-Diᵇ and described two examples in the original paper. One subject had received a blood transfusion 20 years previously and had then had several normal children, although a second transfusion resulted in a delayed hemolytic transfusion reaction. The other subject had given birth to nine normal children but had never received a blood transfusion.

Both anti-Diª and anti-Diᵇ appear to be best detected by the indirect antiglobulin test and appear not to be enhanced by complement. One example of anti-Diᵇ has been shown to be IgG (Feller *et al*, 1970).

The Cartwright (Yt) Blood Group System

Anti-Ytª was first discovered by Eaton *et al* (1956). The corresponding antigen, Ytª, is very common, occurring in approximately 98 per

160

cent of whites. Many examples of anti-Yt^a have subsequently been described in patients who have been transfused or pregnant or both; "naturally occurring" anti-Yt^a has not been reported.

The antithetical anti-Yt^b was described by Giles and Metaxas (1964). The corresponding antigen, Yt^b, is of low frequency in the white population (approximately 8 per cent). The antibody was eluted from cord red blood cells of a baby whose mother possessed both anti-Yt^b and anti-Kell, though clinical evidence of hemolytic disease of the newborn was not detected (Ferguson et al, 1979).

Anti-Yt^a has caused the rapid destruction of transfused red cells (Bettigole et al, 1968; Gobel et al, 1974; Ballas and Sherwood, 1977; Silvergleid et al, 1977). All examples of anti-Yt^b so far described have been accompanied by other red cell antibodies.

Studies by Eaton et al (1956) and by Giles et al (1967) have shown both Yt^a and Yt^b to be inherited as dominant characters.

The Auberger (Au) Blood Group System

The antibody that defined the antigen Au^a was discovered by Salmon et al (1961). A second example was described in 1971 by Dr. Salmon, Dr. Gerbal and Dr. Tippett in a patient's serum that also contained anti-A, anti-Lu^a, anti-K, anti-Fy^b and anti-Yt^b.

Approximately 82 per cent of English and French people are Au(a+). The antigen appears to be a dominant character.

The rare inhibitor In(Lu) inhibits the Au^a antigen as well as the Lu^a, Lu^b, P$_1$ and i antigens (Crawford et al, 1974). (See Chapter 9.)

The Dombrock (Do) Blood Group System

The first example of anti-Do^a was identified by Swanson et al (1965) and the antithetical anti-Do^b by Molthan et al (1973). Approximately 66 per cent of Northern Europeans are Do(a+) and 82 per cent are Do(b+). The frequency of Do(a+) in Japanese people is reported to be much lower, about 18 per cent (Nakajima et al, 1979; Nakajima and Moulds, 1980). Anti-Do^a gives a positive indirect antiglobulin test only with a minority of otherwise good anti-IgG sera; stronger reactions are obtained with enzyme-treated red cells. The antibody does not appear to bind complement, but has

been shown to be responsible for the destruction of small amounts of Do(a+) red cells (Swanson et al, 1965; Polesky and Swanson, 1966).

Only one example of anti-Do^b has so far been reported.

The Colton (Co) Blood Group System

The antibody that revealed the Colton blood group system was described by Heistö et al (1967); three examples of anti-Co^a were described, all probably immune and one, IgG. A further example stimulated by pregnancy was found by McIntyre et al (1976). The infant had a weakly positive direct antiglobulin test, but no signs of hemolytic disease of the newborn.

Anti-Co^b was discovered by Giles et al (1970). Both antigens, Co^a and Co^b, are inherited as dominant characters; about 99.8 per cent of whites are Co(a+) and about 8 per cent are Co(b+), although the frequency of Co(a−) may be lower among U.S. blacks (Race and Sanger, 1975).

Anti-Co^{a}Co^b was found by Rogers et al (1974) in the serum of a woman whose red cells were Co(a−b−).

The Sid (Sd) Blood Group System

The system that came to be called "Sid" was first investigated at Dundee, Oxford and London with the recognition of an antibody that distinguished itself by agglutinating only a portion of red cells, even of strongly positive reactors (Macvie et al, 1967; Renton et al, 1967). The finding of small agglutinates in a sea of free red cells is, in fact, a useful clue to the identity of anti-Sd^a. About 91 per cent of English people are Sd(a+), although only about 10 per cent of samples react strongly with the antibody.

The Sd^a antigen is not demonstrable on cord red cells, appearing from about 7 months onward. Sd(a+) individuals have Sd^a in their saliva — little or none is found in Sd(a−) individuals (Macvie et al, 1967; Renton et al, 1967). The antigen may be suppressed during pregnancy.

The Sd^a antigen is present in most secretions, with the greatest concentration in urine. It is present in the organs of mammals, is particularly abundant in the kidneys and urine of guinea pigs, but is not present in birds (Pickles and Morton, 1977).

There is approximately four times as much Sd^a in the saliva of newborn infants as in that of adults, and approximately 50 per cent of people with Sd(a−) red cells secrete Sd^a in the urine (Morton et al, 1970). About one half of individuals who have Sd(a−) red cells and who also fail to secrete Sd^a in the urine have anti-Sd^a in their serum. The frequency of the antibody, which is IgM, is believed to be about 1 per cent (Renton et al, 1967).

A hemolytic transfusion reaction caused by anti-Sd^a has been described (Peetermans and Cole-Dergent, 1970), though the majority of examples are clinically insignificant.

An autoagglutinin related to the Sid blood group system (anti-Sd^x) was described by Marsh et al (1980a). This antibody has been associated with immune hemolytic anemia (Marsh et al, 1980b).

The antigen Cad, originally described as a low-frequency antigen by Cazal et al (1968), was subsequently shown to be a very strong form of Sd^a (Sanger et al, 1971; Cazal et al, 1971). Race and Sanger (1975) use the notation Sd(a++) for these rare outstandingly strong reactions and suggest the name "super Sid" as convenient laboratory jargon. Cad red cells, even when group O, are agglutinated by an extract of Dolichos biflorus (previously thought to be only anti-A$_1$) (Cazal et al, 1968). Cad red cells are also agglutinated by snail anti-A (Cazal et al, 1971).

The Scianna (Sc) Blood Group System

Schmidt et al (1962) described an antibody, anti-Sm, to a high-frequency antigen that was found to react with all red cells tested but not with those of the person in whom the antibody was found or with those of three of her five sibs. In 1963, Anderson et al described an antibody, anti-Bu^a, which reacted with the red cells of a very small number of people. The realization that one member of the original family who was Sm-negative was Bu(a+) sparked an investigation that revealed that the Sm and Bu^a antigens were probably controlled by allelic genes (Lewis et al, 1964; Lewis et al, 1974). The system was then named Scianna; the antigen Sm became Sc1 and Bu^a became Sc2 (Lewis et al, 1974).

The genes of the Scianna blood group system, Sc^1 and Sc^2, were shown to be inherited independently of all major established blood group systems by Anderson et al (1963), Giles et al (1970) and Lewis et al (1964). Sc1 and Sc2 are inherited as co-dominant characters (see Anderson et al, 1963; Lewis et al, 1974).

The frequency of Sc2 in Canadian subjects was calculated to be 0.12 per cent (Shanahan, 1975). Gene frequencies among subjects of Northern Europe are given as Sc^1:0.992; Sc^2:0.008 (Mollison, 1979).

Little evidence is available concerning the antigenicity of Sc2, although an example of the antibody anti-Sc2 investigated by Shanahan (1975) was found in a patient who had received only three units of whole blood 30 years before the discovery of the antibody in his serum. This finding presents a good indication of the antigenicity of Sc2, since the likelihood of more than one of these units being Sc2 is extremely remote.

The phenotype Sc:−1, −2 was found by McCreary et al (1973) in two members of a family living in Likiep Atoll of the Marshall Islands. An antibody that reacted with all red cells except those that were Sc:−1, −2 was reported by Nason et al (1980). The antibody, called anti-Sc3, was found not to contain separate specificities when absorption studies were performed. It appeared that all Sc1 or Sc2 red cells are also Sc3, while those that are Sc:−1, −2 are Sc:−3.

The Xg Blood Group System

The Xg blood group system is unique among blood groups in that the relevant genes are carried on the X chromosomes so that in this system alone, males have only one gene instead of two. Only one antigen, determined by the gene Xg^a, has been described, though an allele Xg, which may be amorphic, is postulated.

Males can only be of genotype Xg^a or Xg, whereas females may be Xg^aXg^a, Xg^aXg or $XgXg$. The mating of an Xg(a+) man with an Xg(a−) woman therefore must produce all Xg(a+) daughters and Xg(a−) sons. The Xg^a antigen is carried by 89 per cent of females and 67 per cent of males.

Anti-Xg^a was first described by Mann et al (1962), and further examples soon followed (Cook et al, 1963; Sausais et al, 1964). These antibodies were all found in males who had been repeatedly transfused; they were detectable only by the indirect antiglobulin test. The first two antibodies reacted with both anti-IgG and anti-complement and while the third antibody was not tested with specific anti-complement, there was evidence that it did not bind complement (Sausais et al, 1964). Tests performed by Habibi *et al* (1979), using several examples of anti-Xg[a] and absorption-elution tests, showed that the Xg[a] antigen is destroyed by proteases commonly used in blood group serology (bromelyn, ficin, papain, trypsin and pronase) but not by neuraminidase. One example of auto-anti-Xg[a] has been reported (Yokoyama *et al*, 1967; Yokoyama and McCoy, 1967) and one example that appeared to be "naturally occurring" (Fisher, 1965).

The Wright (Wr) Blood Group System

Anti-Wr[a] was first discovered in the serum of a woman who had given birth to two infants affected with hemolytic disease of the newborn; the antibody was detectable only in the indirect antiglobulin test (Holman, 1953). The corresponding antigen, Wr[a], was found in about 1 in 1000 samples in England by Dunsford (1954) and Cleghorn (1960). The antibody, anti-Wr[a], occurs in about 1 in 100 blood samples and is sometimes "naturally occurring." It is commonly found in the serum of patients who have formed other blood group antibodies and in the serum of patients with autoimmune hemolytic anemia (Cleghorn, cited by Mollison, 1979). Two hemolytic transfusion reactions due to anti-Wr[a] have been reported (van Loghem *et al*, 1955; Metaxas and Metaxas-Bühler, 1963).

"Naturally occurring" anti-Wr[a] usually agglutinates Wr(a+) red cells in saline, reacting more strongly at 20° C than at 37° C.

Anti-Wr[b], which may also be found as a warm autoantibody in patients with autoimmune hemolytic anemia, was described by Adams et al (1971).

OTHER ANTIGENS ON THE RED CELL SURFACE

Numerous antigens not related to any existing blood group system occur on the red cells; these may cause difficulties in routine serologic work. Antigens such as Chido, Rogers, Cost, York, Knops and McCoy show a similar pattern of reactions in serologic tests — they react to a varying extent with serum containing the corresponding antibody (particularly Chido and Rogers). It is fairly common to find that a serum that reacts only moderately strongly with these antigens nevertheless has a high titer. (The description "high titer, low avidity" (HTLA) has been used to describe this behavior.) Weaker reactions are not always reproducible.

Newer techniques have helped to demonstrate these antigens, and with them has come a growing realization that the antigens properly belong to the white cells and have merely "spilled over" onto the red cells.

The following is a brief account of some of these antigens. The interested reader is referred to Race and Sanger, *Blood Groups in Man*, 6th Edition, 1975, for more detailed information.

The Bg Antigens

Antigens that were known for many years as "Ot" (Dorfmeier *et al*, 1959) "Ho" (von der Hart *et al*, 1961) and "Bennett-Goodspeed-Sturgeon" or "Donna" (Buchanan and Afaganis, 1963; Chown *et al*, 1963) were shown by Seaman *et al* (1967) to belong to the same complex. Three antibodies were distinguished in the original paper: anti-Bg[a], anti-Bg[a+b] and Bg[a+b+c], recognizing the antigens, renamed Bg[a], Bg[b] and Bg[c]. A fourth antibody, anti-Bg[b+c], was added later (Kissmeyer-Nielsen and Gavin, 1967). There is evidence that the antibody originally called anti-Stobo (Wallace and Milne, 1959) is also part of the Bg complex.

Morton *et al* (1969) showed that the Bg antigens are in reality HLA antigens (on leukocytes) that demonstrate weakly on red cells. Morton *et al* (1971) revealed that Bg[a] corresponded to HLA-A7, Bg[b] corresponded to HLA-Bw17 and Bg[c] to HLA-A28. This was confirmed by Swanson (1973).

Anti-Bg is not uncommonly present as an "unwanted" antibody in commercial blood typing sera, which may lead to the misinterpretation of test results (Marshall, 1973).

The Antigen Chido (Ch[a])

Anti-Ch[a] gives "nebulous" reactions with Ch(a+) red cells (Harris *et al*, 1967) and is neutralized by the plasma and serum but not the saliva of Ch(a+) individuals (Middleton and Crookston, 1972; Swanson *et al*, 1971). It is absorbed by the leukocytes of Ch(a+) individuals (Swanson *et al*, 1971). Chido substance is present in the plasma of all Chido-positive individuals (approximately 98 per cent of the population). This provides a useful test to confirm the red cell phenotype of Ch(a+) and Ch(a−) samples, since anti-Ch[a] gives a wide range of reactions from very strong to very weak (Middleton and Crookston, 1972). Nordhagen *et* al (1979) report that C4 sucrose/low ionic strength (Liss)–coated red blood cells are excellent for the detection of Chido antigens (and Rogers antigens, discussed in a later section). Autoabsorption of anti-Chido using C4-coated red cells has also been reported (Ellisor *et al*, 1980).

The *Chido* and *HLA* loci are linked (Middleton *et al*, 1974).

Anti-Ch^a does not reduce the survival of Ch(a+) red cells *in vivo* (Moore *et al*, 1975; Tilley *et al*, 1977).

The Antigen Rogers (Rg^a)

Approximately 97 per cent of whites are Rg(a+) (Longster and Giles, 1976), and, like Ch^a, Rg^a is present in the plasma of individuals whose red cells carry the antigen. The *Rogers* locus is linked to the *HLA-B* locus (James *et al*, 1976). A gene for C4 (the fourth component of complement) is also close to the *HLA-B* locus. It has been shown that both Ch^a and Rg^a are, in fact, antigens on C4 molecules (O'Neill *et al*, 1978), the antigens being demonstrable on a tryptic C4d fragment (Tilley *et al*, 1978).

The strength of reaction between Rg(a+) red cells and anti-Rg^a is reduced when enzyme-treated red cells are used. Rg(a+) red cells when stored as a clot have been found to react more strongly than "fresh" cells (Giles, 1977). The detection of Rogers antigens (like Chido) antigens) is enhanced by the use of C4 sucrose/low ionic strength (Liss)–coated red cells (Nordhagen *et al*, 1979).

The Antigens Cost (Cs^a), York (Yk^a), Knops (Kn^a) and McCoy (McC^a)

It is possible that the Cs^a, Yk^a, Kn^a and McC^a antigens are related to one another (Molthan and Moulds, 1975). The association between Yk^a and Cs^a was assumed because, while individuals who produced anti-Yk^a were all Cs(a+) Yk(a−), three early examples of anti-Cs^a were from Cs(a−) Yk(a−) individuals (Molthan *et al*, 1969). Approximately 95 per cent of randomly selected US blood donors react with anti-Yk^a; anti-Cs^a reacts with about 97 per cent of unrelated Europeans (Giles *et al*, 1965). Anti-Cs^a can be distinguished from anti-Yk^a because, unlike anti-Yk^a, it reacts with ficin-treated red cells (Giles, 1977).

The Kn^a (Knops) antigen was first reported by Helgeson *et al* (1970). Many examples of anti-Kn^a have been found. The antigen is very common; only 4 Kn(a−) donors were found in tests on 2091 unrelated individuals in Minneapolis (see Race and Sanger, 1975). The antithetical antigen, Kn^b has recently been described (Mallan *et al*, 1980).

Anti-McC^a (McCoy) was reported by Molthan and Moulds (1975), who established its relationship to anti-Kn^a. The antibody has been associated with hemolytic transfusion reactions and probably with hemolytic disease of the newborn. McC^b, McC^c and McC^d antigens have also been documented (Molthan, 1980).

ANTIGENS OF HIGH FREQUENCY

Many antigens that appear to be separate from all known blood group systems are known to occur on the red cells of the vast majority of randomly selected individuals. These include the antigens Vel (Ve^a) (Sussman and Miller, 1952); Gerbich (Ge) (Rosenfield *et al*, 1960); Lan (van der Hart *et al*, 1961); Gregory (Gy^a) (Swanson *et al*, 1967); Holly (Hy^a) (Moulds *et al*, 1975); At^a (Applethwaite *et al*, 1967) and Jr^a (Stroup and MacIlroy, 1970). These antigens are listed at the end of this text under the heading Antigens in Man. All of the corresponding antibodies react with more than 999 out of 1000 blood samples.

ANTIGENS OF LOW FREQUENCY

These so-called "private" antigens are of extremely low frequency in the random population and are not related or controlled by "established" blood group loci. The list of these antigens continues to grow and include, for example, the antigens Sw^a (Swann) (Cleghorn, 1959), Radin (Rd) (Rausen *et al*, 1967), Peters (Pt^a) (Pinder *et al*, 1969). To be placed in this category an antigen must have an incidence of not more than 1 in 400 in the general population, it must be shown to be a dominant character, it must be unrelated to an established blood group system, it must be defined by a specific antibody and it must still be extant (see Race and Sanger, 1975). Many "private" antigens that meet these criteria are known in specialist laboratories, yet accounts of them remain unpublished.

TYPICAL EXAMINATION QUESTIONS

The following questions relate to all the various blood group systems and antigens, to test understanding of their various modes of behavior. Answers to these questions are given in the back of the book.

Section A: Multiple Choice

Choose the phrase, sentence or symbol that completes the statement or answers the question. More than one answer may be correct in each case.

1. Proteolytic enzymes can be of value in enhancing the reactions of antibodies in which of the following blood group systems?
   (a) Kidd
   (b) Duffy
   (c) Lewis
   (d) Rh

2. Which of the following antibodies is likely not to be "naturally occurring"?
   (a) Anti-N
   (b) Anti-Le^a
   (c) Anti-K
   (d) Anti-M
   (e) Anti-Le^b

3. Which of the following antigens occurs in less than 50 per cent of the general Caucasian population?
   (a) K
   (b) E
   (c) k
   (d) Jk^a

4. Select from the following list those antibodies that are capable of crossing the human placenta in the majority of cases
   (a) Anti-E
   (b) Anti-P$_1$
   (c) Anti-A$_1$
   (d) Anti-$\bar{s}$
   (e) Anti-Fy^a

5. Which of the following blood group systems were discovered by the injection of human red cells into animals?
   (a) The ABO blood group system
   (b) The MNSs blood group system
   (c) The Xg blood group system
   (d) The P blood group system

6. The antigens in which of the following blood group systems commonly bind complement?
   (a) The ABO blood group system
   (b) The Kidd blood group system
   (c) The Lewis blood group system
   (d) The Rh/Hr blood group system

7. Substances in which of the following blood group systems are found in saliva?
   (a) The Rh/Hr blood group system
   (b) The Lewis blood group system
   (c) The Duffy blood group system
   (d) The Kell blood group system

8. The first example of autosomal linkage in man was found between which of the following gene complexes?
   (a) *Lutheran* and *Lewis*
   (b) *Rh* and *Duffy*
   (c) *Lutheran* and *Auberger*
   (d) *Lutheran* and *Secretor*

9. Red cells of individuals with the phenotype O$_h$
   (a) are not agglutinated by anti-D even when the D antigen is present
   (b) are strongly agglutinated by anti-H
   (c) give a negative reaction with anti-A and anti-B
   (d) are always Le(a–b–)

10. Which of the following antibodies reacts with approximately eight out of ten donors?
    (a) Anti-K
    (b) Anti-E
    (c) Anti-P$_1$
    (d) Anti-k

Section B: Fill in the Blanks

11. In the spaces provided, enter either "saline 20° C" or "indirect antiglobulin test" as the first choice of technique for the detection of antibodies that correspond to the following blood group antigens:

    (a) B _____

    (b) M _____

    (c) P$_1$ _____

    (d) c _____

    (e) Fy^a _____

    (f) Jk^a _____

    (g) Le^a _____

    (h) D _____

    (i) Le^b _____

    (j) S _____

    (k) $\bar{s}$ _____

    (l) K _____

12. The genes *Lele* interact with the _____, _____ and _____ genes.

13. The genes of the Xg blood group system are carried on the _____ chromosome.

14. In the spaces provided, place the letter "A" for antibodies that commonly bind complement, "B" for antibodies that appear not to bind complement and "C" for antibodies that sometimes bind complement.

(a) anti-f _____

(b) anti-D _____

(c) anti-Fy^a _____

(d) anti-Jk^a _____

(e) anti-B _____

(f) anti-Le^b _____

(g) anti-K _____

(h) anti-Lu^a _____

(i) anti-c _____

(j) anti-P$_1$ _____

15. An individual of group B Le(a–b+) who is a secretor will secrete _____, _____, - and _____ substances in saliva.

Section C: Matching Answers

16. Enter the system name from column two to which the antibodies in column one belong:

COLUMN 1	COLUMN 2
(a) anti-f	Vel
(b) anti-Do^a	Diego
(c) anti-Js^a	Penney
(d) anti-H	S
(e) anti-Fy^a	Lewis
(f) anti-Yt	Rh/Hr
(g) anti-Jk^b	MNSs
(h) anti-Be^a	Cartwright
(i) anti-Di^a	Dombrock
(j) anti-S	Kidd
	Xg
	P
	Kell
	Lewis
	ABO
	Duffy

Section D: True or False

17. Saline-reacting antibodies are always IgG.
18. Complement is required for the antigen-antibody union of most Rh antibodies.
19. The I antigen occurs in almost all individuals.
20. The phenotype Lu(a–b–) may reflect dominant inheritance.
21. Anti-Fy^a commonly occurs as a cold agglutinin.
22. The antibody anti-PP$_1$P^k was originally known as anti-Tj^a.
23. Lewis types are determined by allelic genes Le^a and Le^b.
24. Anti-Jk3 is anti-Jk^a + anti-Jk^b, which are inseparable.
25. The Miltenberger complex of antigens form part of the MNSs blood group system.

GENERAL REFERENCES

1. Boorman, K. E., Dodd, B. E. and Lincoln, P. J.: Blood Group Serology: Theory, Techniques, Practical Applications, 5th Ed. Churchill Livingstone, 1977. (*General text — useful for study in that the "oddities" of each system have been grouped in separate chapters, preceded in earlier chapters by discussion of basic principles.*)
2. Cleghorn, T. E.: A 'new' human blood group antigen, Sw^3. Nature 184:1324, 1959.
3. Erskine, A. G. and Socha, W. W.: Principles and practice of Blood Grouping, 3rd Ed. Blackwell-Mosby, 1980. (*General text — coverage of the blood group systems emphasizes Wiener's approach.*)
4. Issitt, P. D. and Issitt, C. H.: Applied Blood Group Serology. Spectra Biologicals, 1975. (*Comprehensive coverage of the blood group systems. A valuable source of reference.*)
5. Mollison, P. L.: Blood Transfusion in Clinical Medicine, 6th Ed. Blackwell Scientific Publications, 1979. (*Useful reference to the blood group systems. Emphasis on clinical aspects.*)
6. Race, R. R. and Sanger, R.: Blood Groups in Man, 6th Ed. Blackwell Scientific Publications, 1975. (*By far the most extensive coverage of the blood group systems. Invaluable source of reference.*)

WHITE CELL ANTIGENS

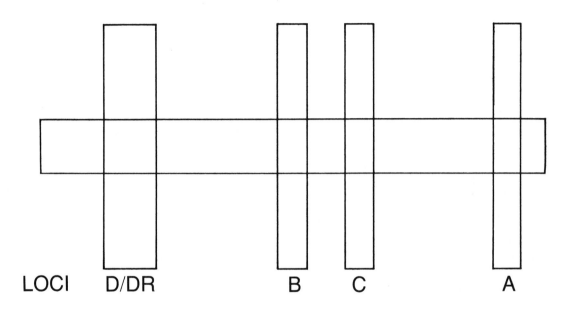

LOCI   D/DR   B   C   A

THE HLA SYSTEM

OBJECTIVES — THE HLA SYSTEM

The student shall know, understand and be prepared to explain:
1. A brief history of the discovery of the HLA system
2. The system of nomenclature in the HLA system, including previous and original nomenclatures
3. The genetics of the HLA system
4. The antigens of the HLA system, specifically to include:
   (a) Frequencies
   (b) Linkage disequilibrium
   (c) Cross reactions
   (d) The HLA antigens and disease
   (e) The HLA antigens on red cells
5. The applications of HLA antigen typing, specifically to include:

(a) Transplantation
(b) Transfusion
(c) Disease
(d) Paternity testing
6. The antibodies of the HLA system, specifically to include:
   (a) Characteristics and occurrence
   (b) The role of HLA antibodies in febrile transfusion reactions
7. Techniques, specifically to include:
   (a) The microlymphocytotoxicity test
   (b) The EDTA leukoagglutination assay
   (c) Tests for leukocyte antibodies

Introduction

Dausset (1954) was first in reporting the presence of antibodies in the serum of multi-transfused patients that agglutinated the lymphocytes of certain individuals (see also Dausset and Nenna, 1952). The first leukocyte antigen, named Mac (now HLA-A2), was described by Dausset (1958) and was found to be present in about 60 per cent of the French population. This, and the discovery that identical twins showed concordant reaction patterns, strongly suggested that the leukocyte markers were genetically controlled. Payne and Rolfs (1958) and van Rood et al (1958) reported the discovery of leukoagglutinating antibodies (leukoagglutinins) and cytotoxic antibodies (cytotoxins) in the sera of pregnant women. Approximately 10 to 25 per cent of all pregnancy sera were found by Nymand et al (1971); Escolar and Mueller-Eckhardt (1971); Bertrams et al (1971) and Wolf (1971) to contain lymphocytotoxic antibodies against HLA antigens inherited from the father. These antibodies revealed further leukocyte antigens, a large proportion of

which were found to be present not only on the white blood cells but also on all nucleated body cells.

Further discoveries about the HLA system came from the introduction of suitable methodology for testing and the development of suitable statistical methods for result analysis. The microlymphocytotoxicity test (see under the heading Techniques) was described by Terasaki and McClelland (1964) and Kissmeyer-Nielsen and Kjerbye (1967).

The HLA system is now recognized as the major histocompatibility system of humans, the antigens being second in importance only to the ABO antigens in organ transplantation. The system is used in clinical medicine and medical research in areas of renal and bone marrow transplantation, platelet and granulocyte transfusion, disease associations and disputed paternity testing. The system is also important to the immunohematologist because HLA antibodies can lead to febrile transfusion reactions and because HLA antibodies can also form troublesome contaminants in blood group typing sera.

169

The Nomenclature of the HLA System

The HLA system is probably the most polymorphic system in man. Its nomenclature has evolved as the genetics have become clarified, and consequently many changes have been made in nomenclature during its relatively short history.

Based on early findings, van Rood (1962) and Payne *et al* (1964) described two loci: 4 (or Four) and LA (respectively), both of which had multiple alleles. In 1967, a nomenclature committee was established by the World Health Organization (WHO), which standardized the nomenclature of the genetic loci and their respective alleles and gene products (antigens). The two loci, Four and LA, were combined into a system called HL-A. The different alleles were assigned numbers, in sequential order of discovery or final definition. This system was slightly modified and expanded in 1970, when numbers began to be assigned to the newly discovered antigens. These numbers were provisional and were preceded by the letter W, indicating "workshop" (e.g., HL-AW15, HL-AW19, etc). When an antigen was converted to a recognized HLA specificity, the prefix W was dropped. The system still caused confusion, however, since it was not immediately obvious whether an antigen belonged to the LA or the Four locus; therefore, the nomenclature committee, which met at the Histocompatibility Testing Workshop in Aarhus (1975), corrected this drawback and introduced the system that is in general use today.

(i) The entire major histocompatibility complex of man was called HLA (Human Leukocyte Antigen). The hyphen between L and A was deleted.

(ii) The gene loci were designated by letters, A, B, C, D. A hyphen was inserted between HLA and the gene locus description (e.g., HLA-A, HLA-B, *etc*). The LA-locus therefore became HLA-A and the Four locus, HLA-B. Two other loci, originally called AJ and MLC, have become HLA-C and HLA-D, respectively.

(iii) The assigned numbers were retained; however, each number was preceded by the letter of the appropriate gene locus (e.g., HLA-A2, HLA-B5).

(iv) The provisional letter W became w (lower case) for antigens that had not been sufficiently defined. This was dropped when the specificity became officially recognized (e.g., HLA-Aw33, HLA-Bw16).

(v) The phenotype of an individual was written as (for example) HLA-A1, 2, B8, 12 or preferably HLA-A1, A2, B8, B12. The genotype of this individual was written as HLA-A2, B8/A1, B12 or HLA-A2, B12/A1, B8 (if only *A* and *B* loci are considered).

The Genetics of the HLA System

The expression of the HLA antigens on the cell surface is controlled by a region on chromosome No. 6 in humans. At the present time, this region appears to be subdivided into four major loci, at each of which are many alleles (Fig. 14–1).

Allelic genes at the HLA-A, HLA-B and HLA-C loci control the expression of antigens that can be detected using serologic methods (e.g., lymphocytotoxicity). The HLA-D locus was first defined using cellular techniques (i.e., proliferation in a primary mixed leukocyte culture). The antigens themselves were termed "lymphocyte defined" (LD) as opposed to the "serologically defined" (SD) antigens produced by genes at the other three loci. More recently, however, it has been found that certain antigens associated with HLA-D can be detected by serological methods, and these are referred to as DR (D-related) antigens.

The presently recognized antigens of HLA, both as detected by serologic methods and by the primary mixed leukocyte culture response to homozygous typing cells, are given in Table 14–1. Each individual possesses a pair of No. 6 chromosomes, like all other autosomes, and each chromosome has four HLA loci. At each locus, any one of the alleles that belong to the corresponding series may be present. If an individual is heterozygous at all four loci, he will have as many as ten HLA antigens (taking both D and DR antigens into account) (Fig. 14–2).

As can be seen (Table 14–1), the HLA-A and HLA-B loci are very markedly polymorphic — the antigens of which can all be recognized by different serums. The HLA-C locus does not appear to be as polymorphic as HLA-A

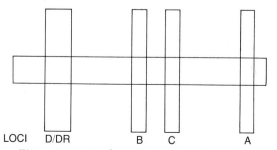

Figure 14–1 A schematic representation of the HLA complex on autosome #6. (From Bach, 1980.)

Table 14–1 THE PRESENTLY RECOGNIZED ANTIGENS OF THE HLA SYSTEM

HLA-A	HLA-B		HLA-Cw1	HLA-D
HLA-A1	HLA-B5	HLA-Bw44	HLA-Cw1	HLA-Dw1
HLA-A2	HLA-B7	HLA-Bw45	HLA-Cw2	HLA-Dw2
HLA-A3	HLA-B8	HLA-Bw46	HLA-Cw3	HLA-Dw3
HLA-A9	HLA-B12	HLA-Bw47	HLA-Cw4	HLA-Dw4
HLA-A10	HLA-B13	HLA-Bw48	HLA-Cw5	HLA-Dw5
HLA-A11	HLA-14	HLA-Bw49	HLA-Cw6	HLA-Dw6
HLA-A25	HLA-B15	HLA-Bw50	HLA-Cw7	HLA-Dw7
HLA-A26	HLA-B17	HLA-Bw51	HLA-Cw8	HLA-Dw8
HLA-A28	HLA-B18	HLA-Bw52		HLA-Dw9
HLA-A29	HLA-B27	HLA-Bw53		HLA-Dw10
HLA-Aw19	HLA-B37	HLA-Bw54		HLA-Dw11
HLA-Aw23	HLA-B40	HLA-Bw55		HLA-Dw12
HLA-Aw24	HLA-Bw4	HLA-Bw56		
HLA-Aw30	HLA-Bw6	HLA-Bw57		HLA-DR1
HLA-Aw31	HLA-Bw16	HLA-Bw58		HLA-DR2
HLA-Aw32	HLA-Bw21	HLA-Bw59		HLA-DR3
HLA-Aw33	HLA-Bw22	HLA-Bw60		HLA-DRw4
HLA-Aw34	HLA-Bw35	HLA-Bw61		HLA-DR5
HLA-Aw36	HLA-Bw38	HLA-Bw62		HLA-DRw6
HLA-Aw43	HLA-Bw39	HLA-Bw63		HLA-DR7
	HLA-Bw41	HLA-Bw4*		HLA-DRw8
	HLA-Bw42	HLA-Bw6*		HLA-DRw9
				HLA-DRw10

*The following are generally agreed inclusions of HLA-B specificities into Bw4 and Bw6:
Bw4: B13, B27, B38 (wlb), Bw44(12), Bw47, Bw49 (w21), Bw51 (5), Bw52 (5), Bw53, Bw57 (17), Bw58 (17), Bw59, Bw63 (15)
Bw6: B7, B8, B14, B18, Bw35, Bw39 (w16), Bw41, Bw42, Bw45 (12), Bw46, Bw48, Bw50 (w21), Bw54 (w22), Bw55 (w22), Bw56 (w22), Bw60 (40), Bw61 (40), Bw62 (15)

and HLA-B. The relationship of the HLA-D to the HLA-DR antigens is not well understood: a given HLA-D antigen is most frequently found in a given population with a given HLA-DR antigen (for the sake of convenience, one refers to an individual having HLA-Dw1 as having HLA-DR1). There is evidence to suggest that the determinants recognized by cellular re-

HLA-A1	A locus	HLA-A9
HLA-Cw2	C locus	HLA-Cw5
HLA-B7	B locus	HLA-B14
HLA-Dw1 ⎫		HLA-Dw4
HLA-DR1 ⎭ D locus		HLA-DRw4

CHROMOSOME PAIR NUMBER 6

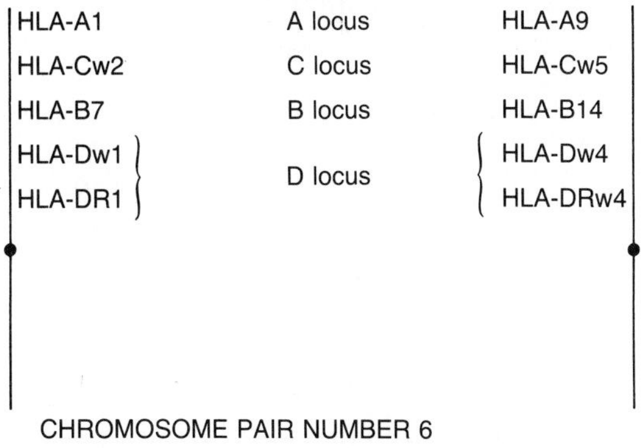

Figure 14–2 A pair of autosomal chromosomes (#6) showing the HLA antigens of an individual.

sponse and by serologic methods are different (see Reinsmoen *et al*, 1979; also *Histocompatibility Testing 1977:* Munksgaard, 1978, p. 360).

The antigens of the HLA system are inherited as mendelian co-dominant characters. Since an individual will inherit one chromosome No. 6 *paternally* and one chromosome No. 6 *maternally*, it follows that five genes (one at each locus, taking into account the DR antigens) will be inherited as a "package" from one parent, and five genes will be inherited as a package from the other parent. Each inherited chromosomal region, composed of five genes, is called a *haplotype*, although this term is also generally used if not all genes are known or tested for. (If only the A and B loci are tested in the example given in Figure 14–2, the results HLA-A1, B7 *and* HLA-A9, B14 would be referred to as "haplotypes".) An individual therefore inherits *two* haplotypes, one from each parent (Fig. 14–3). Considering only the A and B loci illustrated in Figure 14–3 (for the sake of clarity), the child's *phenotype* would be given

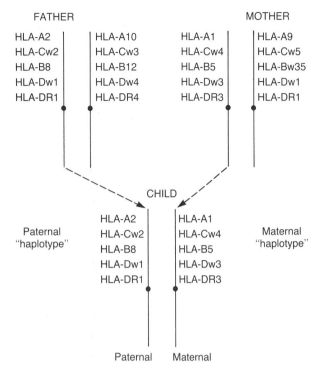

FATHER   MOTHER

HLA-A2 | HLA-A10   HLA-A1 | HLA-A9
HLA-Cw2 | HLA-Cw3   HLA-Cw4 | HLA-Cw5
HLA-B8 | HLA-B12   HLA-B5 | HLA-Bw35
HLA-Dw1 | HLA-Dw4   HLA-Dw3 | HLA-Dw1
HLA-DR1 | HLA-DR4   HLA-DR3 | HLA-DR1

CHILD

Paternal   HLA-A2   HLA-A1   Maternal
"haplotype"   HLA-Cw2   HLA-Cw4   "haplotype"
                HLA-B8   HLA-B5
                HLA-Dw1   HLA-Dw3
                HLA-DR1   HLA-DR3

Paternal   Maternal

Figure 14–3   The inheritance of HLA haplotypes.

as HLA-A2, HLA-A1, A2, B5, B8, HLA-B5. The *genotype* of the child would be HLA-A2, B8/A1, B5, assuming, of course, that parentage is not in question and that recombination (or crossing-over) has not occurred.

The crossing-over rate (frequency) in the HLA system has been variously estimated to be from about 1 in 10,000 (0.011) to about 1 in 18,000 (0.0056) (see Cross *et al*, 1975), although some workers have reported it to be probably as high as 1 per cent (see Boorman *et al*, 1977). This must be borne in mind in theoretic considerations, particularly related to linkage disequilibrium and in paternity testing. An example of crossing-over between the genes of the maternal *A* and *B* loci is shown in Figure 14–4.

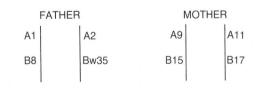

FATHER   MOTHER

A1 | A2   A9 | A11

B8 | Bw35   B15 | B17

Child No. 1   Child No. 2   Child No. 3

A1 | A9   A2   A9 | A1   A11

B8 | B15 Bw35 B17 | B8   B17

Figure 14–4   An example of maternal recombination (crossing-over) between the *A* and *B* loci presenting in child #2.

Besides the *A, B, C, D* and *DR* loci of HLA, there are many other genetic loci within the haplotype or close to it; for example, the genes (structural or regulatory or both) for Bf (the C3 proactivator), C2, C4 and possibly C8. With respect to C4, it is probable that two genes are represented — an allele of one of them determines the blood group antigen Chido and the other, the blood group antigen Rogers (O'Neill *et al*, 1978). There is also a relationship between HLA and Bg antigens (Morton *et al*, 1971). Other genes have also been shown to be linked to HLA (see Amos, 1980) and many diseases have been found to occur most frequently in person carrying a particular allele of HLA-A, B, C, or D/DR (see under the heading The HLA Antigens and Diseases).

THE ANTIGENS OF THE HLA SYSTEM

Frequencies

The antigens currently recognized to be part of the HLA system are given in Table 14–1. Because of the extreme polymorphism of the system (particularly with respect to antigens controlled by the *A* and *B* loci) it follows that the majority of HLA antigens occur infrequently in any given population. Particular HLA haplotypes can all be considered rare.

In addition, there are striking differences in the gene distributions between different races. Table 14–2 gives the frequencies of some HLA genes in three races.

Linkage Disequilibrium

Linkage disequilibrium refers to the *nonrandom* associations of the antigens of the *HLA* loci. This phenomenon also occurs in red cell systems, although it is not assigned the same degree of importance (e.g., the *M* gene tends to occur on the same chromosome as the *S* gene).

In HLA there are striking associations between, for example, A1 and B8 and between A3 and B7. This means that when an individual possesses the HLA-A1 antigen, he or she is likely also to have the HLA-B8 antigen. HLA-A3 and HLA-B7 show a similar association. The mechanism that results in this association is unknown. Linkage disequilibrium has also been shown between the *B* and *C* loci (which is apparently even more marked than between the *A* and *B* loci) and also occurs between the *B* and *D* loci.

An example of linkage disequilibrium can

Table 14–2 GENE FREQUENCIES OF SOME HLA GENES IN WHITES, MONGOLOIDS AND BLACKS*

Gene	Frequency in Whites (%)	Frequency in Mongoloids (%)	Frequency in Blacks (%)
A1	14.76	1.23	3.30
A2	25.68	26.27	14.72
A3	11.56	0.83	8.30
A11	6.21	8.74	0.65
Aw23	2.37	0.48	9.55
Aw24	8.76	32.18	2.80
A25	1.98	0.83	0.33
A26	4.08	8.36	3.81
A28	4.42	1.09	9.01
A29	4.08	0.66	6.20
Aw30	2.60	0.39	14.72
Aw31	2.82	8.36	2.47
Aw32	4.22	0.48	1.47
Aw33	1.71	6.58	4.82
Aw34	0.48	0.96	6.37
Aw36	0.26	0.22	1.97
Ax(Blank)	4.02	2.32	9.52
B7	8.78	5.04	8.51
B8	8.43	0.39	2.14
B13	2.71	1.98	0.65
B18	4.99	0.13	3.82
B27	3.77	0.65	1.81
Bw35	9.31	8.73	7.62
B37	1.52	0.48	0.49
Bw38	3.15	0.83	0.00
Bw39	1.93	3.54	1.81
Bw41	1.50	0.44	0.98
Bx(Blank)	4.41	9.77	6.17
Cw1	3.92	15.74	0.99
Cw2	5.02	0.74	10.70
Cw3	10.61	26.16	9.07
Cw4	12.10	6.20	16.96
Cw5	6.16	1.01	2.48
Cw6	9.12	1.62	9.07
Cx(Blank)	53.07	48.52	50.72

*Information from Eighth International Histocompatibility Workshop— Pre Data Analysis. P. Terasaki, Editor (December, 1979), to be published in *Histocompatibility Testing, 1980.*

be taken from figures reported from the Fourth International Workshop 1970, in which the total chromosomes with HLA-A1 numbered 159 per 1000 and the total chromosomes with HLA-B8 numbered 92 per 1000. If HLA-A1 and HLA-B8 had been randomly associated (i.e., linkage equilibrium), there would have been 14.6 chromosomes with both HLA-A1 and HLA-B8, calculated thus:

$$\frac{159}{1000} \times \frac{92}{1000} \times 1000 = 14.628$$

The number of chromosomes actually observed to have HLA-A1 and HLA-B8 was 67.

It has been postulated that some of the associations between HLA-A and HLA-B antigens and certain diseases may also be the result of linkage disequilibrium between the genes controlling these antigens and genes governing susceptibility to the diseases.

Cross Reactions

Since there is a marked tendency for HLA antigens to stimulate antibodies that react not only with the stimulating antigen, but also with one or more antigens controlled from the same locus, cross reactivity is a common occurrence in practical testing. Some of the common cross-reactive specificities (*HLA-A* and *HLA-B* loci) are given in Table 14–3.

The HLA Antigens and Disease

Correlations of diseases with HLA antigen frequency have recently become the subject of considerable research, the main reasons for this being to obtain pertinent genetic or pathogenic information to be applied clinically to the disease or to obtain biologic information about HLA function.

The incentive to study HLA factors involved in disease susceptibility came from studies by Lilly *et al* (1964), who found that resistance to gross leukemia virus was dependent on the H-2 constitution of the mouse. From these studies, Amiel (1967) and Kourilsky *et al* (1968) undertook the investigation of HLA antigens in patients with acute lymphatic leukemia and Hodgkin's disease. These studies produced evidence of an association between HLA and Hodgkin's disease while the other study yielded no association. Since these early studies, a number of other important associations have been documented for a broad variety of diseases. Table 14–4 lists some of the nonmalignant diseases for which an association has been established with certain HLA antigens, although a detailed compendium listing the worldwide experience from a variety of studies has been compiled by the HLA and Disease Registry of Copenhagen (see Ryder *et al*, 1979). The latest association (at the time of this writing) is between HLA-A2 antigens and chronic lung disease in neonates (Clark *et al*, 1980).

From the information given in Table 14–4 and from other studies, the following generalizations can be made:

1. Disease associations are found primarily with alleles at the B locus (although in certain diseases a stronger association may exist with the HLA-D (HLA-DR) than with the HLA-B

Table 14–3 SOME ANTIGENS OF THE HLA-A AND HLA-B LOCI AND THEIR MOST COMMON CROSS-REACTIVE SPECIFICITIES

HLA-A Antigens	Cross-Reactive Specificities	HLA-B Antigens	Cross-Reactive Specificities
A1	A3, A11	B5	Bw35, B15, B17, Bw21
A2	A28, Aw23, Aw24		B18
A3	A1, A11	B7	Bw22, B27, B40
A9	Aw24(9), Aw23(9), A2	B8	B14
A10	A28(10), A26(10)	B12	Bw21
	A11, Aw32	B13	B40, B7
A11	A3, A26(10), A1	B14	B8, B18
Aw23	Aw24(9), A9, A2	B15	Bw35, B5, B17
Aw24	Aw23(9), A9, A2		Bw21, B18
A25	A10, A26(10), Aw32, Aw33	Bw16	Bw38(16), Bw39(16)
A26	A10, A25(10), A11		Bw22
A28	A2	B17	B15, B5, Bw35, Bw21, B18
Aw30	Aw31, Aw32, Aw33	B18	B5, Bw35, B15, B14, B17
Aw31	Aw30, Aw32, Aw33	Bw21	B15, B5, Bw35, B17
Aw32	Aw30, A25(10), Aw33, Aw31	Bw22	B7, B27, B40, Bw16, Bw38
Aw33	Aw32, Aw31, Aw30, A25(10)	B27	B7, Bw22, B40
		Bw35	B5, B15, B17, B18, Bw21
		B37	
		Bw38	Bw16, Bw39(16), Bw22
		Bw39	Bw16, Bw38(16), Bw22
		B40	B13, B7

alleles). It should be noted that an association with HLA-B7 or HLA-B8 also shows a weak association with HLA-A3 or HLA-A1, respectively, because of the strong A3, B7 and A1, B8 linkage disequilibrium.

2. All of these diseases (Table 14–4) are multifactoral or are dominantly inherited with incomplete penetrance.

3. Most diseases associated with HLA have immunopathological characteristics (i.e., they are either autoimmune diseases or are related to immunodeficiencies).

Table 14–4 SOME NONMALIGNANT DISEASES FOR WHICH AN ASSOCIATION HAS BEEN ESTABLISHED WITH CERTAIN HLA ANTIGENS*

Disease	Relevant HLA Antigen
Ankylosing spondylitis	B27
Reiter's syndrome	B27
Arthritis (following Salmonella infections)	B27
Arthritis (following Yersinia infections)	B27
Rheumatic arthritis	Dw4
Addison's disease	B8
Addison's disease	Dw3
Hemochromatosis	A3
Hemochromatosis	B14
Multiple sclerosis	A3, B7, Dw2
Juvenile diabetes mellitus	B8, B15
Chronic hepatitis	B8 (B8/B8)
Graves disease (in Europeans)	B8
Graves disease (in Japanese)	Bw35
Psoriasis (unspecified)	B13, Bw16, B17

*Information from Grumet, 1977.

The most dramatic association between HLA and disease exists between ankylosing spondylitis and HLA-B27 (Brewerton *et al*, 1973; Schlosstein *et al*, 1973). Approximately 96 per cent of the ankylosing spondylitis patients possessed HLA-B27 as compared to 4 per cent in the control group. HLA-B27 typing is therefore widely used as an aid in the differential diagnosis of the disease (Morris *et al*, 1974a, b), although the association is almost 100 per cent dependent on the diagnostic criteria that are applied (Kissmeyer-Nielsen and Kristensen, 1977).

It is believed that B27 is *directly* involved in the pathogenic mechanism, since neither the B27-associated C alleles nor the associated D-alleles show an influence on the disease; only B27 is associated (Truog *et al*, 1975). Homozygosity for B27 almost always leads to clinical appearance of the disease. With most other HLA-associated diseases it is believed that separate genes are involved that must be closely linked to the *B* or even the *D* locus. The subject of the mechanisms for HLA and disease associations is excellently reviewed by Dupont (1980).

The HLA Antigens on Red Cells

The presence of some HLA antigens on the red cells is important to the immunohematologist because they may interfere with red cell antibody detection and identification; they can cause weak and poorly reproducible reactions with sera containing HLA antibodies. These reactions are particularly notable in saline room temperature, anti-human globulin and especially Autoanalyzer techniques. The antibodies are also troublesome in red cell typing reagents because they are usually difficult to remove by absorption.

Some antigen-antibody reactions that were originally thought to be caused by red cell systems are now known to be caused by HLA antigens. The most notable of these is the Bennett-Goodspeed group of antigens (Morton et al, 1971), which have been shown to be associated with HLA as follows:

1. HLA-B7 positive individuals have red cells possessing Bg^a.

2. HLA-B17 positive individuals have red cells possessing Bg^b.

3. HLA-A28 positive individuals have red cells possessing Bg.

Other antigens that have been correlated with HLA types are Chido (HLA-B12 and HLA-Bw35) and Rogers (HLA-A1, B8 or HLA-A1, Bw35). It is believed that Chido and Rogers alleles may be associated with HLA alleles as a result of linkage disequilibrium, Chido having already been shown to be closely linked with HLA (Middleton et al, 1974).

THE APPLICATIONS OF HLA ANTIGEN TYPING

Transplantation

HLA typing is commonly used to evaluate compatibility between donor and recipient in transplantation. When the donor and the recipient are from the same family, the success of renal transplantation can often be predicted on the basis of HLA-identity matching. Shaw (1975, 1976) reported an 80 to 90 per cent survival rate for HLA-identical siblings and a 58 to 73 per cent survival rate for one-haplotype-related grafts.

The efficacy of HLA matching in genetically *unrelated* or *cadaver* donor transplants (the latter representing about 70 per cent of all renal transplants performed in the US) is still the subject of conflicting reports. The survival rate of cadaver donor transplants is about 47 per cent.

HLA typing of donor and recipient is also used for bone marrow grafting (Thomas, 1975), although at the present time only HLA-identical, genetically related donors are being used to any extent for this purpose.

Table 14–5 INTERPRETATION OF RESULTS OF HLA TYPING

Code	Reaction Observed
1	Negative reaction—viability same as controls.
2	Doubtful negative reactions with a perceptible increase in barely dead cells over the control level.
4	Doubtful positive reaction with a slight detectable change in viability.
6	Positive reaction, clearly different from controls, with 10 to 90% of cells killed.
8	Strong positive reaction with essentially all cells killed (90 to 100%).
0	No reading.

In renal transplantation, compatibilities at the HLA-A and HLA-B loci are the only ones taken into account in most cases, since the clinical significance of HLA-C and HLA-D/DR as related to renal transplantation has not been firmly established. In bone marrow grafting, however, the prospective donors must be identical by both serologic testing and mixed lymphocyte culture testing.

Transfusion

Many patients who are repeatedly transfused with random donor platelets develop a progressive decrease in response to these transfusions, generally attributed to alloimmunization with incompatible HLA antigens. While it is not common practice at the present time to perform HLA typing for routine platelet transfusions, it is obvious that genetically identical platelets would be preferred therapy. Whether platelet therapy would be beneficial to thrombocytopenic patients with lymphocytotoxic antibodies is not yet known (Ahn, 1975).

Transfusions of white blood cells are now commonly used because of the feasibility of collecting and isolating large numbers of granulocytes from single donors through continuous flow techniques (see McCullough, 1974; Graw, 1975). The benefits of granulocyte transfusions are unclear because few thorough, well-controlled studies have been performed. About 27 per cent of patients become sensitized to leukocyte antigens by the fifth transfusion. The importance of HLA matching in granulocyte transfusions was demonstrated by Graw et al (1972), who found that when donor and recipient have identical HLA-A and HLA-B antigens (i.e., four identical HLA loci) the number of donor granulocytes present at 1 hour after transfusion is 50 per cent. (This is considered to be maximum recovery, since 50 per cent of the granulocytes in the blood pool "marginate;" that is, move along or adhere to the walls of venules.) When three out of four HLA loci are identical, the initial survival is 28 per cent, with two it is 17 per cent and with one only, 3 per cent. With randomly selected donors, the initial survival is 5 per cent.

Disease

HLA typing, as mentioned, is used as an aid in the differential diagnosis of certain disease states.

Paternity Testing

HLA typing has become useful in paternity testing, in which it appears to be the most informative tool for excluding parentage in cases of false accusation. The reasons for this include the facts that the antigens are inherited in a mendelian fashion; they are well developed at birth; techniques are accurate, reliable and give reproducible results; and no antigen occurs with high frequency in any given population (see Bryant, 1980).

THE ANTIBODIES OF THE HLA SYSTEM

Characteristics and Occurrence

HLA antibodies are characteristically IgG and have both agglutinating and cytotoxic (complement-activating) properties. "Naturally occurring" HLA antibodies have not been convincingly demonstrated (van Rood and van Leeuwen, 1976). IgM anti-HLA was found by Stocker et al, (1969) in patients who had rejected renal grafts while on immunosuppressive therapy and has also been reported in one multitransfused patient with an IgM level of 6 g/l (Crome and Moffatt, 1971).

Most serologically defined HLA antibodies are reactive in both the leukoagglutination and the lymphocytotoxic techniques, although some may be reactive only in one technique.

Lymphocytotoxic antibodies may be found as early as the twenty-fourth week of pregnancy in primiparae, although the incidence of these antibodies after a first pregnancy has been variously estimated from 4.3 per cent (Ahrons, 1971) to 25 per cent (Goodman and Masaitis, 1967). The incidence of anti-HLA increases with parity; cytotoxic antibodies were found in

55 per cent of women who had had three pregnancies (Goodman and Masaitis, 1967).

The incidence of leukocyte antibodies is relatively high in patients who have received numerous transfusions. Leverenz et al (1974) reported that in patients who had received not more than 10 transfusions, the incidence of lymphocytotoxic antibodies was 25 per cent and in those who had received more than 30 transfusions, the incidence was 44 per cent. Gleichmann and Breininger (1975) reported a series in which patients were tested at 1 week and usually also at 2, 4 and 12 weeks after open heart surgery. These patients received stored blood and most also received 2 to 5 units of fresh blood. As many as 52 out of 54 of these patients developed either a lymphocytotoxic antibody or a leukoagglutinin or both. Fifty patients developed antibody within 1 week of transfusion, but 12 weeks after transfusion antibodies were present in only 62.5 per cent.

Although HLA antibodies are usually IgG, there is no evidence that they damage the fetus.

The Role of HLA Antibodies in Febrile Transfusion Reactions

The incidence of leukocyte antibodies in patients having febrile transfusion reactions is usually reported by most authors to be about 50 per cent (Kissmeyer-Nielsen and Thorby, 1970). Since many antibodies will go undetected unless a panel of leukocytes includes a high proportion of relatively common specificities and unless the tests include lymphocytotoxicity (which is best for anti-HLA) *and* leukoagglutination (which is best for granulocyte-specific antibodies), it is probable that the incidence is much higher than this. Perkins *et al* (1971), for example, found leukoagglutinins in 34 out of 35 patients following a febrile transfusion reaction, using both techniques. This subject is returned to in Adverse Effects of Transfusion, Chapter 25.

TECHNIQUES

The Microlymphocytotoxicity Test (AABB Recommended Technique)*

Preparation of Lymphocytes
1. Place 2 ml of fresh, heparinized blood into two 1-ml centrifuge tubes.

---

*Reprinted with permission from *AABB Technical Manual*, 8th edition. Copyright © American Association of Blood Banks, Washington, D.C., 1981.

2. Centrifuge for 2 min at 3500 g.

3. Remove the buffy coat and place in a centrifuge tube containing 0.3 ml of anti-AB or anti-H, depending on the ABO group.

4. Agglutinate the red blood cells by turning slowly on a vertical wheel at approximately 8 g for 2 to 5 min.

5. Pack the agglutinated red blood cells by centrifuging for 7 sec at 1000 g.

6. Remove the supernatant and gently layer it over 0.3 ml of Ficoll-metrizoate mixture, prepared as follows: (a) Add 9.0 gm of Ficoll to 100 ml of distilled water. (b) Add 20 ml of 75 per cent sodium metrizoate to 24 ml of distilled water to make a 33.9 per cent solution. (c) Mix 24 parts of Ficoll solution with 10 parts metrizoate solution. *Note*: When layering the supernatant, it is important not to mix the Ficoll-metrizoate and lymphocyte suspension.

7. Centrifuge at 3500 g for 3 min. The Ficoll-metrizoate acts as a density gradient. Residual agglutinated red cells and granulocytes are packed at the bottom, lymphocytes remain at the interface, and platelets remain in the anti-ABH supernatant.

8. Take out the white interface and resuspend it in a 1-ml centrifuge tube containing 0.4 ml modified Collins with 0.5 per cent fetal calf serum. It is important to remove all of the interface but a minimum of Ficoll and supernatant. Excess Ficoll will result in granulocyte contamination, whereas excess supernatant will result in platelet contamination.

9. Remove the platelets by centrifugation (1 min at 1000 g). Discard the supernatant and resuspend the lymphocyte pellet in 1 ml of modified Collins with 0.5 per cent fetal calf serum.

10. Centrifuge for 1 min at 5000 g to agglutinate the excess granulocytes and resuspend the pellet.

11. Centrifuge at 1000 g for 4 sec to remove debris. Transfer the supernatant to a new tube.

12. With a blood counting chamber using phase contrast microscopy, adjust the lymphocyte count to 1 million per ml.

Preparation of Testing Trays

1. Dispense all antisera into microdroplet testing trays. To prevent evaporation, add 0.005 ml mineral oil to each well with a multiple needle dispenser attached to a multiple pipetting device. Antisera are dispensed in 0.0001 ml amounts using a 50× multiple repeating dispenser. The trays may be stored at −70° C until ready for use. *Note*: Pre-prepared typing trays can now be purchased from commercial sources.

Test Procedure

1. Thaw antiserum trays immediately before use.

2. Thoroughly mix the lymphocyte suspension. With a 50× multiple repeating dispenser, add 0.001 ml of cell suspension to each well, taking care not to touch the antiserum with the needle.

3. Make certain that cells and antisera are mixed.

4. Incubate at room temperature (approximately 23° C) for 30 min.

5. With a 250× multiple repeating dispenser, add by "soft drop" technique 0.005 ml of rabbit complement to the cell-serum mixtures. Mix if necessary. *Note*: The "soft drop" technique is a gentle layering of reagent onto the cell-serum mixture, so that the cells are not disturbed.

6. Incubate at room temperature for 60 min.

7. Using a multiple needle dispenser by "soft drop" technique, add 0.003 ml of 5 per cent aqueous eosin to each well. Mix if necessary.

8. After 2 min add 0.008 ml of formaldehyde to each well by "soft drop" technique, using a multiple needle dispenser and jet pipette. Mix if necessary.

9. Lower a 50-×75-mm microscope slide onto the wells in order to flatten the top of the droplet.

10. Add heated petrolatum around the rim of the slide to prevent evaporation and siphoning of fluid from individual wells.

Interpretation of Results

Results are interpreted according to the code given in Table 14–5. The presence of antigen is shown by the cell membrane damage, resulting in "killed" cells. If the cells remain viable, the antigen (corresponding to the antibody in a particular well) is not present.

Reactions are read with an inverted phase contrast microscope using a 10× objective. Living (viable) lymphocytes are seen as small and refractile, whereas dead lymphocytes are larger and stained with eosin.

EDTA LEUKOAGGLUTINATION ASSAY

Blood Collection and White Blood Cell Preparation Procedure

All steps in this procedure are performed at room temperature (20° C–24° C).

A negative control consisting of a normal adult male group AB serum that has been shown to contain no leukoagglutinins must be included in each test performed. Males are less likely to possess leukoagglutinins than females because of nonparity. It is advisable to set up tests in duplicate and read the duplicates side by side for immediate comparison.

1. Collect 10 ml venous blood in a 16 × 125

mm tube containing 1 ml of 5 per cent EDTA anticoagulant and thoroughly mix by inversion. Prepare and use cells within 46 hours after blood collection.

2. Add 2.5 ml of Plasmagel. Thoroughly mix by inversion, being careful to avoid bubbles. Allow to stand at room temperature for 20 to 30 minutes for sedimentation.

3. With a Pasteur pipette (14 cm long), remove the supernatant, together with the buffy coat and topmost layer of red blood cells. Transfer equal amounts to two 10 × 75 mm tubes.

4. Centrifuge for 10 minutes at 170 g. The leukocytes and red blood cells with some platelets form a loose button.

5. Transfer the supernatant plasma containing most of the platelets to a 13 × 100 mm tube, leaving an equal volume of the plasma and the cell button in the 10 × 75 mm tubes. Centrifuge the 13 × 100 mm tube at 1,450 g for 30 minutes to pack the platelet-free plasma.

6. Meanwhile, with a clean Pasteur pipette (14 cm long), resuspend the button in the 10 × 75 mm tubes. Exercise care in dislodging the leukocytes clinging to the wall of the tube on top of the red cell button to avoid foaming.

7. Pool the two red blood cell–white blood cell suspensions and carefully place them in a 6 × 50 mm tube, removing any bubbles that may have formed at the top. Resediment the cells for 20 to 30 minutes at room temperature.

8. The white blood cells form a thick creamy layer on top of the sedimented red blood cells. Remove this layer, avoiding the red blood cells, with a clean Pasteur pipette (14 cm long) and transfer it to another 6 × 50 mm tube. Add an equal volume of EDTA buffer and mix the suspension.

9. Place approximately 2 ml of the platelet-free plasma (gradient) from step 5 in a 7 × 100 mm tube. Using a clean Pasteur pipette (23 cm long), carefully layer the leukocyte-EDTA buffer suspension from step 8 on top of the column of platelet-free plasma (gradient) and centrifuge for 2½ minutes at 170 g. The leukocytes pass through the gradient and form a loose pellet at the bottom of the tube. The platelets remain above the column of plasma.

10. With a clean Pasteur pipette (23 cm long), remove the supernatant completely and discard it. Exercise care so that the platelets do not stream down to the leukocyte button. As soon as all the supernatant is removed, invert the tube and, without touching the leukocyte button, swab the inner wall of the tube with 1 or 2 cotton swabs.

11. Place 3 ml of platelet-free plasma from step 5 in a 12 × 75 mm tube. Add 1 ml EDTA buffer and mix.

12. Using a clean Pasteur pipette (23 cm long), resuspend the leukocyte button from step 10 with 2 ml of plasma-buffer diluent from step 11.

13. Perform a white blood cell count on this suspension, adjusting it to 5,000 to 6,000 cells per millimeter with the plasma-buffer diluent from step 11.

Agglutination Test Procedure

1. Heat inactivate sera at 56° C for 30 min.

2. Perform the test in 6 × 50 mm tubes, set up in a convenient arrangement in specially designed blocks. Test each serum in duplicate.

3. Deliver exactly 0.02 ml of undiluted serum to the bottom of the tube using a Hamilton Microsyringe. The same syringe may be used for the addition of all sera, but it must be thoroughly rinsed in saline at least three times between each serum sample.

4. Add one drop of the cell suspension with a Pasteur pipette (23 cm long) held in a vertical position so that all drops will be uniform. Every effort should be made to deliver the drop to the bottom of the tube.

5. Mix each tube individually. If the drop of cell suspension is lodged near the mouth of the tube, gently tap the tube on a firm surface until the drop rolls down into the serum. Holding the top of the tube firmly between the thumb and forefinger, flick the bottom of the tube with each of the three remaining fingers, starting with the little finger. Repeat this snapping gesture until the cells and serum are mixed at least three times.

6. After the contents of all the tubes are thoroughly mixed, cover them all tightly with Saran Wrap and incubate for two hours at room temperature (20° C to 24° C). Prolonged incubation should be avoided. Therefore, when large numbers of sera are being tested, the addition of cell suspensions should be staggered (e.g., add five cell suspensions, wait one hour and add another five cell suspensions, wait one hour and add another five cell suspensions).

7. At the end of the incubation, introduce a clean pipette (14 cm long, smooth tip) to the bottom of the tube and gently aspirate the contents. Place this on a slide and observe microscopically for agglutination, using 150 × magnification.

Tests for Leukocyte Antibodies

Techniques of varying sophistication may be employed to demonstrate the presence of leukocyte antibodies. For example, a panel of ten leukocyte donors may be randomly selected (even if the HLA types are unknown), leukocyte or lymphocyte suspensions may be made and the leukoagglutination or the lymphocytotoxicity test or both may be performed. Ideally both tests should be performed, though this is not always practical. Whereas leukoagglutination is less expensive and is much simpler than lymphocytotoxicity, it is not as reliable, reproducible, sensitive or specific. Preliminary screening and tentative identification of leukocyte antibodies can be performed using frozen lymphocyte panels prepared from continually available donors (see Shaw, 1973).

TYPICAL EXAMINATION QUESTIONS

Choose the phrase, sentence or symbol which completes the statement or answers the question. More than one answer may be correct in each case. Answers are given in the back of this book.

1. With respect to organ transplantation, the antigens of the HLA system are second in importance only to the:
   (a) Kidd blood group system
   (b) ABO blood group system
   (c) MNSs blood group system
   (d) Duffy blood group system
   (Introduction)

2. The genetic locus originally known as Four is now referred to as
   (a) HLA-A
   (b) HLA-B
   (c) HLA-C
   (d) HLA-D
   (The Nomenclature of the HLA System)

3. The expression of HLA antigens on the cell surface is controlled by a region on chromosome No.
   (a) 4
   (b) 1
   (c) 22
   (d) 6
   (The Genetics of the HLA System)

4. Which of the following genetic loci are within the HLA region or close to it?
   (a) *Bf*
   (b) *Bg*
   (c) *C4*
   (d) *Fy*
   (The Genetics of the HLA System)

5. The nonrandom associations of the antigens of the *HLA* loci are known as:
   (a) chromosomal linkage
   (b) linkage equilibrium
   (c) linkage disequilibrium
   (d) association linkage
   (The Antigens of the HLA System)

6. When an individual possesses the HLA-A3 antigen, he or she is also very likely to possess the
   (a) HLA-B8 antigen
   (b) HLA-B5 antigen
   (c) HLA-Bw35 antigen
   (d) HLA-B7 antigen
   (Linkage Disequilibrium)

7. The disease ankylosing spondylitis appears to be associated with

(a) HLA-A3
(b) HLA-B27
(c) HLA-B8
(d) HLA-B14
   (The HLA Antigens and Disease)

8. The HLA-A28 antigen is found in individuals whose red cells possess
   (a) the Bg^a antigen
   (b) the Bg^b antigen
   (c) the Bg^c antigen
   (d) none of the above
   (HLA Antigens on Red Cells)

9. HLA antigen typing is useful in
   (a) renal transplantation
   (b) bone marrow grafting
   (c) granulocyte transfusions
   (d) paternity testing
   (The Applications of HLA Antigen Typing)

10. HLA antibodies are usually
    (a) IgG
    (b) IgM
    (c) IgA
    (d) none of the above
    (The Antibodies of the HLA System –
    Characteristics and Occurrence)

11. In women who have had three pregnancies, the percentage incidence of cytotoxic antibodies is about
    (a) 4.3
    (g) 25
    (c) 55
    (d) 98.2
    (The Antibodies of the HLA System –
    Characteristics and Occurrence)

12. Tests for leukocyte antibodies in patients who have had febrile transfusion reactions should include
    (a) lymphocytotoxicity only
    (b) leukoagglutination only
    (c) lymphocytotoxicity *and* leukoagglutination
    (d) lymphocytotoxicity *or* leukoagglutination, but not both
    (The Role of HLA Antibodies
    in Febrile Transfusion Reactions)

ANSWER TRUE OR FALSE

13. The lymphocytotoxicity test is best for the detection of granulocyte specific antibodies.
    (The Role of HLA Antibodies
    in Febrile Transfusion Reactions)

14. The HLA system is probably the most polymorphic system in man.
    (The Nomenclature of the HLA System –
    General)

15. The locus originally known as "LA" is now known as HLA-A.
    (The Nomenclature of the HLA System)

16. Certain antigens at the *D* locus can be detected using serologic methods and are referred to as D-related (DR) antigens.
    (The Genetics of the HLA System)

17. "Crossing over" does not occur between the loci of the HLA system.
    (The Genetics of the HLA System)

18. Linkage disequilibrium has not been shown to occur between the *HLA-B* and *HLA-C* loci.
    (Linkage Disequilibrium)

19. In general, most of the diseases associated with HLA have immunopathological characteristics.
    (The HLA Antigens and Disease)

20. Lymphocytotoxic antibodies may be found as early as the twenty-fourth week of pregnancy in primiparae, yet do not appear to damage the fetus.
    (The Antibodies of the HLA System –
    Characteristics and Occurrence)

GENERAL REFERENCES

Numerous texts currently available contain useful basic information about the HLA system. The list here provided includes those that should prove most understandable to the immunohematologist.

1. AABB Technical Manual, 7th Ed. American Association of Blood Banks, Washington, 1977. *(One chapter is devoted to the theory of HLA; it includes the same techniques as presented in this text.)*

2. AABB: The Biology and Function of the Major Histocompatibility Complex. Symposium, American Association of Blood Banks. Presented at 33rd Annual Meeting, Washington, November 1980. *(Excellent coverage of genetics, structural definition of serologic specificity, immunogenetics and mechanisms for HLA and disease association, among other topics.)*

3. Bellanti, J. A.: Immunology, Basic Processes. W. B. Saunders Co., Philadelphia, 1979. *(Coverage of HLA system is brief, but makes the subject very understandable. Note that, in spite of the year of publication, old nomenclatures have been used.)*

4. Bender, K.: The HLA System. Biotest Serum Institute, Frankfurt, 1979. *(Extremely useful and thorough coverage of the basic principles of the HLA system.)*

5. Boorman, K. E., Dodd, B. E., and Lincoln, P. J.: Blood Group Serology: Theory, Techniques, Practical Applications. 5th Ed. Churchill Livingstone, 1977. *(The chapter devoted to HLA [p. 243] takes the subject from the viewpoint of the immunohematologist. Alternative techniques are presented.)*

6. Mollison, P. L.: Blood Transfusion in Clinical Medicine, 6th Ed. Blackwell Scientific Publications, Oxford, 1979. *(Contains many references to the HLA system as it affects blood transfusion.)*

HEMOLYTIC DISEASES

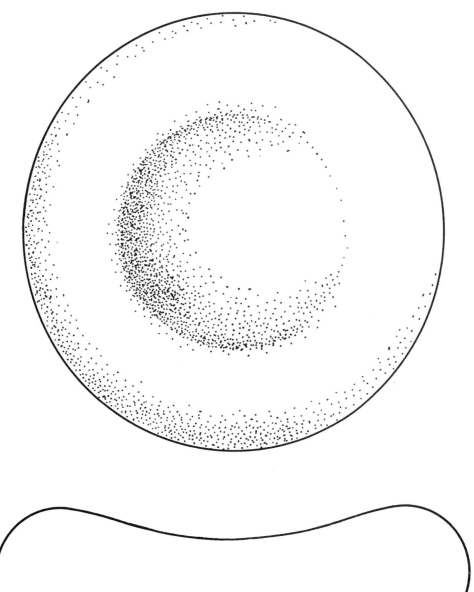

AUTOIMMUNE HEMOLYTIC ANEMIA

OBJECTIVES — AUTOIMMUNE HEMOLYTIC ANEMIA

The student shall know, understand and be prepared to explain:

1. The theories of "self" and "nonself" recognition
2. The possible mechanisms in the initiation of autoimmune diseases, specifically to include:
   (a) The forbidden clone theory
   (b) The sequestered antigen theory
   (c) The immunologic deficiency theory
   (d) The genetic control of the immune system
3. The classifications of autoimmune hemolytic anemia
4. "Warm" antibody autoimmune hemolytic anemia, specifically to include:
   (a) Frequency
   (b) Immunoglobulins involved
   (c) Complement components involved
   (d) Associated diseases
   (e) Specificity of antibodies involved
5. "Cold" antibody autoimmune hemolytic anemia, specifically to include:
   (a) Frequency
   (b) Immunoglobulins involved
   (c) Complement components involved
   (d) Associated diseases
   (e) Specificity of antibodies involved
6. Paroxysmal cold hemoglobinuria, specifically to include:

   (a) General description
   (b) Disease associations
   (c) The Donath-Landsteiner antibody
7. Paroxysmal nocturnal hemoglobinuria, specifically to include:
   (a) General description
   (b) Laboratory investigation
8. Drug-induced hemolytic anemia, including the following mechanisms:
   (a) Immune complexes
   (b) Drug adsorption
   (c) Nonimmunologic protein adsorption
9. Autoimmune hemolytic anemia due to methyldopa (general discussion and proposed mechanisms)
10. Serologic investigation of autoimmune hemolytic anemia, specifically to include:
    (a) Specimen requirements
    (b) The direct antiglobulin test
    (c) Elution
    (d) Identification of antibodies
    (e) The grouping of patients with autoimmune hemolytic anemia
    (f) The transfusion of blood to patients with autoimmune hemolytic anemia

Essential Terms

Adsorption is the take-up of antibody by the cells. *Elution* is the removal of antibody from the cells. *Absorption* is the removal of antibody from the serum, usually by adsorption (see Fig. 15–1).

Introduction

One of the basic phenomena of antigen-antibody interaction is based on the fact that antibodies are formed *only* when an individu-

al's red cells lack the corresponding antigen. This is the basis of Landsteiner's law, and reflects a biologic necessity. Under certain conditions or circumstances, however, the mechanisms that control an individual's immunologic tolerance to antigenic substances that are regarded as "self" appear to fail. The result is the production of an antibody (or antibodies) against the individual's own tissues. Antibodies of this kind are known as *autoantibodies*, and the process is known as *autoimmunization*.

The lack of recognition of "self" is not confined to blood group antigens; a number of

183

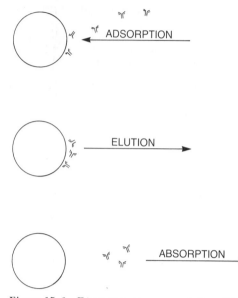

Figure 15–1 Diagrammatic representation of the terms *ADSORPTION, ELUTION* and *ABSORPTION.*

different disease states may be caused partly by tissue autoantibodies. This chapter, however, will be confined to the study of autoimmune hemolytic anemia with respect to autoantibodies that bring about a shortened survival of red cells and thereby an anemic state.

Possible Mechanisms in the Initiation of Autoimmune Diseases

The precise mechanisms that initiate autoimmune diseases are not known. Several hypotheses have been made that include:

The Forbidden Clone Theory. The forbidden clone theory postulates a single clone (i.e., the progeny of a single cell) of changed or altered lymphocytes arising through cell mutation. Mutant cells carrying a "foreign" surface antigen would therefore be destroyed by normal lymphocytes, whereas mutant cells *lacking* foreign surface antigen would not. With the proliferation of these antigen-deficient mutants, so-called "forbidden clones," these cells, because of *genetic* dissimilarity, would be capable of reacting with target cells.

The Sequestered-Antigen Theory. The sequestered antigen theory proposes that during embryonic life, tissues that are anatomically separated or sequestered from the lymphoreticular system are regarded as "nonself." These "nonself" antigens occur in tissues such as the thyroid, the testes, the lens of the eye and the central nervous system. Exposure of the seques-

tered tissue antigen to the lymphoreticular system in later life through trauma or infection then results in autoimmune disease.

The Immunologic Deficiency Theory. The concept of immunologic deficiency proposes that normal individuals who develop autoimmune disease may in fact have an underlying immune deficiency that renders them susceptible to autoimmune states. In this case, injury would occur through the emergence of mutant lymphocytes or as a result of persistence of microbial antigen.

It should be noted that any hypothesis seeking to explain the development of the autoimmune disease state must recognize the *genetic control* of the immune system. It is well documented that autoimmune disorders are characterized by predominance in the female and in families. The immune response gene in humans is closely linked to the *HLA* loci on autosome number 6. Association between certain histocompatibility antigens and a variety of diseases has been reported (see Chapter 14); this offers new potential in understanding the mechanisms of autoimmune diseases.

CLASSIFICATION OF AUTOIMMUNE HEMOLYTIC ANEMIA

Autoimmune hemolytic anemia is normally classified under the following headings, representing clinically distinctive categories:

1. "Warm" antibody autoimmune hemolytic anemia.

2. "Cold" antibody autoimmune hemolytic anemia (also known as cold agglutinin syndrome or cold hemagglutinin disease).

3. Paroxysmal cold hemoglobinuria (PCH).

4. Atypical autoimmune hemolytic anemia.

5. Drug-induced immune hemolytic anemia.

6. Alloantibody-induced immune hemolytic anemia. This includes hemolytic transfusion reactions (discussed in Chapter 25 of this text) and hemolytic disease of the newborn (discussed in Chapter 16 of this text).

Other more complex classifications of autoimmune hemolytic anemia have been suggested, based both on the results of direct antiglobulin tests and on the immunochemical nature of the autoantibody and its serologic behavior; however, these appear to be of no clinical relevance and are generally avoided by most authors (see Dacie, 1975; Mueller-Eckhardt and Kretschmer, 1972; Miescher and Dayer, 1976; Petz and Garratty, 1980).

"Warm" Antibody Autoimmune Hemolytic Anemia

Autoimmune hemolytic anemia of the "warm" type is so called because the causative antibody reacts as well, or better, at 37° C than at lower temperatures. This is by far the most common type of autoimmune hemolytic anemia, accounting for more than 80 per cent of all cases (see Mollison, 1979). The mechanisms of the disease are not fully understood, and some differences may be noted from case to case. In some cases there is no apparent cause for the development of the antibody, and the term *idiopathic* (of unknown origin) is applied. Acquired hemolytic anemia of this type is referred to as *primary*. The term *secondary acquired hemolytic anemia* is applied to cases in which the antibody appears subsequent to a disease state.

Immunoglobulins Involved. In over 80 per cent of cases of autoimmune hemolytic anemia of the warm antibody type, IgG can be detected on the red cells. In almost 50 per cent of cases, complement is also detected and in about 10 per cent of cases, complement alone can be demonstrated. A few cases reveal IgA alone on the red cells, although IgM alone on the red cells has not been reported. In still other cases, various combinations of immunoglobulins and complement are observed. IgG alone is usually reported to be found in less than 50 per cent of cases (see Allgood and Chaplin, 1967; Petz and Garratty, 1975; Worlledge, cited by Mollison, 1979). Issitt *et al* (1976), in reporting the results of a series, however, found the incidence to be about 90 per cent. IgG alone is invariably found in patients with a positive direct antiglobulin test associated with α-methyldopa (Worlledge, 1969; Issitt *et al*, 1976). IgG and complement (sometimes with IgM, with or without IgA) is frequently found on the red cells of patients with autoimmune hemolytic anemia associated with systemic lupus erythematosus (Worlledge, cited by Mollison, 1979). A few cases have been described in which the serum contained both IgM and IgG autoantibodies (Moore and Chaplin, 1973; Freedman and Newlands, 1977), and both IgM warm hemolysins (enzyme reactive) and IgM warm autoagglutinins have been reported in cases of warm autoimmune hemolytic anemia (Dorner *et al*, 1968). For example, Freedman *et al* (1977) described a case of autoimmune hemolytic anemia associated with a complement-binding IgM antibody of anti-I^T specificity, reacting optimally at 37° C.

Complement. C3d is the only subcomponent of C3 present on circulating red cells in patients with warm-type autoimmune hemolytic anemia (Engelfriet *et al*, 1970) and similarly C4d is the only subcomponent of C4 present (Stratton, 1975; Michael *et al*, 1976; Freedman and Newlands, 1977), thus stressing the importance of anti-C3d in routine antiglobulin sera. C5 and C6 can also be detected on the red cells of patients with warm-type autoimmune hemolytic anemia (Kerr *et al*, 1971), although anti-C5 and anti-C6 are usually not present in routine antiglobulin sera. Complement *alone* is regularly found on the red cells of patients whose serum contains IgM hemolysins reacting *in vitro* only with enzyme treated red cells (von dem Borne *et al*, 1969).

Associated Diseases. Autoimmune hemolytic anemias are classified as "secondary" to certain diseases for any of the following reasons: (1) The frequency of autoimmune hemolytic anemia associated with a particular underlying disease is greater than can be explained by chance alone. (2) The reversal of the hemolytic anemia simultaneous with the cure of the associated disease. (3) Evidence of immunologic aberration as part of the underlying disorder, especially if the associated disease is thought to have an autoimmune pathogenesis.

Warm-type autoimmune hemolytic anemia is reasonably classified as secondary when associated with the diseases listed in Table 15–1, although other diseases that do not show as significant a relationship have been reported (see Dacie, 1975).

Table 15–1 DISORDERS FREQUENTLY ASSOCIATED WITH WARM ANTIBODY AUTOIMMUNE HEMOLYTIC ANEMIA[*]

Reticuloendothelial neoplasms
   Chronic lymphocytic leukemia
   Hodgkin's disease
   Non-Hodgkin's lymphomas
   Thymomas
   Multiple myeloma
   Waldenström's macroglobulinemia
Collagen diseases
   Systemic lupus erythematosus
   Scleroderma
   Rheumatoid arthritis
Infectious diseases, especially childhood viral syndromes
Immunologic diseases
   Hypogammaglobulinemia
   Dysglobulinemias
   Other immune deficiency syndromes
Gastrointestinal disease
   Ulcerative colitis
Benign tumors
   Ovarian dermoid cyst

[*]From Petz and Garratty, 1980.

Table 15–2   CLASSIFICATION OF AUTOANTIBODIES IN WARM AUTOIMMUNE HEMOLYTIC ANEMIA*

Specificity	*Normal D-Positive*	*Partially Deleted e.g., −D−*	*Deleted Rh$_{null}$*
Anti–nl	Pos	Neg	Neg
Anti–pdl	Pos	Pos	Neg
Anti–dl	Pos	Pos	Pos

*According to Wiener and Vos, 1963.

Specificity of Antibody.   The associated antibodies in warm-type autoimmune hemolytic anemia often show an association with Rh. Some examples are specific for one particular Rh antigen, such as e (Wiener *et al*, 1953) or D (Höllander, 1954). Others react more strongly with e-positive than with e-negative red cells (Dacie and Cutbush, 1954). Wiener and Vos (1963) found that, in two thirds of cases, the antibody reacted well with all cells except those of type Rh$_{null}$. They classified their patients according to whether their sera reacted with normal D-positive cells (nl = not deleted) or also with Rh positive cells that were "partially deleted" (pdl = partially deleted e.g., −D−) or with both of these types of cells and also with "dl" (deleted) cells (i.e., Rh$_{null}$) (see Table 15–2).

In 1967, Celano and Levine concluded that three specificities could be recognized: (1) anti-LW, (2) an antibody reacting with all samples except Rh$_{null}$, and (3) an antibody reacting with all samples including Rh$_{null}$.

There remains some uncertainty whether the specificity of antibodies that react with all cells including Rh$_{null}$ (i.e., anti-dl) is related in any way to the Rh structure. Marsh *et al* (1972), in testing 50 patients, found three with specificity involving both Rh and U. Forty per cent of the antibodies were classified as anti-dl (i.e., no recognizable specificity). Issitt *et al* (1976) absorbed sera containing anti-dl with Wr(a+b−) red cells to remove the anti-dl and found that anti-Wr^b remained as the sole antibody in two out of 64 cases. In 23 out of 33 cases, anti-dl was found in association with alpha-methyldopa; the same antibody was also found in 23 out of 30 "normal" individuals with a positive direct antiglobulin test (Issitt *et al*, 1976). Leddy and Bakemeier (1967) found that (with one exception) antibodies reacting weakly or not at all with Rh$_{null}$ red cells failed to bind complement, whereas 70 per cent of antibodies reacting as well with Rh$_{null}$ red cells as with Rh-positive red cells did bind complement, strongly suggesting a relationship between specificity and complement binding.

A minority of warm antibodies that at first appear to have the specificity of an Rh alloantibody can be absorbed completely by red cells *lacking* the corresponding antigen. Issitt and Pavone (1980) suggest that the specificity of these antibodies is anti-Hr or anti-Hr$_0$.

Several other specificities have been associated with warm autoimmune hemolytic anemia, and this list appears to be far from complete. These include auto-anti-Jk^a (van Loghem *et al*, 1954), auto-anti-K (Flückiger *et al*, 1955; Dausset *et al*, 1957), auto-anti-U (Nugent *et al*, 1971), auto-anti-I^T (Garratty *et al*, 1974; Freedman *et al*, 1977), auto-anti-A (Szymanski *et al*, 1976), auto-anti-N (Dube *et al*, 1975), auto-anti-Gerbich (Reynolds *et al*, 1980) and many others. (The interested reader is referred to Petz and Garratty, 1980, pp. 237–246, for complete coverage of this subject.)

"COLD" ANTIBODY AUTOIMMUNE HEMOLYTIC ANEMIA (COLD HEMAGGLUTININ DISEASE, COLD AGGLUTININ SYNDROME)

In contrast to "warm" autoimmune hemolytic anemia, "cold" antibody autoimmune hemolytic anemia is so called because the associated antibody reacts best at lower temperatures (i.e., room temperature or below) or has a very wide thermal range. Cold autoimmune hemolytic anemia is relatively uncommon compared with warm autoimmune hemolytic anemia, the incidence being about 15 to 20 per cent of all cases (Dacie, 1962; Dausset and Colombani, 1959; van Loghem *et al*, 1963; Petz and Garratty, 1975). However, it occurs much more frequently than paroxysmal cold hemoglobinuria.

Like the "warm" antibody type of autoimmune hemolytic anemia, the "cold" type can be idiopathic or secondary to certain diseases (see under the heading Associated Diseases).

Immunoglobulins Involved.   The antibodies in cold-type autoimmune hemolytic anemia are commonly IgM and can be of very high titer. Anti-Pr represents an antibody that reacts equally well with adult and cord red cells and detects a receptor that is destroyed by proteolytic enzymes. Anti-Pr can be IgA or IgM, though IgA antibodies tend to be of specificity anti-Pr$_1$ and IgM antibodies tend to be of specificity anti-Pr$_2$ or anti-Pr$_3$ (see Angevine et al, 1966; Garratty et al, 1973; Roelcke et al, 1974a; Tonthat et al, 1976; Roelcke et al, 1976). Occasionally, "cold" IgM antibody is accompanied by a warm IgG autoantibody of the same or another specificity. Cold agglutinins that are solely IgG have also been described (Ambrus and Bajtai, 1969; Mygind and Ahrons, 1973). It has been suggested that patients in whom IgM antibodies predominate, autoantibodies of classes IgG and IgA are also regularly present, though in lower titer (Ratkin et al, 1973).

Complement. While sera containing cold autoagglutinins may fail to agglutinate red cells at temperatures in the range 30 to 37° C, they may still bring about the attachment of complement to them. C4c, C3d, C3c and C3d can all be detected when fresh serum is used, but in the circulation (because of the action of C3b− and C4b− inactivator, only C3d and C4d are detectable on the red cells (Englefriet et al, 1970, Stratton, 1975; Michael et al, 1976).

Disease Associations. In approximately half of patients with infection from *Mycoplasma pneumoniae*, increased titers and thermal range of cold hemagglutinins are observed. Subclinical hemolysis may be common and in occasional patients there is an episode of hemolytic anemia (see Tanowitz et al, 1978). In patients in whom cold agglutinin syndrome occurs in association with *Mycoplasma pneumoniae* infection, it usually occurs in the second or third week of the patient's illness when recovery from the respiratory infection may be complete. A rapid onset of hemolysis is frequently observed and abnormal IgM cold agglutinins, which characteristically have anti-I specificity, are present. These cold autoagglutinins are transient and the hemolysis is therefore self-limiting, usually resolving in two to three weeks. The hemolytic anemia, however, may rapidly proceed and several fatalities have been reported (see Dacie, 1962; Tanowitz et al, 1978).

The increased titer of anti-I following infection with *M. pneumoniae* suggests that the organism possesses an I-like antigen. Lipopolysaccharide prepared from *M. pneumoniae* inhibits anti-I, although the intact organism does not. The organism also inhibits the cold agglutinins produced in rabbits following an injection of the organism (Costea et al, 1972).

Acute hemolytic anemia complicating infectious mononucleosis is a well described though infrequent occurrence. Anti-i is frequently present in patients with this disorder as a transient phenomenon (Jenkins et al, 1965; Rosenfield et al, 1965). While the antibody is reported to be present in about 50 per cent of cases, less than 1 per cent of these patients develop a hemolytic syndrome (Worlledge and Dacie, 1969). In patients in whom a hemolytic syndrome does *not* develop, the anti-i is seldom detectable *in vitro* at a temperature higher than 25° C, whereas when it does develop, the antibody is active *in vitro* up to a temperature of at least 28° C (Worlledge and Dacie, 1969).

Occasional cases of association of hemolytic anemia and high titer cold agglutinins with chronic lymphatic leukemia, "lymphosarcoma," "reticulum cell sarcoma," Hodgkin's disease and multiple myeloma have been reported (Pirofsky, 1969). A number of other disorders (e.g., cirrhosis, malaria, septicemia) have also been reported to be associated with cold agglutinin syndrome, although the significance of the relationship is questionable.

Finally, cold agglutinin syndrome has been compared with Waldenström's macroglobulinemia because of similar clinical findings and course. The relationship is unclear, though it is perhaps best to consider them as distinct disorders, or perhaps to think of Waldenström's macroglobulinemia as a *variant* of cold agglutinin syndrome (for discussion see Petz and Garratty, 1980).

Specificity of Antibody. Most antibodies in cold-type autoimmune hemolytic anemia are considered to have I specificity because they react more strongly with adult red cells than with cord red cells, although it would perhaps be more correct to use the term "I-like." Less commonly, the antibody has anti-i specificity (Marsh and Jenkins, 1960) and in a small number of cases, anti-Pr, which includes several slightly different receptors, all of which are determined by N-acetyl-neuraminic acid (Roelcke et al, 1974; Roelcke et al, 1974a).

PAROXYSMAL COLD HEMOGLOBINURIA

Paroxysmal cold hemoglobinuria (PCH) is also associated with cold antibodies. The antibody, which is often referred to as the Donath-Landsteiner antibody, was first described in a patient with tertiary syphilis, although the majority of cases seen nowadays are associated with viral infections, particularly in children. Patients with the disease suffer from hemoglobinuria (i.e., hemoglobin in the urine) in cold weather, with severity ranging from an isolated attack to repeated attacks over several years.

The DL antibody has anti-P specificity (see The P Blood Group System, Chapter 11, and Techniques, Chapter 23).

PAROXYSMAL NOCTURNAL HEMOGLOBINURIA

Paroxysmal nocturnal hemoglobinuria (PNH) is a rare acquired condition in which there is a deficiency of red cell acetylcholinesterase and some abnormality in the phospholipids of the cell. These red cells hemolyse as a result of complement activation.

Many of the patients suffering from this disease are middle-aged, although all age groups can be affected. The passage of dark urine (hemoglobinuria) in the morning after a night's sleep is characteristically the first sign of the disease. In addition, there may be slight splenomegaly, jaundice, back ache and anemia.

The peripheral blood picture in patients with paroxysmal nocturnal hemoglobinuria is relatively normal except for anemia, but there may be slight macrocytosis with reticulocytosis. Thrombocytopenia and leukopenia also sometimes occur. The Ham's test may show positive results in patients with any condition with spherocytosis (but not in those with paroxysmal nocturnal hemoglobinuria if complement is excluded), and therefore the examination of the peripheral blood film is very important.

Paroxysmal nocturnal hemoglobinuria has a complex relationship to aplastic anemia, myelofibrosis, and myeloblastic leukemia. For this reason, it is important to exclude these and other systemic conditions (Whitehead, 1973). Since the condition is accompanied by chronic intravascular hemolysis with resultant hemosiderinuria, it is not uncommon for the disease to present as an iron deficiency anemia with mild reticulocytosis that shows evidence of increased hemolysis upon the initiation of appropriate iron therapy. The hemolysis is probably the result of new "complement-sensitive" erythrocytes entering the circulation from the bone marrow.

It has been shown that if a sufficient volume of normal red cells is transfused to a patient with paroxysmal nocturnal hemoglobinuria, the number of the patient's own cells in the circulation falls to a low level and hemoglobinuria temporarily ceases (Dacie, 1948). These transfused red cells survive normally in the circulation of the patient (Dacie and Firth, 1943; Dacie, 1948; Mollison, 1947). It is not uncommon, however, for patients with paroxysmal nocturnal hemoglobinuria to react adversely to transfusion. The reaction is characterized by chills and fever accompanied by diarrhea, abdominal pain and headache. While the hemoglobinuria ceases (if initially present) during the chills and fever phase, afterwards there is intense hemoglobinuria that may last for several hours (Crosby and Stefanini, 1952). The mechanism of these reactions is unknown, although it would appear that an antigen-antibody reaction is involved, leading to the activation of complement, to which PNH cells are highly sensitive. These reactions are not diminished by the use of washed red cells (Sherman and Taswell, 1977). However, since it has been shown that the interaction of leukocyte antigens and antibodies can cause lysis of PNH red cells *in vitro*, it would seem to be good practice to use leukocyte-poor red cells for transfusion. The activation of complement in cases of paroxysmal nocturnal hemoglobinuria is by the alternative pathway, apparently by the red cell membrane itself (see Götze and Müller-Eberhard, 1970).

The Laboratory Investigation of Paroxysmal Nocturnal Hemoglobinuria

A variety of methods exist for the laboratory investigation of paroxysmal nocturnal hemoglobinuria, all of which serve to increase the sensitivity of the defective red cell membrane to the action of complement. No one test should be relied upon to detect this condition, which usually requires serial testing.

The Ham's Test

Principle. When serum is acidified, it enhances the binding of complement to the red cells. Red cells from patients with paroxysmal nocturnal hemoglobinuria are more susceptible to hemolysis under these conditions.

Method

1. Wash the patient's red cells in isotonic saline.
2. Prepare a 40 to 50 per cent suspension of red cells in saline.
3. To 1 ml of fresh normal serum, add 0.1 ml of N/5 HCl.
4. Mix well.
5. To the acidified serum, add two drops of the patient's red cell suspension.
6. As controls, set up (a) the patient's red cells with unacidified normal serum, and (b) normal red cells with acidified patient's serum.
7. Mix well.
8. Incubate at 37°C for one hour.

9. Centrifuge and examine the supernatants. A positive reaction is indicated by definite hemolytic staining of the supernatant in the test with, at most, slight staining of the supernatant in control (a) and a clear supernatant in control (b).

Note: The only other condition that gives this positive result is marked erythrospherocytosis, which will be obvious in the blood smear.

It should also be noted that the addition of 0.003 to 0.005 M magnesium to the serum prior to testing greatly enhances the sensitivity of the test owing to the activation of the alternate complement pathway (May *et al*, 1973). 0.1 M magnesium is prepared from a stock solution of 2.8 M magnesium chloride. Add 0.1 ml of 0.1 M magnesium chloride to 1.9 ml of serum prior to testing.

The Sucrose Hemolysis Test
(Sugar-Water Test)

Principle. The sucrose hemolysis test is based on an empiric observation that red cells from patients with paroxysmal nocturnal hemoglobinuria are hemolyzed when incubated with autologous or isologous compatible normal serum or plasma in low ionic strength sucrose conditions.

Reagents

1. Sucrose, reagent grade   92.4 g
   0.005 M monobasic sodium
      phosphate   910.0 ml
   0.005 M dibasic sodium phosphate   90.0 ml
   Adjust the pH to 6.1 (if necessary).
2. Serum: type compatible normal serum either fresh or stored at −20°C for not longer than 2 weeks in order to retain full complement activity. (The test serum is not satisfactory.)
3. Cells: fresh EDTA or ACD anticoagulated test blood. Wash the red cells at least three times with normal isotonic saline and make up to a final 50 per cent suspension.

Method

1. Set up the following tubes:

	1	*2*	*3*	*4*	
Sucrose	0.90	0.95	0.95		ml
Cells	0.05	0.05		0.05	ml
Serum	0.05		0.05		ml
0.04% Ammonia in					
distilled water				0.95	ml

2. Incubate at room temperature for one hour.
3. Centrifuge to obtain a cell-free supernatant.
4. Transfer the supernatant and add 4 ml of 0.9% NaCl to each tube.

5. Read the optical density (OD) against a water blank at 540 nm.
6.

$$\% \text{ lysis} = \frac{OD_1 - (OD_2 + OD_3)}{OD_4 - OD_2} \times 100$$

Interpretation. Over 5 per cent lysis indicates paroxysmal nocturnal hemoglobinuria.

DRUG-INDUCED HEMOLYTIC ANEMIA

The administration of drugs may lead to the development of a wide variety of hematologic disorders, including autoimmune hemolytic anemia. Petz and Garratty (1980) report that 12.4 per cent of patients with acquired immune hemolytic anemia out of 347 investigated by them had anemias that were caused by drugs. There appear to be at least four ways in which drugs cause autoimmune hemolytic anemia, and each will be examined in turn.

Autoimmune Hemolytic Anemia and Methyldopa

Certain drugs cause a positive direct antiglobulin test with or without attending hemolytic anemia by a mechanism that is not clearly understood. Most important in this group is the antihypertensive drug alpha-methyldopa (Aldomet). Of patients receiving this drug, 15 to 20 per cent develop a positive direct antiglobulin test after about 3 to 6 months of treatment (this development being dose-dependent), though only about 1 per cent develop hemolytic anemia. In most cases the immunoglobulin on the red cells is solely IgG1 (van der Meulen, 1978), although complement was also found on the red cells in a few cases (Eyster and Jenkins, 1970). The antibodies often appear to have Rh specificity (see Worlledge *et al*, 1966).

Although the precise mechanism by which methyldopa causes autoimmune hemolytic anemia is not known, it is believed (among other hypotheses) that the drug alters the red cell membrane in some way or possibly damages suppressor T cells, in either case promoting the formation of autoantibodies. (For complete discussion of the mechanisms currently proposed, see Petz and Garratty, 1980, page 286.)

Worlledge (1969) reported that the total of alpha-methyldopa–induced cases exceeded the total of all other drug-induced autoimmune hemolytic anemias so far described. It is important to note, however, that when the drug is discontinued, the red cell autoantibodies usually dis-

Table 15–3 DRUGS THAT HAVE BEEN
REPORTED TO CAUSE A POSITIVE DIRECT
ANTIGLOBULIN TEST AND HEMOLYTIC ANEMIA*

Stibophen (Fuadin)
Quinidine
P-aminosalicylic acid (PAS)
Quinine
Phenacetin
Penicillins
Insecticides (chlorinated hydrocarbons)
Antihistamine (Antazoline, Antistine)
Sulfonamides
Isoniazid (INH, Rifamate, Nydrazid)
Chlorpromazine (Thorazine)
Pyramidon (Aminopyrine)
Dipyrone
Methyldopa (Aldomet, Aldoril, Aldoclor)
Melphalan (Alkeran)
Cephalosporins
Mefenamic acid (Ponstel)
Carbromal (Carbrital, Carbropent)†
Sulfonylurea derivatives (Diabinese, Dymelor, Orinase,
    Tolinase)
Insulin
Levodopa (Sinemet)
Rifampin (Rifadin, Rifamate, Rimactane)
Methadone†
Tetracycline
Methysergide (Sansert)
Acetaminophen
Hydrochlorothiazide
Streptomycin
Procainamide (Pronestyl, Sub-Quin)
Ibuprofen (Motrin)
Hydralazine (Apresoline, Hydralazide, Unipres)

---

*From Petz and Garratty, 1980.
†Reported to cause positive direct antiglobulin test,
but not hemolytic anemia.

appear and the direct antiglobulin test becomes
negative. It may take a long time for this to
occur — in some cases even up to two years.

Immune Complexes

The "immune complex" mechanism was
originally described to explain the basis of
thrombocytopenia, yet this same mechanism
appears also to be responsible for erythrocyte
sensitization and hemolysis in some patients.

Table 15–3 lists drugs that have been reported to cause a positive direct antiglobulin
test and hemolytic anemia. It is probable that
the immune complex mechanism is responsible
for the hemolytic anemia caused by most of
these drugs.

In brief, the mechanisms of immune complexes are as follows:

1. Administration of the drug results in the
production of an antibody directed against the
drug.

2. The antibody combines with the drug to
form an immune complex.

3. The antibody-drug complex is then adsorbed onto red cells (or white cells or platelets).

4. The cell-bound antibody-drug complex
may activate complement, resulting in intravascular hemolysis (Fig. 15–2).

Note: The red blood cells in this reaction can be
considered to be "innocent bystanders" and for
this reason, the immune complex mechanism is
sometimes referred to as the *innocent by-
stander mechanism.*

Drug Adsorption

Penicillin can cause a positive direct antiglobulin test and hemolytic anemia by the
drug adsorption mechanism, as follows: (1) The
drug itself is nonspecifically bound to the red
cells and remains firmly bound regardless of
whether the patient develops an antibody to the
drug. (2) If antibody is formed, it will react with
the cell-bound drug, giving a positive direct
antiglobulin test — and may result in hemolytic
anemia. (*Note:* Complement is not usually activated by antipenicillin antibodies.)

Cephalosporins can also act in the same
way (see Fig. 15–3).

Nonimmunologic Protein Absorption

Cephalosporins can cause a positive direct
antiglobulin test by three different mechanisms:

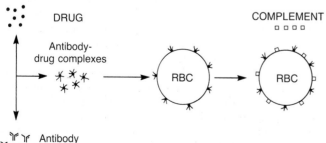

Figure 15–2 The immune complex mechanism.

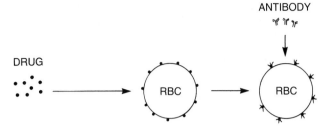

Figure 15–3 The drug adsorption mechanism.

1. The drug (cephalothin) may combine with the red cell membrane and then react with anti-cephalothin antibody (i.e., drug adsorption mechanism) (Abraham *et al*, 1968; Gralnick *et al*, 1967; Spath *et al*, 1971).

2. The cephalothin-coated red cell may react with cross-reacting penicillin antibodies (Abraham *et al*, 1968; Gralnick and McGinniss, 1967; Gralnick *et al*, 1967; Nesmith and Davis, 1968; Spath *et al*, 1971).

3. Cephalothin may modify the red cell membrane so that the cells adsorb proteins nonimmunologically (Gralnick *et al*, 1967; Molthan *et al*, 1967; Spath *et al*, 1971).

The nonimmunologic characteristics of cephalosporin-induced abnormalities include a positive direct antiglobulin test to a variety of proteins (e.g., gamma, beta, alpha globulins; albumin and fibrinogen; a nonreactive red cell eluate; serum may contain low-titer anticephalosporin or cross-reacting antipenicillin antibodies). Hemolytic anemia has not been described in this type. If the abnormalities are immunologic, however, the direct antiglobulin test will be positive due to sensitization *mainly* with IgG. The red cell eluate will react with cephalosporin-treated but not untreated red cells, and the serum usually contains high titer antibodies against cephalosporin-treated cells. In this type, hemolytic anemia may occur, though it is rare.

ATYPICAL AUTOIMMUNE HEMOLYTIC ANEMIA

Several unusual findings in cases of autoimmune hemolytic anemia have been reported, including:

1. Autoimmune hemolytic anemia with a negative direct antiglobulin test.

2. Autoimmune hemolytic anemia during pregnancy (its effects on the fetus).

3. The development of autoimmune hemolytic anemia following blood transfusion.

A full discussion of these and other abnormalities is beyond the scope of this book; interested students will find an excellent review

of the subject in Petz and Garratty (1980), pp. 305–357.

SEROLOGIC INVESTIGATION OF AUTOIMMUNE HEMOLYTIC ANEMIA

The actual techniques used in the investigation of autoimmune hemolytic anemia are given in other sections of this text and will not be repeated here. A basic format for investigation, however, is presented.

Specimen Requirements

Two specimens of blood should be collected from the patient: one in a "dry" tube (without anticoagulant) to provide serum and a second in EDTA to provide red cells for the direct antiglobulin test and the preparation of an eluate (see Chapter 23). If it is not known whether the hemolytic anemia is of the "warm" or "cold" type, the specimens should be collected and separated at 37° C. However, Petz and Garratty (1980) state that, unless a severe case of cold agglutinin syndrome is being dealt with, warming the samples at 37° C for 10 to 15 minutes produces reliable results in most cases.

EDTA is the anticoagulant of choice, since if blood is cooled to below body temperature, it will prevent the binding of complement to the cells by "insignificant" cold agglutinins, *in vitro*.

The Direct Antiglobulin Test (see Chapter 21)

The direct antiglobulin test is an extremely important diagnostic aid in cases of autoimmune hemolytic anemia. A negative result, however, does not exclude the diagnosis if the patient has other symptoms of the disease. A negative direct antiglobulin test may be caused by:

1. Antiglobulin reagents (i.e., "broad-spectrum") that are not able to detect the partic-

ular proteins involved. As discussed, certain rare patients with autoimmune hemolytic anemia have been found to possess only IgA or IgM on their red cells. Some commercial "broad-spectrum" antiglobulin reagents will not detect IgA and IgM and occasionally they will not detect C3d sensitization. In cases such as these, a direct antiglobulin test using monospecific antisera (anti-IgA, anti-IgM, etc.) may prove helpful.

2. Sensitization of the cells with small numbers of IgG molecules such that the degree of sensitization is below the threshold of the antiglobulin test. In cases such as these, more sensitive methods can be used; for example, the detection of agglutination augmented by polyvinylpyrrolidone (PVP) performed on the Auto-Analyzer (see Burkhart *et al*, 1974) or the complement-fixing antibody consumption test (see Gilliland *et al*, 1970; Gilliland *et al*, 1971).

Elution

Although the direct antiglobulin test provides useful information, the definitive diagnosis of autoimmune hemolytic anemia is dependent upon the characterization of the antibodies present in the patient's serum (see under the heading Identification of Antibodies) and in the red cell eluate. Therefore, if the direct antiglobulin test is positive, it is essential to remove the antibody from the cells (i.e., elute) in order to determine the specificity. Occasionally, red cells with a negative antiglobulin test will provide a strongly reactive eluate. Complement components causing a positive direct antiglobulin test will result in a negative eluate; however, if IgG is present on the cells, it can be eluted by simple methods using heat or ether (see Chapter 23) and identified by testing the eluate against a panel of phenotyped red cells.

If the direct antiglobulin test is positive due to IgG sensitization yet the eluate shows no activity against normal red cells, then drug-induced autoimmune hemolytic anemia can be suspected.

Identification of Antibodies (see Chapter 22)

In cases of "warm" antibody autoimmune hemolytic anemia, the panel of cells for identification should be set up with both eluate and serum. It is important that the nature of the autoantibody be identified if possible and also that the specificity of alloantibodies be iden-

tified in case a transfusion becomes necessary. It is desirable to test the serum and eluate in several dilutions against panel cells, because the specificity sometimes becomes apparent only after the "nonspecific" element has been diluted out.

In cases of "cold" antibody autoimmune hemolytic anemia, the antibody usually has anti-I specificity; therefore, the investigation should include several cord samples. Note, however, that if the anti-I is extremely powerful, cord cells may also give a positive result and the temperature of testing may have to be raised to obtain a typical anti-I pattern of reactivity.

Identification may require titration of the antibody against cord red cells and adult red cells to show a difference in reactivity.

Grouping of Patients with Autoimmune Hemolytic Anemia

ABO and Rh typing of patients with autoimmune hemolytic anemia is frequently complicated by the presence of autoagglutinins and sensitized red cells. If autoagglutinins are present, the patient's red cells should be collected into EDTA and washed at 37° C with warm saline before being tested. $Rh_o(D)$ typing should be performed using saline-reactive rather than slide-and-rapid-tube reagents. The same is true for other Rh phenotyping.

It is also wise to phenotype the patient as completely as possible before transfusion. Accurate testing of antiglobulin-reactive antibodies with the patient's red cells may be complicated by a positive direct antiglobulin test; however, if the autoantibody is eluted and the phenotyping performed on the resultant red cells, accurate results can often be obtained.

Transfusion of Blood to Patients with Autoimmune Hemolytic Anemia

Generally, transfusion should be avoided if possible in patients with autoimmune hemolytic anemia, since the donor cells will almost certainly be rapidly destroyed. If transfusion is essential, blood may be selected that is compatible with any alloantibodies that the patient may possess — after which the reactions that are obtained with this blood are compared with those obtained between the patient's serum and his own cells from which autoantibody has been eluted. As an alternative, "*in vivo* compatibility testing" may be utilized using ^{51}Cr-tagged donor cells to determine the rate of destruction (see Mayer *et al*, 1968, Mollison, 1979; see also Chapter 23). It should be noted, however, that this approach should not be used as a substitute for serologic evaluation of the patient.

When patients with autoimmune hemolytic anemia are transfused, the initial rate of destruction of the transfused red cells may be greater than that of the patient's own red cells. Later, however, rates of destruction will equalize. This may result from the fact that the average age of red cells in the donor unit is likely to be greater than that of the red cells of the patient, and "old" cells are more susceptible to damage both *in vivo* and *in vitro* by hemolytic heteroantibodies (Cruz and Junqueira, 1952; London, 1961; Gower and Davidson, 1963; de Wit and van Gastel, 1969) and to destruction *in vivo* by nonhemolytic IgM alloantibodies (Burton and Mollison, 1968) than are "young" cells.

TYPICAL EXAMINATION QUESTIONS

Select the phrase, sentence or symbol that completes the statement or answers the question. More than one answer may be acceptable in each case. Answers are given in the back of this book.

1. "Adsorption" refers to
   (a) removal of antibody from the serum
   (b) removal of antibody from the cells
   (c) take-up of antibody by the cells
   (d) none of the above
   (Essential Terms)

2. The process whereby an antibody is produced against an individual's own tissues is known as
   (a) alloimmunization
   (b) heteroimmunization
   (c) nonself-immunization
   (d) autoimmunization
   (Introduction)

3. The immune response gene is closely linked to
   (a) the *Rh* loci
   (b) the *HLA* loci
   (c) the *ABO* loci
   (d) the *MNSs* loci
   (Possible Mechanisms in the Initiation of Autoimmune Diseases)

4. Autoimmune hemolytic anemia of the "warm" antibody type
   (a) accounts for more than 80 per cent of all cases
   (b) involves, in most cases, IgG antibody
   (c) is sometimes "secondary" to cases of systemic lupus erythematosus
   (d) often shows antibody specificity associated with Rh
   ("Warm" Antibody Autoimmune Hemolytic Anemia)

5. "Cold" antibody autoimmune hemolytic anemia
   (a) is associated with *Mycoplasma pneumoniae*
   (b) usually involves I-like antibodies
   (c) is never "idiopathic"
   (d) usually involves IgM antibody, although IgG and IgA antibodies could also be present, though in lower titer
   ("Cold" Antibody Autoimmune Hemolytic Anemia)

6. The antibody most often present as a transient phenomenon in cases of infectious mononucleosis is
   (a) anti-I
   (b) anti-i
   (c) anti-Pr
   (d) anti-e
   ("Cold" Antibody Autoimmune Hemolytic Anemia — Disease Associations)

7. Paroxysmal cold hemoglobinuria
   (a) involves the DL antibody, which has anti-P_1 specificity
   (b) is frequently associated with viral infections, particularly in children
   (c) was first described in a patient with tertiary syphilis
   (d) is usually associated with warm antibodies
   (Paroxysmal Cold Hemoglobinuria)

8. The mechanism of autoimmune hemolytic anemia due to methyldopa is
   (a) the immune complex mechanism
   (b) unknown
   (c) the Drug Adsorption mechanism
   (d) the nonimmunogenic protein adsorption mechanism
   (Drug-Induced Hemolytic Anemia)

9. When there is no apparent cause for the development of the antibody in autoimmune hemolytic anemia, the applied term is
   (a) secondary
   (b) specific
   (c) idiopathic
   (d) autoimmunization
   ("Warm" Antibody Autoimmune Hemolytic Anemia)

10. The test for the detection of the hemolysin involved in paroxysmal cold hemoglobinuria is
    (a) the Mendel test
    (b) the Landsteiner test
    (c) the direct antiglobulin test
    (d) the Donath-Landsteiner test
    (Paroxysmal Cold Hemoglobinuria)

11. If the direct antiglobulin test is positive due to IgG sensitization yet the eluate shows no activity against normal red cells,
    (a) drug-induced hemolytic anemia can be suspected

(b) the patient probably has "cold" autoimmune hemolytic anemia

(c) the elution procedure should be considered unreliable

(d) none of the above   *(Elution)*

12. In the investigation of "cold" antibody autoimmune hemolytic anemia

(a) several cord samples should be set up with the patient's serum

(b) specimens should be collected and separated at 37° C, or warmed at 37° C for 10 to 15 minutes before testing

(c) titration of the antibody may be necessary against cord and adult red cells to determine specificity

(d) the ABO and Rh typing will not be affected by the presence of autoagglutinins

(The Serologic Investigation of Autoimmune Hemolytic Anemia)

ANSWER TRUE OR FALSE

13. The term "elution" refers to the removal of antibody from the red cells.

(Essential Terms)

14. IgG alone is invariably found in patients with a positive direct antiglobulin test due to α-methyldopa.

("Warm" Antibody Autoimmune Hemolytic Anemia — Immunoglobulins Involved)

15. In "warm" antibody autoimmune hemolytic anemia, the complement components C5 and C6 are not present on the patient's red cells.

("Warm" Antibody Autoimmune Hemolytic Anemia — Complement)

16. Anti-pdl refers to an antibody against "partially deleted" Rh-positive red cells.

("Warm" Antibody Autoimmune Hemolytic Anemia — Specificity of Antibody)

17. "Cold" antibody autoimmune hemolytic anemia is always idiopathic.

("Cold" Antibody Autoimmune Hemolytic Anemia)

18. The receptor for anti-Pr is enhanced by proteolytic enzymes.

("Cold" Antibody Autoimmune Hemolytic Anemia — Specificity of Antibody)

19. Penicillin can cause a positive direct antiglobulin test and hemolytic anemia by the drug adsorption mechanism.

(Drug-Induced Hemolytic Anemia)

20. "Broad-spectrum" antiglobulin reagents will always detect IgA and IgM sensitized red cells.

(The Direct Antiglobulin Test)

GENERAL REFERENCES

1. Boorman, K. E., Dodd, B. E. and Lincoln, P. J.: Blood Group Serology; Theory, Techniques, Practical Applications, 5th Ed. Churchill Livingston, New York, 1977. *(Chapter devoted to autoimmune hemolytic anemia is concise, yet written in a way that is easy to understand. Contains several appropriate techniques.)*

2. Mollison, P. L.: Blood Transfusion in Clinical Medicine. 6th Ed. Blackwell Scientific Publications, Oxford, 1979. *(Discussion is divided in many sections of this text, yet is thorough and places the emphasis on the clinical aspects, although the laboratory aspects are well covered.)*

3. Petz, L. D. and Garratty, G.: Acquired Immune Hemolytic Anemias. Churchill Livingstone, New York, 1980. *(An excellent book, containing complete and thorough coverage of the subject. Highly recommended for all students and all blood banks involved in the investigation of autoimmune hemolytic anemia.)*

HEMOLYTIC DISEASE OF THE NEWBORN

OBJECTIVES — HEMOLYTIC DISEASE OF THE NEWBORN

The student shall know, understand and be prepared to explain:

1. A brief history of the discovery of hemolytic disease of the newborn
2. The mechanisms of sensitization of Rh hemolytic disease of the newborn
3. The mechanisms of sensitization of ABO hemolytic disease of the newborn
4. The influence of ABO incompatibility on Rh immunization
5. Prenatal investigations, including:
   (a) Tests on the mother
   (b) Tests on the father
   (c) Amniotic fluid examination (amniocentesis)
   (d) Intrauterine transfusion
6. Postnatal investigations, including:
   (a) ABO grouping of the cord blood
   (b) Rh typing of the cord blood
   (c) The direct antiglobulin test
   (d) Specific antiglobulin test
   (e) Elution
   (f) Hematologic tests
7. The most common clinical features of hemolytic disease of the newborn
8. The treatment of infants suffering from hemolytic disease of the newborn, including the selection of blood for exchange transfusion
9. The prevention of hemolytic disease of the newborn (the use of $Rh_0(D)$ immune globulin), specifically to include:
   (a) Dose
   (b) Preinjection of $Rh_0(D)$ immune globulin
   (c) Antibodies in the maternal serum after injection
   (d) Antenatal treatment
   (e) Other indications for the use of $Rh_0(D)$ immune globulin

Introduction

Hemolytic disease of the newborn (originally known as erythroblastosis fetalis) is a disease which starts *in utero* and causes jaundice, anemia and enlargement of the liver and spleen of the infant.

The cause of the disease is blood group incompatibility in which antibody, originating in the maternal circulation as a direct result of antigenic stimulation by fetal red cells, enters the fetal circulation through the placenta and attaches to the blood group antigens on the infant's red cells, resulting in the destruction of those cells. The severity of the effects of the disease ranges from mild anemia to mental retardation, brain damage, kernicterus or still-birth. The severity depends on the number of fetal red cells destroyed and the ability of the fetus to compensate by increased production of new cells.

ABO antibodies, which occur as IgG in some group O subjects, and $Rh_0(D)$ antibodies are most commonly implicated as the cause of hemolytic disease of the newborn, although in the case of ABO antibodies the disease is rarely severe. Other blood group antibodies seldom cause hemolytic disease of the newborn; the least uncommon as a cause is anti-c and after that anti-E and anti-K. It is important to realize, however, that the list of other antibodies that have been shown to be responsible for the disease includes virtually every blood group antibody that can occur as IgG. It should also be noted that the severity of the disease is not influenced by the specificity of the antibody involved.

Rh Hemolytic Disease of the Newborn: Mechanisms of Sensitization

The human placenta consists of blood vessels, vascular spaces and small amounts of supportive tissue. Its prime function is the exchange of substances between mother and fetus (the simple diffusion of gases, water and electrolytes and the active transportation of nutritional materials).

The fact that hemolytic disease of the newborn is caused by the passage of *antibodies* from mother to fetus was first demonstrated by Levine and Stetson (1939), who described how the mother of a stillborn fetus suffered a hemolytic transfusion reaction to the transfusion of her husband's blood. The mother's serum was subsequently found to agglutinate the red cells of her husband and about 80 per cent of other randomly selected ABO compatible donors (see The Rh/Hr Blood Group System, Chapter 5). Levine and Stetson interpreted their findings by postulating that the mother, who lacked this "new" antigen, had become immunized by the red cells of her fetus that possessed the antigen, having inherited it from the father. This interpretation is now known to have been entirely correct, confirmed in the now-classic paper of Levine *et al* (1941).

When hemolytic disease of the newborn due to anti-$Rh_o(D)$ occurs, mother and infant are always incompatible with respect to the Rh factor: the mother is $Rh_o(D)$-negative and the infant has inherited the $Rh_o(D)$ factor from the father and is $Rh_o(D)$-positive.

The first Rh-incompatible infant is usually unaffected. While fetal cells do cross the placenta during the pregnancy (though usually not before the 24th week of gestation) the number of cells is usually small and insufficient to cause antibody production. This is known because Rh antibodies are seen in the maternal circulation in only about 2 per cent of cases at the end of a first pregnancy with an ABO-compatible, Rh-positive fetus. In addition to this fact, elevated steroid levels and other factors associated with pregnancy may suppress the mother's primary immune response (Fig. 16–1).

At term, however, a so-called "transplacental hemorrhage" is not uncommon — at which time the amount of fetal blood entering the maternal circulation varies between a trace and 10 ml or more. It should be noted that amniocentesis, cesarean section and manual removal of the placenta increases the risk of appreciable leakage of fetal cells into the maternal circulation, as do stillbirth, spontaneous miscarriage and D&C (dilation and curettage) (Fig. 16–2).

Within about six months after delivery, about 7 per cent of these $Rh_o(D)$-negative women have produced detectable antibodies. There is now known to be a relationship between the *number* of fetal cells in the maternal circulation and the chance of the appearance of an antibody (Fig. 16–3).

When pregnancy with a second $Rh_o(D)$-positive fetus occurs, small numbers of fetal

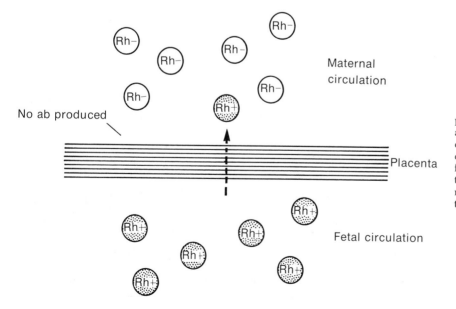

Figure 16–1 First incompatible pregnancy. Small amounts of blood from the fetal circulation enter the maternal circulation after the twenty-fourth week of gestation, yet they are usually in insufficient numbers to cause the production of antibody in the mother.

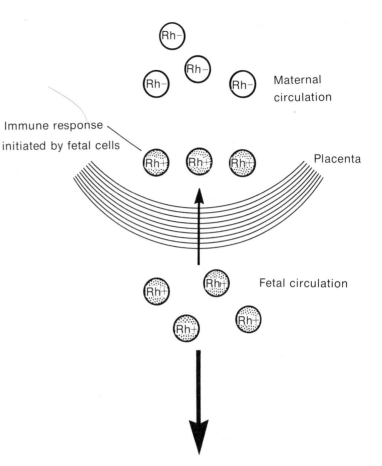

Figure 16–2 First pregnancy — term. A fetomaternal transfusion (transplacental hemorrhage) has occurred, initiating an immune response in the mother.

cells cross the placenta into the maternal circulation again from about the 24th week of gestation onward, but this time, since they are secondary doses of antigen, they are capable of stimulating the antibody to high titers (Fig. 16–4).

The anti-Rh_o(D) formed is IgG, and, as discussed in Chapter 2, is the only immunoglobulin transferred across the placenta. This antibody therefore crosses back into the fetal circulation. In the first 12 weeks of gestation only small amounts of IgG are transferred, although evidence of the passage of anti-Rh has been reported in fetuses of 6 and 10 weeks' gestation, respectively (Chown, 1955; Mollison,

1951). In the fetal circulation, this antibody combines with fetal Rh_o(D)-positive red cells, leading to their destruction (Fig. 16–5). It should be noted that sufficient anti-Rh can cross the placenta by the 16th to 20th week of gestation to cause intrauterine death, although this is uncommon before about the 20th week.

ABO Hemolytic Disease of the Newborn: Mechanisms of Sensitization

The mechanisms of hemolytic disease of the newborn caused by ABO incompatibility are similar to those of Rh incompatibility in that

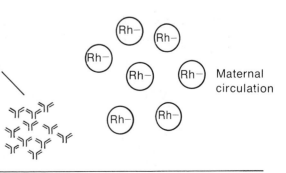

Figure 16–3 Antibody production —post-term.

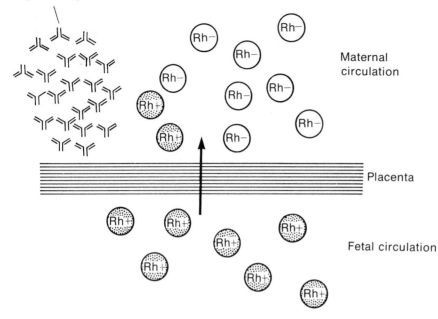

IgG anti-Rh$_o$(D) stimulated to
high titers by fetal cells

Maternal
circulation

Placenta

Fetal circulation

Figure 16–4 Second incompatible pregnancy. Small amounts of fetal cells crossing into the maternal circulation during the pregnancy provoke a secondary response, stimulating the existing antibody to high titers.

the passage of fetal red cells into the maternal circulation provokes an immune response in the mother.

Unlike Rh hemolytic disease of the newborn, the ABO form of the disease can and does occur in the first pregnancy. The mother is invariably group O and therefore possesses anti-A and anti-B in her plasma. It has been demonstrated that the "immune" anti-A and anti-B in group B and A subjects respectively is usually IgM, whereas the "immune" anti-A, B in group O subjects is more often partly IgG (Rowson and Abelson, 1960; Kochwa *et al*, 1961), which is capable of crossing the placenta.

It is not surprising that ABO hemolytic disease of the newborn may affect the first pregnancy when one considers that anti-A and anti-B are always present and therefore readily stimulated. In spite of the fact that there is a

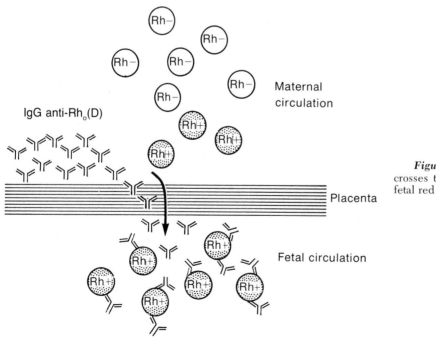

Rh−

Rh−

Rh−

Rh−

Rh−

Rh+

Rh+

Rh+

IgG anti-Rh$_o$(D)

Maternal
circulation

Placenta

Rh+

Rh+

Rh+

Rh+

Rh+

Fetal circulation

Figure 16–5 Maternal antibody crosses the placenta and combines with fetal red cells.

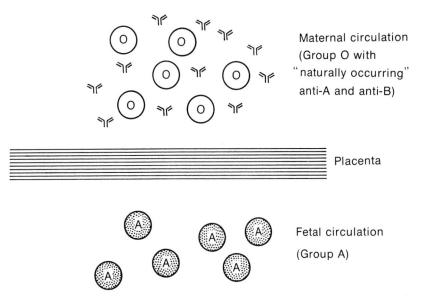

Figure 16–6 ABO incompatible pregnancy.

high incidence of heterospecific pregnancies (based on the high frequency of group O mothers in the population), ABO hemolytic disease of the newborn that is severe enough to warrant treatment occurs only in about one in 3000 births (Ames and Lloyd, 1964; Voak and Bowley, 1969). Mild forms of the disease are more common. It is interesting to note that ABO disease is between two and six times commoner in blacks than in whites (Kirkman, 1977). This rarity of the disease is thought to be due to the presence of A and B substances in the fetal tissues and fluids that will neutralize the anti-A and anti-B antibodies before they can attack the fetal red cells. Since there is no association of the disease with infants who are nonsecretors, however, either this is not the whole explana-

tion or the amount of substance in the tissues and the trace amounts in the fluids of nonsecretor infants are a sufficient protection.

An example of the mechanism of ABO hemolytic disease of the newborn is as follows: A mother of blood group O becomes pregnant with a fetus of blood group A (Fig. 16–6). The fetal red cells cross the placenta into the maternal circulation from about the 24th week of gestation, stimulating the existing anti-A to high titers. The "immune" anti-A thus stimulated is largely IgG (Fig. 16–7). The "immune" IgG anti-A then crosses the placenta into the fetal circulation, where it combines with fetal red cells, leading to their destruction (Fig. 16–8).

While severe forms of ABO hemolytic disease of the newborn are rare, when they do

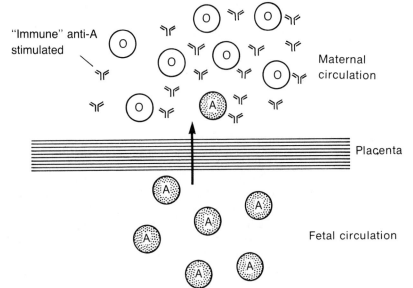

Figure 16–7 Fetal red cells cross the placenta into the maternal circulation, stimulating the formation of immune IgG anti-A.

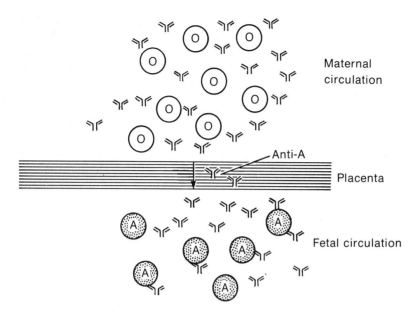

Figure 16–8 IgG anti-A crosses the placenta into the fetal circulation, where it combines with fetal red cells, leading to their destruction.

occur some of the infants suffering from the disease require exchange transfusion, some are kernicteric and some are stillborn.

The Influence of ABO Incompatibility on Rh Immunization

Immunization due to Rh through pregnancy (and transfusion) is less common when the fetus is ABO incompatible with the mother — although once the mother does become immunized to the Rh antigen, further ABO-incompatible infants in the family are not protected. The reason for this could be that when the $Rh_o(D)$-positive fetal red cells are ABO incompatible, they are destroyed immediately upon entering the maternal circulation by the existing ABO antibodies. As a result, all of the D antigenic sites are presented at one time and as a single dose to the immunocytes, which is less likely to induce an immune response than a series of small, repeated immunizing doses over a long period of time.

PRENATAL INVESTIGATIONS

Tests on the Mother

Prenatal investigations of the blood of the mother are routinely performed to identify those women at risk of having a child affected with hemolytic disease of the newborn. Once these women are identified, regular screening tests can be utilized to ascertain the degree of involvement. A mother's first prenatal specimen should be taken at or before the 13th week of pregnancy; that is, at the first obstetrical visit. An obstetric and transfusion history should be taken and relevant laboratory tests should include a full ABO grouping, Rh typing and antibody screening. If the mother is $Rh_o(D)$ positive or $Rh_o{}^u(D^u)$ positive, a further specimen should be requested at 32 weeks' gestation to ensure that antibodies of other specificities have not been formed. Antibody screening using enzyme and antiglobulin techniques is recommended on both $Rh_o(D)$-positive and Rh_o(D)-negative mothers for this purpose. It is well to note that antibodies such as anti-Lewis, anti-IH, anti-H and anti-I are relatively common during pregnancy but do not cause hemolytic disease of the newborn because, being IgM, they are not able to cross the placenta. Treatment of the serum with 2-mercaptoethanol or dithiothreitol (see Special Techniques, Chapter 23) will aid in distinguishing IgM from IgG antibodies.

If the mother is $Rh_o(D)$-negative, her red cells should be routinely tested for the Rh_o variant (D^u). The results of this test should be read macroscopically. If results are read microscopically, the record should indicate this. If the original antibody screening test is negative, the test should be repeated at about 32 weeks' gestation — and if still negative at this time, no further prenatal tests need be made. However, if an antibody is detected by screening tests, specificity should be established using a panel of eight or more cells (see Chapter 22).

All significant antibodies should be monitored at least monthly. At each of these visits, the mother's serum should be retested using a full panel. The antibody should be titrated by doubling dilutions of serum, using the technique in which the antibody reacts best. Titrations must always be run in parallel with the previous sample to determine if there has been a significant change in titer. A change in titer of more than two tubes (i.e., over fourfold) or a score change of more than 10 is significant. Score changes of 5 to 10 and titer changes of less than two tubes are equivocal and could be the result of variation in technique between different technologists. (Titration is described in Chapters 22 and 23.)

The correlation of the titer of maternal antibody and the severity of the disease are often inaccurate. Titration, however, does serve to identify those women who are candidates for amniocentesis. While it is true that a rising titer in the first affected pregnancy indicates that the baby probably will be affected with hemolytic disease of the newborn, serial titers in subsequent pregnancies have only limited prognostic value.

Tests on the Father

If a mother is $Rh_0(D)$-negative yet demonstrates no irregular antibodies, a specimen of blood from the father may be helpful in establishing the risk of immunization, and also in predicting the outcome of future pregnancies. If the father is also $Rh_0(D)$-negative (cde/cde), then hemolytic disease of the newborn caused by Rh immunization can be discounted. In other types of hemolytic disease of the newborn, the father's red cells can be tested to determine if he is homozygous or heterozygous for the gene producing the immunizing antigen.

Amniotic Fluid Examination (Amniocentesis)

Amniocentesis is the technique of withdrawing amniotic fluid (which surrounds the fetus in utero) through the mother's abdominal wall for laboratory analysis. As described, antibody formed by the mother will cause the destruction of fetal red cells after crossing the placenta. As a result of this destruction, excess bilirubin-like pigment is produced and is cleared from the fetal circulation via the placenta and amniotic fluid. This bilirubin-like pigment causes the amniotic fluid to be stained yellow; the greater the intensity of yellow color exhibited by the fluid, the more severe will be the affliction of the fetus. The intensity of this yellow color in the amniotic fluid can be measured spectrophotometrically; this measurement gives an indirect indication of the degree of red cell destruction being manifested by the fetus. (A method of quantitation of this bilirubin-like pigment is given in Chapter 23.)

The first amniotic fluid examination is usually done at about 26 weeks' gestation but may be performed earlier if there is a past history of a baby with hemolytic disease of the newborn. There are two main indications for amniocentesis: The first is an antiglobulin titer of 32 or higher for an atypical antibody known to be capable of causing hemolytic disease of the newborn. (*Note:* this minimal critical titer may vary slightly in different laboratories.) The second is a history of hemolytic disease of the newborn.

Amniocentesis should not be performed without clear indications because of the inherent risks associated with the procedure (the possibility of infection, the possibility that more severe sensitization may occur if the needle allows the escape of fetal red cells into the maternal circulation and the possibility that labor may be induced or that fetal death may occur). Amniocentesis is *never* indicated in ABO hemolytic disease of the newborn.

The amniotic fluid sample should be free of fresh blood or hemoglobin or both. A small number of red cells, however, will always be present in the fluid, and these can be typed after centrifugation of the fluid for ABO and Rh. The direct antiglobulin test can also be performed on these red cells. The adult or fetal origin of these cells can be determined with the use of the Kleihauer test (see Chapter 23) and in this way the infant's blood type may be predicted.

In principle, spectrophotometric examination involves the passing of a light path through the amniotic fluid. When no bilirubin-like pigment is present, the light will pass directly through the fluid. When the pigment is present, a certain amount of light will be absorbed by the yellow color at the specific wavelength of 450 nm ($\Delta OD450$). Since "trends" are much more valuable than isolated points, sequential studies are performed at two-week intervals, or closer if necessary. A special absorbance curve from 350 to 750 nm is made of the amniotic fluid; a line is then projected from 375 to 525 nm and the change in absorbance seen at 450 nm is plotted on a Liley graph according to the appropriate week of gestation (Liley, 1961) (see Figs. 16–9, 16–10).

If the $\Delta OD450$ is in the low zone on the Liley graph (Fig. 16–10), or if it falls into the

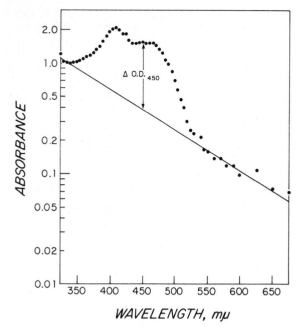

Figure 16–9 Visible absorption spectrums of amniotic fluid. The log absorbance has been plotted against the wavelength. The peak at ΔOD450 above the tangent (which corrects for background absorbance) is directly related to the severity of the disease. (From *AABB Technical Manual*, 7th edition, copyright © 1977, American Association of Blood Banks, Washington, D.C.)

zone (or if there is a trend from the middle zone to the upper zone as the pregnancy progresses) fetal death can be considered to be imminent. In "early" pregnancy (prior to 32 to 34 weeks) an intrauterine transfusion may be indicated. After 32 to 34 weeks' gestation, the pregnancy is usually interrupted to deliver the baby. Before premature delivery is undertaken, a determination of the lecithin/sphingomyelin (L/S) ratio on the amniotic fluid may be valuable in predicting fetal lung maturity, and therefore the ability of the fetus to survive (Bryson *et al*, 1972).

Intrauterine Transfusion

Intrauterine transfusion is the technique of introducing red cells, which find their way into the fetal circulation, into the fetal peritoneal cavity while the fetus is still *in utero*. The technique was evolved by Liley (1963). While there are several modifications, the one in fairly general use is the insertion of a needle into the fetal abdominal cavity with the position being checked by x-ray (Holman and Karnicki, 1964).

The amount of fresh blood transfused depends on the size of the fetus. Group O Rh-negative blood is normally used, which is cross-matched with the maternal serum. If ABO grouping of the fetus has been established from a sample of amniotic fluid, blood of the same group as the fetus can be used.

Intrauterine transfusion is usually not performed later than the 34th week of gestation.

low zone as the pregnancy progresses, the infant will be unaffected or will have only mild hemolytic disease. A "middle" zone pattern suggests moderate affliction, which may require exchange transfusion after an early delivery. If the ΔOD450 values are above 0.3 in the upper

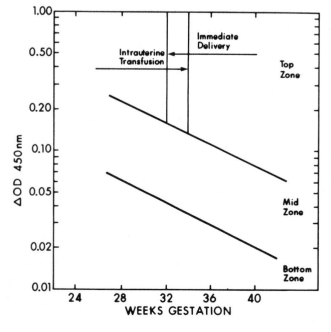

Figure 16–10 Liley graph. The absorbance value at ΔOD450 is plotted on this graph to indicate the degree of affliction with hemolytic disease and to indicate whether intrauterine transfusion or immediate delivery is indicated (see text). (From *AABB Technical Manual*, 7th edition, copyright © 1977, American Association of Blood Banks, Washington, D.C.)

Delivery is usually at about the 36th week, often by lower segment cesarean section.

At birth, infants with hemolytic disease of the newborn caused by anti-$Rh_o(D)$ who have been recipients of intrauterine transfusions often type as Rh negative with a negative direct antiglobulin test. This is due to the fact that 90 per cent of the baby's blood may be that of the donor.

POSTNATAL INVESTIGATIONS

Immediately after birth, a clotted sample of blood is taken from the placental vein ("cord" blood). Examination of all cord bloods is important, even when hemolytic disease of the newborn is not anticipated or even suspected. The infant's blood should undergo the following tests: ABO, $Rh_o(D)$ type and D^u if $Rh_o(D)$ is negative, direct antiglobulin test, specific antiglobulin test, elution if the result of the direct antiglobulin test is positive and identification of antibody in the eluate.

ABO Grouping

Anti-A and anti-B agglutinins do not usually develop until a few months after birth, and therefore any such agglutinins in the cord serum are probably of maternal origin. The ABO group of the baby, therefore, is based entirely on cell (forward) grouping. It should be noted that if the baby has received repeated intrauterine transfusions, erroneous results may be found in ABO grouping, Rh typing and the direct antiglobulin test.

Rh Typing

Some considerable difficulty may be experienced with respect to accurate Rh typing of babies with hemolytic disease of the newborn. In addition to the causes of false positive and false negative $Rh_o(D)$ typing already discussed (Chapter 5), the presence of Wharton's jelly in the sample and the coating of Rh-negative red cells by an antibody other than anti-$Rh_o(D)$ may cause false positive reactions — while the saturation of cord red cells with maternal anti-$Rh_o(D)$ may cause false negative reactions.

Wharton's jelly is the mucoid connective tissue that makes up the matrix of the umbilical cord. Contamination of the cord sample with Wharton's jelly often results in the spontaneous agglutination of red cells. This agglutination may be enhanced by the potentiating media that is added to slide-and-rapid-tube test anti-$Rh_o(D)$ serum. The use of an albumin control or saline-reactive anti-$Rh_o(D)$ serum will aid in detecting the anomaly. The effects of contamination by Wharton's jelly can be avoided by carefully washing the cord cells before testing, three to six times with warm saline, or by insisting that the sample be obtained by venipuncture from a placental vein.

If the cord red cells have been sensitized *in vivo* by maternal antibody other than anti-$Rh_o(D)$, for example, anti-hr'(c), false positive results may be obtained — especially when albumin typing antisera are used. Again, the use of an 8 per cent albumin control or saline anti-$Rh_o(D)$ will aid in resolving the problem.

False negative (or weak positive) results are sometimes encountered when a newborn is Rh positive and the red cells are saturated with maternal anti-$Rh_o(D)$ so that all of the $Rh_o(D)$ sites are "blocked." If the mother is $Rh_o(D)$ negative and the baby appears also to be $Rh_o(D)$ negative yet with a strongly positive direct antiglobulin test, the condition can be suspected. Elution of the anti-$Rh_o(D)$ from the cord red cells will confirm that the infant is $Rh_o(D)$ positive.

Direct Antiglobulin Test

The direct antiglobulin test is usually strongly positive in $Rh_o(D)$ and other forms of hemolytic disease of the newborn, yet may be weak or negative in the ABO variety.

Elution

Whenever the results of the direct antiglobulin test are positive, identification of antibody in the eluate of cord cells should be performed. If the mother's serum contains no unexpected antibody, yet the mother and infant are ABO incompatible, the eluate should be tested against A_1, B and O red cells by the saline and antiglobulin techniques. The procedure must be used to diagnose ABO hemolytic disease of the newborn. If no antibodies are demonstrated in the mother's serum or in the eluate from the cord cells, yet the direct antiglobulin test is positive, hemolytic disease of the newborn resulting from a "private," or low-incidence, factor can be suspected. This can be confirmed by testing the mother's serum with the father's red cells (if ABO compatible) or by absorbing the anti-A or anti-B from the mother's serum and then testing with the father's red cells (if ABO incompatible).

Additional Tests

In addition to the blood bank tests described, the following hematologic tests should be performed on the cord blood whenever the mother is known to be immunized to *any* red cell antigen: hemoglobin, hematocrit, serum bilirubin and blood smear evaluation.

Clinical Aspects

A detailed account of the clinical aspects of hemolytic disease of the newborn is beyond the scope of this book, and therefore only the most common clinical features of the disease are discussed here. The interested reader is referred to Mollison (1979) for comprehensive coverage of this subject.

The most common clinical features of hemolytic disease of the newborn are *anemia* and *jaundice*, which usually occur together. The anemia is usually accompanied by an increase in reticulocytes and nucleated red cells. The jaundice usually is apparent at birth or within 24 hours of birth. If jaundice occurs at a later period of neonatal life, then it is usually "physiologic" and not due to hemolytic disease of the newborn.

THE TREATMENT OF INFANTS SUFFERING FROM HEMOLYTIC DISEASE OF THE NEWBORN

Not all infants suffering from hemolytic disease of the newborn require treatment. In each case, the clinical, hematologic and serologic findings must all be considered, although the finding of anemia or raised serum bilirubin or both would indicate the need for treatment even if the serologic findings were unimpressive.

Treatment of hemolytic disease of the newborn is by transfusion to the infant of blood that lacks the antigen corresponding to the causative antibody.

Selection of Blood for Exchange Transfusion

Exchange transfusion is performed to lower the serum bilirubin concentration, to remove the baby's red cells that have been coated with antibody, to provide substitute compatible red cells with adequate oxygen-carrying capacity and to reduce the amount of irregular antibody

in the baby. To meet these objectives, donor blood should lack the red cell antigens corresponding to the maternal antibodies — it should be crossmatched with the maternal serum (because antibodies in the infant will be of maternal origin and will therefore be in greater concentration in the mother's serum). It should be less than five days old to ensure maximum red cell viability, to minimize the extra pigment and potassium loads released from nonviable red blood cells, to ensure immediate and good hemoglobin function through maximum 2,3 DPG levels and to ensure minimum plasma potassium, which could lead to cardiac irregularities.

ABO Hemolytic Disease of the Newborn. Group O red cells of the same Rh type as the baby should be used. Concentrated red cells or frozen deglycerolyzed red cells used in combination with compatible plasma (e.g., group AB) is most satisfactory, since this will avoid the transfusion of anti-A and anti-B.

Rh_0 and "Other" Forms of Hemolytic Disease of the Newborn. Blood of the same ABO group as the baby can be used when the mother and infant are ABO compatible. If the donor unit is prepared before delivery of an infant with Rh hemolytic disease of the newborn, a group O Rh(D)-negative unit that lacks excessive hemolytic activity (or concentrated red cells or frozen deglycerolyzed red cells) can be selected. O Rh_0(D)-negative blood that lacks the corresponding antigen to the causative antibody is selected in hemolytic disease of the newborn caused by antibodies other than anti-Rh_0(D). Again either the blood selected should be low in hemolytic anti-A or anti-B activity or it should be given as concentrated or frozen deglycerolyzed red cells. If the transfusion can be delayed until the ABO and Rh group of the infant is determined, then group-specific blood that lacks the antigen to the causative antibody is preferable.

It should be noted that if the clinical situation is critical, blood that is slightly older than five days may be used for transfusion.

In cases in which exchange transfusion is required more than once, subsequent units should be of the same ABO and Rh type as the first unit. The presence in the maternal serum of antibodies that are additional to the causative antibody (e.g., anti-Lewis, anti-I) may require the use of blood that is incompatible with the maternal serum. Since these antibodies do not cross the placenta, the transfusion can be considered "safe" provided that the blood lacks the antigen corresponding to the maternal IgG antibody. Alternatively, the maternal serum can be treated with 2-mercaptoethanol or dithio-threitol and then used in the compatibility test. After delivery, compatibility tests can be performed using the cord cell eluate in this situation.

If the antibody involved is reactive against a high-frequency antigen and compatible blood cannot be found, the following alternatives may be considered:

1. The mother's siblings (if available) may be tested for suitability.

2. A unit of blood may be collected from the mother. The plasma is removed and the red cells resuspended in group AB plasma.

3. Incompatible blood may be used (see Allen, 1968).

PREVENTION OF HEMOLYTIC DISEASE OF THE NEWBORN (USE OF $Rh_o(D)$ IMMUNE GLOBULIN)

The initial experiments revealing that passively administered anti-Rh could interfere with primary Rh immunization were performed by Stern *et al* (1961). Finn (1960) had postulated that fetal red cells in the maternal circulation might be destroyed by the administration of a suitable antibody; experiments in an attempt to prove this were made by that worker and his colleagues during the year that followed.

It is now well known that when an adequate dose of IgG anti-D (about 20 μg per/ml Rh-positive red cells) is given to an Rh-negative woman within 72 hours after delivery of an Rh-positive infant, Rh immunization is usually prevented. Candidates for this prophylaxis are (1) $Rh_o(D)$-negative and D^u-negative mothers who have no detectable anti-$Rh_o(D)$ in their serums and have an Rh-positive or D^u-positive infant and (2) women who have abortions, first trimester amniocentesis, antepartum hemorrhage or ectopic pregnancies. $Rh_o(D)$ immune globulin is not given to $Rh_o(D)$-negative women who deliver $Rh_o(D)$-negative infants, to $Rh_o(D)$-negative women whose serum contains anti-$Rh_o(D)$ or to $Rh_o(D)$-positive or D^u-positive women.

Dose. $Rh_o(D)$ immune globulin is supplied as a sterile, clear injectable for intramuscular administration. The usual recommended dose (contained in one vial) is about 300 μg, which is believed to offer protection against a fetomaternal hemorrhage of 30 ml (15 ml packed cells) or less (Pollack *et al*, 1971), although not all workers agree with these figures (see Mollison, 1979 p. 340 for detailed discussion). A "massive" fetomaternal hemorrhage

can be confirmed by the acid-elution test of Kleihauer-Betke (see Chapter 23). When such a hemorrhage has occurred, one vial of $Rh_o(D)$ immune globulin may not be enough to suppress alloimmunization from this large challenge. If massive fetomaternal hemorrhage is confirmed, the volume of the hemorrhage must be determined in order to calculate the number of vials of $Rh_o(D)$ immune globulin to administer. This volume can be calculated by multiplying the percentage of fetal cells (seen in the acid-elution stain) by 50. Since each dose of $Rh_o(D)$ immune globulin protects against sensitization from about 30 ml of fetal blood, the volume is divided by 30 and multiplied by 2. The "2" is a correction factor, since the accuracy of the acid-elution test is poor and the actual fetomaternal hemorrhage may be twice that of the estimate. Therefore, if 1.2 per cent fetal cells are seen in the acid-elution smear after counting of 2000 cells, 4 vials of $Rh_o(D)$ immune globulin are required, calculated as follows:

$$1.2 \times 50 = 60 \text{ ml (fetomaternal hemorrhage)}$$

$$\frac{60}{30} \times 2 = 4 \text{ vials}$$

Preinjection Tests on the Mother. Before $Rh_o(D)$ immune globulin is administered to the mother, the following serologic tests should be performed:[*] (1) ABO grouping, (2) $Rh_o(D)$ typing of the mother (including D^u test, which should be read microscopically), (3) serum tests for irregular antibodies, and (4) direct Coombs test. Some laboratories perform a compatibility test between the mother's red cells and the sample of $Rh_o(D)$ immune globulin on each vial of $Rh_o(D)$ immune globulin. This test can be considered optional.

The Injection of $Rh_o(D)$ Immune Globulin. In normal situations, the entire contents of one vial of $Rh_o(D)$ immune globulin is injected intramuscularly into the buttock. When multiple vials are to be administered to the mother, baseline studies of hemoglobin and bilirubin should be obtained. Several vials of $Rh_o(D)$ immune globulin can be pooled in one syringe for a single injection, but not more than 5 ml should be injected at one time into each buttock. If more than 10 doses are required, the injections should be spaced over a 72-hour period.

Antibodies in Maternal Serum After Injection. Anti-$Rh_o(D)$ and any other antibodies that may be present in the immune globulin

---

*AABB recommendations.

(e.g., anti-C, anti-E) can usually be detected in the mother's serum 12 to 60 hours after injection and may continue to be detectable for as long as five months. Antibodies detected in the mother's serum six months after delivery probably represent *active* immunization, and may indicate the failure of the $Rh_0(D)$ immune globulin to block alloimmunization. Such failures are rare and may be the result of prior undetected anti-$Rh_0(D)$ in the maternal serum before administration of $Rh_0(D)$ immune globulin. *Note:* The administration of $Rh_0(D)$ immune globulin can prevent the occurrence of Rh sensitization but cannot reverse it.

Antenatal Treatment. Since primary Rh immunization occurs *during* pregnancy in at least 0.78 per cent of Rh-negative women carrying an Rh-positive fetus, several workers now administer $Rh_0(D)$ immune globulin antenatally *and* postnatally. Trials conducted in Canada (Bowman *et al*, 1978) and in Australia (Davey, 1976) have shown that the combined antenatal-postnatal treatment is more effective than postnatal treatment alone in suppressing Rh immunization. While it may appear that the injection of anti-$Rh_0(D)$ into an $Rh_0(D)$-negative woman pregnant with an Rh-positive fetus is potentially dangerous (the antibody being IgG

and therefore capable of crossing the placenta), practical experience has shown this not to be so. The reason for this is that even if the antibody does cross the placenta, IgG is transferred relatively slowly and not more than 30 μg of a 300 μg dose will reach the infant, most having been catabolized by the mother by the time that equilibrium is reached.

Other Indications. The value of $Rh_0(D)$ immune globulin in preventing sensitization for first trimester amniocentesis, antepartum hemorrhage and ectopic pregnancy has not been established. The American College of Obstetricians and Gynecologists, however, has recommended its administration to such patients. In addition, Rh-negative women who have abortions (spontaneous or induced) are candidates for $Rh_0(D)$ immune globulin unless the father or fetus is known to be Rh negative. This is because the $Rh_0(D)$ antigen has been demonstrated on fetal red cells as early as 38 days after conception (Bergstrom *et al*, 1967). A method of determination of the Rh blood group of fetuses in abortion by suction curettage was proposed by Greendyke *et al* (1976). A modification of this technique using the enzyme papain in a rapid-tube technique was proposed by Bryant et al (1979).

TYPICAL EXAMINATION QUESTIONS

Choose the phrase, sentence or symbol that completes the statement or answers the question. More than one answer may be correct in each case. Answers are given in the back of this book.

1. The severity of hemolytic disease of the newborn is influenced by
   (a) the number of fetal red cells destroyed
   (b) the specificity of the antibody involved
   (c) the ability of the fetus to compensate for red cell destruction by increased production of new cells
   (d) none of the above
   (Introduction)

2. When hemolytic disease of the newborn occurs owing to anti-$Rh_0(D)$
   (a) the mother is always $Rh_0(D)$ negative
   (b) the father is always $Rh_0(D)$ positive
   (c) the mother is always $Rh_0(D)$ positive
   (d) the infant is always $Rh_0(D)$ positive
   (Rh Hemolytic Disease of the Newborn: Mechanisms of Sensitization)

3. In ABO hemolytic disease of the newborn, the mother is invariably of blood group
   (a) AB
   (b) B

   (c) A
   (d) O
   (ABO Hemolytic Disease of the Newborn: Mechanisms of Sensitization)

4. Which of the following tests are performed on a mother's first prenatal specimen?
   (a) ABO grouping
   (b) $Rh_0(D)$ typing
   (c) Antibody screening
   (d) Kleihauer test
   (Prenatal Investigations: Tests on the Mother)

5. Inherent risks associated with amniocentesis include the possibility of
   (a) infections
   (b) more severe sensitization if maternal red cells escape into the fetal circulation
   (c) fetal death
   (d) induction of labor
   (Amniotic Fluid Examination)

6. Fresh blood used for intrauterine transfusion is normally
   (a) group AB $Rh_0(D)$ positive
   (b) the same group as the fetus
   (c) crossmatched with the maternal serum
   (d) group O $Rh_0(D)$ negative
   (Intrauterine Transfusion)

7. Cord blood should routinely undergo the following serologic tests
   (a) ABO typing
   (b) $Rh_o(D)$ typing
   (c) direct antiglobulin test
   (d) elution if direct antiglobulin test is positive
   (Postnatal Investigation)
8. If a baby has received repeated intrauterine transfusions before birth, erroneous results may occur in which of the following postnatal tests?
   (a) ABO grouping
   (b) Rh typing
   (c) direct antiglobulin test
   (d) all of the above
   (Postnatal Investigations: ABO Grouping)
9. False positive Rh typing on cord samples may result from
   (a) saturation of fetal $Rh_o(D)$-positive red cells with maternal anti-$Rh_o(D)$
   (b) the presence of Wharton's jelly in the sample
   (c) the coating (sensitization) of cord red cells *in vivo* by a maternal antibody other than anti-$Rh_o(D)$
   (d) all of the above
   (Postnatal Investigation: Rh Typing)
10. Hematologic tests on cord blood should include
    (a) haptoglobin
    (b) hemoglobin
    (c) hematocrit
    (d) serum bilirubin
    (Postnatal Investigations: Additional Tests)
11. Blood for exchange transfusion should be less than five days old
    (a) to ensure maximum red cell viability
    (b) to ensure minimum plasma potassium
    (c) to minimize hemoglobin function
    (d) none of the above
    (Selection of Blood for Exchange Transfusion)
12. The usual recommended dose of $Rh_o(D)$ immune globulin to prevent Rh immunization is:
    (a) 900 μg

(b) 20 μg
(c) 300 μg
(d) 600 μg
(Prevention of Hemolytic Disease of the Newborn)

ANSWER TRUE OR FALSE

13. Hemolytic disease of the newborn can be caused by virtually every blood group antibody that can occur as IgG.
    (Introduction)
14. Rh hemolytic disease of the newborn commonly affects the first infant (i.e., the first incompatible pregnancy).
    (Rh Hemolytic Disease of the Newborn: Mechanisms of Sensitization)
15. The lecithin/sphingomyelin ratio performed on amniotic fluid gives an indication of the severity of hemolytic disease of the newborn.
    (Amniotic Fluid Examination)
16. The most common clinical features of hemolytic disease of the newborn are anemia and jaundice.
    (Clinical Aspects)
17. In selecting blood for exchange transfusion in ABO hemolytic disease of the newborn, group O red cells of the same Rh type as the mother should be used.
    (Selection of Blood for Exchange Transfusion)
18. $Rh_o(D)$ immune globulin should be given to women who have first trimester amniocentesis.
    (Prevention of Hemolytic Disease of the Newborn)
19. The injection of $Rh_o(D)$ immune globulin antenatally is potentially dangerous to an $Rh_o(D)$-positive fetus because the antibody is IgG and therefore capable of crossing the placenta.
    (Prevention of Hemolytic Disease of the Newborn)
20. The direct antiglobulin test may be weak or negative in ABO hemolytic disease of the newborn.
    (Postnatal Investigations: Direct Antiglobulin Test)

GENERAL REFERENCES

1. Boorman, K. E., Dodd, B. E., and Lincoln, P. J.: Blood Group Serology: Theory, Techniques, Practical Applications, 5th Ed. Churchill Livingstone, 1977. *(Emphasis on serologic aspects of hemolytic disease of the newborn. Includes techniques.)*
2. Issitt, P. D., and Issitt, C. H.: Applied Blood Group Serology. Spectra Biologicals, 1975. *(Good general coverage of hemolytic disease of the newborn* *(Chapter 26). Includes some discussion of clinical features).*
3. Mollison, P. L.: Blood Transfusion in Clinical Medicine, 6th Ed. Blackwell Scientific Publications, Oxford, 1979. *(Extremely comprehensive coverage of hemolytic disease of the newborn. Particularly useful with respect to clinical aspects.)*

Section Six

PRACTICAL ASPECTS

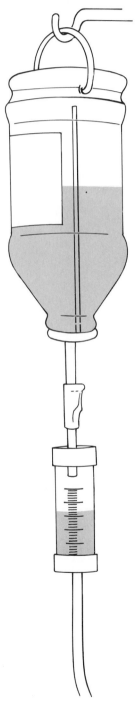

THE DONATION OF BLOOD

OBJECTIVES — THE DONATION OF BLOOD

The student shall know, understand and be prepared to explain:

1. The regulations and requirements for the collection and processing of blood as outlined by the American Association of Blood Banks, specifically to include:
   (a) The selection of blood donors: physical requirements, including weight, temperature, pulse, blood pressure; absence of skin lesions; age requirements; interval between donations; state of health and absence of disease; taking of drugs; vaccinations; history of hepatitis or malaria; hemoglobin (hematocrit)
   (b) The collection of blood, specifically:
      (1) Donor registration (information required)
      (2) Routine fingerprick grouping
      (3) Hemoglobin estimation (methods used)
      (4) Method of blood collection
   (c) Reactions during or after donation (types and treatment)
2. The process of plasmapheresis, specifically to include:
   (a) Selection of donors for plasmapheresis
   (b) Consent requirements
   (c) Method of plasmapheresis
   (d) Hazards of plasmapheresis
3. The use of cell separators, specifically to include:
   (a) Types of cell separators available
   (b) Uses of such machines (fraction collection and therapeutic)
   (c) Adverse effects to patients undergoing cell separation

4. The process of plateletpheresis (thrombapheresis) specifically to include:
   (a) Selection of donors for plateletpheresis
   (b) Method of plateletpheresis
   (c) Hazards of plateletpheresis
5. The process of leukapheresis, specifically to include:
   (a) Selection of donors for leukapheresis
   (b) Method of leukapheresis
   (c) Hazards of leukapheresis
6. The process of autologous transfusion, to include:
   (a) Methods of collection
   (b) Uses of autologous blood
   (c) Hazards of autologous transfusion
   (d) Serologic testing of autologous blood
7. The methods of collecting blood for testing purposes, including:
   (a) Fingerprick (microsampling)
   (b) Venipuncture, to include the preparation of the patient, equipment required, and a full understanding of the technique
8. The testing of blood donations
9. Anticoagulants, specifically to include:
   (a) Definition
   (b) Tubes available (CPD, ACD, EDTA, heparin)
   (c) The addition of adenine

Introduction

Regulations and requirements for the collection and processing of blood are established in the United States by the American Association of Blood Banks, the Food and Drug Administration of the US Government and the American National Red Cross and must be adhered to by all blood banks. The discussion that follows is based on the requirements as outlined in the *Technical Manual of the American Association of Blood Banks*, 8th Edition, 1981.

SELECTION OF BLOOD DONORS

Physical Requirements

Blood donors must meet several physical requirements to be eligible to donate.

211

Weight. A full blood donation (450 ± 45 ml of blood in addition to processing tubes not exceeding 30 ml) may be taken from otherwise eligible donors weighing 110 lbs (50 kg) or more. If a prospective donor weighs less than 110 lbs, a lesser amount of blood may be collected, calculated as follows:

$$\frac{\text{Donor's weight}}{110 \text{ (lbs)}} = \frac{\text{Amount to collect}}{450 \text{ (ml)}}$$

It should be noted that if a lesser amount of blood is to be drawn, the amount of anticoagulant in the collection bag must be reduced proportionally. Anticoagulant may be transferred to an integral satellite bag and then sealed. The amount of anticoagulant to withdraw is calculated as follows:

$$\frac{\text{Amount of anticoagulant (CPD)}}{63 \text{ (ml)}} = \frac{\text{Amount to draw}}{450 \text{ (ml)}}$$

In this as in all blood collection, the amount of blood drawn should be at least 90 per cent of the amount recommended for the volume of anticoagulant.

Temperature. The prospective donor should not have an oral temperature in excess of 37.5° C.

Pulse. The pulse rate of the prospective donor should be between 50 and 100 beats per minute and there should be no pathologic irregularity. Irregularities in the pulse or blood pressure must be referred to the attending physician whose duty it is to determine the acceptability of the donor.

Blood Pressure. The blood pressure of the prospective donor should be between 90 mm and 180 mm Hg (systolic) and between 50 mm and 100 mm Hg (diastolic). Blood pressure readings outside these parameters should be investigated through referral to the attending physician who will determine the acceptability of the donor.

Absence of Skin Lesions. Prospective donors with boils, open wounds or any severe skin infections or with mild skin disorders in the antecubital area (the site of venipuncture) must be deferred.

General Appearance. Prospective donors who appear ill, who appear to be under the influence of alcohol or drugs or who are excessively nervous are best deferred temporarily.

Age Requirements

Blood donations may be taken from individuals between the ages of 17 and 65, although donors in the age group 17 to 21 should produce a letter of consent signed by a parent or legal guardian unless state law defines the legal age for blood donation to be less than 21. After the 66th birthday, donors may be accepted if they have specific written consent from a physician dated not more than two weeks before the date of donation. Acceptability in this instance will be at the discretion of the attending physician and provided that all other criteria have been met.

Other Requirements

1. The interval between donations must be eight weeks (except in special circumstances and with the written consent of a physician).
2. The donor should be deferred if pregnant and for six weeks after the termination of pregnancy (unless possible autologous or exchange transfusion is planned).
3. The donor should be in general good health. In cases of minor illness (cough, sore throat, headache, etc.) deferment will depend on the degree of severity at the discretion of the attending physician. Acutely ill patients must be deferred or rejected. Chronic conditions should be evaluated by a physician.
4. The donor should have no history of rheumatic heart disease or coronary heart disease.
5. Donors with active pulmonary tuberculosis must be rejected.
6. Donors who have had major surgery should be deferred for at least six months. Minor surgery (hernia repair, appendectomy) is disqualifying only until healing is complete. A donor who has had tooth extraction or oral surgery should be deferred for at least 72 hours.
7. The taking of most medications is not a cause for rejection or deferment of the donor (oral contraceptives, mild analgesics, minor tranquilizers), although donors presently under the influence of marijuana should be deferred. Donations from individuals who have taken aspirin or aspirin-containing compounds should not be used as the *only* source for platelet preparations (plateletpheresis). A history of recent or present therapy with antibiotics, insulin

and so forth should be evaluated by a physician.

8. Donors who have recently been immunized yet who show no symptoms would be accepted after the following time limits:
    (a) Smallpox: Two weeks after an immune reaction or after the scab has fallen off.
    (b) Measles, mumps, yellow fever, oral polio vaccine, animal serum products: two weeks after last immunization.
    (c) German measles: two months after last injection.
    (d) Rabies (therapeutic): one year after last injection.
9. Donors with symptomatic bronchial asthma should be rejected.
10. Donors with a history of convulsion or fainting spells (unless confined to childhood) should be rejected.
11. Donors with a tendency toward abnormal bleeding should be rejected.
12. Donors who have recently traveled in areas considered endemic by the Malaria Program Center for Disease Control, US Department of Health and Human Services, may be accepted as regular blood donors six months after return to a nonendemic area, provided that they have been free of symptoms and have not taken antimalarial drugs in the interim. Donors who have had malaria should be deferred for three years after becoming asymptomatic or after therapy is discontinued. Immigrants or visitors from endemic areas should be deferred for three years after departure from the area, provided that they have been asymptomatic; those who have been military personnel in an endemic area should likewise be deferred for three years after therapy is discontinued or after departure from the area, provided that they have been asymptomatic during that time. (*Note:* Donations from these individuals are acceptable if they are used *only* for the preparation of fractions that are *devoid of red blood cells* (plasma, plasma components).)
13. Since the presence of the agent of viral hepatitis cannot as yet be detected with *certainty* by any available means, including laboratory tests for HBsAG, the following regulations should be strictly enforced:
    (a) Donors with a history of viral hepatitis must be rejected permanently.
    (b) Donors who at any time have had a confirmed positive test for HBsAg must be rejected permanently.
    (c) Donors whose blood, blood component or derivative resulted in post-transfusion hepatitis in the recipient within six months after transfusion must be rejected permanently if that donor's blood is shown to be causative or if it was the only unit given to the recipient.
    (d) A donor who at any time has been a drug addict (involving the injection of drugs) must be rejected permanently.
    (e) Recipients of blood, blood components or derivatives, including those in blood group immunization programs, should be deferred as donors for at least six months.
    (f) Donors who have had skin allographs or tattoos or both (including those who have undergone ear-piercing or acupuncture under questionable conditions) should be deferred for at least six months.
    (g) Donors (excluding hospital personnel) who have had close contact with a patient with viral hepatitis should be deferred for at least six months. Hospital personnel in areas in which hepatitis is endemic (e.g., in renal dialysis units) should be deferred for six months after employment in such areas.
    (h) Inmates of penal or mental institutions should be deferred until six months after release.
14. Prospective donors who do not meet minimum hemoglobin or hematocrit requirements (see under the heading Hemoglobin or Hematocrit Estimation) should be rejected.

It should be noted that "special" donors (for therapeutic purposes, autologous transfusion, plasmapheresis, donor immunization and hyperimmunizations) may be exempt from most of the usual requirements.

THE COLLECTION OF BLOOD

Donations of blood must be collected only by trained personnel working under the direction of a qualified licensed physician. The donor record must be signed by the phlebotomist who performs the procedure.

Since blood donations are voluntary, it is essential that the procedure be as pleasant, safe and convenient as possible for donors if new donors are to be attracted and if continued participation is to be encouraged. To this end, donor clinics should be attractive, well-lighted, well-ventilated and open at convenient hours.

Staff should be courteous, friendly, understanding and professional.

Donor Registration

In order that it be reasonably possible to identify and recall a donor, the following information must be obtained from each donor and updated each time a donation is made:

1. Date of donation
2. Name (in full), including last and first and middle initial
3. Address (in full), residence or business or both
4. Telephone number, residence or business or both
5. Age (see Age Requirements) and date of birth
6. Sex

This information is kept on file in the blood bank for at least five years. The donor should sign a consent form, giving permission to take and use his or her blood. This form should be explained in simple terms — as should the basic procedure of blood collection — and the signature of the donor should be witnessed by a qualified person. The donor should in no way be coerced into signing the form.

Information concerning the time of the donor's last meal (which should have been within the last four to six hours), the name of the intended recipient (if applicable), the blood group of the donor (if known), the race of the donor (which may be useful if blood of a specific phenotype is needed) and the donor's occupation may prove useful. In some occupations there may be the possibility of a safety hazard to the donor or his or her co-workers if adequate time has not elapsed between the donation and return to work. If additional identification is required, the donor may be asked to produce his or her social security card or driver's license and these numbers may be recorded.

Routine Grouping

Although the procedure is not essential, some donor clinics perform a slide ABO grouping from blood obtained by fingerprick after the donor has been registered. This serves as a double-check on the group when full grouping is later performed on the donated blood.

Hemoglobin Estimation

In order to be eligible to donate, donors must meet minimum hemoglobin (or hematocrit) requirements. The hemoglobin shall be no less than 12.5 gm/dl for female donors and no less than 13.5 gm/dl for male donors. While determination of the hemoglobin concentration is preferred, some donor clinics prefer to substitute the hematocrit value, which should be no less than 38 per cent for females and no less than 41 per cent for males.

The usual method for the determination of hemoglobin concentration is the "copper sulphate method," although spectrophotometric methods may also be used (see Todd and Sanford, 1974).

The copper sulfate method of hemoglobin determination is based on the relationship of specific gravity to hemoglobin concentration. A drop of blood dropped into copper sulfate solution is encased in a sac of copper proteinate, which prevents any change in specific gravity for about 15 seconds. If the drop of blood has a satisfactory hemoglobin concentration and therefore a satisfactory specific gravity, it will sink in the solution within 15 seconds. If not, the drop will hesitate, will remain suspended or will rise to the top of the solution within 15 seconds.

The copper sulfate solution used should have a specific gravity of 1.053 to test female donors (equal to 12.5 gm/dl hemoglobin) and 1.055 to test male donors (equal to 13.5 gm/dl hemoglobin). The solutions should be stored at room temperature and should be tightly capped to prevent evaporation.

The test procedure is as follows:

1. Dispense 30 ml of copper sulfate solution into appropriately labeled, clean, dry tubes or bottles. (*Note:* The solution must be changed daily or after each 25 tests.)
2. Clean the site of skin puncture thoroughly with antiseptic solution and wipe dry with sterile gauze.
3. Puncture the finger or ear lobe with sufficient force to allow a free flow of blood using a sterile disposable lancet. (Do not squeeze the site of puncture, as this may dilute the drop with excess plasma tissue and give false results.)
4. Collect the blood in a capillary tube, avoiding air in the tube, and allow the drop of blood to fall gently into the tube from a height of about 1 cm above the surface of the solution.
5. Observe for 15 seconds.
6. Record result (>12.5 gm/dl, <12.5 gm/dl or >13.5 gm/dl, <13.5 gm/dl).

It should be noted that this is *not* a quantitative test and will only show that the hemoglobin is equal to, above or below acceptable limits. It should also be noted that a donor with abnormally high serum protein (or one with multiple myeloma) will pass the copper sulfate test, however low the hemoglobin. The test may therefore be considered of dubious value in some instances.

BLOOD COLLECTION METHOD

1. Choose the site of venipuncture. Apply a tourniquet or a blood pressure cuff inflated to 50 mm to 60 mm of mercury and select a large firm vein in an area that is free of skin lesions. Having the donor make a fist is usually helpful in making the veins more prominent.
2. Release the tourniquet and thoroughly cleanse the proposed site of venipuncture and an area of at least 1¼ inches in all directions from the site. This can be done by scrubbing the area with aqueous soap or detergent solution for at least 30 seconds, removing the soap with 10 per cent acetone in 70 per cent alcohol and allowing to dry. Apply tincture of iodine (3 to 3¼ per cent in 70 per cent ethyl alcohol), and after it has dried remove iodine with 10 per cent acetone in 70 per cent alcohol. Another method of cleansing is to scrub the area for 30 seconds with 0.75 per cent aqueous scrub solution of Iodophor compound (e.g., PVP-iodine or Poloxamer-iodine complex) and then apply Iodophor complex solution and allow 30 seconds before venipuncture. The site, once prepared, may be covered with dry sterile gauze until venipuncture is performed, and should *not be touched again*.
3. Inspect the collection bag for defects. Ensure that anticoagulant solution is clear.
4. Reapply tourniquet or blood pressure cuff inflated to 50 mm to 60 mm of mercury.
5. When the selected vein is again prominent, uncover the sterile needle and perform venipuncture immediately. The tubing may be taped to hold the needle in place and covered with dry sterile gauze.
6. Release any temporary closure in the tubing to allow the blood to flow into the bag.
7. Have the donor open and close his or her hand, squeezing a rubber ball or other resilient object slowly and continuously during donation.
8. Mix the anticoagulant with the blood as it flows into the bag. This should be done continuously until collection is complete, either manually by placing the bag on a rotator or by using a vacuum-assist device.
9. During the donation, the bag should be weighed using spring scales and the flow stopped when the weight of the bag is 425 to 520 gm. Since 1 ml of blood equals 1.053 to 1.055 gm, this represents 405 to 495 ml of blood. Note that this weight does *not* include the weight of the container with its anticoagulant, which must be compensated for. If the balance or vacuum-assist methods are used, blood flow will stop automatically when the proper amount of blood has been collected.
10. The entire bleeding procedure should take no more than eight minutes to prevent the triggering of the clotting mechanism, although units that have taken more than eight minutes are still satisfactory if adequate blood flow is maintained and the bag is constantly agitated.
11. When donation is complete, seal the tubing 4 to 5 inches from the needle by using a metal clip or by making a knot.
12. Grasp the tubing on the donor side of this seal, press to remove the blood for a distance of no more than an inch, clamp with a hemostat and cut the tubing between the seal and the hemostat.
13. Fill processing tubes for laboratory tests by releasing the hemostat and allowing the blood to flow directly from the vein. *Ensure that all tubes are properly identified with the bag.*
14. Remove the tourniquet. Remove the needle from the donor's arm and apply pressure to the phlebotomy site using sterile, dry gauze. (The donor may assist by holding gauze in place with his or her other hand). Discard the needle and assembly into a special container to prevent accidental contamination to personnel.
15. Strip donor tubing, forcing the blood back into the bag; invert the bag several times to ensure thorough mixing, then allow the tubing to refill with anticoagulated blood from the bag.
16. Seal tubing into segments suitable for compatibility testing using knots, metal clips or a dielectric sealer. Make a double seal about two inches from the bag to allow segments to be separated from the container without breaking the sterility of the container.
17. Reinspect the bag for defects. Recheck all identity numbers on bag, processing tubes and donor record.
18. Store whole blood or red blood cell concentrates at a temperature of 2 to 6° C. If platelets are to be harvested from the donation, blood should be maintained at room temperature (20 to 24° C) until platelets are separated. This must be completed no longer than four hours after donation is complete.

Reactions During or After Donation

Donor reactions are rare; yet when they do occur, personnel must be prepared to recognize and treat such reactions without delay. Typical donor reactions include syncope (fainting or vasovagal syndrome), weakness, excessive perspiration, dizziness, pallor and nausea. Occasional donors may have convulsions, loss of consciousness or involuntary bowel or urinary passage.

At the first sign of reaction, the phlebotomist should stop the phlebotomy, lower the donor's head and elevate the feet (if possible), loosen restrictive clothing and ensure that the donor has adequate airway.

The following are preliminary measures that can be taken by the phlebotomist in the case of specific reaction, although in all cases the attending physician should be summoned.

1. Syncope: Administer aromatic spirits of ammonia by inhalation (*Note*: Do not hold vial too close to nose). Apply cold compresses to the donor's forehead.

2. Weakness, excessive perspiration, dizziness, pallor: Apply cold compresses to the donor's forehead.

3. Nausea: Instruct the donor to breathe slowly. Have emesis basin and tissues available.

4. Convulsions: Prevent donor from injuring himself or herself by attempting to control movements. Note that sometimes during seizures, people exhibit great muscular strength — obtain assistance.

5. Hyperventilation: Have donor rebreathe into a paper bag.

If donor does not respond rapidly or exhibits more serious symptoms, call for medical aid.

PLASMAPHERESIS

Plasmapheresis is the procedure whereby a unit of blood is withdrawn from the donor to obtain *plasma*, followed by reinfusion of the donor's own red blood cells. The technique is performed either for source plasma (not intended for intravenous infusion) or for fresh frozen plasma. The plasma can also be used for fractionation into products such as serum albumin and gamma globulin.

Plasmapheresis is usually performed using multibag systems, although it is also possible to use centrifugal blood-separation devices (discussed under the headings Plateletpheresis and Leukopheresis).

Selection of Donors for Plasmapheresis

Before each plasmapheresis, the donor's weight, total serum protein and hemoglobin

concentration (and/or hematocrit) must be determined and recorded. If the plasma is intended for transfusion or for preparation of fractionation products for transfusion, the same standards apply for the selection of blood donors as discussed. If, however, the plasma is not intended for transfusion and is clearly labeled to indicate this, then the criteria for donor selection may be limited to those designed for the safety of the donor. In special circumstances (e.g., when plasma or platelets from a donor who *does not* meet the usual requirements are of unusual value) plasmapheresis may be performed *only* upon the advice and written consent of a physician who is familiar with the health status of the donor. In *all* cases the suitability of a donor for source plasma (human) must be determined by a physician or qualified designate.

A donor's continued suitability for a plasmapheresis program should be reviewed by a qualified, licensed physician. If a participant in such a program donates a unit of whole blood (or if, for technical reasons, it is not possible to return the red cells to the donor following plasmapheresis), he or she should be removed from the program either for 72 hours (AABB regulations) or for eight weeks (Code for Federal Regulations). A donor must allow 72 hours to elapse after plasmapheresis before donating whole blood.

Consent

The procedure of plasmapheresis and the attendent risks must be fully explained to the prospective donor *in lay terms* before any procedures are performed. The donor should be asked to sign a consent form that clearly outlines the procedure and states the potential hazards in simple language. This form must conform to local law and should be approved by an attorney before use.

METHOD OF PLASMAPHERESIS

Precise methodology for plasmapheresis will depend on the equipment being used and the recommendations of the manufacturer for such equipment. The method that follows is stated in general terms. Students requiring a more detailed procedure are referred to the *Technical Manual of the American Association of Blood Banks*, page 19.

1. Whole blood is taken in the amount of 500 ml into a "double bag" (or a "quadruple bag" for double plasmapheresis), which is a special set with a main bag containing anticoagulant for

blood collection and a "dry" satellite bag into which the plasma can be squeezed. The system is closed so as to eliminate the risk of contamination. The same procedures and precautions used in general blood collection apply also to plasmapheresis. Suitable tubes and connectors allow the blood collection bag and "dry" bag to be disconnected from the tubing leading to the donor's vein when the donation is completed.

2. Saline is run into the donor's vein while the double bag is centrifuged at 4100 rpm for 5 min at 4° C.

3. After centrifugation, the plasma is expressed into the dry satellite bag. The satellite bag is then separated from the packed red blood cells that are returned to the donor. If double plasmapheresis is to be performed, a second unit of blood is collected as soon as all of the red blood cells from the first unit have been returned to the donor.

Hazards of Plasmapheresis

The greatest hazard of plasmapheresis (especially when more than one donor is being bled at the same time) is the possibility of accidental exchange of the red blood cells so that the donor receives red cells that are not his or her own. Stringent measures must be taken to prevent this, including getting the donor to sign his or her name on the blood collection bag and ensuring that the donor identifies the signature before the red cells are returned to his or her circulation.

Not more than 500 ml of blood should be taken at one time to minimize the chance of acute circulatory effects and because there is always some possibility that it will not be possible to return the red cells. Once the red cells from the first unit have been returned, however, a second unit of 500 ml may be collected. Erythrocyte loss (including blood taken for testing purposes) should not exceed 25 ml per week during serial plasmapheresis. To avoid protein depletion, the maximum amount of plasma removed in a 48-hour period should not exceed that contained in one liter of whole blood. In a seven-day period, the plasma from no more than two liters of whole blood may be removed.

USE OF CELL SEPARATORS

Large quantities of platelets or leukocytes can be collected from single donors using either intermittent-flow centrifugation (Tullis *et al*, 1971; Huestis *et al*, 1975; Mishler *et al*, 1976) or continuous-flow centrifugation (Cooper *et al*,

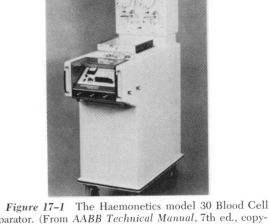

Figure 17–1 The Haemonetics model 30 Blood Cell Separator. (From *AABB Technical Manual*, 7th ed., copyright © 1977, American Association of Blood Banks, Washington, D.C.)

1975). The machine in most common use is the Haemonetics Model 30 Blood Cell Processor (described by Tullis *et al*, 1971) (Fig. 17–1), which involves intermittent-flow centrifugation and uses a Latham bowl (Fig. 17–2). In principle, this device involves the drawing of blood into the rotating Latham bowl. After separation of the components of the blood into layers, different fractions are harvested sequentially into separate plastic bags. The required fraction is retained and the remaining components are returned to the donor, after which the whole operation may be repeated.

Continuous-flow centrifugation is offered by the IBM separator (described by Judson *et al*, 1968), which has been used for plateletpheresis although it is primarily designed for the harvesting of leukocytes to be transfused to leukopenic patients. Also used is a simplified version of the IBM separator, known as the Aminco Celltrifuge (Fig. 17–3). In this system, blood is fed into a rapidly revolving bowl (Fig. 17–4) in which red cells, leukocytes, platelets and plasma are separated into layers. Any layer can be removed while the remainder of the blood is continuously returned to the donor.

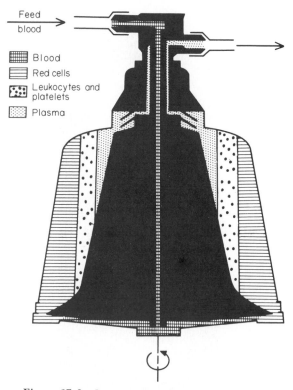

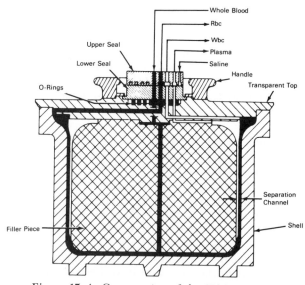

Figure 17–4 Cross-section of the IBM-Aminco bowl used in IBM-Aminco Cell Separator (see Fig. 17–3). (From *AABB Technical Manual*, 7th ed., copyright © 1977, American Association of Blood Banks, Washington, D.C.)

Figure 17–2 Cross-section of the Latham Haemonetics bowl (used in Haemonetics model 30 — see Fig. 17–1). (From Mollison, P. L.: *Blood Transfusion in Clinical Medicine*, 6th ed., London, Blackwell Scientific Publications, 1979, p. 12.)

Cell separators are also used for the *removal* of some unwanted elements of the blood. Therapeutic uses of blood cell separators have undoubtedly not yet been fully explored, yet this therapy has proved useful in several circumstances.

The Hyperviscosity Syndrome. This is most commonly caused by an increase of serum IgM (Waldenström's disease), though it is sometimes caused by higher molecular weight polymers of IgG or IgA in patients with myelomatosis. Intensive plasma exchange to reduce plasma viscosity to within normal limits has proved successful. After this, patients can be maintained on a 5-liter plasma exchange every 4 to 6 weeks (Buskard *et al*, 1976).

Goodpasture's Syndrome. Successful results have been reported from the exchange of

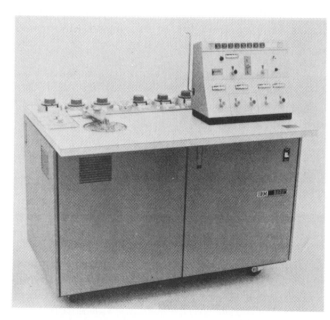

Figure 17–3 The IBM-Aminco Cell Continuous–Flow Blood Cell Separator. (From *AABB Technical Manual*, 7th ed., copyright © 1977, American Association of Blood Banks, Washington, D.C.)

4-liter volumes of plasma (see Lockwood *et al*, 1976).

Familial Hypercholesterolemia. In the homozygous form, this condition is characterized by a high level of low-density lipoprotein that is virtually confined to the plasma. Repeated plasma exchange at 3-week intervals for 4 to 8 months has proved extremely successful in two patients with this disorder (Thompson *et al*, 1975).

Autoimmune Hemolytic Anemia. Plasmapheresis is of no value in warm autoimmune hemolytic anemia and of little value in cold autoimmune hemolytic anemia (see Rosenfield and Jagathambal, 1976). An almost complete remission maintained for three years was, however, observed in a patient with sickle cell trait and autoimmune hemolytic anemia associated with a mixed cryoglobulin consisting of IgG anti-i complexed with IgM and IgA following plasmapheresis (Rosenfield and Jagathambal, 1976).

Thrombotic Thrombocytopenic Purpura. A remission was induced in 8 out of 14 patients treated by exchange transfusion (in some instances with steroids) by Bukowski *et al* (1976).

Severe Thrombocytosis. Plateletpheresis has proved successful on a patient with polycythemia vera whose platelet count rose following splenectomy (Greenberg and Watson-Williams, 1975).

Chronic Lymphocytic Leukemia. Continuous-flow leukapheresis may be very effective in reducing the size of the spleen and lymph nodes in patients with chronic lymphocytic leukemia. Sézary syndrome may also be effectively treated by leukapheresis (Lowenthal, 1977b).

Chronic Granulocytic Leukemia. In patients with chronic granulocytic leukemia, leukapheresis performed two or three times a week using a suitable sedimenting agent can abolish symptoms, reduce the size of the liver and spleen and restore the peripheral blood leukocyte count to normal (see Goldman *et al*, 1975, Lowenthal, 1977a).

Cancer Immunotherapy. See review by Hobbs *et al* (1977).

Scleroderma and Raynaud's Phenomenon. Plasma exchange has been found to be beneficial in the treatment of patients with Raynaud's phenomenon secondary to scleroderma, although the effects are short term (see McCune *et al*, 1980).

Note: Leukapheresis has also been found to be successful as an alternative to marrow for autologous transplantation after chemotherapy (Stiff *et al*, 1980). Partial plasma exchange and immunosuppression, however, have proved un-successful in affecting the course of lower motor neuron disease (Keleman *et al*, 1980).

Adverse Effects to Patients Undergoing Cell Separation

Patients undergoing cell separation may experience chills, nausea and vomiting and syncope (fainting). Citrate toxicity, which has been noted in 58 per cent of donors undergoing discontinuous leukapheresis or plateletpheresis (Huestis *et al*, 1975), can be avoided by using half-strength ACD-A or sodium citrate, which appears to be adequate to prevent coagulation in plastic containers (Olson *et al*, 1977; Mishler *et al*, 1976) and does not appear to affect platelet function (Mishler *et al*, 1976).

The giving of blood on a cell separator can result in air embolism and large amounts of cooled or overheated blood being returned to the donor (unless the temperature of the blood is carefully monitored). The possibility of electrocution must also be considered — a possibility that emphasizes the need to check for electrical safety. Finally, it is probably wise to use cell separators only in places in which a cardiac arrest team is immediately available because of the possibility that the donor may collapse during donation.

PLATELETPHERESIS (THROMBAPHERESIS)

Plateletpheresis, or thrombapheresis, is the procedure whereby platelets are separated centrifugally from whole blood with the continuous or intermittent return of platelet-poor red cells and plasma to the donor. The procedure makes it possible to use the same donor repeatedly at short intervals, so that it may be possible to supply, for example, a patient's entire needs for platelets from a single HLA-compatible donor (e.g., a sibling of the patient). As discussed, plateletpheresis also has therapeutic uses. Hazards of plateletpheresis are discussed under the preceding heading.

Plateletpheresis may be performed using multiple-bag systems (for methodology, see Technical Manual of the American Association of Blood Banks, 1977, page 24), although this is rare now since the advent of blood cell separators.

Selection of Donors for Plateletpheresis

The same standards that apply to whole blood donations and plasmapheresis apply to donors undergoing plateletpheresis. In serial pheresis programs, the donor's hemoglobin, platelet count and total serum protein should be monitored between phereses to prevent significant thrombocytopenia and hypoproteinemia. If the platelet count is below 150,000 per mm³ immediately before plateletpheresis, donation should be deferred except upon the specific advice of the attending physician. If a pheresis donor gives a unit of blood or if it becomes technically impossible to return the donor's red cells during plateletpheresis, the same standards apply as for plasmapheresis (see p. 216). Donors who have ingested aspirin within 72 hours before plateletpheresis are unsuitable and must be deferred.

Method of Plateletpheresis

The method for plateletpheresis will depend on the type of equipment used. The *Technical Manual of the American Association of Blood Banks* (1977) offers a methodology for use of the Haemonetics Model 30, which should be used in conjunction with the manufacturer's instructions.

LEUKAPHERESIS

Leukapheresis is the harvesting of granulocytes with the return of the rest of the blood to the donor. The procedure is performed to obtain large amounts of granulocytes from a single compatible donor for transfusion and for therapeutic reasons.

To increase the yield of granulocytes, donors may be given steroids (e.g., prednisolone), which increase the peripheral granulocyte count, or a rouleaux-forming agent (cell sedimenting agent). For example, hydroxyethyl starch, dextran or modified gelatin may be introduced into the donor or cell separator, which improves the separation between red cells and leukocytes because the specific gravities of red cells and granulocytes are very similar and centrifugation alone is an inefficient means of separation (Huestis *et al*, 1975; Mishler *et al*, 1975).

Selection of Donors for Leukapheresis

The standards for the selection of donors for leukapheresis are the same as those for plateletpheresis, except that since the donors receive *heparin,* which can cause adverse donor reactions or bleeding, they must be evaluated by a physician to determine their suitability.

Method of Leukapheresis

Procedures for leukapheresis will depend on the type of equipment used, the details of which are available from the instrument manufacturer. Chosen procedures should include criteria for and dosages of any ancillary agents used and the prevention and treatment of reactions in the donor. These procedures should be approved by the committee on human subjects experimentation of the particular institution before routine use.

Hazards of Leukapheresis

These are discussed under Adverse Effects to Patients Undergoing Cell Separation. With both continuous-flow centrifugation and intermittent-flow centrifugation, the risks include the possibility of hypovolemic hypotension, citrate toxicity, chills, embolism, extracorporeal hemolysis, drug toxicity and thrombocytopenia. With continuous-flow centrifugation, there is a slight risk of hemorrhage, depending on the specific protocol used. This risk does not exist with intermittent-flow centrifugation. If filtration leukapheresis is performed using the Fenwal filtration-elution pump, the same risks apply (the risk of hemorrhage being greater), with the exception of citrate toxicity.

AUTOLOGOUS TRANSFUSION

By definition, autologous transfusion is the transfusion of blood or blood products that are derived from the recipient's own circulation. The procedure eliminates many of the hazards of homologous blood transfusion, particularly the risk of hepatitis transmission.

Autologous blood can be collected by conventional procedures or through salvage of blood lost during surgery or following trauma. Using conventional collection drawing and storage procedures, patients may be bled in advance of intended transfusion, the units or products then being available when needed. The criteria for this type of "predeposit" phlebotomy are largely the decision of the attending physician. In general, no more than 450 ml (±45 ml) or 12 per cent of estimated blood volume, whichever is the lesser, should be withdrawn at a single donation, and the hemoglobin should be 11 gm/dl or greater. Donations should be no more frequent than once every four days. Predeposit phlebotomy should not be performed within 72 hours of major surgery

Table 17–1 SCHEDULE FOR THE "LEAPFROG TECHNIQUE" TO MAKE FIVE UNITS OF BLOOD (NOS. 5, 6, 7, 8, 9) AVAILABLE FOR SURGERY*

Withdrawal Time	Unit Withdrawn	Unit Reinfused	Unit Withdrawn
Day 1	Unit 1		
Day 8	Unit 2	Unit 1	Unit 3
Day 15	Unit 4	Unit 2	Unit 5
Day 22	Unit 6	Unit 3	Unit 7
Day 29	Unit 8	Unit 4	Unit 9

*From *Technical Manual of the American Association of Blood Banks*, 1977.

without at least partial replacement of plasma proteins using plasma protein fraction (PPF) and albumin.

There is evidence that up to eight units of whole blood can be removed from an individual within 20 days without ill effects if daily iron supplements are given orally (Newman *et al*, 1971; Hamstra and Block, 1969). The storage duration for these units should not exceed that recommended for the anticoagulant used. If the procedure for which the predeposits were made is postponed or when fresher units are required, the so-called "leapfrog" or "piggyback" system can be used whereby older units are reinfused to the donor immediately following the withdrawal of a fresh unit (Ascari *et al*, 1968). A suggested schedule for the "leapfrog" technique is given in Table 17–1.

Autologous blood may be obtained through the *salvage* of blood lost during surgery or following trauma. This blood is merely collected from the interior of the body by instrumentation and returned to the patient immediately after filtration.

Uses of Autologous Blood

Autologous transfusion is indicated in the following circumstances: (1) To provide blood products to patients who react adversely to all homologous blood. (2) To provide blood to patients of extremely rare blood type, or to patients with unexpected antibodies for which compatible blood cannot be found. (3) To provide blood products to patients who refuse blood from homologous donors because of religious beliefs.

Hazards of Autologous Transfusion

Perhaps the most significant hazard of autologous transfusion is that of mistaken reinfusion to another recipient, which may result in a hemolytic transfusion reaction, hepatitis trans-

mission or any of the other adverse effects of homologous transfusion. In order to avoid this possibility, positive identification of both the recipient and the predeposited blood products is essential. Forms of identification used should include the patient's full name, signature, hospital registration number (or social security number, birth date or other similar identifying number if the individual is an outpatient) and the date of donation. In addition to these minimum requirements, because of the importance of identification many laboratories also record the integral tubing segment numbers that are matched with the unit prior to transfusion and attach a photograph of the patient to the unit. Also, an identification card with the donor numbers on the predeposited units is issued to the patient. This card must be presented on admission to the hospital.

In general, blood or blood products intended for autologous transfusion should not be reassigned for homologous use. In the event that the need for blood or blood products for autologous use is not realized, however, such products may be released for homologous use if all of the criteria for donor selection for homologous products have been fulfilled. If these products do not meet these requirements, they must be discarded in an appropriate manner.

In the case of intraoperative autotransfusion, several complications have been documented (see Ochsner *et al*, 1973; Lawson *et al*, 1974; Pliam *et al*, 1975). Microemboli (fat, denatured protein and platelet-leukocyte microaggregates) have been reported. These may lead to post-traumatic pulmonary insufficiency. Hemolysis with increased plasma hemoglobin levels has been reported. Another complication is thrombocytopenia, probably due to consumptive coagulopathy initiated by release into the recovery system of thromboplastic substances from tissue trauma. Air embolism, probably due to technical errors, has also been documented.

In addition, intraoperative autotransfusion is said to be contraindicated in patients with malignant conditions (Yaw *et al*, 1975) or perforated viscera, in the presence of gross contamination or infection, in hepatic or renal dysfunction and when a significant preoperative coagulopathy exists.

Serologic Tests

In general, predeposited blood products intended for autotransfusion should be handled and processed as similarly as possible to products intended for homologous use. If the autologous blood is to be available for homologous use, all serologic tests normally performed on blood for homologous transfusion must be performed. (See under the heading The Testing of Blood Donations.)

Immediately before release of autologous blood for transfusion to the donor-recipient, ABO grouping should be performed on a fresh specimen from the recipient to ensure that it agrees with the typing of the predeposited blood. Compatibility testing between the freshly drawn recipient's sample and the autologous blood products is desirable, but optional.

COLLECTION OF BLOOD FOR TESTING PURPOSES

Fingerprick (Microsampling)

Microsampling is indicated for the testing of blood of a newborn infant, usually taken from the toe or heel, for very young children when only a small amount of blood is required and from adults when veins are very poor or cannot be used because of the simultaneous administration of intravenous fluids. Microsampling is also used in some donor clinics to obtain a preliminary ABO grouping and on patients requiring uncrossmatched blood in an emergency situation in which for some reason a venipuncture cannot be performed. The microsample is then used for ABO grouping to provide the patient with group-specific blood.

METHOD OF MICROSAMPLING

1. Select the site for puncture (finger, toe, heel, ear lobe). Rub the chosen site vigorously with a gauze pad moistened well with 70 per cent alcohol to cleanse the area and increase the circulation.
2. Wipe the area dry with sterile gauze.
3. Hold the finger (or other chosen site) firmly

above the intended site of puncture, but do not squeeze as this may cause tissue fluids to mix with and dilute the blood.
4. Using a sterile blood lancet, make a deep puncture in the skin. (Note: the puncture should be deep enough to ensure adequate blood flow and to ensure against the need to repeat the procedure.)
5. Wipe away the first drop of blood using dry sterile gauze.
6. Apply moderate pressure about 1 cm above the site of puncture to obtain a drop of blood. Once this drop has been collected, release the pressure to allow recirculation of the blood and repeat until sufficient blood has been collected.
7. Apply a piece of dry sterile gauze to the site of puncture, using slight pressure, until the bleeding has stopped.

Venipuncture

The venipuncture (puncture of the vein) is the technique most often used to obtain blood from a patient or donor for serologic testing purposes. It should be noted that the veins are also the entry point for medications, intravenous solutions and blood transfusions. Because there are only a limited number of easily accessible veins in a patient, great care should be taken to preserve their condition and availability.

Preparation of the Patient. Since many individuals are afraid of venipuncture, it is important that the procedure be performed quickly, efficiently and with an attitude of professionalism. In general it is best for the patient to be lying down. If this is not possible, the patient should be seated in a sturdy, comfortable chair with the arm firmly supported on a table or chair arm that is easily accessible to the venipuncturist. Under no circumstances should the subject be standing or sitting on a high stool during any process of blood collection (including microsampling) because of the possibility of syncope. All equipment for the procedure should, if possible, be prepared in advance, or at least be easily accessible to the venipuncturist. (*Note*: in this preparation, care should be taken to preserve the sterility of the equipment.)

Equipment. A venipuncture may be performed using syringe and hypodermic needle or a Vacutainer holder and needle. The Vacutainer system is most often used now except in individuals who have very small veins (e.g., young children) or veins that "collapse" easily under

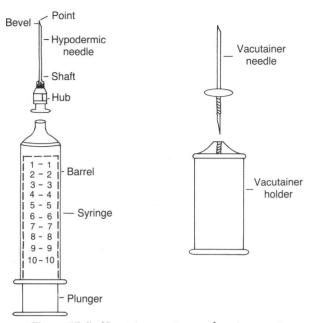

Bevel — Point

— Hypodermic needle

— Shaft

— Hub

— Barrel

— Syringe

— Plunger

Vacutainer needle

Vacutainer holder

Figure 17–5 Vacutainer system and syringe system basic equipment for blood collection by venipuncture.

the pressure of the vacuum in the test tube. These two types of equipment are shown in Figure 17–5.

In addition, the following equipment is required: (1) Gauze pad or cotton ball soaked in 70 per cent alcohol (v/v). (2) Appropriate test tubes. A color code is used for Vacutainer tubes. The color of the *stopper* indicates the anticoagulant that is in the tube. Red-stoppered tubes, which are most often used in blood banking, are "dry" (free of anticoagulant). (3) Tourniquet (or blood pressure cuff). A soft rubber tourniquet is most often used. (4) Band-Aid (see Fig. 17–6).

The choice of needle used will depend on the type of vein the subject has. The *gauge* of the needle refers to the diameter (or bore) of the needle. The higher the gauge number, the smaller will be the bore. The most commonly used needle is 20 gauge. However, if the subject's veins are small, a 21- or 22-gauge needle is recommended. The length of the needle used is a matter of personal choice. The two most commonly used lengths are 1 inch and 1½ inches.

Method of Venipuncture*

Identification of the Subject. Perhaps the major source of error in any laboratory lies in the misidentification of the patient. Blood taken from the wrong patient or labeled incorrectly can lead to serious, even fatal, consequences. For this reason, before venipuncture is performed it is important to ensure accuracy of the identification. For hospital patients, this can be

---

*Methods of performing venipuncture vary widely according to the preferences of the individual worker. The method presented here will serve as a guide to the uninitiated, yet it is conceded that many slight variations exist and few can be said to be superior or inferior to any other.

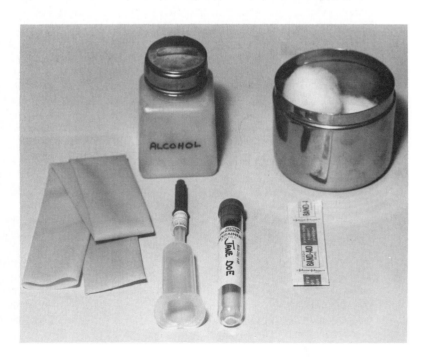

Figure 17–6 The equipment required for venipuncture using the Vacutainer system.

done by checking the wrist band on the patient's arm, checking all information (full name, hospital number, date of birth) and ensuring that this information corresponds with that on the requisition. All specimen tubes should be carefully and accurately labeled before the blood is drawn. The patient should be addressed directly, if conscious, and asked "What is your name?" It is not good enough to say to the patient: "Is your name _____?" because a patient who is under the influence of sedatives or who has just been awakened may mumble a reply that could be taken as an affirmative answer. It is also wise to have the patient spell his or her last name. If the first name is an unusual one, the spelling of this name should also be ascertained.

Applying a Tourniquet. When adequate identification has been completed, a tourniquet (or blood pressure cuff) is placed on the upper arm about two inches above the elbow. When using a soft rubber tourniquet, stretch both ends around the arm to obtain the correct amount of tension, grasp both ends with the right hand and reach through the loop with the left hand to grasp the left side of the tourniquet. Then, with the left hand, pull the tourniquet halfway through the loop and release carefully (Fig. 17–7). The tourniquet should be just tight enough to be slightly uncomfortable (but not

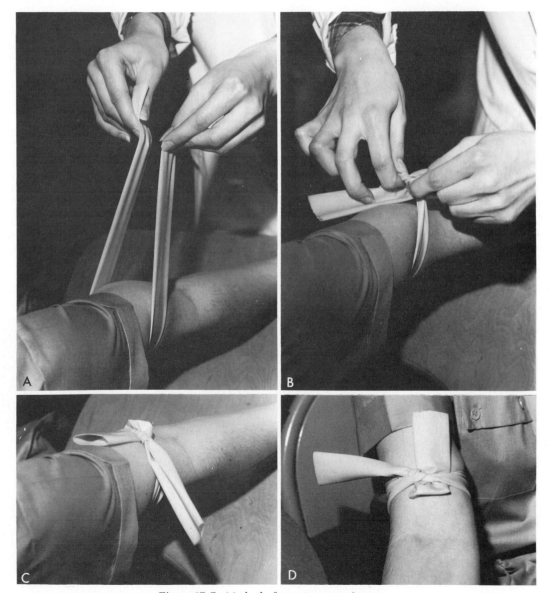

Figure 17–7 Method of tourniquet application.

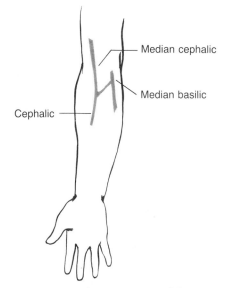

Figure 17–8 The major veins of the arm.

painful) to the patient. When it is securely in place, the patient should be asked to make a tight fist. This will make the veins more easily palpable.

Selection of a Vein for Venipuncture. The three major veins of the arm are the cephalic, median cephalic and median basilic (Fig. 17–8). While all three are suitable for venipuncture, the median cephalic is usually the vein of choice because in most cases it is well anchored in tissue and will not move when punctured, unlike the median basilic vein, which does have a tendency to move in many patients. The cephalic vein is generally not the first choice because it is located on the edge of the outer part of the arm where the skin tends to be a little tougher.

Using the left index finger, palpate the arm until the best vein, which should feel similar to an elastic tube, is found. (Note: Be sure that you cannot feel a pulse, as this indicates that the vessel is an artery and not a vein.)

In some cases it is almost impossible to locate a vein in one arm, though there may be a suitable one in the other arm. It is good general practice to check both arms in every case unless large good veins are found, in which case the choice of which arm to use may be left to the patient. If no vein can be located in either arm, the veins of the lower arm, wrist or hand may be used or, as a last resort, an ankle vein. In these cases, a syringe or microVacutainer assembly should be used for venipuncture because the use of standard-sized Vacutainers may tend to collapse these veins.

Preparation of the Site. Cleanse the in-

tended site of venipuncture well with the gauze pad or cotton ball soaked in 70 per cent alcohol, then wipe the area dry with a dry gauze pad. If a venipuncture is performed without removing the excess alcohol, small amounts of alcohol may penetrate the skin with the needle and cause stinging pain to the patient. The cleansed area should not be touched again with the finger or any other unsterile object (Fig. 17–9).

Insertion of the Needle. Grasp the patient's arm just below the intended site of venipuncture, pulling the skin tight with the thumb. If a syringe is being used, the plunger should first be moved up and down the barrel once or twice to ensure that it will move freely. (*Note:* Be sure that all air is expelled from the syringe before proceeding.)

The syringe (or vacutainer assembly) is held with the free hand between the thumb and the last three fingers. The index finger may be rested against the hub of the needle to serve as a guide. The needle must point in the same direction and in line with the vein and should be at an appropriate 15° angle to the arm (Fig. 17–10).

In order to provide more tissue to serve as an anchor for the needle, the vein should be entered slightly below the area where it is visible. If the chosen vein is prominent, it may be entered directly, puncturing the skin and the vein in one movement. If, however, the veins are deeper and therefore more difficult to locate, the skin may be punctured first and then, if necessary, the left index finger may be used to palpate above the puncture site to locate the vein before entry into the vein.

If a syringe is used, the blood will begin to

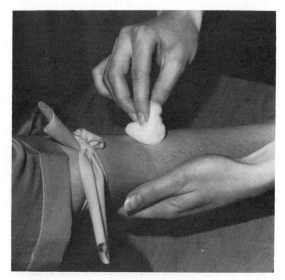

Figure 17–9 Preparing the intended site of venipuncture.

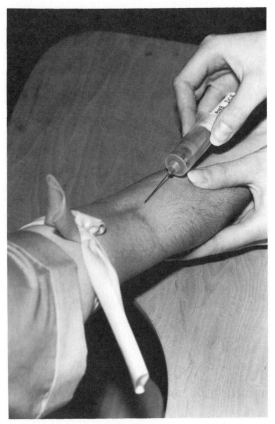

Figure 17–10   Performing the venipuncture.

flow into the barrel as soon as the vein has been entered. The plunger is then slowly drawn back until the required amount of blood has been collected. Care should be taken not to pull too hard on the plunger, as this may cause the blood to hemolyze, or the applied force may pull the wall of the vein down onto the bevel of the needle, causing the blood flow to cease. Also, when the plunger is pulled back, care must be taken not to inadvertently pull the needle out of the vein.

If a vacutainer assembly is used, the test tube is pushed firmly but carefully into the back of the holder such that it is punctured by the inner needle as soon as the main needle is in the vein. The vacuum in the tube will cause the blood to be drawn up into it.

As soon as the blood begins to flow into the tube, the patient may open his or her fist. The tourniquet may be released or it may be left on until the required amount of blood has been collected. If the venipuncture is being performed on a small child or on an adult with very small veins, it may be necessary to remove the tourniquet to prevent the vein from collapsing owing to the fact that blood is being removed

faster than it is entering the vein. It should also be noted that if the tourniquet is left on too long, the blood in the area will have an increased concentration of cells (so-called *hemoconcentration*).

Failure to Obtain Blood. In the event that blood cannot be obtained in a venipuncture, any of three explanations may apply.

1. The vein has been "missed." This can be caused by not inserting the needle deep enough or inserting it slightly to the left or the right of the vein. The index finger may be used to locate the vein; however, no attempt should be made to effect the puncture from where the still-placed needle is located, as this will be painful to the patient and could cause tissue damage. The needle should be withdrawn until the point is almost to the surface of the skin, and then redirected. In some instances, it may be necessary to perform a second venipuncture.

2. The needle has gone through the vein. The first indication of this is usually that the area surrounding the puncture site begins to swell owing to leakage of blood into the tissues. In this event, the tourniquet should be released and the needle withdrawn immediately, with pressure applied to the site.

3. Loss of vacuum. If air has entered the Vacutainer collection tube, there will be no vacuum to draw the blood from the vein. Occasional tubes, too, will not have a satisfactory vacuum because of leakage or manufacturer error. If this is suspected, the tube should be removed and a new tube inserted in its place.

Removal of the Needle. The tourniquet must be released before the needle is removed from the vein. A piece of dry sterile gauze or cotton ball is applied to the puncture site, and the needle withdrawn quickly and in a straight line. Pressure is immediately applied to the venipuncture site for several minutes until the bleeding has stopped. (The patient may be asked to hold the gauze in place with his or her free hand.) The arm may be kept straight, bent at the elbow or elevated above the heart (Fig. 17–11).

If a syringe has been used, the needle should be removed before expelling the blood into appropriate tubes. This should be performed without delay so that the blood does not begin to clot in the barrel.

All disposable equipment should be discarded immediately. The needle (if disposable) should be cut in half and placed in a special container provided for this purpose. Under no circumstances should needles be thrown into a wastebasket.

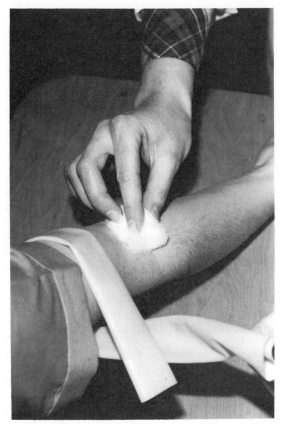

Figure 17-11 Applying pressure to the site of veni-puncture.

TESTING OF BLOOD DONATIONS

The donor's red cells and serum should be tested in all blood donations.

Donor's Red Cells

(a) ABO grouping — forward, using anti-A, anti-B and Anti-A,B serums that meet FDA standards.

(b) Rh typing — using anti-Rh_o(D) serum that meets FDA standards. Rh-negative samples must be tested for Rh_o variants (D^u). Routine phenotyping of other antigens (C and E) should also be performed on Rh_o(D)-negative and D^u-positive donors.

Donor's Serum

(a) ABO grouping — reverse, using known group A_1 red cells and known group B red cells.

(b) Antibody screen — using methods that will demonstrate hemolyzing, agglutinating and coating antibodies expected to be clinically significant. Units containing such antibodies should only be issued as red blood cells (packed cells).

(c) Syphilis test — as required by the FDA

using an acceptable serologic test. If the test is positive, the blood may not be issued for transfusion. Blood may, however, be issued in an emergency situation *before* the test is completed, provided the records and labels so indicate.

(d) Hepatitis tests — for HB_SAg, using reagents and techniques specified by the FDA, or proved equally sensitive and specific. If the test is positive, the blood or components may not be issued for transfusion. Blood may, however, be issued in an emergency situation before the test is completed. However, if the test is subsequently found to be reactive, the recipient's physician must be notified.

(e) Hemolysin tests — performed only if other than group-specific units of whole blood are issued.

The details of these tests are given in other sections of this text.

ANTICOAGULANTS

An anticoagulant is a substance that acts to prevent the clotting of red cells. The substance often also contains a preservative to provide proper nutrients for continuing metabolism in the red cell during storage. The anticoagulant is mainly used in blood donations to ensure proper maintenance of red blood cell hemoglobin function and viability and to maintain the delicate biochemical balance of certain elements such as glucose, pH, ATP (adenosine triphosphate) and 2, 3-DPG (diphosphoglycerate). This is to ensure that the red cells, once transfused, will provide the recipient with the means of delivering oxygen to the tissues — this being the major purpose of transfusion.

Occasionally, anticoagulated specimens are used in special serologic investigations. However, they are never used for crossmatching because of the effect of anticoagulants on complement binding.

CPD (Citrate Phosphate Dextrose)

This is the anticoagulant most often used in blood donations at the present time. Compared with ACD, CPD, which contains less acid, gives slightly less hemolysis, a slightly smaller "leak" of potassium from the red cells and a prolonged post-transfusion survival of the red cells (Table 17–2) (see Gibson *et al*, 1957). Several comparisons have so far been published that support the indication of better viability of

Table 17–2 SOME OF THE BIOCHEMICAL AND VIABILITY CHANGES
OF BLOOD STORED IN CITRATE PHOSPHATE DEXTROSE (CPD)*

Biochemical Substance	Days of Storage				
	0	7	14	21	28
Viable cells (24 hours after transfusion) (%)	100	98	85	80	75
Plasma pH (at 37° C)	7.20	7.00	6.89	6.84	6.78
ATP (% of initial value)	100	96	83	86	75
2,3-DPG (% of initial value)	100	99	80	44	35
p50 (pO$_2$ at Hb = HbO$_2$)	23.5	23	20	17	17
Plasma Na (sodium) (dl)	168	166	163	156	154
Plasma K (potassium) (dl)	3.9	11.9	17.2	21.0	22.5
Plasma hemoglobin (mg%)	1.7	7.8	12.5	19.1	28.9
MCHC (Coulter counter)	33.5	33.1	32.6	—	32.8
Whole blood NH$_3$ (mg%)	282	300	447	500	705
Plasma dextrose (mg%)	345	312	282	231	230
Hematocrit	36.3	35.8	36.5	34.7	35.7
Inorganic PO$_4$ (mM/liter)	3.6	3.6	4.2	4.9	5.5
WBC (× 10^9)	4.9	4.4	4.1	3.2	2.9

*Modified from *Technical Manual of the American Association of Blood Banks,* 1977.

red cells in CPD as opposed to ACD (e.g., see Orlina and Josephson, 1969; Dern *et al,* 1967; Dern, 1970; Warner, 1970).

Commonly used CPD solution has the following composition: trisodium citrate, 26.3 gm; citric acid, 3.27 gm; dextrose, 25.5 gm; monobasic sodium phosphate, 2.22 gm; and water for injection (sterile water) to make 1000 ml.

To prevent the clotting of 100 ml. of blood, 14 ml of this solution is required.

The maximum allowable storage time (so-called "shelf-life") for blood stored at 2 to 6° C in CPD is presently 21 days. This shelf-life is determined by the requirement that at least 70 per cent of the transfused red cells must remain in the circulation 24 hours after transfusion. As will be noted (Table 17–2), the average survival of red cells in CPD 24 hours after transfusion is 75 per cent after 28 days, a fact that should allow the shelf-life of blood stored in CPD to be extended. This has not been done because there is a wide range in survival values, particularly after storage for long periods of time (see Gibson *et al,* 1957; Dern *et al,* 1970; Bowman, 1963).

Red cells are not in a suspended normal physiologic state during storage. Several changes occur, but these do not reduce the effectiveness of transfusion because of the recipient's ability to remove the severely damaged cells from the circulation and to restore the others to a normal state — a process that normally takes about 24 hours (Benesch and Benesch, 1967; Chanutin and Curnish, 1967). Certain measurable biochemical changes occur when blood is stored at 2 to 6° C for up to 28 days (see Table 17–2). The most important of

these changes when compared with blood stored in ACD are discussed later.

ACD (Acid Citrate Dextrose)

Up until recently, acid citrate dextrose (ACD) was the anticoagulant of choice in blood donations. Compared with CPD, ACD is slightly less efficient in maintaining red cell viability, ATP and 2, 3-DPG content, although Prins and Loos (1970) found no difference between the viability of packed red cells from ACD blood and CPD blood after 14 days' storage.

The ACD solution most often used is NIH-A, often referred to as ACD-A. It has the following composition: trisodium citrate, 22.0 gm; citric acid, 8.0 gm; dextrose, 24.5 gm; and water for injection (sterile water) to make 1000 ml.

To prevent the clotting of 100 ml. of blood, 15 ml. of this solution is required.

Conflicting values have appeared in the literature with respect to the average survival of red cells stored in ACD-A. For example, Orling and Josephson (1969) found average survival of 74.8 per cent after 21 days' storage for red cells stored in ACD-A compared with 79.4 per cent for red cells stored in CPD, whereas Högman *et al* (1974) found the survival after the same time period to be 82 per cent with both ACD and CPD. Dern *et al* (1967) found the average survival of ACD blood to be 60 per cent after 28 days' storage. In a later study, the average value was reported at 72 per cent, compared with 77 per cent for CPD (Dern, 1970).

As with CPD, certain measurable biochemical changes occur when blood is stored at 2 to

6° C for up to 28 days in ACD. Some of these are compared with CPD blood in the following discussion.

In both ACD and CPD, the dextrose acts as a nutrient and as a preservative. Both solutions act as an anticoagulant by binding calcium. The pH of CPD blood is higher than ACD blood, since CPD itself has a higher pH. It should be noted that the pH of blood-citrate mixtures is much affected by temperature and is about 0.5 units greater at 4° C that at 37° C. The pH of ACD blood at 4° C is initially about 7.4 to 7.5 (Beutler, 1972) but it usually falls to below 7.0 in the first few days of storage. After 28 days the pH of CPD plasma is 6.78 compared with 6.71 in ACD plasma (Gibson *et al*, 1961).

Important Biochemical Changes in CPD- and ACD-Stored Blood

Adenosine Triphosphate (ATP). ATP is a nucleotide compound occurring in all cells; it represents the energy reserve of the cells. There is good correlation between ATP levels and the post-transfusion viability of stored red cells (see also Chapter 18). ATP concentrations are initially better maintained in ACD because of the lower pH of this anticoagulant, which favors its maintenance. Late in storage, however, ATP concentrations are frequently higher in CPD-stored blood, probably because of the extra 2 millimoles of phosphate present in CPD solutions. ATP content is regenerated *in vivo* after transfusion and can also be regenerated *in vitro* by incubating the cells at 37° C with adenosine. It should be noted that many red cells *are* eliminated from the circulation after transfusion before there is time for them to acquire a normal ATP content *in vivo*.

2, 3-Diphosphoglycerate (2, 3-DPG). In human red cells, 2, 3-DPG and hemoglobin (Hb) are nearly equimolar; 2, 3-DPG profoundly lowers the affinity of Hb for oxygen at concentrations commonly found in the red cells. One mole of 2, 3-DPG combines with one mole of deoxy-Hb to form a complex that is highly resistant to oxygenation; 2, 3-DPG must be displaced for oxygen to be bound.

2, 3-DPG concentrations are better maintained in CPD-stored blood throughout the storage period than in ACD-stored blood because of the higher pH. Hemoglobin function expressed as p50 (an inverse function of oxygen affinity) is maintained at near-normal values for about two weeks in CPD-stored blood, whereas the p50 in ACD-stored blood decreases to values below normal during the first week of storage (Dawson, 1970).

It takes from three to eight hours for severely depleted red cells to regenerate one half of their 2, 3-DPG levels after transfusion and approximately 24 hours for complete restoration of 2, 3-DPG and normal hemoglobin function (Benesch and Benesch, 1967; Chanutin and Curnish, 1967).

Sodium and Potassium. When blood is stored at 4° C, the normal physiologic transport of sodium and potassium across the red cell membrane is almost stopped; intracellular and extracellular concentrations of sodium and potassium, however, tend toward equilibrium as storage continues.

Within 24 hours after transfusion, red cells stored in CPD correct their sodium imbalance. The potassium content, however, does not become normal for more than six days (Mollison, 1972).

The Addition of Adenine

Several studies have been performed that demonstrate the beneficial effects of adenine on red cell preservation (de Verdier *et al*, 1964a; Akerblom *et al*, 1967; Wood and Beutler, 1967; Warner, 1970; Shields, 1968; Shields, 1969a, 1969b; Strumia *et al*, 1970). Some of the survival studies indicate that, on the average, post-transfusion survival falls to 80 per cent after about 3 weeks in ACD but falls to this level only after about 5 weeks in ACD to which adenine has been added.

The addition of adenine (in a final concentration in the blood mixture of 0.5 mM) to ACD hastens the loss of 2, 3-DPG, although it helps to maintain ATP (Chanutin, 1967). 2, 3-DPG levels, however, can be improved without markedly reducing the ATP levels in ACD-adenine blood by adjusting the pH from 5.0 to 5.5 — a pH that is only very slightly below that of CPD (Dawson *et al*, 1975).

The results of numerous studies have shown that the best preservative solution currently available for red cells stored as whole blood is CPD-adenine (17 mg adenine per unit of blood). This solution gives approximately 80 per cent red cell survival *in vivo* after four weeks' storage and 75 to 80 per cent survival at 5 weeks with more than 60 per cent maintenance of 2, 3-DPG levels at 2 weeks. Storage of packed red blood cells in CPD-adenine provides survival of the red cells that is entirely satisfactory after periods up to four weeks. In addition, no adverse clinical reactions have been noted that are attributable to adenine (see de Verdier *et al*, 1966) even in exchange transfusion to newborn infants (Kreuger, 1976).

EDTA (Ethylenediaminetetraacetic Acid)

This anticoagulant is rarely used in blood transfusion work because it has displayed no distinct advantages over citrate and because it has been shown to damage platelets and greatly inhibit the action of complement.

The sodium salts of EDTA are strong chelating agents that bind calcium and thereby prevent coagulation. Thirty ml of 1.36 per cent Na_2H_2EDTA, which provides 1.1 mmol EDTA, will prevent the clotting of 500 ml of blood.

Heparin

Heparin is a natural anticoagulant that affects the clotting of blood by neutralization of thrombin. Fifteen mg of heparin is sufficient to prevent the clotting of 500 ml of blood.

Because the anticoagulant lacks dextrose and has a higher pH than ACD or CPD, which stimulates glycolysis, heparin serves only as an anticoagulant and not as a preservative. Blood collected into heparin must be used within 48 hours — preferably within 24 hours. Heparin is not recommended for routine blood collection but is commonly used in specimens for HLA typing. It has been used for collecting blood for cardiopulmonary bypass surgery and for exchange transfusions.

TYPICAL EXAMINATION QUESTIONS

Choose the phrase, sentence or symbol that completes the statement or answers the question. More than one answer may be acceptable in each case. Answers are given in the back of this book.

1. Individuals who have been immunized against smallpox and show no symptoms can be accepted as blood donors
   (a) two weeks after immunization
   (b) two weeks after an immune reaction
   (c) two weeks after the scab has fallen off
   (d) one week after immunization
   (*Selection of Blood Donors — Other Requirements*)

2. The minimum hemoglobin requirement for female blood donors is
   (a) 10.5 gm/dl
   (b) 12.5 gm/dl
   (c) 12.0 gm/dl
   (d) 13.5 gm/dl
   (*Hemoglobin Estimation*)

3. The specific gravity of the copper sulfate solution used to estimate the hemoglobin concentration in male blood donors should be
   (a) 1.053
   (b) 1.056
   (c) 1.052
   (d) 1.055
   (*Hemoglobin Estimation*)

4. At the first sign of a reaction to blood donation, the phlebotomist should
   (a) stop the phlebotomy
   (b) lower the donor's head and elevate the feet, if possible
   (c) loosen restrictive clothing
   (d) leave the donor to summon help
   (*Reactions During and After Donation*)

5. The greatest hazard of plasmapheresis is
   (a) collection of 500 ml of blood at one time
   (b) erythrocyte loss
   (c) accidental exchange of red blood cells so that the donor receives the wrong blood
   (d) none of the above
   (*Hazards of Plasmapheresis*)

6. The use of half-strength ACD-A or sodium citrate in patients undergoing leukapheresis or plateletpheresis
   (a) is adequate to prevent coagulation in plastic containers
   (b) is inadequate to prevent coagulation in plastic containers
   (c) reduces the incidence of citrate toxicity
   (d) appears to affect platelet function
   (*Adverse Effects to Patients Undergoing Cell Separation*)

7. A potential plateletpheresis donor should be deferred (except upon the specific advice of the attending physician) if his or her platelet count is below
   (a) 500,000 per mm³
   (b) 350,000 per mm³
   (c) 150,000 per mm³
   (d) none of the above
   (*Selection of Donors for Plateletpheresis*)

8. Predeposit phlebotomy for autotransfusion purposes should not be performed
   (a) more frequently than once every eight days
   (b) if the hemoglobin is less than 13.5 gm/dl
   (c) within 72 hours of major surgery without at least partial replacement of plasma proteins
   (d) more frequently than once every four days
   (*Autologous Transfusion*)

9. Complications with respect to intraoperative autotransfusion include the possibility of
   (a) thrombocytopenia
   (b) hemolysis
   (c) microemboli
   (d) air embolism
   (e) all of the above
   (*Autologous Transfusion*)

10. The anticoagulant most often used in blood donations at the present time is
    (a) citrate phosphate dextrose
    (b) acid citrate dextrose
    (c) ethylenediaminetetraacetic acid
    (d) heparin   *(Anticoagulants)*
11. The maximum shelf-life of blood stored in CPD at 2 to 6° C is presently
    (a) 28 days
    (b) 21 days
    (c) 4 weeks
    (d) 42 days
                    (CPD [Citrate Phosphate Dextrose])
12. After 28 days' storage in CPD, the percentage of viable red cells measured 24 hours after transfusion is approximately
    (a) 85
    (b) 60
    (c) 95
    (d) 75   *(CPD [Citrate Phosphate Dextrose])*

ANSWER TRUE OR FALSE

13. A full donation of blood may be taken from donors who are in all other respects eligible weighing 100 lbs or more.
                    *(Selection of Blood Donors —
                    Physical Requirements)*

14. Blood cell separators may be used for therapeutic purposes as well as for the collection of specific cellular elements.
                    (Use of Cell Separators)
15. Thrombapheresis is the collection of platelets from a donor with subsequent return of platelet-poor red blood cells and plasma to the donor.
                    (Plateletpheresis)
16. The gauge of a blood-taking needle refers to the diameter (or bore) of the needle. The lower the gauge number, the smaller is the bore.
                    (Venipuncture)
17. In both ACD and CPD, the dextrose acts as a nutrient for the red cells and therefore as a preservative.
                    (ACD [Acid Citrate Dextrose])
18. 2, 3-DPG concentration is better maintained in ACD-stored blood than in CPD-stored blood because ACD solutions have a higher pH.
                    *(Important Biochemical Changes in CPD-
                    and ACD-Stored Blood)*
19. The addition of adenine to ACD in a final concentration in the blood mixture of 0.5 mM hastens the loss of 2, 3-DPG.
                    (The Addition of Adenine)
20. Heparin is commonly used in routine blood collection (blood donations).
                    (Heparin)

GENERAL REFERENCES

1. Mollison, P. L.: Blood Transfusion in Clinical Medicine, 6th Ed. Blackwell Scientific Publications, Oxford, 1979. *(Contains extensive coverage of the donation of blood, the use of cell separators and anticoagulants. Standards for blood donation are based on the British experience, and as such provide a useful source of comparison. Covers the therapeutic uses of cell separators and the clinical advantages and disadvantages of recommended anticoagulants.)*
2. Standards for Blood Banks and Transfusion Services, 8th Ed. American Association of Blood Banks, Washington, D. C., 1977.
3. Technical Manual of the American Association of Blood Banks, 7th Ed. American Association of Blood Banks, Washington, D.C., 1977. *(Contains all of the information covered in this text, including the standards and requirements for blood donations, plasmapheresis, plateletpheresis and leukapheresis, autotransfusion, venipuncture and anticoagulants. Should be considered essential reading for all individuals involved in blood transfusion work.)*

BLOOD COMPONENTS

OBJECTIVES — BLOOD COMPONENTS

The student shall know, understand and be prepared to explain the preparation, storage requirements and clinical indications of the following blood components:

1. Whole blood
2. Red blood cells (red cell concentrates — packed cells)
3. Platelet concentrates
4. Leukocyte concentrates
5. Leukocyte-poor red cells
6. Washed red blood cells
7. Frozen-thawed red blood cells
8. Fresh-frozen plasma
9. Stored plasma
10. Human serum albumin
11. Fibrinogen
12. Immune serum globulin (gamma globulin)
13. Cryoprecipitated antihemophilic factor (factor VIII concentrate)
14. Factor IX complex

Introduction

Selective transfusion of specific blood components is preferable to the routine use of whole blood, since a concentrated form of the required fraction can be administered, thus reducing the risk of circulatory overload, and thereby allowing for the efficient treatment of many patients from a single donation.

The collection of blood components was made possible by the development of plastic multiple bags with integral tubing as well as by technical advances in high speed temperature-controlled centrifugation. It is now possible to collect from a single unit of whole blood these components: red blood cells (packed cells), platelets, leukocytes, plasma, cryoprecipitate as well as plasma derivatives such as albumin, factor VIII concentrate, fibrinogen, gamma globulin, factor IX concentrate and factor II, VII, IX, and X concentrates.

In this section, the preparation, storage and clinical indications of the various blood components will be discussed.

CELLULAR COMPONENTS: WHOLE BLOOD

Preparation

Whole blood, by broad definition, is that which is taken from the donor, with none of the various components removed. In a standard donation, whole blood contains 450 ml of blood and 63 ml of citrate phosphate dextrose (CPD). A 10 per cent leeway is permitted; that is, units are considered satisfactory if they contain between 405 and 495 ml of blood. Units that contain less than 405 ml are usually not issued as whole blood (see The Donation of Blood, Chapter 17).

Storage

Blood is usually stored at a temperature in the range 2 to 6° C. When blood is collected, the unit should be placed at this temperature as soon as possible — within one hour at the latest. Freshly drawn blood contains viable phagocytes that provide some bactericidal power; therefore, if necessary, the unit may be kept at room temperature for a short period of time before being refrigerated.

Proper storage conditions are essential if the survival time of stored red cells is to be kept at the maximum. Within the temperature range 2 to 6° C, the rate of glycolysis is some 40 times slower than it is at 37° C (see Strumia, 1954; Chaplin *et al*, 1954; Maizels, 1954; Hughes-Jones *et al*, 1957). At temperatures below 2° C, red cells are swollen by the effects of dextrose; they become extremely fragile and are likely to hemolyze. At temperatures above 6° C, bacterial growth is increased and red cell survival is decreased.

In spite of the reduction of the rate of glycolysis in blood stored at about 4° C, sufficient lactic acid is produced to cause a progressive fall in pH, which in turn interferes with the function of enzymes such as hexokinase and phosphofructokinase, leading to the halting of glycolysis. In addition, the post-transfusion survival time of the cells is reduced as the period of storage increases: 5 per cent of the red cells are lost after one week of storage, 10 to 15 per cent after two weeks and 15 to 30 per cent after three weeks.

In addition to this loss of red cell viability, red cell organic phosphates, adenosine triphosphate (ATP) and 2,3-diphosphoglycerate (DPG) become depleted on storage. The fall in red cell ATP is associated with a change in the shape of the red cells from discs to spheres, a loss of membrane lipid, a decrease in the critical hemolytic volume and a striking increase in cellular rigidity (Haradin *et al*, 1969). An ATP level of about one third of normal is believed to correspond to a red cell viability of 50 per cent (Akerblom *et al*, 1967).

The decrease in the level of 2,3-DPG, which is significant during the first week of storage, has been shown to impair the ability of the red cells to release oxygen to the tissues (Chanutin and Curnish, 1967; Benesch and Benesch, 1967). It appears, however, that in most cases the 2,3-DPG level of transfused red cells is of no clinical significance (see Mollison, 1979, p. 60; see also Anticoagulants, Chapter 17).

Other changes in blood stored at 4° C include the halting of the active transport of potassium and sodium across the red cell membrane, with the intracellular and extracellular concentrations tending to come into equilibrium. In addition, red cells become agglutinable by a specific antibody on storage. This agglutination appears to be closely related to loss of viability (Brendemoen, 1952) (see Chapter 24).

Clinical Indications

Whole blood is indicated when a patient has blood loss severe enough to cause symptoms of hypovolemia (i.e., when restoration of blood *volume* attains the same degree of importance as restoration of actual cellular elements). Less acute hemorrhage, anemia and replacement of blood loss during most surgical or obstetric procedures can usually be treated effectively with red blood cells (packed cells).

In general, there is little justification for the routine use of whole blood for transfusion. If all of the constituents of blood are required clinically, these constituents are provided more effectively by the judicious *combination* of components than by a unit of stored whole blood in which the labile contents are reduced.

RED BLOOD CELLS (RED CELL CONCENTRATES — PACKED CELLS)

Preparation

Red blood cells is the term used to describe blood from which much of the plasma has been removed. Other terms used are *red cell concentrates* and *packed cells*. Units intended for use as red blood cells should be collected in blood collection units with integral transfer containers. On a routine basis, blood may be allowed to sediment at 4° C, or it may be centrifuged in a high-speed refrigerated centrifuge such as RC–3 with a swinging bucket for 5 minutes at 4100 rpm (5000 g) at 5° C. The plasma is then expressed into the transfer container and the two containers (primary pack and transfer pack) are separated by sealing and then cutting the integral tubing in such a way that neither pack will be contaminated.

Single units of whole blood may be used as red blood cells by using a sterile transfer container and aseptically inserting the cannula of the transfer container into the outlet site of the bag of blood, then expressing the plasma into the container. In this case it should be remembered that the unit has been entered, is therefore open to possible contamination and must be transfused within 24 hours.

Approximately 25 per cent of the plasma-citrate should be left on the cells when preparing red blood cells to ensure that the blood will still flow through a "giving" set.

Storage

Red blood cells must be stored at 2 to 6° C after the plasma has been separated. If a "closed" system has been used in the preparation of the concentrate, the same expiration time as for whole blood applies. If, however, the hermetic seal has been broken during processing (i.e., when the packed cells are prepared from single units of whole blood by entering the pack), the red blood cells must be transfused within 24 hours or be discarded. Storage of the plasma as "fresh frozen" or "stored" is discussed later.

Clinical Indications

The use of red cell concentrates offers several advantages over the use of whole blood. Their use:

1. Minimizes the possibility of circulatory overload.

2. Reduces the incidence of transfusion reactions from donor antibodies.

3. Reduces the volume of anticoagulant and electrolytes needed in transfusion.

4. Minimizes the incidence of transfusion reactions to plasma components.

5. Permits each blood donation to be used as components and fractions, thereby serving the needs of more than one recipient.

Because of these advantages, red blood cell concentrates are useful in all situations in which it is important to increase the hematocrit level with the least disturbance of blood volume; that is, in cases of anemia as well as many other conditions. In fact, it is good general practice to use red cell concentrates in *all* cases unless there is a *specific* indication for the use of whole blood.

Table 18–1 CHARACTERISTICS OF WHOLE BLOOD AND "PACKED" RED CELLS PER SINGLE UNIT*

Characteristic	*Whole Blood*	*"Packed" Red Cells*
Volume (ml)	500 ± 25	300 ± 25
Hematocrit (%)	40 ± 5	70 ± 5
Red cell volume (ml)	200 ± 25	200 ± 25
Plasma volume (ml)	300 ± 25	100 ± 25
Albumin content (gm)	10 – 12	4 – 5

*Modified from Herst, R., and Shepherd, F. A., 1980.

The characteristics of whole blood and red blood cell concentrates are compared in Table 18–1.

PLATELET CONCENTRATES

Preparation

Platelet concentrates are prepared from individual units of fresh whole blood, with each unit containing on the average 6×10^6 platelets suspended in approximately 50 ml of plasma. This represents about 60 per cent of the platelets contained in one unit of blood.

The preparation procedure is as follows:

1. A donation for use in the preparation of platelet concentrate (or platelet rich plasma) is collected either in ACD or CPD using a blood collection unit with integral transfer bags.

2. The unit is centrifuged at 2500 rpm (1740 g) for 3 minutes in the RC–3 at 20° C. This should be done as soon as possible after donation (no more than 4 hours) and the unit should not be chilled below room temperature (20 to 24° C) at any time before or during platelet separation.

3. The platelet-rich plasma is expressed into a satellite pack and separated. The red cells are then refrigerated.

4. The platelet-rich plasma is centrifuged at 4100 rpm for 5 minutes in the RC–3 at 20° C.

5. The platelet-poor plasma is expressed into a second satellite pack, leaving about 50 ml of plasma on the platelet button. The platelet-poor plasma may be frozen and stored as fresh frozen plasma if desired, provided this can be accomplished within six hours of collection.

6. The platelet button should be resuspended, either by leaving the container undisturbed at room temperature for about one hour and then gently manipulating to allow uniform resuspension *or* by placing the container at room temperature on a slow rotator that will allow for gentle agitation until the platelets are uniformly resuspended (about two hours). *Note*: Platelet concentrates must be handled gently at all times; rough handling or agitation may result in irreversible aggregation of the platelets.

See also Plateletpheresis, Chapter 17.

Storage

The optimal conditions for platelet storage appear to be a temperature of 22° C and constant agitation. For up to 24 hours under these conditions, stored platelets have an overall recovery and survival time after transfusion that is almost as good as that for fresh platelets (50 per cent as opposed to 63 per cent) (Murphy *et al*, 1970). After 72 hours of storage, recovery is reduced to 40 per cent and total survival time is 7.9 days (Slichter and Harker, 1976).

Blood stored at 4° C for 24 hours in ACD is a poor source of viable platelets (Jackson *et al*, 1956; Baldini *et al*, 1960), with a survival time reduced to 1 to 4 days after transfusion (Morrison and Baldini, 1967; Slichter and Harker, 1976; Valeri, 1976). With platelet concentrates and platelet-rich plasma, the diminished number of viable platelets may be due to platelet aggregation on warming. It has been suggested that warming platelets in a water bath at 37° C for 45 minutes *without stirring* results in minimal aggregation (Kattlove and Alexander, 1971).

One of the limiting factors in platelet storage at 22° C is the fall in pH (Murphy *et al*, 1970) caused by lactate production from platelet glycolysis. A dramatic change in platelet morphology with loss of viability is noted when the pH reaches 6.0. The rate of fall of pH is governed by the number of platelets and the volume of plasma in which they are stored. If 50 ml of plasma is used (if the platelet count is greater than $1600 \times 10^9/l$) the pH will be less than 6.0 after 3 days. A more rapid fall in pH with reduction in viability by an unknown mechanism, independent of pH, is caused by failure to agitate the platelets during storage (Murphy and Gardner, 1976).

In addition to this, platelets stored at 22° C can produce infection, although the risk is evidently a small one. Not a single case of infection was noted by Aster *et al* (1976) in an experience of over 4000 transfusions of platelet concentrates. If the hermetic seal is broken during preparation, however, the risk of contamination is great. The platelets should be used as soon as possible — no longer than 24 hours from opening the bag — or discarded.

Platelets may be frozen in dimethyl sulfoxide (DMSO) using carefully controlled conditions (see Kim *et al*, 1976; Schiffer *et al* 1976), and transfusion of frozen platelets has been reasonably successful when all of these conditions have been met.

Clinical Indications

Platelet transfusions are given to patients suffering from thrombocytopenia when the platelet count has fallen below about $20 \times 10^9/l$

and when this is associated with failure of platelet production. Platelet transfusions are also commonly given to patients with acute leukemia and other neoplastic conditions involving the bone marrow and in the treatment of depression of hemopoiesis by infections, drugs or unknown causes.

The Platelet Transfusion Subcommittee of the Acute Leukemia Task Force (1968)[*] listed the following indications for platelet transfusions in cases of leukemia: (1) in the treatment of hemorrhage when the platelet count is below $50 \times 10^9/l$, including any overt bleeding such as epistaxis or hematuria or suspected or proved internal bleeding (intracranial, intracutaneous or intramuscular). (2) If the platelet counts falls to below $10 \times 10^9/l$, because the risk of hemorrhage is then high.

Platelet transfusions may also be indicated in patients in whom the hemostatic defect is due to some abnormality of platelet *function* rather than to thrombocytopenia. For example, transfusion of normal platelets may be beneficial in the case of troublesome bleeding following cardiac bypass in patients with a platelet count of more than $50 \times 10^9/l$, apparently caused by damage to platelets by the oxygenator (Moriau *et al*, 1977).

It should be noted that platelet transfusions are seldom useful for patients with idiopathic thrombocytopenic purpura, since in that condition transfused platelets are so rapidly destroyed.

LEUKOCYTE CONCENTRATES

Preparation

It is generally not practical to obtain granulocytes from single units of blood because 30 to 50 units of *fresh* blood are required for a single infusion. Leukapheresis techniques are preferable (see Chapter 17).

Storage

Generally, granulocyte preparations should not be stored but should be infused as soon as possible after collection. If storage is necessary, it should never be for longer than 24 hours because after that time survival of the trans-

---

[*]Platelet Transfusion Subcommittee of the Acute Leukemia Task Force: Platelet transfusion procedures. Cancer Chemother. Rep. Part 3, 1, 1, 1968.

fused cells is greatly reduced (see Price and Dale, 1976) and also because the cells are prepared in an open system and therefore sterility cannot be assured beyond that time.

Clinical Indications

Leukocyte concentrates (primary granulocytes) may be of value for selected patients with granulocyte counts below $500 \times 10^6/l$ and evidence of continuing infection uncontrolled by antibiotics.

SPECIAL RED CELL PREPARATIONS: LEUKOCYTE-POOR RED BLOOD CELLS

Preparation

There are several methods of preparing leukocyte-poor red blood cells. The methods in most common use include inverted centrifugation, filtration, and reconstitution of frozen red blood cells. None of these techniques can remove *all* leukocytes, yet transfusion reaction caused by leukocyte antibodies can usually be avoided if the total number of granulocytes is reduced to 25 per cent of the original number (Perkins *et al*, 1966).

Inverted Centrifugation Method. Blood may be collected into citrate-phosphate-dextrose (CPD) or acid-citrate-dextrose (ACD) and should be prepared within 24 hours of collection, as follows:

1. Centrifuge the blood bag with integral transfer container(s) at approximately 4100 rpm (5000 g) (RC–3, horizontal head) for 5 minutes at 5° C.

2. Hang the centrifuged, inverted bag on a ring stand or inverted plasma expressor for several minutes. (*Note*: The temperature of the blood must not exceed 10° C during this procedure.)

3. Place the *transfer* container on a scale such as a dietary scale below the primary blood bag and adjust the scale to zero.

4. Penetrate the closure of the primary bag, avoiding agitation of the contents, and allow about 80 per cent of the red blood cells to flow into the transfer bag. The amount to be transferred can be calculated by estimating the amount of blood in the bag (excluding the anticoagulant) and multiplying this number by the donor's hematocrit (assume 40 per cent for females and 43 per cent for males). The total weight of red blood cells to be transferred can

then be calculated, using the figure 1.06 gm as the weight of 1 ml of red blood cells.

Example:

460 ml. of blood in bag × donor hematocrit (43 per cent)
$$= 460 \times 0.43$$
$$= 197.8$$

197. 8 ml of red cells in bag × percentage of red cells to be transferred (80 per cent)
$$= 197.8 \times 0.80$$
$$= 158.24$$

158.24 ml of red cells to be transferred × weight of 1 ml of red cells (1.06)
$$= 158.24 \times 1.06$$
$$= 167.7344$$

This number may be corrected to the nearest whole number; therefore the total weight of the red blood cells to be transferred can be taken as 168 gm.

Filtration Method. Original methods of preparing leukocyte-poor red blood cells involved passing the blood, which had been collected in heparin, through a nylon filter, prewarmed to 37° C. Leukocyte-poor red blood cells can now be prepared by passing the blood through a microaggregate filter either in the laboratory or at the patient's bedside. Blood is collected into citrate-phosphate-dextrose (CPD) or acid-citrate dextrose (ACD) and the plasma is removed (see under the heading Preparation of Red Blood Cells). The unit is centrifuged at 5000 g (4100 rpm in horizontal head RC–3) for 10 minutes at 4° C. The blood is then filtered through a microaggregate filter with a standard pore size of 40 microns. Filtrate may be collected into a transfer pack and then transfused, or the microaggregate filter is attached directly to the blood pack during administration of blood to the patient (Wenz *et al*, 1979).

Freezing Method. Leukocyte-poor red cells result from the freezing and thawing of red blood cells (see Frozen Red Cells, below). Leukocyte-poor red blood cells can also be prepared by manually washing the red cells 4 to 6 times in normal saline, or by using special automated cell-washing equipment.

Storage

Leukocyte-poor red blood cells must be stored at 2 to 6° C after preparation. If a closed system has been used in preparation, the same 21-day expiration time as for whole blood applies. If the pack has been entered, however, allowing for the possibility of contamination, the unit must be infused as soon as possible after processing (within 24 hours) or be discarded.

Clinical Indications

Leukocyte-poor red blood cells are indicated for patients who have repeated febrile reactions due to the presence of leukocyte antibodies. The preparation is also used for patients undergoing renal dialysis to reduce the risk of alloimmunization to leukocyte and platelet antigens.

WASHED RED BLOOD CELLS

Preparation (Manual Washing)

This method of washing red blood cells is recommended by the American Association of Blood Banks.

1. Centrifuge whole blood at 2500 rpm (1740 g) for 3 minutes at 5° C using horizontal head RC–3

2. Express the plasma and buffy coat into the satellite bag and seal.

3. Place a temporary clamp on a plasma transfer set. Insert one end of this set into the injection site of a 250 ml bottle of cold (5° C) normal saline (sodium chloride injection, U.S.P.) intended for intravenous use. Insert the other end into one of the outlet sites of the primary pack, release the temporary clamp and drain the saline into the pack.

4. Place a temporary clamp on the tubing.

5. Remove the cannula from the saline bottle and replace the cannula's original plastic cover. Cover the exposed site of the saline bottle with sterile gauze.

6. Bind the transfer set tubing to the outside of the primary pack with tape. The cannula should be in a vertical position at the top of the pack to prevent leakage or damage to the pack.

7. Resuspend the red cells in the saline and mix thoroughly.

8. Centrifuge the pack at 4100 rpm (5000 g) for 5 minutes at 5° C using horizontal head RC–3.

9. Place the bag on the expressor, carefully release the taped tubing and uncover the cannula.

10. Place the cannula back into the injection site of the empty saline bottle and express the saline and residual buffy coat into the empty bottle. Keep the bottle inverted and below the level of the blood bag outlet site during this procedure.

11. Transfer the cannula to another bottle of cold sterile saline and repeat steps 3 through 10 until the blood cells have been washed a total of three times.

12. Seal the tubing close to the blood bag.

Many continuous-flow washing systems are now available for the washing of red blood cells.

Storage

Washed red blood cells should not be stored. They should be prepared especially for a proposed transfusion, because extra manipulations and the absence of a preservative lead to poor red cell survival *in vitro*, and because the risk of contamination is increased.

Clinical Indications

Clinical disorders requiring saline-washed red blood cells are rare, but their use is indicated in paroxysmal nocturnal hemoglobinuria, transfusion of out-of-group red blood cells, and hypersensitivity to plasma proteins. A more efficient product in these cases is frozen-thawed red blood cells, which should be chosen when practical.

FROZEN-THAWED RED BLOOD CELLS

Preparation

There are several variations in the technique of preparing frozen-thawed red blood cells — the major variations involving the thawing procedure. There are at present two *basic* methods available, one of which uses a high concentration of glycerol (about 40 per cent W/V) while the other uses a lower concentration (about 14 per cent W/V). Several instruments are available for the purpose and are used according to the specific instructions of the manufacturer.

Method of Preparation Using a High Concentration of Glycerol

1. The unit may be collected into CPD or ACD and can be stored as whole blood or as red cell concentrate for up to six days before processing (Valeri, 1974).

2. Remove as much of the plasma as possible. If the unit is "fresh," platelets should also be removed. Use standard techniques as discussed in this chapter for the preparation of a platelet concentrate, frozen plasma or cryoprecipitate.

3. Use 6.2 M glycerol (available commercially) that is approximately 57 per cent, giving a final glycerol concentration of approximately 40 per cent. The glycerol and the red blood cells should be at room temperature so that diffusion of the glycerol into the red cells is not delayed.

4. For standard-sized units of blood, add 100 ml of glycerol *while the red cells are being agitated.*

5. Allow five minutes for equilibration.

6. Add the remaining 300 ml of glycerol, while continuing to agitate the red cell and glycerol mixture.

7. Place the glycerolized red cells into a cardboard or metal canister from the freezer and immerse it in a 37° C water bath for approximately 10 minutes. (*Note:* Handle the unit very gently when it is frozen to avoid breaking the container.)

8. Deglycerolize the unit using one of the four instruments available commercially to provide semiautomated, continuous-flow or batch washing. The Elutramatic, Haemonetics Model 17 and IBM Model 2291 involve a similar basic procedure in which the first wash is 12 per cent sodium chloride, the second is 1.6 per cent sodium chloride and the third is 0.8 per cent sodium phosphate. The protocol recommended by the manufacturer should be carefully followed.

Method of Preparation Using a Low Concentration of Glycerol

1. Steps 1 and 2 are the same when using high or low concentrations of glycerol.

2. Use a 35 per cent glycerol solution to give a final red cell concentration of 14 per cent glycerol. The amount used is equal to the volume of red cells packed to a 90 per cent hematocrit.

3. Add all the glycerol to the red cells and mix well.

4. Place the glycerolized red cells into a cardboard or metal canister.

5. Freeze the unit by immersing it directly into liquid nitrogen (−196° C) for approximately three minutes, then store in the vapor phase of liquid nitrogen at −150° C.

6. When the unit is to be thawed for use, remove the canister from the liquid nitrogen and immerse it in a 37° C water bath for approximately 10 minutes.

7. Deglycerolization can be carried out using batch-washing techniques in a standard refrigerated centrifuge or by using a commercial continuous flow or semiautomated batch-washing instrument (see Rowe, 1973).

Storage

Red blood cells with high-concentration glycerol must be stored at −65° C or below and preferably at −80° C. The length of time units can be thus stored is limited (by FDA regulations) to three years, although this time could probably be greatly extended.

Red blood cells with low concentration glycerol must be stored in the vapor stage of liquid nitrogen at −150° C. The maximum storage time has not been established, but units so stored for three years or longer have been satisfactory.

After thawing, the red cells should be stored (at 2 to 6° C) for no longer than 24 hours. The system is open during reconstitution and there is therefore a possibility of bacterial contamination.

Clinical Indications

Because of the marked reduction of plasma proteins, platelets and leukocytes, frozen-thawed red cells are indicated and desirable in the following circumstances:

1. To minimize severe allergic transfusion reactions

2. For patients who have IgA-anti-IgA reactions

3. For patients with paroxysmal nocturnal hemoglobinuria

4. To minimize sensitization to leukocyte and platelet antigens in prospective transplant patients

5. For the provision of "rare" blood

6. For the provision of blood for autologous transfusion.

It has been postulated that frozen-thawed red blood cells may have a reduced risk of transmitting hepatitis (see Carr *et al*, 1973; Tullis *et al*, 1970).

PLASMA COMPONENTS: FRESH-FROZEN PLASMA

Preparation

When units of whole blood are to be used for the preparation of fresh-frozen plasma, it is important that the anticoagulant be constantly and thoroughly mixed with the blood during donation, because any activation of the coagulation factors will lower the yield of these factors in the plasma.

If difficulty is experienced in venipuncture, or if the donation time exceeds eight minutes, the unit should not be used for the preparation of fresh-frozen plasma.

Plasma from whole blood can be used as "fresh-frozen" plasma provided it is processed within six hours after collection, using the following suggested procedure:

1. Remove any attached pilot tubes and centrifuge the blood (collected in double or triple plastic containers) at 4100 rpm (5000 g) in the horizontal head RC–3 for 5 minutes at full speed at 5° C.

2. Place the unit on a plasma expressor, clamp the tubing with a hemostat and dislodge the bead from the tubing at the satellite pack.

3. Release the hemostat and express up to 225 ml of plasma into the satellite pack.

4. Seal the tubing with a dielectric sealer if available or with metal clips 2 to 3 cm apart, taking care not to obliterate the segment number of the primary pack. Place another seal near the satellite pack.

5. Cut the tubing between the two seals close to the red blood cell container. The tubing may be coiled and placed against the plasma container where it will be available for cross-matching the plasma.

6. The plasma pack should be labeled with the following information: volume of plasma, ABO and Rh types, antibody screening results, HBsAg test result and expiration date.

7. Freeze immediately. The plasma must be frozen solid within six hours after collection from the donor.

Storage

In order to ensure that the stability of coagulation factors V and VIII is maintained, plasma must be frozen solid as rapidly as possible after preparation. This can be achieved in a dry ice–ethanol bath or in a mechanical freezer maintained at −30° C or lower. (*Note*: if a liquid freezing bath is used, the plasma pack must be placed in a polyethylene overwrap for protection from chemical alteration.)

Fresh-frozen plasma may be stored for up to 1 year if maintained constantly at −18° C or lower, then converted (redesignated) as stored plasma. Beyond this period the plasma should not be used for the treatment of hemophilia A because of decrease of factor VIII (antihemophilia A factor) in some units. Immediately before use, the plasma should be thawed with

agitation at 30 to 37° C, and must be infused within two hours after thawing.

Clinical Indications

Fresh-frozen plasma is used primarily for administration to patients with clotting factor deficiencies; e.g. factor IX (Christmas factor), factor VIII (antihemophilia A factor), factor II, factor V, factor VII and factor XI.

Cell-free plasma is also useful in the treatment of IgA and IgM deficiencies, burns and complement (C5) dysfunction or in other abnormalities of complement-mediated functions.

When fresh blood is ordered, fresh-frozen plasma may also be used with packed red blood cells, provided that thrombocytopenia is not the problem.

It should be noted that recipients should always receive group-specific fresh-frozen plasma; in special circumstances, however, plasma from group AB donors may be given to recipients of all other blood groups.

STORED PLASMA

Preparation

Stored plasma is obtained from whole blood during the first 72 hours of storage at 4° C or derived from the supernatant plasma after cryoprecipitate production.

Storage

Plasma stored in a liquid state between 2 and 6° C may be kept for no longer than 26 days from phlebotomy, or for 5 years at −18° C or lower. *Note:* Fresh-frozen plasma after one year of storage at −18° C may be redesignated as stored plasma and given four more years of freezer shelf life at −18° C or lower.

Clinical Indications

Stored plasma contains reduced levels of labile clotting factors but is clinically effective in patients requiring volume or protein replacement. Stored plasma may also be indicated in the treatment of:

1. Burns
2. Hypovolemic shock
3. Coagulation factor deficiencies (other than factor V and factor VIII
4. Anticoagulant (vitamin K antagonist) reversal.

In addition, stored plasma may be used as a pump prime for extracorporeal circulation and for the reconstitution of concentrated red cells if clinically necessary.

HUMAN SERUM ALBUMIN

Preparation

Human serum albumin is prepared from normal human plasma by cold ethanol plasma fractionation. In very general terms, the ionic strength of the supernatant left after the other fractions have been removed is varied, and the pH is adjusted to 4.8 This allows for the formation of a fraction V precipitate. Human serum albumin is prepared by "reworking" the fraction V. Two hundred ml of 25 per cent human serum albumin can usually be prepared from three liters of plasma. Human serum albumin is also prepared in concentrations of 5 per cent. Both preparations have a physiologic pH and a sodium content of approximately 145 ± 15 mEq/l.

Storage

Human serum albumin can be stored for up to three years at room temperature. At no time should the storage temperature exceed 37° C — and freezing of the component must be avoided. Under no circumstances should human serum albumin be used beyond the expiration date as stated by the manufacturer.

Clinical Indications

Human serum albumin is indicated in the following situations:
1. In the treatment of hypovolemic shock due to hemorrhage or surgery
2. In the treatment of burns as a protein and fluid replacement
3. As a fluid replacement during manual or automated therapeutic plasma exchange
4. To promote a diuresis in edema due to hypoproteinemia
5. In neonatal hyperbilirubinemia, to assist in binding unconjugated bilirubin.

Note: Human serum albumin is *not* indicated in chronic nephrosis or in hypoproteinemia associated with chronic cirrhosis, malabsorption, protein-losing enteropathies, pancreatic insufficiency and undernutrition. Human serum albumin is also contraindicated for patients in whom a rapid increase in circulating blood volume may be deleterious (e.g., in congestive cardiac failure, renal insufficiency or stabilized chronic anemia) or for patients who have a history of allergic reaction to albumin.

FIBRINOGEN

Preparation

1. Plasma is pooled in batches of 100 to 150 liters.
2. The pH of the plasma is adjusted to 7.2 and the temperature to −3° C.
3. A precise volume of chilled ethanol is added.
4. The mixture is stirred and the resultant precipitate separated.
5. The precipitate is fraction I and yields human fibrinogen.

Storage

Human fibrinogen can be stored for five years at 4° C without showing notable deterioration. It can also be lyophilized, though in this state it is often difficult to reconstitute.

Clinical Indications

Human fibrinogen is rarely used because it has a post-transfusion hepatitis risk of at least 25 per cent (Mainwaring and Brueckner, 1966). Cases of hypofibrinogenemia may occur as an isolated inherited deficiency or may be acquired associated with obstetric complications, disseminated intravascular coagulation and some forms of cancer. In these situations treatment is best directed toward the underlying *cause* of the disease rather than toward replacement of fibrinogen, although some physicians provide fibrinogen replacement during correction of the underlying disorder.

For those rare clinical circumstances in which fibrinogen is indicated, cryoprecipitate or plasma may be substituted, because these

Table 18–2 FIBRINOGEN CONTENT OF VARIOUS BLOOD COMPONENTS*

	Plasma Per Bag	Fibrinogen Per Bag
Plasma (fresh frozen or stored)	200 ml	500 mg
Cryoprecipitate	5 ml	250 mg
Platelet concentrate	50 ml	125 mg
Whole blood	250 ml	625 mg

*Modified from Herst, R., and Shepherd, F. A., 1980.

possess a high fibrinogen content. The choice of product will depend on the other clinical requirements of the patient. Table 18–2 gives the average fibrinogen content of various blood components.

IMMUNE SERUM GLOBULIN (GAMMA GLOBULIN)

Preparation

Immune serum globulin (also known as gamma globulin) is prepared by cold ethanol fractionation from the supernatant remaining after the preparation of human fibrinogen. This supernatant is cooled to −5° C, the pH and ionicity are reduced slightly and the ethanol concentration is raised. Under these conditions, a precipitate (fractions I and III) forms. The precipitate is "reworked" and fraction II — immune serum globulin — is separated and purified.

Storage

Immune serum globulin is stored at 2 to 8° C for two years without notable deterioration.

Clinical Indications

Immune serum globulin, which is an aqueous solution of the gamma globulin fraction of human plasma, is used to provide passive antibody protection after exposure to certain diseases and for prophylaxis in congenital antibody and immune deficiency disorders. The preparation consists mainly of IgG, but IgA is usually present in variable amounts and IgM may also be detectable.

Immune serum globulin provides passive antibody protection in cases of measles (rubella), hepatitis A, and hypogammaglobulinemia. (Congenital immune deficiency disorders can be treated by monthly injections of immune serum globulin; the effect in *acquired* hypogammaglobulinemia is less well documented.)

CRYOPRECIPITATED ANTIHEMOPHILIC FACTOR (FACTOR VIII CONCENTRATE)

Preparation

Blood donations to be used in the preparation of cryoprecipitated antihemophilic factor are collected into a blood-collection unit with two integral transfer bags. Both ACD and CPD (or sodium citrate) are suitable as anticoagulants. When the blood is collected, adequate mixing is essential. If the collection takes more than eight minutes, the unit should be considered to be unsatisfactory for the preparation of the component, since some clotting may occur that will consume coagulation factors.

Within four hours of collection, centrifuge the unit at 4000 rpm (4470 g) for 10 minutes at 8° C, using an RC–3 refrigerated centrifuge with a horizontal head. Express about two thirds of the plasma into one of the satellite packs, taking care to ensure that no red cells are expressed. Seal the tubing between the plasma and the red blood cells; separate the red blood cells and store at 2 to 6° C.

Within two hours of separation from the red blood cells, the plasma must be frozen. This can be done by placing the unit in a mechanical freezer capable of maintaining −30° C or below. If such a freezer is not available, an ethanol–dry ice bath is also satisfactory (95 per cent ethanol and chipped dry ice) and will freeze the unit solid in about 15 minutes. (*Note*: Before immersing the plasma in the ethanol–dry ice, it is important to protect the plasma bag by placing it in a polyethylene overwrap that should be sealed as tightly as possible.) The frozen plasma may be stored at −18° C or lower until the cryoprecipitate is prepared: it may be kept for up to three months in this state without significantly decreasing the factor VIII yield.

When preparing cryoprecipitate, the frozen plasma is thawed at 2 to 6° C until it has a "mushy" consistency (16 to 18 hours), at which time one of two procedures may be used to obtain the concentrated factor VIII.

Procedure A

1. Centrifuge the plasma at 2 to 4° C at 4,100 rpm (5000 g) for 5 minutes in the RC–3.

2. Hang the inverted bag and allow the supernatant plasma to flow rapidly into the second satellite bag, leaving the cryoprecipitate sticking to the wall of the bag in which the frozen plasma was stored.

3. Seal and separate promptly to prevent the cryoprecipitate from melting and flowing out of the bag.

4. Ten to fifteen ml of the supernatant plasma may be left in the bag to aid in resuspension of the cryoprecipitate after thawing. Alternatively, 10 to 15 ml of saline may be added to the bag after thawing for this purpose.

Procedure B

1. Place the thawing plasma on a hook (holder) when approximately one tenth of the plasma is still frozen.

2. With this bag in an upright (inverted)

position, allow the supernatant plasma to flow slowly into the satellite bag, using the ice crystals at the outlet as a filter.

3. Seal the bag when 90 to 95 per cent of the cryoprecipitate-poor plasma has been removed. The cryoprecipitate paste will stick to the bag wall or to the ice.

4. Freeze the cryoprecipitate within four hours and store as recommended under the heading Storage.

5. When the product is to be used, it may be rapidly reconstituted by thawing in a 37° C water bath. The plastic bag should be carefully kneaded to ensure that the precipitate is fully resuspended. The contents from each bag can also be pooled, sequentially using an ever-increasing volume of plasma to flush each subsequent bag.

6. Once thawed, the component should be maintained at room temperature and administered within six hours. It may not be refrozen.

Storage

Cryoprecipitate may be stored at $-18°$ C or lower for up to 12 months from the date of blood collection. Losses in potency can be reduced by storage at $-30°$ C, if available.

Clinical Indications

Cryoprecipitate (factor VIII concentrate) is indicated in cases of hemophilia A (congenital factor VIII deficiency), von Willebrand's disease, and acquired factor VIII deficiency (disseminated intravascular coagulation, transfusional dilution in massive transfusion).

Dosage

The amount (measured in units) of factor VIII in various blood components and fractions is given in Table 18–3. One so-called "unit" of factor VIII equals the factor VIII activity of 1 ml of fresh normal pooled plasma. Factor VIII levels are usually reported as a percentage of normal.

The amount of factor VIII required for transfusion can be calculated as follows:

1. Weight (kg) × 70 ml/kg = blood volume (ml)

2. Blood volume (ml) × (1 − hematocrit) = plasma volume (ml)

3. Plasma volume (ml) × (desired factor VIII level (per cent) − initial factor VIII level (per cent) = units of factor VIII required.

If the factor VIII level is not known, it can be assumed to be zero per cent in a patient with severe hemophilia A.

Factor VIII has a half-life after transfusion of 8 to 12 hours, and therefore it is necessary to elevate the factor VIII level to twice that which is required to attain the desired factor VIII level just before the next dose is administered.

FACTOR IX COMPLEX

Preparation

Factor IX complex is prepared by fractionation of pooled plasma and contains factors II, VII, IX and X with a minimal amount of total protein. The amount of factor IX differs with different lots and is stated on the vial. Trace amounts of anticoagulant may be present.

Storage

Factor IX is supplied as a lyophilized product and must be stored at 2 to 8° C. The expiration date recommended by the manufacturer must be observed.

Clinical Indications

Factor IX complex is indicated for the prevention and control of hemorrhagic episodes in

Table 18–3 THE AMOUNT OF FACTOR VIII IN VARIOUS BLOOD COMPONENTS AND FRACTIONS*

Blood Component (Fraction)	Volume	Units of Factor VIII Per Container	Units of Factor VIII Per ml
Fresh whole blood (24 hr)	517.5 ml	225	1.0
Stored plasma	225 ml	225	1.0
Fresh-frozen plasma	225 ml	190	0.8
Cryoprecipitate	10 ml	100	10.0
Commercial cryoprecipitate	20–30 ml	200–1000	10–33

*Modified from AABB Technical Manual, 1977.

congenital factor IX deficiency (hemophilia B), congenital factor VII deficiency, and congenital factor X deficiency.

Acquired deficiencies of factors II, VII, IX and X should *not* generally be treated with factor IX complex, because these conditions can be effectively treated with plasma with less risk.

The risk of hepatitis virus transmission is high when using factor IX complex (see Factor IX Complex and Hepatitis, *FDA Drug Bulletin*, 1976).

Factor IX complex is contraindicated for the treatment of patients with liver disease and in neonates because of the risk of thrombosis or disseminated intravascular coagulation.

TYPICAL EXAMINATION QUESTIONS

Choose the phrase, sentence or symbol that completes the statement or answers the question. More than one answer may be correct in each case. Answers are given in the back of the book.

1. Within a temperature range of 2 to 6° C, the rate of glycolysis in whole blood is
   (a) the same as it is at other temperatures
   (b) 40 times slower than it is at 37° C
   (c) 40 times faster than it is at 37° C
   (d) 10 times slower than it is at 37° C
   (Storage — Whole Blood)

2. In whole blood stored at 2 to 6° C
   (a) there is a progressive fall in pH
   (b) the post-transfusion survival time of the cells is reduced
   (c) ATP levels are increased
   (d) 2,3-DPG levels become depleted
   (Storage — Whole Blood)

3. The optimal condition for platelet storage appears to be
   (a) 22° C
   (b) 40° C
   (c) 4° C with constant agitation
   (d) 22° C with constant agitation
   (Storage — Platelets)

4. Platelet concentrates are usually requested for administration to patients with
   (a) hemophilia
   (b) hemorrhage when the platelet count is below $50 \times 10^9/l$
   (c) thrombocytopenia associated with failure of platelet production
   (d) hemostatic defects due to an abnormality of platelet function
   (Clinical Indications — Platelet Concentrates)

5. Washed red blood cells, once prepared, should be
   (a) stored at 2 to 6° C
   (b) stored at room temperature
   (c) given as soon as possible and not stored
   (d) stored at 37° C
   (Storage — Washed Red Blood Cells)

6. Patients with paroxysmal nocturnal hemoglobinuria may benefit from the administration of
   (a) whole blood
   (b) cryoprecipitate
   (c) washed red blood cells
   (d) frozen-thawed red blood cells
   (General)

7. When it is important to increase a patient's hematocrit level with the minimum disturbance of blood volume, it is best to use
   (a) leukocyte-poor whole blood
   (b) washed red blood cells suspended in fresh plasma
   (c) platelet concentrate
   (d) concentrated red blood cells
   (General)

8. Cryoprecipitate (factor VIII concentrate)
   (a) is useful in treatment of patients with hemophilia A
   (b) is useful in treatment of patients with hemophilia B
   (c) is useful in treatment of patients with von Willebrand's disease
   (d) may be used for treatment of patients with hypogammaglobulinemia
   (Cryoprecipitated Antihemophilic Factor — Factor VIII Concentrate)

9. Below is a list of conditions that require therapeutic administration of blood, blood fractions or components. Name the product that would be of value in these circumstances in the spaces provided.
   (a) Thrombocytopenia _____

   (b) Granulocytopenia _____

   (c) Patients with repeated febrile reactions due to leukocyte antibodies _____

   (d) Transfusion of "out-of-group" red blood cells _____

   (e) Clotting factor deficiencies _____

   (f) Neonatal hyperbilirubinemia _____

(g) Hypogammaglobulinemia _____

(h) Factor VIII deficiency _____

(i) von Willebrand's disease _____

(j) Congenital factor X deficiency _____

10. Give the optimal storage temperature for the following components and the recommended length of storage:
    (a) Whole blood _____

(b) Concentrated red blood cells in which the hermetic seal has been broken during preparation_____

(c) Platelet concentrates _____

(d) Leukocyte-poor red blood cells, prepared in a "closed" system _____

(e) Red blood cells frozen in high-concentration glycerol _____

(f) Fresh-frozen plasma _____

(g) Stored plasma (frozen) _____

(h) Human serum albumin _____

(i) Fibrinogen _____

(j) Cryoprecipitate _____

GENERAL REFERENCES

The following texts provide useful coverage of the subject of blood components and may be referred to by the interested student.

1. A Seminar on Blood Components. Myhre, B. A. (Ed.) American Association of Blood Banks, Washington, 1977.

2. Mollison, P. L.: Blood Transfusion in Clinical Medicine. Blackwell Scientific Publications, Oxford, 1979.
3. Technical Manual, American Association of Blood Banks, Washington, D.C., 1977.
4. Technical Manual, American Association of Blood Banks, Washington, D.C., 1981.

Section Seven

TECHNIQUES

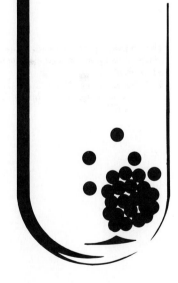

MATERIALS

OBJECTIVES — MATERIALS

The student shall know, understand and be prepared to explain the mode of action and laboratory uses of the following materials in the blood transfusion laboratory:
Saline
Bovine albumin
Low ionic-strength solution (LISS)

Proteolytic enzymes
Complement
Reagents
Lectins (*Dolichos biflorus, Ulex europaeus, Vicia graminea, Iberis amara, Arachis hypogea, Salvia sclaera*)

Some knowledge of the various materials used for practical work in the blood transfusion laboratory is essential for technologists engaged in such work. The following discussion will emphasize the most common materials, their mode of action and laboratory uses.

SALINE

A 0.85 per cent solution chloride in distilled water is of the same osmotic pressure as the contents of the human red cell (i.e., isotonic). The solution is known as *isotonic saline* and is used in the laboratory as a general cell-suspending medium.

Isotonic saline is prepared by dissolving 8.5 g of sodium chloride in one liter of distilled water. The solution should be freshly prepared but need not be sterile. Alternatively, commercial pre-prepared saline is available, as are commercially produced tablets of NaCl of various weights.

BOVINE ALBUMIN

Bovine albumin is one of the plasma proteins obtained from beef blood; when processed it is a useful high-protein medium used for the enhancement of certain blood group antibodies. Processing includes the biochemical control of protein concentration, pH and specific conductivity.

Preparations of bovine albumin vary greatly in their potentiating effect, apparently depending on the polymer content; that is, the proportion of polymers present (Jones *et al*, 1969; Goldsmith *et al*, 1971; Goldsmith, 1974; see also report by working party to ICSH, 1976). There is a tendency for batches of bovine albumin to be better at potentiating agglutination when they contain 85 per cent of the albumin in the monomer form with the remainder in dimer or polymer forms than are those with 95 per cent in monomer form. However, it appears that the correlation is not strong. It was concluded, therefore, that aliquots of a successful batch of albumin should be retained and used as a standard in testing new batches of albumin (Report to ICSH, 1976). Excess of polymerized material, it was found, leads to "false" agglutination of unsensitized red cells.

It is believed that bovine albumin and other colloid media enhance agglutination by reducing the electrical repulsion between red cells. The concentration of colloid is of some importance, and generally the higher the concentration, the greater the effect. (Twenty-two per cent albumin is better than normal serum in enhancing agglutination by IgG anti-Rh.) One exception to this is found with respect to IgG

247

anti-A and anti-B, in which a medium of 7 per cent albumin is better than one of 22 per cent and normal serum is better still (J. F. Mohn, cited by Mollison, 1979). Concentrations of 30 per cent albumin may have a tendency to cause rouleaux, although for the detection of weak atypical antibodies — particularly Rh — reactions are often somewhat stronger if this concentration is used. Bovine albumin also potentiates agglutination by some IgM antibodies; for example, autoanti-I (Haynes and Chaplin, 1971; Garratty et al, 1977) and anti-i (Burnie, 1973).

In the indirect antiglobulin technique, it has been found that the sensitivity of the test is increased by sensitizing red cells in the presence of albumin rather than saline (Stroup and Macilroy, 1965) (see *The Antiglobulin Technique*, Chapter 21).

With the use of bovine albumin there is an occasional problem of an *albumin autoagglutinating factor,* an antibody found in the serum of some "normal" individuals that agglutinates unsensitized red cells in the presence of most but not all batches of bovine albumin. Golde *et al* (1969) found the problem to be caused by sodium caprylate, which is used in some preparations of bovine albumin to ensure that over-polymerization does not occur. The "autoagglutination" is believed to be due to a nonspecific adsorption of an antigen-antibody complex onto red cells. The antibody, therefore, appears to be a gamma globulin directed against albumin that has been altered by caprylate.

In addition to this, Gunson and Phillips (1975) reported the presence of an agglutination inhibitor in 3 out of 28 commercial preparations of bovine albumin. This inhibitor causes a reduction in sensitivity of a standard assay technique on the AutoAnalyzer and is also apparent using manual methods. The inhibition is not related to the degree of polymerization of the albumin — and the reason for the inhibiting effect is not yet known. Yet it offers another reason for the careful standardization of batches of bovine albumin before they are put into general use.

Besides these complications, the possibility of bacterial contamination also has to be considered. Bovine albumin is not necessarily maintained in a sterile condition throughout its production; therefore, it may contain bacterial metabolites that could have adverse effects on agglutination tests. The refractive indices of bacteria and albumin are very similar. For this reason it is difficult to detect bacterial contamination visually because no cloudiness appears. The solution should be kept in the refrigerator whenever it is not in actual use, and the manu-

facturer's instructions as to the expiration of the product should be closely followed.

Bovine albumin is commercially available as a 22 per cent or a 30 per cent solution. It usually contains sodium azide as a preservative and should be stored at about 4° C and should not be frozen.

LOW-IONIC-STRENGTH SOLUTION (LISS)

As discussed in Chapter 2, the uptake of antibody by red cell antigens is much more rapid in low-ionic-strength suspending solution. Low-ionic-strength solutions are available commercially, but can be easily prepared in the laboratory by adding 20 ml of 0.15 M phosphate buffer (pH 6.7) and 800 ml of 0.3 M sodium glycinate (pH 6.7). The latter is prepared by dissolving 18 g of glycine in approximately 500 ml distilled water and adding 1.0M NaOH until the pH is 6.7 (approximately 0.35 ml.) to 180 ml. of 0.17M saline.

The low-ionic-strength solution may be used instead of isotonic saline as a suspending medium for red blood cells in antibody detection tests by using equal volumes of serum and 3 to 5 per cent red cells (one drop of each). Isotonic saline is still used for *washing* the red blood cells, and the low-ionic-strength solution is used as the *final* suspending medium.

The primary advantage of suspending red cells in low-ionic-strength solution rather than in saline lies in the increased rate of uptake of certain antibodies, particularly selected Rh antibodies believed to be of low affinity, which allows for a shortened incubation time. While maximum antibody coating may be observed after incubation for as little as 5 minutes, a 10-minute incubation is usually recommended because reactions are sometimes stronger at 10 minutes than at 5 minutes (Moore and Mollison, 1976). LISS may be stored at 4° C and, unless previously sterilized, should be discarded after a few days.

PROTEOLYTIC ENZYMES

The treatment of red cells with certain enzymes may cause them to be agglutinable by so-called "incomplete" red cell antibodies. The enzymes in common use in blood transfusion laboratories include papain, trypsin, ficin and bromelin. The choice of enzyme used is largely a matter of convenience, since there does not appear to be any important qualitative difference between them.

The mode of action of these enzymes varies with antigenic specificity. They react by reducing the net surface charge density by splitting off negatively charged carboxyl groups of sialic acid and thus reduce the zeta potential. Pollack *et al* (1965) demonstrated that red cells treated with ficin show the greatest reduction of zeta potential — papain follows closely and trypsin has the least effect.

Tests with enzyme-treated red cells are more sensitive than any other in detecting Rh antibodies, although they tend to give false positive results (Moore, 1970; W. J. Jenkins, cited by Mollison, 1979). Additional Rh specificities are often revealed when using enzyme-treated red cells, so that a "pure" anti-D, for example, may be found to contain anti-C or anti-E (see Giles, 1960). Other antibodies that are enhanced in their reactions when enzyme-treated red cells are used include:

1. Anti-Le[a] and anti-Le[b] (Rosenfield and Vogel, 1951). Some Lewis antibodies lyse enzyme-treated red cells but fail to lyse untreated red cells.

2. Anti-P[1] (Rosenfield and Vogel, 1951)

3. Anti-Jk[a] in the indirect antiglobulin test (van der Hart and van Loghem, 1953), which may lyse ficin-treated red cells and characteristically show a "dosage" effect (Haber and Rosenfield, 1957)

4. Anti-I and anti-i.

The reactions of anti-K and anti-k are not enhanced when the red cells are treated with enzymes (Unger and Katz, 1952; Haber and Rosenfield, 1957), and impure preparations of trypsin may inactivate K (Morton, 1957).

Antigens that are weakened or inactivated by proteolytic enzymes include:

1. M and N (Morton and Pickles, 1951; Mäkelä and Cantell, 1958; Springer and Ansell, 1958)

2. S (Morton and Pickles, 1951; Morton, 1957)

3. Fy[a], Fy[b] (Unger and Katz, 1952; Morton, 1957; Haber and Rosenfield, 1957)

4. Ch[a] (Middleton and Crookston, 1972)

5. Rg[a] (Longster and Giles, 1976)

6. Sp[1] (Pr) (Marsh and Jenkins, 1968)

7. Tn (Issitt *et al*, 1972)

Note: Although the T antigen is not inactivated by the concentrations of enzymes used in ordinary blood grouping techniques, it is inactivated by 3 to 4 per cent papain or ficin (Issitt *et al,* 1972).

As discussed in Chapter 2, if serum is incubated for a sufficient length of time with papain or with certain other enzymes, immunoglobulin molecules will be cleaved. For this reason, so-called "two-stage" techniques, in which red cells are first treated with an enzyme and then washed and incubated with antibody, are more sensitive in detecting low concentrations of antibodies than "one-stage" techniques. In these, red cells, enzyme and antibody are incubated together (see Kissmeyer-Nielsen, 1964; Dybkjear, 1965).

The sensitivity of enzymes in detecting certain antibodies has the disadvantage of also readily detecting "cold" alloagglutinins that are of no clinical importance. For this reason, and also because certain blood group antibodies of clinical importance may not be detected when enzyme-treated red cells are used, the enzyme test should under no circumstances be used as the sole test for compatibility.

Details of one- and two-stage enzyme tests are given in Chapter 23; the preparation method of enzyme solutions is also given in Chapter 23.

Of the enzymes in common use, papain, from the pawpaw (*Corica papaya*), is claimed to be cheaper and to give increased sensitivity when compared with trypsin. Trypsin, which is prepared from pig's stomach, has the distinct disadvantage of agglutinating most red cells after brief periods of incubation with normal serum, although after one hour at 37° C, 99 per cent of these will have become negative (Rosenthal and Schwartz, 1951; Rosenfield and Vogel, 1951). In addition to this, the serum of some normal donors contains a hemolysin that is capable of reacting with the donor's own trypsinized red cells (Heistö et al., 1965) (see Chapter 24).

Ficin is an extract from the fig (*Ficus corica*) and is about as effective as, though more noxious than, bromelin, which is an extract from the pineapple (*Ananas sativus*). While ficin is not used as commonly as the other enzymes, bromelin is often used in the AutoAnalyzer, where it is mixed with polyvinylpyrrolidone (PVP) and is useful for the routine detection of irregular antibodies in blood donors.

COMPLEMENT

If serum is being examined for the presence of a *hemolytic* antibody a freshly drawn sample of blood will normally contain an adequate amount of complement. In some instances, however, as when it is not possible to obtain a fresh blood sample, it may be necessary to add complement to the test system in order to demonstrate the hemolytic antibody. A source of complement is also required in HLA testing

(Chapter 14) and in the complement fixation test (Chapter 2).

Human Serum. This may be used as a source of complement, provided that proper storage conditions have been maintained. It has been reported that serum kept at 4° C for 24 hours or for 1 week at −50° C provides a source of complement that is indistinguishable from that in fresh serum. Serum stored at 20° C for 24 hours, at 4° C for 1 week, at −20° C for 4 weeks or at −50° C for 2 months provides a source of complement that is only slightly inferior to that found in fresh serum (Polley and Mollison, 1981).

Serum from a group AB subject is best used as a source of human complement, since it will not itself contain hemolytic anti-A or anti-B. If serum from subjects of other groups is used, it is necessary to remove the anti-A or anti-B or both by absorption at zero degrees C with an equal volume of packed, washed A_1B red cells (Thomsen and Thisled, 1928).

It should also be remembered, however, that the human serum used as a source of complement may contribute blood group *substances* that can directly inhibit the hemolytic antibody. For example, if A serum is mixed with O serum, the lysis of A red cells may be inhibited (Moss, 1910). Similarly, Le^a substance in the serum of a Le(a+b−) or Le(a−b+) subject may inhibit hemolysis by anti-Le^a (Cutbush et al, 1956). The choice of serum used as a source of complement will, in these cases, be dependent on the specificity of the particular hemolytic antibody.

Animal Serum. This may also be used as a source of complement as an alternative to using absorbed group O serum for the detection of all human complement-binding blood group antibodies (Mollison and Thomas, 1959). The use of horse serum in this regard has been reported to give exactly the same results as those obtained when human serum is used (Dennis and Konugres, 1959). Rabbit serum may even be somewhat superior in obtaining hemolysis with some anti-A sera that fail to lyse when horse serum or human serum is used as a source of complement (Dennis and Konugres, 1959).

When animal serum is used as a source of complement, it is essential that it be free of heteroagglutinins. This can be achieved by absorbing the animal serum three times at 0° C (each for 15 minutes) with an equal volume of human A and O red cells that have been washed six times. The cells and serum should also be cooled to zero degrees C before being mixed to avoid hemolysis. The red cells are first incubated with antibody-containing serum and then washed and incubated with fresh (absorbed) animal serum (a two-stage technique) (Mollison and Thomas, 1959).

REAGENTS

Reagents for use in the blood transfusion laboratory are available from several commercial companies. They also may be prepared in the laboratory if the appropriate facilities and equipment are available.

Provided that contamination is prevented, blood grouping sera will retain their potency for long periods of time when stored at 4° C. The half-life of antibodies in gamma globulin solution stored at 4° C has been reported to be not less than 20 years (Gerlough, 1958), although IgM antibodies appear to be less stable than IgG antibodies.

To prevent bacterial contamination, sera stored at 4° C require some sort of bacteriostatic agent such as 0.1 per cent sodium azide, which in a *final* concentration of 0.01 per cent is bacteriostatic (J. H. Humphrey, cited by Mollison, 1979). It should be noted that concentrations of sodium azide greater than 0.3 per cent have been shown to affect the titer of Rh antibodies and the electrophoretic pattern of serum (Saravis, 1959).

Reagent antisera can be stored at −20° C and as such do not require the addition of any bacteriostatic agent. Repeated thawing and freezing of antisera, however, should be avoided. Antisera containing high concentrations of albumin should be stored at 4° C and should *not* be frozen. Frozen sera that contains antibodies must be completely thawed and inverted several times before use, because antibodies are usually concentrated in the lower portion of frozen sera and may be attached to ice crystals.

Antisera for use as laboratory reagents may be obtained from individuals (patients or donors) whose serum contains high-titered antibodies. When procuring donations for antisera, it is preferable to obtain *serum* rather than plasma. This can be accomplished as follows:

1. Bleed the donor into a sterile container without anticoagulant.

2. Place the container at 37° C for 1 hour to ensure good clot retraction.

3. Leave the clotted blood at 4° C overnight to allow the absorption of cold autoagglutinin onto the red cells.

4. Centrifuge the container.

5. Aspirate the serum into a second sterile container.

Blood grouping reagents, however, are now most frequently obtained by plasmapheresis, which yields plasma. Serum can be obtained from this by the addition of calcium, as follows:

1. Centrifuge the blood at 500 g for 15 minutes.

2. Recover the supernatant platelet-rich plasma into a second sterile container and return the red cells to the donor (plasmapheresis).

3. Add 15 ml. of a solution containing 5.5 g $CaCl_2 \cdot 6H_2O$ and 1.6 g $MgCl_2 \cdot 6H_2O$ in 100 ml of sterile water (distilled) to the plasma. (*Note:* This amount of calcium-magnesium solution is correct when the maximum amount of plasma, containing virtually all the original citrate, is harvested. The calcium-magnesium solution should be reduced in proportion for lesser amounts of citrate-plasma).

4. Place the mixture at room temperature or at 37° C for 15 minutes.

5. Centrifuge the resulting serum at 5000 rpm for 8 minutes to clarify the serum.

6. Recover the serum into a third sterile container.

Note: Serum obtained in this way may contain residual fibrin and also contain excess calcium that will form calcium complexes on storage and will precipitate. A method for the removal of this excess calcium was described by Moghaddam *et al* (1971, 1976).

Red cells used as laboratory reagents (A_1 cells, A_2 cells, B cells, O cells, screening cells, panel cells and control cells) are usually stored at 4° C in a modified Alsever's solution, the composition of which is as follows:

Trisodium citrate (dihydrate), 8.0 g

Dextrose, 19.0 g

Sodium chloride, 4.2 g

Citric acid (monohydrate), 0.5 g

Distilled water to 1 liter

One volume of this solution is added to one volume of blood. When stored in this manner, reagent red cells are usually sufficiently reactive for three to four weeks, although their antigenic and serologic reactivity gradually decreases during this time. The rate of deterioration differs from one antigenic determinant to another and is dependent, to some extent, on the medium in which the cells are stored. Careful monitoring of reactivity is therefore desirable (see Quality Control, Chapter 20). It should be noted that stored reagent red cells should be free of hemolysis when used. However, freedom from hemolysis is *not* an indication of reactivity, and controls should be considered essential.

Anti-human globulin reagent is discussed in Chapter 21.

LECTINS

Since the last century it has been known that certain seed extracts have the ability to agglutinate human and animal red cells. Mäkelä (1957) reports that the first attempts to find *specific* blood group agglutinins in these extracts, which were unsuccessful, were made by Marcusson-Begun in 1926 and by Sievers in 1927. This discovery was made by Renkonen (1948) and Boyd and Reguera (1949), working independently.

Since that time, numerous studies have produced a wealth of knowledge and a seemingly endless list of seed extracts that have blood group specificity. A complete summary of these is well beyond the scope of this book; therefore, only the most common examples will be considered.

Two names have been suggested for plant agglutinins: phytagglutinins and lectins. The name lectin would be used for those agglutinins that show specificity.

Dolichos biflorus (Anti-A₁)

The *Dolichos biflorus* lectin was found by Bird (1951, 1952). The extract from the seeds of this plant agglutinates A_1 and A_1B red cells and is practically negative with A_2 and A_2B red cells. Since the reaction is over 500 times stronger with A_1 than with A_2 red cells, allowing the A_2 reaction to be diluted out very easily, the lectin is of considerable practical use in making the A_1A_2 distinction.

Solutions of *Dolichos biflorus* are readily available from commercial companies; however, they can be very easily prepared in the laboratory if the seeds are available.

The *Dolichos biflorus* extract does not react with group O or group B red cells suspended in albumin or treated with enzymes as other seed anti-A preparations tend to do. It does not react with the Forssman antigen (Bird, 1952) nor with the T antigen of "changed" red cells (Bird, 1954). It does, however, react with O and B cells of the very rare Sd(a++) phenotype (see Chapter 13) and with red cells that are Tn-activated (Chapter 24) and with Sd(a+) red cells.

Once prepared, *Dolichos biflorus* solutions retain their avidity for three years at 4° C. The solutions should not be kept at room temperature, nor should they be frozen.

Ulex europaeus (Anti-H)

The seeds of *Ulex europaeus* (common gorse) in solution have anti-H specificity. This was discovered by Cazal and LaLaurie (1952) and was soon recognized to be extremely useful with respect to the determination of secretor status (Boyd and Shapleigh, 1954). It is routinely used by most workers in the detection of H substance in saliva, by testing the ability of the saliva to inhibit (neutralize) the reaction of the lectin with group O red cells.

Anti-H from the seeds of *Ulex europaeus* is prepared in much the same way as anti-A_1 is prepared from the seeds of *Dolichos biflorus*.

If the extract is stored at 4° C, its shelf-life is at least one year.

Other Lectins

Vicia graminea (Anti-N). The extracts of this lectin provide a powerful and specific anti-N reagent, reacting best with saline-suspended red cells (Ottensooser and Silberschmidt, 1953; Uhlenbruck and Krupe, 1965). The reagent parallels anti-N in its cross-reactivity, but there is evidence to indicate that it combines with a receptor in the N antigen structure that is different from that which reacts with anti-N antibody. For example, as mentioned in Chapter 10, treatment of red cells with neuraminidase inactivates this reactivity with hetero-anti-M and -N as well as allo-anti-M and -N, but enhances their reactivity with *Vicia graminea* (Huprikar and Springer, 1970).

Anti-N specificity is also exhibited by extracts of the plant *Bauhinia purpura*, which reacts better in serum and in colloidal diluents (Boyd *et al*, 1958) than in saline.

Iberis amara (Anti-M). Extracts of the seeds of this plant have anti-M specificity and react best with saline-suspended red cells at room temperature (Mäkelä, 1952). The lectin is not as satisfactory for use in laboratory tests as human antisera with titers of 64 or more.

Arachis hypogea (Anti-T). Extracts of raw peanuts (*Arachis hypogea*) contain a powerful anti-T agglutinin for neuraminidase-treated red cells (Bird, 1964). The lectin can also be useful in detecting contamination as a cause of unusual blood group reactions given by old or much-traveled samples (see Polyagglutination, Chapter 24).

Salvia sclaera (Anti-Tn). Extracts of *Salvia sclaera* contain a useful anti-Tn (Bird and Wingham, 1973). The lectin must be diluted to avoid nonspecific activity but then reacts strongly with Tn red cells and not at all with T-activated cells (see Polyagglutination, Chapter 24).

TYPICAL EXAMINATION QUESTIONS

Choose the phrase, sentence or symbol that completes the statement or answers the question. More than one answer may be correct in each case. Answers are given in the back of this book.

1. Isotonic saline is prepared using
   (a) 8.5 g of sodium chloride in 2000 ml of distilled water
   (b) 0.9 g of sodium chloride in 1000 ml of distilled water
   (c) 0.85 g of sodium chloride in 1000 ml of distilled water
   (d) 8.5 g of sodium chloride in 1000 ml of distilled water

   (Saline)

2. Bovine albumin potentiates agglutination by which of the following antibodies?
   (a) anti-D
   (b) anti-M
   (c) anti-I
   (d) anti-i

   (Bovine Albumin)

3. The advantages of low ionic-strength solution in comparison with normal saline include
   (a) increased incubation time
   (b) decreased incubation time
   (c) increased rate of uptake of certain antibodies
   (d) decreased rate of uptake of certain antibodies, which increases the sensitivity of the test for such antibodies.

   (Low-Ionic-Strength Solution (LISS))

4. Which of the following antibodies are weakened or inactivated by proteolytic enzymes
   (a) anti-K
   (b) anti-Rg^a
   (c) anti-P_1
   (d) anti-Tn

   (Proteolytic Enzymes)

5. Serum stored under which of the following conditions will provide a source of complement that is almost indistinguishable from that in fresh serum?
   (a) 4° C for 24 hours

(b) 1 week at −50° C

(c) 4° C for 2 months

(d) −50° C for 6 months

(Complements)

6. A satisfactory bacteriostatic agent for use in blood grouping reagents is sodium azide in a final concentration of

(a) 0.1 per cent

(b) 0.3 per cent

(c) 0.01 per cent

(d) 0.001 per cent

(Reagents)

7. Extracts from the seeds of *Salvia sclaera* are a source of

(a) anti-T

(b) anti-N

(c) anti-A

(d) Anti-Tn

(Lectins)

8. An extract from the seeds of *Dolichos biflorus* will react with

(a) B cells that also react with anti-Sd (a++)

(b) A₂ cells when the lectin is undiluted.

(c) O cells that are Tn-activated

(d) A₁ cells

(Lectins — Dolichos biflorus)

9. Anti-N specificity is found in extracts of seeds of which of the following plants?

(a) *Arachis hypagea*

(b) *Bauhinia purpura*

(c) *Vicia graminea*

(d) *Iberis amara*

(Other Lectins)

10. *Dolichos biflorus* solutions should be stored at

(a) 22° C

(b) 4° C

(c) 37° C

(d) −20° C

(Dolichos Biflorus)

ANSWER TRUE OR FALSE

11. A 0.85 per cent solution of sodium chloride in distilled water is isotonic.

(Saline)

12. A medium of 30 per cent bovine albumin is better for the detection of IgG anti-A and anti-B than 22 per cent bovine albumin.

(Bovine Albumin)

13. A 5-minute incubation is usually recommended for the detection of antibodies suspended in low-ionic-strength solution.

(Low-Ionic-Strength Solution (LISS))

14. The reactions of anti-Leᵃ with Le (a+) red cells is enhanced when enzyme-treated red cells are used.

(Proteolytic Enzymes)

15. Trypsin will agglutinate most red cells after brief periods of incubation with normal serum.

(Proteolytic Enzymes)

16. Heteroagglutinins can be considered unimportant when animal serum is used as a source of complement.

(Complement)

17. Freedom from hemolysis is an indication of red cell reagent reactivity.

(Reagents)

18. Plant agglutinins that show no blood group specificity are known as phytagglutinins.

(Lectins)

GENERAL REFERENCES

Most blood transfusion texts contain some information regarding the materials used in the routine laboratory. Those that provide the most comprehensive coverage include the following:

1. Boorman, K. E., Dodd, B. E., and Lincoln, P. J.: Blood Group Serology: Theory, Techniques, Practical Applications, 5th ed. Churchill Livingstone, New York, 1977. *(Appendix II, pp. 462–473, is devoted to Reagents.)*

2. Mollison, P. L.: Blood Transfusion in Clinical Medicine, 6th Ed., Blackwell Scientific Publications, Oxford, 1979.

3. Race, R. R. and Sanger, R.: Blood Groups in Man, 6th ed. Blackwell Scientific Publications, Oxford, 1979. *(Particularly useful coverage of lectins.)*

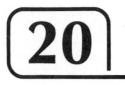

QUALITY CONTROL

OBJECTIVES — QUALITY CONTROL

The student shall know, understand and be prepared to explain:
1. The quality control of reagents, specifically to include:
   (A) Reagent antisera (new batches and daily quality control)
   (B) Reagent red cells (new batches and daily quality control)
   (C) Anti-human globulin (Coombs) reagent (evaluation and daily quality control)
2. The quality control of equipment, specifically to include:
   (A) Centrifuges
   (B) Automatic cell washers
   (C) Rh viewing boxes
   (D) Thermal equipment
3. The quality control of personnel
4. The quality control of blood components, specifically to include:
   (A) Platelet concentrates
   (B) Cryoprecipitate
   (C) Fresh frozen plasma
   (D) Frozen-thawed red cells
   (E) Leukocyte-poor red cells
5. The quality control of receiving and issuing procedures

Routine quality control of reagents, equipment and personnel is essential in any laboratory if the highest standards of blood transfusion practice and technology are to be maintained. While careful adherence to standard procedure will for the most part assure safety, quality control programs constantly reinforce the importance of these standards and offer indications of where these standards need to be upgraded.

The single most common cause of transfusion disasters is inaccurate identification — either of the patient, the patient's blood specimen, the donor's blood specimen, the donor unit or the requisition. This should be kept in mind at all times; meticulous accuracy must be insisted upon and carefully monitored. It is disarming to realize that the most elaborate, most complete quality control program with respect to laboratory reagents, equipment and personnel is no safeguard at all against an incorrectly labeled specimen or requisition.

Several standards exist for laboratory quality control. In this text, the requirements of the American Association of Blood Banks have been used as a guide. Students requiring more detailed coverage on the subject are referred to the *Technical Manual of the American Associa-*

tion of Blood Banks and also to the list of general references at the end of this chapter.

QUALITY CONTROL OF REAGENTS

It is often difficult to determine just how comprehensive a quality control program should be in order to be regarded as satisfactory. In general, quality control should not be excessively time-consuming; it should be so planned such that a technologist can easily complete the essential tests without too much interference with the regular workload. In particular it should not result in the accumulation of unnecessary data. In other words, quality control programs should be practical and realistic.

Reagent Antisera

New Batches. In the US, commercial reagent antisera (and red blood cell products) are licensed by the Bureau of Biologics (BoB) for sale *only* if they meet minimum standards for specificity and potency. Evaluation of these products by individual laboratories (by testing the titer, avidity, specificity and so forth) can be considered unnecessary. The manufacturer's instructions should be reviewed, however, with each new lot number to ensure that locally used procedures do not conflict with the directions of the manufacturer.

Daily Quality Control. Reagent antisera (both commercially prepared and prepared from locally collected sera) may suffer a loss of specificity or potency or both as a result of deterioration during shipping or storage, or as a result of contamination during preparation or use by other antisera, blood products or microorganisms. Specificity, in particular, can be lost through recrudescence of anti-A or anti-B activity after an absorbed serum has been stored.

For these reasons, individual laboratories must confirm that each reagent, on each day of use, is suitably reactive when used according to the manufacturer's directions.

The following antisera should be tested each day of use, using a known positive and a known negative control.

Anti-A
Anti-B
Anti-A,B
Anti-Rh$_o$(D)
All other blood grouping sera
Anti-human globulin serum
Lectins
Enzymes
Hepatitis test reagents
Syphilis serology reagents

Careful records must be maintained of these controls. Records must include the name of the individuals who will be using the reagents through the day, the commercial source and identification numbers of the reagents tested, the date of testing and the source and nature of the positive and negative cells used.

Using these positive and negative controls, the reactivity and specificity of the reagents may be established. When the activity of previously absorbed anti-A or anti-B is tested, it is important to remember that the behavior of these antibodies must be compared with A$_1$ and B cells against their behavior with O cells, since the return of anti-A or anti-B activity will not be apparent against group O cells.

Reagent antisera that are in common use may be tested on the day of use before the day's tests begin. Reagents that are seldom used are best tested in parallel with the actual test using positive and negative control cells. It is best to choose red cells with a weakly reactive antigen as a positive control, since these will provide a better indication of antiserum potency. If control red cells are chosen from a panel of cells

(group O), a specimen that is *heterozygous* for the antigenic determinant should be routinely selected, as a positive control.

To guard against deterioration, loss of potency or specificity in reagent antisera, the following precautions are suggested:

1. Store all antisera at 2 to 6° C when not in actual use.

2. Freeze all rare sera or in-house reagents for extended storage. Thaw at 37° C and thoroughly mix before use.

3. Avoid repeated thawing and refreezing. (Antisera are best divided into aliquots before freezing so that only the volume to be used need be thawed.)

Reagent Red Cells

New Batches. Like reagent antisera, commercial reagent red cells are licensed by the BoB for sale only if they meet minimum standards for specificity and potency. Evaluation of new batches, therefore, need not be performed. The manufacturer's directions, however, should be reviewed with each new lot.

Daily Quality Control. Reverse grouping cells (i.e., A$_1$, A$_2$ and B cells) and antibody detection (screening) cells should be tested on each day of use using a positive and a negative control. Reverse grouping cells should be tested for specificity with undiluted anti-A and anti-B. This will, in fact, serve as a control of both the antisera and the reagent red cells, and therefore need be performed only once to serve both purposes. Should a discrepancy be found, the cells and the serum should be tested independently with a panel of reagents of known reactivity.

With respect to antibody detection (screening) cells and antibody identification (panel) cells, it is impractical to perform daily tests on each sample — and virtually impossible to test each antigen for change in reactive strength. Antibody detection (screening) cells can, however, be checked with a weak saline-reactive antibody and a weak antiglobulin-reactive antibody. If possible, special attention should be given to the reactivity of labile antigens (e.g., P$_i$ and Le^a). The use of the corresponding antibodies in this case is especially likely to reveal loss of antigenic strength.

Of particular importance in the daily quality control of reagent red blood cells is to check each vial visually for evidence of hemolysis. If the supernatant fluid is hemoglobin-tinged and a single wash removes this, the cells can be used as a freshly prepared saline suspension. Many laboratories prefer to use a saline suspension of washed reagent red blood cells —

especially if there is a problem in antibody identification — because some patients have antibodies directed against antibacterial agents or other materials in commercially used suspending media (Gray, 1964; Gillund *et al*, 1972; Beattie *et al*, 1976).

Anti-Human Globulin (Coombs) Reagent

The antiglobulin test (direct and indirect) is described in Chapter 21. The reagent used in the test contains anti-IgG activity (required by Bureau of Biologics standards) and also some element of anticomplement activity. The anti-IgG is the most important component, since it will detect most antibodies likely to cause *in vivo* hemolysis. The anticomplement component is most useful in detecting immune sensitization of circulating red cells, although some antibodies (notably examples of Lewis and Kidd) react only with the anticomplement component.

Evaluation of Antiglobulin Reagents. Antiglobulin reagents are available from several different commercial suppliers; because the preparation of good antiglobulin sera is a highly complicated task, it is often desirable to run evaluation studies on those sera that are available to determine which will be most satisfactory in the test system used by the individual laboratory.

Anti-IgG. Blood group antibodies occur as IgG1, IgG2, IgG3, IgG4 (see Chapter 2). Unfortunately, at the present time it is not possible to evaluate antiglobulin reagents for anti-IgG1, 2, 3 and 4 content. Instead, the antiglobulin reagents should be tested against as many different IgG blood group antibodies as possible (e.g., anti-Fy^a, anti-Fy^b, anti-Jk^a, anti-Do^a, anti-K). Red blood cells should be *sensitized* with these antibodies so that they produce a 1+ reaction. (This is achieved by serial dilution of the antibody; see Titration, Chapter 23.) Aliquots of the various sensitized red cells are then tested against the various antiglobulin sera under consideration using standard procedures (Chapter 21) and their reactivities are compared.

Note: It is extremely important to remember when evaluating the anti-IgG content of antiglobulin sera that many IgG antibodies bind complement, and therefore the evaluation tests may be detecting a mixture of IgG antibody and complement. To prevent such sera from binding complement, EDTA may be added to the sera, as follows:

1. Prepare a solution containing 4.0 g dipotassium EDTA and 0.3 g NaOH in 100 ml of distilled water. The final pH of the solution should be between 7.0 and 7.4.

2. To 1 ml of diluted serum, add 0.1 ml of EDTA solution, to produce a final concentration of 4 mg per 1 ml serum.

3. Allow the EDTA and serum mixture to stand for 10 minutes at room temperature.

4. To a dry button of red cells (possessing the antigen corresponding to the antibody in the diluted serum) add 4 drops of the EDTA-tested serum and mix well.

5. Incubate at 37° C for 60 to 90 min.

6. Wash the red cells three times in large volumes of isotonic saline. After each wash, drain off as much saline as possible and blot the mouth of the tube. The red cells will now be sensitized with IgG, but no complement will be bound to the red cells.

7. Perform the direct antiglobulin test (as described in Chapter 21) with each antiglobulin serum under consideration.

8. Record results.

Anticomplement. Probably the most satisfactory method of testing for the anticomplement levels in antiglobulin sera is to use the two-stage EDTA procedure using Lewis antibodies, which readily bind complement. The most important complement component in antiglobulin sera is anti-C$\overline{3}$ (anti-C$\overline{3b}$ and anti-C$\overline{3d}$), and the two-stage EDTA procedure allows the binding of specific C$\overline{3b}$ and specific C$\overline{3d}$ to red cells when performed as follows:

1. Perform steps 1 through 6 as just described for the prevention of complement binding (first stage).

2. After the cells have been washed three times and completely drained (step 6) add two drops of fresh compatible serum to each tube as a source of complement.

3. Incubate for 15 minutes at 37° C.

4. Wash the red cells three times in large volumes of isotonic saline. After each wash, drain off as much saline as possible and blot the mouth of the tubes.

The short incubation time in the second stage causes the red cells to bind intact C$\overline{3b}$ and allows too little time for the cleavage of C$\overline{3b}$.

5. Perform the direct antiglobulin test (as described in Chapter 21) with each antiglobulin serum under consideration.

6. Record results. The strength of the reaction will give an indication of the amount of anti-C3b in the antiglobulin sera.

This technique is also used to determine the amount of anti-C$\overline{3d}$ in the antiglobulin sera by using a 24-hour incubation in the second stage. This allows enough time for the C$\overline{3b}$INA present in the serum used as a source of complement to cleave the C$\overline{3b}$ and leave only C3d on the red cells. (*Note:* Sodium azide, 0.1 per cent, should be added to the fresh serum to prevent bacterial growth during this incubation.)

Some antiglobulin reagents also contain anti-C$\overline{4}$. This can be tested for by using the low-ionic-strength medium method (commonly known as the sugar water test) (see under the heading Daily Quality Control).

With the use of these methods, red cells coated with C$\overline{3d}$ alone, C$\overline{3b}$ alone, C$\overline{3d}$ and C$\overline{3c}$ and C$\overline{4}$, C$\overline{3c}$ and C$\overline{3d}$ (using the low-ionic-strength medium method) can be prepared. By the process of elimination, it then is possible to show with reasonable certainty which antiglobulin reagents contain which anticomplement antibodies and approximately how much.

(*Note:* The anti-C$\overline{3d}$ component of antiglobulin sera can also be tested for using red cells from a patient with cold hemagglutinin disease where only complement is present on the red cells.)

Unwanted Agglutinins. There are several methods available to ensure that antiglobulin sera do not contain any "unwanted" agglutinins. Issitt *et al* (1974) suggested the use of A, B and O red cells, unwashed and suspended in their own serum, in agglutination tests at room temperature and at 4° C. These have the effect of neutralizing antiglobulin antibodies so that any agglutination observed can be attributed to unwanted antibodies. Use of A, B and O red cells ensures that anti-A, anti-B and anti-H and anti-species antibodies, all of which can be present in animal sera, will be detected. (*Note:* If autologous serum is used in this test, it is important to include controls to show that autoagglutinins are not present in the serum.)

Daily Quality Control. For routine daily quality control of antiglobulin sera, it is sufficient to use Rh$_o$(D)-positive red cells sensitized with IgG anti-Rh$_o$ (D), which is diluted so as to give no more than a 2+ reaction with antiglobulin serum. These sensitized red cells can be prepared by selecting a dilution of anti-Rh$_o$(D) that coats but does not agglutinate Rh$_o$(D)-positive red cells. While a patient's serum sample with a weakly reactive anti-Rh$_o$(D) can be used, it is usually necessary to dilute a stronger antibody. This can be accomplished by titrating the antibody (see Chapter 23) and selecting the dilution that shows 1+ macroscopic agglutination.

As an alternative, the diluted anti-Rh$_o$(D) can be used to prepare a batch of sensitized red cells that can be stored either at 4° C (in CPD, ACD or Alsever's solution) or frozen, for example, in liquid nitrogen, in small aliquots until needed.

Evaluation of antiglobulin serum daily for anticomplement activity is considered unnecessary (*Technical Manual, AABB,* 1977). The reason for this is that antiglobulin reagent that is damaged by improper storage conditions will show comparable loss of both anti-IgG and anticomplement activity (Garratty, cited by *AABB Technical Manual,* 1977).

If it is considered desirable for the individual laboratory to perform daily quality control for the anticomplement component in antiglobulin serum, the simple low-ionic-strength medium method can be used as follows:

1. Add red cells obtained from a fingerprick to a solution of 6 per cent sucrose and 0.15 per cent sodium chloride in distilled water.

2. Incubate the mixture at 37° C for 15 minutes.

3. Wash the red cells three times in large volumes of isotonic saline.

4. Test the washed cells by the direct antiglobulin test (see Chapter 21). A positive reaction indicates that anti-C$\overline{3}$ or anti-C$\overline{4}$ or both are reactive in the antiglobulin reagent.

Quality control of antiglobulin testing should extend to *each test* by the addition of sensitized red cells to each "negative" antiglobulin test. This control is discussed in more detail in Chapter 21.

QUALITY CONTROL OF EQUIPMENT

All instruments and equipment used in the laboratory must be properly maintained and monitored to ensure accurate testing. The equipment that should be regularly checked includes all centrifuges, automatic cell washers, Rh view boxes and thermal equipment.

Centrifuges

The purpose of the centrifuge in serologic testing is to wash red blood cells and to enhance red cell antigen-antibody reactions *in vitro*. In both of these applications centrifugation should pack the red cells into a well-defined cell button — but not so tightly that unagglutinated red cells cannot be resuspended with gentle manipulation. The supernatant fluid should be clear after centrifugation, and the red cell button should be "clean" (not jagged or fuzzy).

To ensure that a centrifuge is working efficiently, the following calibrations should be performed upon receipt of the instrument, after adjustments or repairs and annually when the instrument is in routine use:

1. Check the speed indicator and actual revolutions per minute (rpm) using an optical electronic device (tachometer) to ensure corre-

lation between the two. Mark any discrepancy on the face of the speed indicator.

2. Using a stopwatch, check the accuracy of the timer and the actual time of centrifugation, which includes the time of acceleration but not of deceleration. If there is discrepancy between the two, mark the correction on the face of the timer. (*Note:* Since timers are rarely completely reliable, it is wise to run this check every three months.)

3. Determine the optimal speed and time of centrifugation to satisfy the criteria given previously. This can be achieved as follows:

Saline Reactive Antibodies. Use serum from a group A individual diluted with bovine albumin or human group AB serum to give a 1+ agglutination reaction. Use group B red cells (2 to 5 per cent saline suspension) as a positive control and group A red cells (2 to 5 per cent saline suspension) as a negative control.

Albumin-Reactive Antibodies. Use anti-Rh_o(D), diluted in bovine albumin or human group AB serum to give a 1+ agglutination reaction. Use a 2 to 5 per cent saline suspension of Rh-positive red cells as a positive control and a 2 to 5 per cent saline suspension of Rh-negative red cells as a negative control.

Antiglobulin-Reactive Antibodies. Use unmodified antiglobulin serum. As a positive control, use a 2 to 5 per cent saline suspension of Rh-positive red cells incubated at 37° C for 15 minutes with diluted anti-Rh_o(D) (in bovine albumin or human AB serum) 1:100, and then washed three times in saline. As a negative control, use a 2 to 5 per cent saline suspension of Rh-negative red cells treated in the same way.

For each of the above, prepare five 10 × 75 or 12 × 75 mm test tubes for positive reactions. The serum and test cells should be added to each tube just before centrifugation.

In pairs (one positive and one negative) centrifuge the tubes for different times (e.g., 10 seconds, 15 seconds, 20 seconds, 30 seconds, 45 seconds) and record the results. If a variable-speed centrifuge is being tested, both time and speed must be varied. For each spin, record whether the supernatant fluid is clear, whether the cell button is clearly delineated, whether the red cells are easily dispersed, whether the negative reactions are clearcut and the degree of agglutination observed in the positives. The centrifugation time and speed selected should be the minimum required to fulfill these criteria. The optimal time and speed of centrifugation should be marked on the outside of the centrifuge, and all observations should be recorded permanently in the quality control records.

Automatic Cell Washers

Automatic cell washers are primarily designed for use in the washing phase of the antiglobulin test. These machines, which are available from several commercial suppliers in variously modified styles, automatically wash, decant, mix and rewash red cells from one to four times. Some systems also add the antiglobulin reagent to each tube.

Careful quality control of these machines is essential to ensure accurate results and to prevent malfunction. As with ordinary centrifuges, the following checks should be performed upon receipt of the machine, after adjustments or repairs and annually when the instrument is in routine use:

1. Ensure that an equal volume of saline is being added to each tube. To do this, stop the machine after the saline addition is complete and examine the amount of saline in each tube. If the volume is not uniform, consider the possibility that air is in the system, that saline delivery holes or lines are plugged, that the carriage is improperly aligned, or that the saline pump is defective. Since the obvious is most often overlooked, also consider the possibility that the saline bottle is empty.

2. Ensure that the red cell buttons are properly resuspended. Again, this is accomplished by stopping the machine after the addition of saline is complete and examining the tubes. Since in most cell washers the cell button is resuspended by the force of the saline hitting it in a constant stream, if the cell buttons are not properly resuspended, the saline addition nozzle may need adjustment or the centrifuge carrier may need to be realigned. If neither of these adjustments solves the problem, the force of the saline addition pump should be examined.

3. Be sure that the total volume of saline added to each tube is less than 80 per cent of the volume of the tube to guard against crosscontamination caused by foaming as a result of forceful saline addition to tubes containing protein. In procedures utilizing a large volume of protein during incubation (e.g., pools for screening) the ratio of saline to serum can be critical. This ratio can be determined by using a hemolysate of known concentration in a volume equal to the expected serum volume and measuring the hemoglobin concentration after the saline addition phase.

4. Verify that the time and speed of centrifugation are correct. The same quality control procedures recommended for regular centrifuges can be used. If adjustments are required, a service call may be necessary.

5. Be sure that the automatic braking sys-

tem is operative. This can be done by noting how long the centrifuge takes to come to a stop after spinning. If the system is inoperative it should be repaired, because the head may take from one to three minutes to coast to a stop and this will throw off the timing of other cycles.

6. Inspect the decant cycle to be sure that it is adjusted correctly. An almost dry cell button with no loss of red cells is the ideal. To determine if there has been a loss of red cells, a carefully measured volume of a well-mixed red blood cell suspension can be added to each tube. When the wash cycle is complete, perform a red blood cell count or hemoglobin on a dilution of the recovered cells with a similar dilution of the initial cell suspension. Alternatively, isotopically (^{51}Cr) labeled washed red cells can be used and initial counts in the tube can be compared with recovered counts after the wash cycle.

7. Be sure that the washing of the cells is efficient and thorough. Since even a small amount of serum remaining after the red cells have been washed can neutralize the antiglobulin serum, it is essential that the wash cycle be as efficient and as thorough as possible. This can be accomplished as follows:

    a. Set up test mixtures of serum and red cells according to the method in routine use.

    b. Stop the machine after each saline addition and spin *before decantation begins*, then obtain an aliquot of the supernatant saline from each tube.

    c. Test the supernatant saline for protein *either* by adding an equal volume of 5 per cent sulfosalicylic acid (turbidity indicates the presence of protein in a concentration of 1 mg to 25 mg per cent) *or* by determining its optical density at 280 mm. If a UV spectrophotometer is not available, a crystal of bromphenol blue added to the serum will bind to albumin and by reading the optical density (OD) or per cent turbidity (% T) between 600 and 625 nm, the amount of remaining protein can be determined.

(*Note:* Similar evaluations should be performed using serum-cell mixtures fortified with albumin and high protein techniques that are converted to the antiglobulin test. This same procedure can also be used in the evaluation of manual (nonautomatic) centrifuges.)

If protein is present after three washes, it may be necessary to increase the volume of saline in each wash, to decrease the volume of serum or albumin in the test mixture or to increase the number of wash cycles.

8. Be sure that the antiglobulin serum addition is working satisfactorily. Systems that automatically add the antiglobulin serum to the test tubes after the final wash-decant cycle should be checked periodically as follows:

    a. Visually inspect the tubes before and after the antiglobulin serum is added to be sure that the tubes have been properly agitated and that the contents are properly mixed.

    b. Visually inspect the tubes after the cycle is complete to verify that an *equal volume* of antiglobulin serum is present and that it has been delivered to the *bottom* of the tube. If the antiglobulin serum has run down the side of the tubes, adjustment of the delivery probe will be necessary. The amount (volume) of antiglobulin serum added to each tube can be determined by substituting a dye (e.g., 1 per cent crystal violet) for the antiglobulin serum and measuring the amount of dye in the tubes after the cycle is complete. Unequal antiglobulin serum addition may be caused by loss of antiglobulin serum from the probe resulting from suction during centrifugation cycles (which causes less than the full volume to be added to the first tube) by a bad probe or a blocked line or by air in the system. Obviously one should also check to be sure that the vial of antiglobulin serum is not empty.

During routine use of the machine, tubes should be visually inspected after each complete cycle to verify that they contain an equal volume of antiglobulin serum. The addition of presensitized red cells after the test has been read to all "negative" tubes is of particular importance when using automatic systems.

9. On a routine basis, the manufacturer's directions should be followed with respect to cleaning of the equipment and to periodic maintenance. Records should be kept of all calibrations, service calls, problems and maintenance of the machines.

Rh Viewing Boxes

The purpose of lighted viewing boxes, when Rh testing is performed on a slide or plate, is not only to facilitate reading of the test but also to provide sufficient heat so the temperature of the reaction mixture is approximately 37° C. The surface of the view box should remain between 40 and 50° C and this temperature should be checked routinely before use. Slides should be placed in the middle part of the surface to avoid possible cold spots.

Thermal Equipment

Water baths or heat blocks are used in the laboratory to achieve a temperature of 37° C for the detection of warm-reacting antibodies. (*Note:* Hot air or bacteriologic incubators are generally not suitable because reagents tend to evaporate.)

The temperature of each piece of equipment should be constantly monitored by placing a thermometer in the equipment and allowing it to remain there permanently. Each temperature should be checked and recorded when the instrument is received in the laboratory, after repairs, and on each day of use. These records must be retained for five years.

Blood bank refrigerators and freezers should be equipped with an alarm system and a temperature recording device. In addition, they should be connected to an emergency power system. The temperature of refrigerators and freezers should be checked daily and the alarm systems should be tested periodically to ensure that they are working satisfactorily.

QUALITY CONTROL OF PERSONNEL

The area of quality control of personnel is probably the most important of all aspects, yet it is also the most difficult to monitor. The following are suggested safeguards that will help to ensure a high standard of transfusion practice.

1. Be sure that all persons employed in the laboratory are properly qualified, dedicated and able to withstand stressful situations.

2. Do not hesitate to remove from the laboratory any person who, for whatever reason, cannot be trusted to perform the work safely and effectively.

3. Provide staff members with an organizational chart with accurate job descriptions. See that administrative, technical, clerical and supervisory responsibilities are clearly assigned.

4. Provide a written procedures manual (which should be reviewed and updated yearly) including all procedures, policies and the uses of all record forms. See that each staff member is familiar with those portions of the manual that pertain to his or her assigned duties.

5. Develop comprehensive orientation programs for new employees.

6. Develop continuing education programs for all employees.

7. In the event of an error, review and document pertinent procedures in retrospect and discuss the error and corrective action with the staff.

8. Ensure that all changes in instructions regarding procedures are brought to *all* employees' attention.

9. Provide written or pictorial descriptions or both of how to read, score and record test results. Verify that all personnel adhere to these instructions by running periodic duplicate, independent or blind testing.

10. Become involved in proficiency testing programs (e.g., AABB, CAP or governmental), which will provide comparisons with other institutions as well as evaluation of procedures, equipment, materials and personnel. These tests should be performed on rotation basis by all personnel who routinely perform the specific procedures.

QUALITY CONTROL OF BLOOD COMPONENTS

Blood components prepared, used or stored by individual laboratories should undergo periodic quality control both *in vitro* to document the effective separation of specific elements or coagulation factors and *in vivo* to evaluate the clinical effectiveness of the preparation.

Platelet Concentrates

Centrifuge Calibration. If platelet concentrates are being prepared by a laboratory, the centrifuge(s) used for this purpose must be calibrated to determine the optimal centrifugation time and speed to produce an acceptably high yield of platelets from platelet-rich plasma. This can be done by preparing platelet-rich plasma from four units of whole blood (see Chapter 18) using a selected speed and time of centrifugation, performing a platelet count on the sample of platelet-rich plasma from each unit and computing the average platelet count obtained. This procedure is then repeated using different centrifugation times and speeds, and the mean yields for each set of centrifuge conditions are compared in order to select the best. The centrifuge is then tested with a tachometer at the selected speed setting; the reading is recorded. The revolutions per minute (rpm) should be measured monthly. If they do not vary, the centrifuge need not be recalibrated. Centrifuge recalibration should, however, be repeated annually, and if the centrifuge is repaired. All records of calibration data, tachometer readings, maintenance and repairs must be maintained.

In Vitro Assay. Platelet counts should be performed on at least four platelet concentrates on a monthly basis. Either an electronic particle counter or phase microscopy can be used for this purpose. Phase microscopy has the advantage of permitting simultaneous observation of platelet morphology. Platelet counts should be performed from a specimen of blood taken from the donor into an EDTA tube and also on a segment from the unit of platelet concentrate after processing. When these counts are complete, calculate the per cent yield and record results. Determination of the number of platelets in each concentrate can be calculated using the following formula:

Platelet count/mm^3 × 1000 × volume of platelet concentrate = number of platelets in platelet concentrate

At 72 hours after preparation, prepare two segments (one long and one short) from the unit of platelet concentrate. The long segment is used for the platelet count and the short segment is used to determine the pH. The volume of concentrate can be measured by expressing the contents of the unit into a graduated cylinder. These three determinations (pH, platelet count and volume) are recorded.

The FDA and the AABB standards require $5.5 × 10^{10}$ platelets in 75 per cent of the platelet concentrates tested after 72 hours of storage (see Code of Federal Regulations, Title 21, Food and Drug Administration, parts 640.20 to 640.26, and Standards for Blood Banks and Transfusion Services, 8th Ed. Washington, D.C., American Association of Blood Banks, 1976).

The pH must remain above 6.0 throughout the storage period. Platelets stored at 22 ± 2° C should be suspended in at least 50 ml of plasma (AABB standards) or in 30 to 60 ml of plasma (FDA regulations); platelets stored at 2 to 6° C should be suspended in at least 20 ml of plasma (AABB standards) or this may be increased to 30 ml of plasma (FDA regulations). At least four units of platelets should be examined each month (FDA regulations). Outdated platelets may be used for this purpose.

In Vivo Quality Control. Two methods can be used to measure the clinical effectiveness of platelet transfusions. The first is to measure the patient's platelet count before and after transfusion (e.g., at one hour and/or 24 hours). The second is to evaluate the bleeding time at a set time before and after transfusion.

Cryoprecipitate

In Vitro Assay. At least four bags of cryoprecipitate should be assayed each month to determine the *in vitro* activity of factor VIII. The method for this type of assay is explained in detail in the *Technical Manual of the American Association of Blood Banks*, p. 351, 1977. On the average, each unit should contain a minimum of 80 units of factor VIII activity, or 40 units of factor VIII activity for every 100 ml of plasma processed.

In Vivo Quality Control. To measure the clinical effectiveness of cryoprecipitate, the patient's factor VIII levels before and after the transfusion can be compared. Alternatively, the effect of the transfusion on the patient's partial thromboplastin time (PTT) provides a quick index of effective activity. In a patient without anti-AHF inhibitor, the *in vivo* recovery can be calculated by measuring the increase in circulating factor VIII activity one hour after infusion, using the formula:

$$\frac{\text{Platelet plasma volume (ml)} × (\text{Postinfusion Factor VIII level–Pretransfusion Factor VIII level})}{\text{Number of units infused} × 100}$$

= Units of factor VIII per unit

Fresh-Frozen Plasma

Units of fresh-frozen plasma should be prepared and stored in such a manner as to indicate if thawing and refreezing has occurred. This is done by pressing a tube into a bag during freezing so that it leaves on the bag an impression that will disappear if thawing occurs, or by freezing a few test tubes of colored water on a slant and then storing them upright in different parts of the freezer. If thawing occurs, the slant of the frozen liquid will become straight. Alternatively, plasma that was originally frozen horizontally can be stored in an upright position, or a recording thermometer in a container in the freezer can provide adequate evidence of maintenance of freezer temperature.

Quality control of fresh-frozen plasma should be performed after 12 months of storage at −18° C (or lower) by assaying the appropriate coagulation factors.

Frozen-Thawed Red Cells

In the deglycerolization of frozen red blood cells, the final wash solution should periodically be tested by colorimetric or spectrophotometric measurement to ensure that free hemoglobin does not exceed 200 mg/dl. The recovery of red blood cells after thawing should also be calculated regularly, using the formula:

$$\frac{\text{Grams of red cells after processing}}{\text{Grams of red cells before processing}} \times 100$$

$$= \% \text{ red cell recovery}$$

Recoveries of 80 to 90 per cent of the erythrocytes should be obtained using most current techniques with the exception of the agglomeration method in which recoveries are often only 60 to 70 per cent.

Leukocyte-Poor Red Cells

To determine the percentage of white cells remaining in a unit of leukocyte-poor red cells, the following technique is recommended in the *AABB Technical Manual*, p. 293, 1977.

1. Weigh the unit of leukocyte-poor red cells and attached tubing. Subtract the weight of the empty bag (usually 26 g) and record the weight.

2. Strip the tubing, mix the red cells well and refill the tubing. Repeat this five times.

3. Segment the tubing, making a small segment at the end to be used for counting.

4. Prepare a 1 to 500 dilution by pipetting 10 lambda (0.020 ml) of leukocyte-poor red cells into 10 ml of isotonic saline. This must be done immediately after segmenting the tubing. If several units are being counted, complete this step on them all before continuing.

5. Perform counts.

6. Calculate the percentage of white cells remaining in the unit as follows:

Volume of product (in ml) = weight in grams ÷ 1.09 (this being the weight of 1 ml of red cells)

Total white cells (expressed as count $\times 10^9$) = Volume of unit (in ml) × white count per mm³ × 1000

Percentage of white cells remaining =

$$\frac{\text{Total white cells of leukocyte-poor product}}{\text{Total white cells of unit of whole blood}} \times 100$$

A commonly used goal is for the removal of at least 75 per cent of the initial white blood cells, although if the donor had an unusually high leukocyte count, this figure would not be realistic. A residual count of fewer than 1.0×10^9 white blood cells in the entire unit is probably a more sensible goal, although no specific standards for this exist. Results of these determinations can be recorded as the percentage of initial white cells removed or as the total leukocyte count in the final product.

QUALITY CONTROL OF RECEIVING AND ISSUING PROCEDURES

The majority of errors in blood transfusion work result from improper labeling and identification. Errors can be made from the time the unit is collected all the way through to administration of that unit to a recipient. Wherever possible, two people should check the identification of all steps involved in collection, pretransfusion testing and administering blood and blood products in order to minimize this risk. The following is a list of procedures in which incorrect identification can occur. These activities require careful checks and confirmation.

1. Recording of donor identification number
   (A) On record card at time of phlebotomy
   (B) Attached to blood bag
   (C) On all blood samples used for processing
   (D) In laboratory records of blood processing
2. Application of ABO and Rh labels to blood bag
3. Recording of patient's name and identifying number
   (A) On the requisition (request) for cross-match
   (B) On patient's wristband when the sample is drawn
   (C) At the patient's bedside: donor blood and labels (forms)
4. Recording the name of person administering the transfusion
5. Recording the name of person who discontinues the transfusion

---

TYPICAL EXAMINATION QUESTIONS

Choose the phrase, sentence or symbol that completes the statement or answers the question. More than one answer may be correct in each case. Answers are given in the back of this book.

1. If control red cells from a panel of cells (group O) are selected as a positive control in routine testing for red cell antigens, the cells should be
   (a) homozygous for the antigenic determinant

(b) heterozygous for the antigenic determinant
(c) either homozygous or heterozygous for the antigenic determinant
(d) stored at 37° C before use

(Reagent Antisera)

2. Antibody identification (panel) cells
   (a) should be quality-controlled every day
   (b) should be tested for changes in reactive strength daily
   (c) should be quality-controlled once a month
   (d) none of the above

(Reagent Red Cells)

3. The most important complement component in antiglobulin serum is
   (a) anti-C$\bar{1}$
   (b) anti-C$\bar{3}$
   (c) anti-C$\bar{4}$
   (d) anti-C$\overline{3b}$ and anti-C$\overline{3d}$

(Anti-Human Globulin (Coombs) Reagent)

4. Test for the anti-C3d component of antiglobulin serum by using
   (a) the two-stage EDTA procedure, using a 24-hour incubation in the second stage
   (b) the one-stage EDTA procedure
   (c) red cells from a patient with cold hemagglutinin disease
   (d) red cells from a patient with anti-Rh$_o$(D)

(Anti-Human Globulin (Coombs) Reagent)

5. The low-ionic-strength medium method will detect
   (a) either anti-C$\bar{3}$ or anti-C$\bar{4}$ in antiglobulin serum but not both
   (b) anti-C$\bar{4}$ (only) in antiglobulin serum
   (c) anti-C$\bar{3}$ (only) in antiglobulin serum
   (d) anti-C$\bar{3}$ or anti-C$\bar{4}$ or both in antiglobulin serum

(Anti-Human Globulin (Coombs) Reagent)

6. If protein is detected in the saline after three washes in an automatic cell washer, which of the following adjustments can be made?
   (a) Increase the volume of saline in each wash
   (b) Decrease the volume of saline in each wash
   (c) Decrease the volume of serum or albumin in the test mixture
   (d) Increase the number of wash cycles

(Automatic Cell Washers)

7. The surface of an Rh viewing box should be kept at a temperature of

(a) 37° C
(b) 40 to 50° C
(c) 22° C
(d) 100° C

(Rh Viewing Boxes)

8. In the quality control of platelets concentrates, *in vitro* assays should be performed on at least four units of platelet concentrates
   (a) daily
   (b) weekly
   (c) monthly
   (d) yearly

(Platelet Concentrates)

9. After 72 hours of storage, the number of platelets in 75 per cent of platelet concentrates should be at least
   (a) 1.0×10^9
   (b) 2.5×10^{10}
   (c) 5.5×10^{10}
   (d) 20.0×10^{10}

(Platelet Concentrates)

10. On the average, the amount of factor VIII activity in cryoprecipitate should be
    (a) 80 units per bag
    (b) 160 units per bag
    (c) 8 units per bag
    (d) 40 units per 100 ml of plasma

(Cryoprecipitate)

ANSWER TRUE OR FALSE

11. Specificity of reagent antisera can be lost through recrudescence of anti-A or anti-B activity after an absorbed serum has been stored.

(Reagent Antisera)

12. Reagent red cells should be checked visually each day for evidence of hemolysis

(Reagent Red Cells)

13. The most important component of antiglobulin sera is anti-C$\bar{3}$.

(Anti-Human Globulin (Coombs) Reagent)

14. Hot air incubators are suitable for the detection of warm-reacting antibodies

(Thermal Equipment)

15. Free hemoglobin in the final wash after deglycerolization of frozen red blood cells should not exceed 200 mg/dl.

(Frozen-Thawed Red Cells)

GENERAL REFERENCES

1. Code of Federal Regulations, Title 21, Food and Drugs, Parts 640.20–640.26.
2. Myhre, B.: Quality Control in Blood Banking. John Wiley and Sons, New York, 1974.
3. Standards for Blood Banks and Transfusion Services, 8th Ed. American Association of Blood Banks, Washington D.C., 1976.
4. Quality Control in Blood Banking. American Association of Blood Banks, Technical Workshop, 1973.

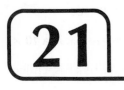

THE CROSSMATCH

OBJECTIVES — THE CROSSMATCH

The student shall know, understand and be prepared to explain:

1. The various techniques used in crossmatching, including:
   (A) Saline techniques
   (B) Albumin techniques
   (C) Enzyme techniques
   (D) The antiglobulin technique (direct and indirect)
2. The selection of blood for transfusion in:
   (A) Routine situations
   (B) Emergency situations
   (C) When group-specific blood is not available
   (D) When Rh-type specific blood is unavailable
3. Massive transfusion
4. Crossmatching of patients with coagulation abnormalities
5. Crossmatching of patients after the infusion of synthetic plasma expanders
6. The issuing of blood

Introduction

The crossmatch (or "compatibility test") is the most important and most frequently performed procedure in the blood transfusion laboratory. In general terms, the crossmatch consists of a series of procedures performed before transfusion to ensure the proper selection of blood for a patient and to detect any irregular antibodies in the serum of the recipient that would reduce or adversely affect the survival of the donor's red cells after transfusion.

There are two kinds of crossmatch: the so-called "major" crossmatch, which involves the testing of the donor's red cells with the recipient's serum, and the "minor" crossmatch, involving testing of the donor's serum with the recipient's red cells. The standards of the American Association of Blood Banks and the regulations of the FDA (BoB) require that pretransfusion testing include the major crossmatch by a method or methods that will demonstrate agglutinating, sensitizing and hemolyzing antibodies — and that it will include the antiglobulin test. Pre-transfusion testing need not, however, include the minor crossmatch, because this is performed as a routine test on donor units after collection (see Chapter 17).

In general, the crossmatch should detect most recipient antibodies directed against antigens on the donor red cells as well as major errors in ABO grouping, labeling and identification of donors and recipients. It is important to note, however, that the crossmatch will *not* guarantee normal donor cell survival or prevent recipient immunization. Nor will it detect all ABO grouping errors, Rh typing errors (unless the recipient's serum contains previously formed Rh antibody) or *all* irregular antibodies in the recipient's serum.

Many procedures are available that, in combination, constitute a satisfactory crossmatch. The techniques outlined in this text do not necessarily constitute all of the known procedures in use. However, they do offer the majority of possibilities through the thermal ranges that provide for the detection of most clinically significant antibodies.

SALINE TECHNIQUES

Applications and Limitations in Crossmatching

Certain blood group antibodies react at body temperature *in vivo*; however, they may

264

give optimal reactions *in vitro* at temperatures below that of the body. Saline techniques are designed to detect IgM antibodies that react optimally at room temperature (22° C) or lower. These include, for example, anti-M, anti-N, anti-Le^a, anti-Le^b, anti-Lu^a and anti-P$_1$. The technique also serves to detect major ABO grouping errors, since incompatibility in this phase will result (in potentially serious situations) if red cells of an incorrect ABO group have been mistakenly selected for crossmatching.

As a sole compatibility test, saline techniques are, of course, inadequate, since clinically significant IgG antibodies are not detected in this phase. Note that agglutination in the saline crossmatch may indicate the presence of cold agglutinins (e.g., anti-I) which will often increase in strength with reduction in temperature.

Technique 1: Saline (Immediate Spin)

1. **Place two drops of the patient's serum in a 10 × 75 mm test tube.**
2. **Add one drop of a washed 5 per cent suspension of the donor's red cells.**
3. **Centrifuge immediately at 3400 rpm (Serofuge) for 15 seconds.**
4. **Read macroscopically. (Examine negative reactions microscopically.) An optical aid (e.g., an illuminated concave mirror) can be used in the reading of the test.**
5. **Record results.**

Note. In emergency situations, this technique will detect major ABO grouping errors or the presence of strong antibodies, so that the time of incubation can be saved. Immediate-spin techniques are not generally used in routine situations.

Technique 2: Saline (22° C Incubation)

1. **Place two drops of the patient's serum in a 10 × 75 mm test tube.**
2. **Add one drop of a washed 5 per cent suspension of the donor's red cells.**
3. **Incubate at room temperature for 15 to 30 minutes.**
4. **Centrifuge at 3400 rpm (Serofuge) for 15 seconds.**
5. **Examine macroscopically for hemolysis and for agglutination using an optical aid. (Examine negative reactions microscopically.)**
6. **Record results.**

Technique 3: Saline (37°C)

1. **Place two drops of the patient's serum in a 10 × 75 mm test tube.**
2. **Add one drop of a washed 5 per cent suspension of the donor's red cells.**
3. **Incubate at 37° C in heat blocks or in a water bath for 15 to 30 minutes.**
4. **Centrifuge at 3400 rpm (Serofuge) for 15 seconds.**
5. **Examine macroscopically for hemolysis and for agglutination using an optical aid. (Examine negative reactions microscopically.)**
6. **Record results.**

ALBUMIN TECHNIQUES

Applications and Limitations in Crossmatching

The addition of bovine albumin to the crossmatch presents ideal conditions for the detection of Rh/Hr and certain other blood group antibodies (see Materials — Bovine Albumin, Chapter 19). Bovine albumin acts to increase the dielectric constant of the medium, thereby reducing the zeta potential and allowing IgG antibodies to be demonstrated. The majority of IgG antibodies are detectable in this way, although some may only agglutinate very weakly (e.g., anti-Fy^a).

The sensitivity of the antiglobulin test can be increased through the addition of bovine albumin. This is discussed in the section The Antiglobulin Technique, later in this chapter.

One of the main disadvantages of albumin techniques is the presence of nonspecific aggregates revealed in microscopic reading, especially when 30 per cent albumin is used. While these aggregates are rarely a problem for the experienced worker, the inexperienced may be confused by them. In appearance, they have smooth edges and leave a trail of unagglutinated red cells. While a drop of saline will often help to disperse them, it should be noted that this may also disrupt weak agglutination.

A further disadvantage of albumin techniques is the occasional presence in the serum of *albumin autoagglutinating factor* (AAAF). This is a rare type of autoagglutinin that reacts with red cells only when they are suspended in bovine albumin and not when they are suspended in saline (Wiener *et al*, 1956). In fact, the antibody responsible for this phenomenon is not directed against albumin at all (Beck *et al*, 1976) but rather against sodium caprylate (which is used as a stabilizer in some preparations of bovine albumin) or other fatty acid salts. (For further discussion, see Chapter 24.)

Technique 4: Albumin (Immediate Spin or 37° C Incubation)

1. Place four to six drops of the patient's serum in a 10 × 75 mm test tube.
2. Add one drop of a washed 5 per cent suspension of the donor's red cells.
3. Add two to three drops of 22 to 30 per cent bovine albumin, according to the manufacturer's directions, and mix well.
4. Incubate at 37° C in heat blocks or in a water bath for 15 to 30 minutes (37° C incubation method). This step is omitted in the immediate-spin method.
5. Centrifuge at 3400 rpm (Serofuge) for 15 seconds or for one minute at 1000 rpm.
6. Examine macroscopically for hemolysis and for agglutination using an optical aid. (Examine negative reactions microscopically.)
7. Record results.

Note. Albumin techniques provide a satisfactory back-up test for the indirect antiglobulin technique in routine crossmatching. Slide (or tile) techniques using bovine albumin are not generally recommended, since they encourage the formation of rouleaux (see Chapter 24) and since questionable reactions may appear as the mixture dries on the slide.

The albumin-enhanced antiglobulin procedure is discussed under the Antiglobulin Technique, later in this chapter.

Additional albumin tests are described in Chapter 23.

ENZYME TECHNIQUES

Applications and Limitations in Crossmatching

Like albumin techniques, enzyme techniques can provide a satisfactory back-up test for the indirect antiglobulin technique in routine crossmatching, because they are capable of detecting many clinically significant IgG and saline-inactive IgM antibodies. Both one- and two-stage methods are available. The two-stage technique (red cells pretreated with enzyme and then tested with the patient's serum) is most widely used. One-stage techniques (enzyme, patient's serum and donor's red cells incubated together) are easiest to apply in the crossmatch situation and therefore are convenient. However, they are less sensitive than two-stage techniques (see Kissmeyer-Nielsen, 1964).

The major limitation of enzyme techniques is their inability to detect certain antibodies in the MNSs and Duffy blood group systems. This fact immediately precludes the use of enzyme techniques as a sole test for compatibility. Other limitations include the inactivation of certain enzymes if improperly stored (e.g., papain) and the incidence of "nonspecific" agglutinins as a result of the method's high sensitivity. Moreover, false results can be obtained if red cells are "overtreated" with certain enzymes such as papain owing to fragmentation of the immunoglobulin molecules by the enzyme (see Chapter 2).

On the positive side, enzymes occasionally allow for the detection of some antibodies not demonstrated by other techniques — notably some early Rh/Hr antibodies and certain rare examples in the Kidd system.

Enzyme tests may be carried through the antiglobulin technique if required (see under the heading The Antiglobulin Technique.) Since cold autoagglutinins are enhanced by enzyme techniques, a patient autocontrol should always be run with each test.

The enzymes commonly used in the blood transfusion laboratory are bromelin, trypsin, papain, and ficin, each of which have certain individual characteristics.

A specific technique often used in crossmatching is the one-stage bromelin technique, which is described later. It should be noted that the inclusion of this method should not be taken as an indication that it is in any way superior to other available methods. When commercially produced enzymes are used, the manufacturer's instructions should always be followed.

Further techniques involving enzymes are described in Chapter 23.

Technique 5: The One-Stage Bromelin Technique

1. To each of two 10 × 75 mm test tubes, add two drops of the patient's serum. (The first tube should be labeled "test" and the second "auto control".)
2. To the tube labeled "test," add one drop of washed 2 to 5 per cent suspension (in saline) of the donor's red cells.
3. To the "auto control" tube, add one drop of a washed 2 to 5 per cent suspension (in saline) of the patient's own red cells.
4. Add one drop of bromelin to each tube and mix well.

5. Incubate both tubes at room temperature for 15 minutes.
6. Centrifuge at 3400 rpm (Serofuge) for 15 seconds.
7. Examine for agglutination and for hemolysis using an optical aid and record the results.
8. Resuspend the red cells completely and incubate both tubes at 37° C for 15 minutes.
9. Centrifuge at 3400 rpm (Serofuge) for 15 minutes.
10. Examine for agglutination and for hemolysis using an optical aid and record the result.
11. Follow with the antiglobulin technique (described later).

THE ANTIGLOBULIN TECHNIQUE

Applications and Limitations in Crossmatching

The antiglobulin test is probably the most important and most widely used serologic procedure in modern blood banking. The test has a wide range of applications, as is evidenced by the frequent references to it in many parts of this text. The antiglobulin technique will be discussed in some detail here because it represents the most essential part of any crossmatch procedure.

In principle, the antiglobulin test involves red cells coated with so-called "incomplete" antibodies; that is, those that fail to agglutinate red cells suspended in saline. These antibodies are usually IgG and are agglutinated by the *anti-IgG* in antiglobulin serum through the "linking" of the IgG molecules on neighboring red cells. This basic principle was described by Moreschi (1908), who used rabbit red cells incubated with goat anti-rabbit red cell serum.

Coombs *et al* (1945) rediscovered the test and introduced it into clinical medicine. These workers showed that the test could be used to detect both IgG antibodies in serum (the *indirect* antiglobulin test) and the *in vivo* sensitization of red cells (the *direct* antiglobulin test) (Coombs *et al*, 1946). Both these tests are described later.

As mentioned, the majority of incomplete antibodies are IgG and are detected using anti-IgG serum. Some incomplete antibodies are IgM (e.g., Lewis antibodies) or may be partly IgA. These antibodies may be detectable by the indirect antiglobulin test using anti-IgM (Polley *et al*, 1962) or anti-IgA (Adinolfi *et al*, 1960), respectively, although in the case of Lewis antibodies, they are usually best detected using anti-complement.

Dacie *et al* (1957) first recognized the fact that antiglobulin serum might react with complement components on red cells. It was subsequently shown that the main complement components detected were C4 (Jenkins, G. C. *et al*, 1960; Pondman *et al*, 1960) and C3 (Harboe *et al*, 1963).

Of all compatibility tests, the antiglobulin test probably comes closest to approaching the ideal, and its inclusion in a crossmatch is required by AABB standards and by FDA (BoB) regulations. It is capable of detecting many IgG antibodies that do not react in either saline or high-protein media or that react weakly or variably in these media. It also detects antibodies that bind complement but that may not be capable of binding to red cells in sufficient amounts to give a positive test. The main limitation of the test is the large number of factors that may influence or affect the reaction (see Causes of False Positive Reactions and Causes of False Negative Reactions, later in this section).

Preparation of Antiglobulin Reagent

The antiglobulin reagent used in routine laboratory work is a pool of serum usually made from two different colonies of rabbits, although goats and sheep can also be used. One colony of rabbits is immunized with highly purified IgG to produce anti-IgG and the other with human beta globulins to produce anti-complement.

Anti-IgG Antiglobulin Reagent. In the preparation of specific anti-IgG antiglobulin reagent, highly purified IgG from pooled plasma is used, prepared as follows:

1. Pooled plasma is encouraged to precipitate through the addition of ammonium sulfate.

2. The antiglobulin fraction is cycled twice through a DEAE cellulose column with only the 0.01 molar fraction being collected on each occasion.

3. The final preparation is mixed with Freund's complete adjuvant.

Rabbits are immunized by deep intramuscular injection of this preparation into four different sites with a total of 8 mg of IgG. Intravenous injection does not produce a good antibody response (Biro and Garcia, 1965). Six weeks later, a booster shot of 15 mg of alum-precipitated IgG is given and the animal is bled three weeks later.

In most cases, the only antibody produced following the injection of IgG is anti-γ chain, which is specific for IgG. Some animals also produce anti-L chain, and the serum then crossreacts with other immunoglobulins. While the presence of anti-L chain in antiglobulin serum is of no significance in routine clinical use, it obviously causes problems if an attempt is being made to determine the immunoglobulin class of blood group antibodies. If anti-L chain is produced, it can subsequently be neutralized by the addition of purified L chains.

The anti-IgG in hyperimmunized animals is all 7S fraction (IgG), although early in immunization, appreciable amounts of IgM anti-IgG (19S antibody) are produced. The serologic characteristics of IgG anti-IgG and IgM anti-IgG are slightly different (see Haynes and Chaplin, 1971).

Anti-Complement Antiglobulin Reagent. Several methods may be used to prepare anti-complement reagent, depending on which components are required. If a reagent containing a mixture of anti-complement antibodies is satisfactory, this can be simply and conveniently prepared as follows:

1. Wash zymosan in saline, then heat in a boiling water bath for 30 minutes.

2. Centrifuge and wash the zymosan three times in veronal buffered saline with added Ca^{++} and Mg^{++}.

3. Resuspend the zymosan in veronal-buffered saline to 30 mg/ml.

4. Add 0.2 ml of this suspension to 2 ml of fresh serum, diluted 1 in 20.

5. Incubate the mixture for one hour at 37° C.

6. Centrifuge and wash three times in veronal buffer.

7. Resuspend in 2 ml of normal saline.

8. This suspension is then injected intravenously into the rabbit. It contains 6 mg of coated zymosan.

The antibody produced is predominantly anti-C3, though probably some anti-C4 is also made (Stratton, 1966). Other antibodies are also made, including anti-IgG (Mollison, 1979), but the addition of purified human IgG to the product provides a satisfactory anti-complement reagent.

Methods of preparing anti-complement reagents that are more "pure" than that described and that do not depend on the purification of the relevant proteins, were proposed by Freedman et al (1977). In brief, these are performed as follows:

Method 1. Monkey red cells are coated with human C4d by exposure to EDTA-treated human serum at low ionic strength, followed by trypsinization. The cells are then reinjected into the donor monkey. The antibody that results from this agglutinates red cells sensitized with C4d and C4b, but not those sensitized with C4c, C3d or C3b.

Method 2. Rabbit red cells are incubated with MgEDTA-treated human serum so as to block activation of the classic complement pathway but permit activation of the alternative pathway. The cells are trypsinized and then injected into the donor rabbit. The resulting antiserum contains anti-C3d and some anti-C3c but does not contain anti-C4.

In the laboratory, anti-complement can be prepared by the addition of a precise volume of IgG to broad-spectrum antiglobulin reagent, which causes the neutralization of the anti-IgG yet leaves the anti-complement unaffected. The role of anti-complement in antiglobulin reagents is described later.

Anti-IgM and Anti-IgA. These monospecific antiglobulin reagents can be prepared by the injection of IgM or IgA myeloma proteins into rabbits. Alternatively, a sample of the rabbit's red cells can be incubated with human saliva, which is then reinjected intravenously into the animal (see Tönder and Larsen, 1970).

Preparations of anti-IgM and anti-IgA are often contaminated with some anti-IgG, and the resulting antiserum usually has to be absorbed with IgG to obtain a specific reagent.

Broad-Spectrum Antiglobulin Reagent. This is the reagent used in routine blood bank work. It is prepared by combining anti-IgG and anti-complement, prepared as described. As such it contains both components and can be used to detect antibodies that do or do not initiate complement sensitization of red cells (see under the heading Role of Anti-Complement in the Antiglobulin Reaction).

Use of Monospecific Antiglobulin Reagents

Several monospecific antiglobulin reagents can be prepared by injecting animals with highly purified proteins such as IgG, IgM, IgA, C3 or C4, or by the absorption of unwanted antibodies from broad-spectrum antiglobulin reagent.

These monospecific reagents are most frequently used to determine which protein is responsible for a positive *direct* antiglobulin test. Monospecific anti-IgG and anti-C3 may also be of value in the indirect antiglobulin test in the identification of mixtures of noncomplement-binding and complement-binding antibodies.

Techniques used when testing red cells with these reagents are exactly the same as for broad-spectrum reagents (see under the heading Methods).

Note: Anti-IgA, -IgM, -C3 and -C4 must

never be used *alone* for crossmatching or for antibody detection.

Role of Anti-Complement in the Antiglobulin Reaction

The necessity for anti-complement components in antiglobulin serum used for pretransfusion testing has been the subject of some considerable controversy and discussion for a number of years. During the last meeting of the Working Party on the standardization of antiglobulin reagents (International Society of Blood Transfusion, 1980), it was agreed that antiglobulin reagents containing anti-complement will detect potentially significant antibodies that are undetectable by pure anti-IgG using a routine centrifugation antiglobulin test. It was therefore agreed unanimously that anti-complement should be present in antiglobulin reagent. The decision was further supported by two observations:

1. In the routine hospital laboratory, the enhanced reactions seen with complement-binding antibodies when anti-complement is present in the antiglobulin reagents are more easily detected than the sometimes rather weak reactions with pure anti-IgG. Therefore, with the inclusion of anti-complement, the crossmatch can be considered "safer."

2. A long-term study of antibodies detected in the crossmatch using monospecific anti-IgG and anti-complement reagents in parallel was conducted by Dr. L. D. Petz. The study revealed that with fresh serum the incidence of antibodies reacting only with anti-complement is as high as 1 in every 3000 patients. Kidd specificities were commonly found in such cases.

The role of anti-complement in the antiglobulin reaction can be summarized as follows:

1. To detect complement-binding clinically significant antibodies that may be missed by pure anti-IgG in routine testing.

2. To enhance the reactions of complement-binding antibodies.

3. To detect IgM antibodies, which invariably bind complement yet which may elute off the red cells with increase in temperature, leaving complement components *alone* on the red blood cells.

It is generally agreed that anti-C4 is less important than anti-C3 for the detection of clinically significant complement-binding antibodies. Since red cells stored in CPD have higher than normal levels of C4 and C3 bound to their membrane, antiglobulin serum should have low levels of anti-C4. Anti-C3d levels must be high enough to detect C3d on red cells that have been sensitized with complement-binding antibodies *in vitro* but not so high as to cause "false positive" reactions with CPD stored blood.

In the direct antiglobulin test, the presence of anti-complement in the antiglobulin serum is of even greater importance for two reasons.

1. In cold hemagglutinin disease (cold antibody autoimmune hemolytic anemia) the patient's cold antibody reacts up to 30 to 32° C. The patient's red cells therefore become sensitized with antibody in the peripheral circulation when the skin temperature drops to this range. The antibody, which usually binds complement, may cause hemolysis of the red cells; however, if the cells escape hemolysis, they will recirculate and be warmed to 37° C. At this temperature the cold antibody elutes off the cells into the plasma, leaving only complement components (primarily C3d) attached to the red cells. These complement components are detected only by the anticomplement component in antiglobulin serum.

2. In as many as one-fifth of patients with warm antibody autoimmune hemolytic anemia, only complement is demonstrable on the red cells. It is believed that IgG is present on the red cells of these patients but in amounts below the threshold of the antiglobulin test as routinely performed (Gilliland *et al*, 1970).

It should also be remembered that red cells can become sensitized with complement because of the initiation of the complement cascade by *immune complexes*, which may be attached to or remote from the red cell. An example is the formation of immune complexes due to drugs, in which the drug–anti-drug complex can attach nonspecifically to the red cell membrane and cause the activation of complement with subsequent attachment of complement components to the red cell membrane (see Immune Complexes, Chapter 15.)

THE INDIRECT ANTIGLOBULIN TEST

The indirect antiglobulin test is used for the detection of antibodies that may cause red cell sensitization *in vitro*. If both IgG antibody and the corresponding antigen are present in a serum–red cell mixture, incubation will cause the antibody to attach to the specific antigenic receptors on the red cell. After washing to dilute the excess antibody in the serum, the addition of antiglobulin serum will "link" the IgG molecules on neighboring red cells, producing agglutination (Fig. 21–1).

In addition to crossmatching, the indirect

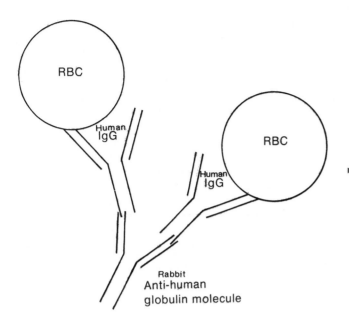

Figure 21–1 Reaction of the anti-human globulin molecule.

antiglobulin test is also used for the detection and identification of unexpected antibodies — for detecting red cell antigens not demonstrable by other techniques and for special studies, such as the antiglobulin consumption test, mixed agglutination reactions and leukocyte and platelet antibody tests.

Technique 6: The Indirect Antiglobulin Technique

1. **Place two to six drops of the serum under test (patient's serum) in a 10 × 75 mm test tube.**
2. **Add one drop of washed 5 per cent suspension of the test cells (donor's red cells, screening red cells, etc.) *Optional*: Two drops of bovine albumin may be added to the mixture; see under the heading The Addition of Bovine Albumin to the Indirect Antiglobulin Test.**
3. **Mix well.**
4. **Incubate at 37° C for 15 to 30 minutes.**
5. **Centrifuge immediately upon removal from the incubator for 15 seconds at 3400 rpm (Serofuge); examine for hemolysis and agglutination using an optical aid; record results.**
6. **Wash three or four times in large amounts of saline. Decant each wash as completely as possible.**
7. **Add one to two drops of antiglobulin reagent.**
8. **Mix well.**
9. **Centrifuge at 3400 rpm (Serofuge) for 15 seconds.**
10. **Examine for agglutination using an optical aid.**
11. **Record results.**

12. ***Optional*: Add one drop of known sensitized red cells to all negative tests. Centrifuge at 3400 rpm for 15 seconds; examine for agglutination. If no agglutination is seen, the test result is invalid and must be repeated.**

Addition of Bovine Albumin to the Indirect Antiglobulin Test

The sensitivity of the indirect antiglobulin test can be increased by sensitizing the red cells in the presence of albumin rather than saline (Stroup and Macilroy, 1965). These workers suggested that the incubation time of the test could be reduced to 15 minutes in this way. With full incubation (30 minutes or longer), the use of bovine albumin is of less importance, since parallel tests reveal no obvious difference in sensitivity with or without the use of albumin after this incubation time.

Bovine albumin appears to be less effective in accelerating antibody uptake than low ionic-strength medium (Moore and Mollison, 1976). In fact, the simplest and most effective way of increasing sensitivity is to increase the ratio of serum:cells (see under the heading Serum to Cell Ratio in Compatibility Tests).

Use of Enzyme-Treated Cells in the Indirect Antiglobulin Test

The "enzyme" antiglobulin test is performed by first enzyme-treating the red cells (see Chapter 23) and then using these cells in the indirect antiglobulin test exactly as described. Unger (1951) showed that some antibodies will be detected in the antiglobulin test only if enzyme-treated red cells are used. Van der Hart and van Loghem (1953) reported the enzyme-antiglobulin test to be particularly suitable for the detection of anti-Jk[a]. It will also detect the presence of the Le[a] antigen on red cells that by other methods appear as O Le(a−b+) (Cutbush et al, 1956).

It should be noted, however, that "false positive" results can be obtained with enzyme-treated red cells. This may be due to the presence of heteroagglutinins in the antiglobulin sera or to overtreatment with the enzyme.

Use of Low Ionic-Strength Medium in the Indirect Antiglobulin Test

As discussed in Chapter 19, the suspension of red cells in low ionic-strength solution rather than saline increases the rate of uptake of antibody, which allows for a greatly reduced incubation time. In routine situations, it has been recommended that incubation time may be reduced to 10 minutes. This is also valuable in cases of great urgency.

In the use of low ionic-strength solution, it is recommended that only *equal* volumes of serum and a 3 to 5 per cent suspension of red cells be used in a ratio of 1:1. The low ionic-strength solution is only used as the final suspending medium — isotonic saline is still used for washing the red cells (AABB recommendation, 1977).

Various Phases of the Antiglobulin Test

Sensitization Phase (Indirect antiglobulin test only)

Effect of the Suspending Medium. As discussed, the suspending medium for the red cells in the antiglobulin test may be saline, albumin, serum or low ionic-strength solution. Each of these have, to varying extents, an influence on the rate of antibody uptake by the red cells, which affects the required incubation time. Of the four, low ionic-strength solution appears to have the most dramatic influence, allowing incubation time to be reduced to 10 minutes (see Elliot et al, 1964; Hughes-Jones et al, 1964; Low and Messeter, 1974).

Effect of the Serum:Red Cell Ratio. Hughes-Jones et al (1964) showed that the amount of antibody taken up per red cell is at a maximum when the ratio of serum to red cells is about 1000:1. Under standard conditions, the ratio is much lower. In manual compatibility tests, a positive antiglobulin test will be obtained *only* when the test red cells are coated with 100 to 500 antibody molecules per cell. Besides the serum to red cell ratio; the amount of antibody uptake is also influenced by a number of other factors such as pH, temperature, ionic strength and so forth.

The best serum to red cell ratio that is within the realm of practical application has been reported to be 80 to 1 (Wright, 1967). In order to achieve this ratio, the following variables must be considered.
1. Number of drops of serum used
2. Volume delivery of the Pasteur pipette
3. Dropper volume delivery
4. Per cent concentration of the red cells used

In order to determine if an 80:1 serum to red cell ratio is being used, perform a three-part calculation.
1. Measure the number of drops per ml delivered by five randomly selected Pasteur pipettes. Calculate the ml per drop delivered by the Pasteur pipette using the formula

$$\frac{1}{\text{Number of drops per ml}}$$

2. Repeat this procedure with the red cells and perform a hematocrit to determine per cent concentration. Use the highest number of drops/ml and the highest packed cell volume obtained by testing several red cell samples and apply the formula

$$\frac{1}{\text{Number of drops per ml} \times \text{per cent concentration}}$$

3. The number of drops of serum needed to provide an 80:1 serum to red cell ratio is then determined using the formula

$$80 \div \frac{\text{ml/drop of serum}}{\text{ml/drop of packed red cells}}$$

Effect of the Temperature of Incubation. Complement sensitization and most IgG antibody reactions occur optimally at 37° C. Hughes-Jones et al (1964) reported that variation in temperature over the range 2 to 40° C has little effect on the equilibrium constant, although at 37° C the reaction is 20 times faster than at 4° C.

Effect of Incubation Time. An incubation time of 15 to 30 minutes at 37° C permits the detection of most clinically significant antibodies. Hughes-Jones et al (1963) reported that when five volumes of serum containing anti-Rh are incubated at 37° C with one volume of a 20 per cent suspension of Rh-positive red cells, it take about six hours for the maximum amount of antibody to be taken up by the red cells (i. e., for equilibrium to be reached). About 25 per cent of this maximum amount is taken up in the first 15 minutes, about 75 per cent within the first hour and about 95 per cent within the first two hours. As has been discussed, the suspending medium greatly increases the rate of antibody uptake. Incubation time, therefore, is somewhat arbitrary, although extension of the time to one hour or two hours appears to have very few disadvantages and may detect a few weaker examples of antibodies undetected after 15 minutes of incubation.

Washing Phase

In the vast majority of cases large amounts of immunoglobulin still remain in the serum after incubation is complete. This excess must be removed, because antiglobulin reagent will combine with the free globulin and there may be insufficient antibody remaining to combine with that attached to the red cells. Washing is, in fact, a *diluting process* that reduces the amount of free globulin to a point at which it will not interfere with the reaction. Inadequate washing can lead to false negative reactions in the test. To ensure that washing is adequate, the following is recommended:

1. Washing must be rapid and uninterrupted to minimize loss of cell-bound antibody by elution.

2. Saline should be decanted as completely as possible after *each* wash.

3. Red cells should be completely resuspended after each wash.

4. Saline should be added in a forceful stream.

5. The mouth of the test tube should not be covered with the finger or the palm of the hand when mixing. Serum on the hands or fingers can inactivate the antiglobulin serum.

6. Adequate volumes of saline should be used. Three or four washings are usually sufficient if 10×75 mm or 12×75 mm test tubes are filled at least three quarters full of saline.

7. After adding antiglobulin reagent, mix well.

8. Add antiglobulin reagent immediately following the completion of washing.

The centrifugation phase is discussed in Chapter 20.

THE DIRECT ANTIGLOBULIN TEST

The direct antiglobulin test is used to demonstrate whether or not red cells have been coated (sensitized) with antibody *in vivo*. The test is useful in the diagnosis of hemolytic disease of the newborn and autoimmune hemolytic anemia and in the investigation of red cell sensitization caused by drugs and of immediate and delayed transfusion reactions.

Positive direct antiglobulin tests are often confusing because they can be the result of a wide variety of causes such as disease states, drugs or contamination (see Chapter 15).

It should be noted that an individual who has a positive direct antiglobulin test, regardless of cause, cannot be typed with any antisera that react in the antiglobulin test, since a positive reaction will not necessarily indicate the presence of antigen.

Technique 7: The Direct Antiglobulin Test

1. **Place one drop of a 2 to 5 per cent saline suspension of red cells to be tested in a labeled 10×75 mm test tube.**
2. **Wash the red cells four times in large volumes of saline. Care should be taken for adequate removal of the supernatant after each wash. Note that washing results in dilution rather than removal of free globulin.**
3. **Add one or two drops of antiglobulin reagent.**
4. **Mix well.**
5. **Centrifuge at 3400 rpm (Serofuge) for 15 seconds.**
6. **Examine for agglutination using an optical aid and record results. *Note*: The manner in which the red cells are dislodged from the bottom of the tube is of great importance. The tube should be held at an angle and shaken *gently* until all cells are dislodged, then tilted gently back and forth until an even suspension of cells or agglutinates is observed.**
7. **Add IgG-sensitized red cells as a control, centrifuge and read. If a negative result is obtained, the test result is invalid. If monospecific anticomplement reagents are used, complement-sensitized red cells should be substituted for IgG-sensitized red cells.**

Controls for Direct and Indirect Antiglobulin Tests

Probably the best general control for the direct or indirect antiglobulin test is the addition of IgG-sensitized red cells after reading. A positive result indicates the following:

1. The antiglobulin reagent has remained active and has not been neutralized.

2. The red cells have been adequately washed.

3. The final volume of saline did not excessively dilute the antiglobulin serum.

4. Antiglobulin reagent was added to the test tubes.

A negative result invalidates the test.

Commercially prepared presensitized red cells can be used for this purpose, or they can be prepared in the laboratory by titrating an IgG antibody (anti-Rh$_0$ (D)) and using the dilution that results in a 2+ agglutination. Diluted serum is then prepared and incubated (at 37° C) with enough Rh$_0$ (D)-positive red cells to provide one drop of sensitized red cells for every negative antiglobulin test in the day's workload.

SOURCES OF ERROR IN THE ANTIGLOBULIN TEST

Causes of False Positive Reactions

1. Traces of species-specific antibodies (heteroagglutinins) due to improper preparation of the antiglobulin serum.

2. Enzyme-treated red cells (because of greater sensitivity) reacting with residual antispecies antibodies.

3. Test cells that have a positive direct antiglobulin test.

4. Anti-T or anti-Tn in the antiglobulin serum reacting with T-activated or Tn red cells (see Beck *et al*, 1976). This can be caused by bacterial contamination of the test cells or by septicemia in the patient.

5. Extreme reticulocytosis due to transferrin bound to reticulocytes reacting with anti-transferrin in the antiglobulin serum. *Note*: most antiglobulin reagents today have little antitransferrin activity (see Mollison, 1979).

6. Colloidal silica in saline stored in *glass bottles* that is leached from the container.

7. Metallic ions in saline stored in *metal* containers or used in equipment with metal parts. This may bring about nonspecific protein sensitization of the red cells.

8. Improperly cleaned glassware or other forms of contamination of cells, serum or reagents.

9. Overcentrifugation.

10. Autoagglutination before washing that may persist through the washing phase.

11. Uptake of complement onto the red cells *in vitro*. After a period of storage, clotted blood samples may react with anti-complement in the antiglobulin serum (anti-C3 and/or anti-C4). A small percentage of samples from segments of plastic tubing (i.e., containing blood stored at 4° C with anticoagulant) will react with anti-C4d (Garratty and Petz, 1976). The cause of these false positives has not been definitely established.

Causes of False Negative Reactions

1. Incorrect technique for the particular antibody involved.

2. Inadequate washing of the red cells causing neutralization of the antiglobulin serum by trace amounts of residual globulin (as little as 2 μg of IgG/ml as a final concentration).

3. Insufficient active complement when the particular antibody is detectable only in the presence of active complement or insufficient anti-complement in the antiglobulin reagent.

4. Improper storage of test cells, test serum or antiglobulin reagent or all of these, resulting in loss of reactivity.

5. Delays or interruptions in the test procedure, particularly during the washing phase, which may result in the elution of the antibody from the red cells.

6. Failure to add antiglobulin reagent.

7. Red cell suspensions that are too heavy (which may not permit optimum coating with antibody) or too weak (which may make reading difficult).

8. Undercentrifugation or overcentrifugation. The latter because of the excessive force required to resuspend the red cells.

9. Contamination of the antiglobulin reagent with human serum.

10. Incorrect incubation temperature (not allowing for maximum coating of the red cells) or fluctuating incubation temperature.

11. Insufficient incubation time.

12. Prozone. (*Note*: This should not be a problem with licensed products provided that the manufacturer's directions are followed.)

13. Failure to check negative reactions microscopically.

SELECTION OF BLOOD FOR TRANSFUSION

Routine Situations

ABO. When whole blood is to be transfused, the blood selected for crossmatch should be of the same ABO group as that of the recipient. In cases in which group-specific and type-specific blood is unavailable, as in transfusing group A blood to an AB recipient or in cases of ABO and/or Rh hemolytic disease of the newborn, it may be acceptable or even advisable to transfuse *packed red cells* of a different ABO group, provided they are compatible.

It is considered unnecessary to be concerned with subgroups of A unless the patient has a clinically significant anti-A_1 or anti-HI (anti-O), in which case the following should be kept in mind:

1. Anti-A_1 in patient serum: Examples of anti-A_1 that are active *in vitro* at 30° C or higher have been shown to be capable of extensive red cell destruction. These patients should receive blood of subtype A_2.

2. Anti-HI(O) in patient's serum: Examples of anti-HI (anti-O) that are *not* inhibited by H substance are occasionally active at temperatures above 30° C and have been known to cause rapid destruction of transfused (incompatible) red cells. These patients should receive blood of group A_1 since there is less H substance on A_1 cells than on A_2 cells.

Rh. As a general rule, the blood selected for crossmatch should also be the same $Rh_0(D)$ type as that of the recipient. Matching for the Rh/Hr antigens *other* than $Rh_0(D)$ is considered unnecessary. This holds true unless, of course, the patient has a known Rh/Hr antibody, in which case blood lacking the corresponding antigen must be selected. $Rh_0(D)$-negative recipients should receive blood that, in addition to being $Rh_0(D)$-negative, should also be rh'(C)-negative and rh''(E)-negative. In cases of shortage or emergency, rh''(E)-positive (D^u-negative) blood may be substituted when transfusing adult $Rh_0(D)$-negative recipients. This should be avoided for the transfusion of women in child-bearing age except in cases of dire urgency. Generally, rh''(E)-positive (D^u-negative) blood is preferable to rh'(C)-positive (D^u-negative) blood under these circumstances. The latter, when transfused to an $Rh_0(D)$-negative recipient, could stimulate the formation of anti-G.

For D^u-positive recipients, the transfusion of $Rh_0(D)$-positive blood appears to involve very little risk of immunization to anti-Rh_0 (D).

Emergency Situations

In cases in which there is insufficient time to determine the patient's blood group, blood of group O $Rh_0(D)$-negative (rh'(C)-negative, rh''(E)-negative) may be used if *most* of the plasma is removed, or if it has been tested and been found to be free of hemolytic anti-A and anti-B. Blood of group O $Rh_0(D)$-positive may be used *only* if O Rh-negative blood is unavailable.

In the vast majority of circumstances in which blood is required in an emergency situation, there is time to perform a routine ABO and $Rh_0(D)$ typing. If time permits, an emergency crossmatch can be performed (discussed later). In cases such as these (even when crossmatching has not been performed), group- and type-specific blood should be given. It is best to perform all tests in the transfusion facility without relying on previous records. Evidence of the patient's blood group *must not be* taken from cards, dog tags, driver's licenses or other such records.

When Group-Specific Blood Is Not Available

Transfusion of blood of a group that is not the same as that of the recipient is acceptable when the required group is not available under two conditions: (1) Blood must be issued as packed red cells, wherever possible. (2) If whole blood is issued, it must be shown to *lack* hemolysins directed against cells of the recipient's group.

The choice of alternative blood groups that are acceptable is summarized in Table 21–1.

In cases when groups A_1 (or A_2) or B are both acceptable as an *alternative* first choice for transfusion (see Table 21–1), either group may be chosen, but only *one of the two* should be used for a given recipient. If a patient has received one of these two and blood of yet another group is needed, it is best to use blood of group O. Generally in these circumstances, group A blood is chosen preferentially because it is more readily available than group B blood.

The decision to change back to group-specific blood should be based on the presence or absence of anti-A or anti-B or both in subsequent samples of the recipient's blood. If the crossmatch of a *freshly drawn* sample from the

Table 21–1 CHOICE OF ALTERNATIVE BLOOD GROUPS THAT ARE ACCEPTABLE FOR RECIPIENTS OF PARTICULAR BLOOD GROUPS*

Patient's Blood Group	Alternative Blood Group	
	First Choice	Second Choice
A_1	O	None
A_2 (with anti-A_1)	O	None
A_1 (with anti-HI(O))	None	None
B	O	None
A_1B	A or B†	O
A_1B (with anti-HI(O))	A_1 or B†	None
A_2B (with anti-A_1)	A_2 or B†	O

*Modified from Technical Manual, AABB, 1977.
†See text.

patient with group-specific blood indicates compatibility (especially in the saline room-temperature phase), this blood can be issued. In the case of incompatibility, transfusion with red cells of the previously chosen ABO group should be continued. (*Note*: Group-specific transfusions should *not* be given through the same infusion set as was used for transfusion of red cells of a different ABO group.) The effect of transfused alloantibodies should be evaluated when the emergency is over, since these antibodies may cause hemolysis of the recipient's red cells.

When Rh Type-Specific Blood is Unavailable

When Rh-negative blood is unavailable, Rh-positive blood may be transfused rather than withhold blood from a patient whose need is critical, provided the blood is compatible and provided that anti-Rh antibodies have not been detected at any time in the patient's serum (as revealed by previous records). If at all possible, this should be avoided in female recipients who are of child-bearing age.

It should be noted that up to 70 per cent of Rh-negative recipients who receive Rh-positive blood may form anti-$Rh_o(D)$. If only one unit of Rh-positive blood has been given in error, large doses of $Rh_o(D)$ Immune Globulin may be given in an attempt to prevent immunization. Approximately 15 to 20 ml of $Rh_o(D)$ Immune Globulin may be required for this purpose (Pollack *et al*, 1971).

Rh-negative blood may be given to an Rh-positive recipient provided the crossmatch shows compatibility, if Rh-positive blood is unavailable.

SUGGESTED CROSSMATCH PROCEDURE*

Before a specimen of blood from the intended recipient is accepted for crossmatch, all clerical details regarding identification must be checked. The patient's full name, hospital number, address and date of birth must coincide on the specimen tube and on the requisition. Specimens that are unlabeled must be rejected. Under no circumstances should the clerical details be written on the specimen tube after it has been received by the blood bank or after the blood has been taken. Specimens should also be rejected on the basis of clerical error, hemolysis, appearance of contamination and so forth. In doubtful cases such as when the patient cannot be identified owing to uncon-

*AABB-recommended techniques.

sciousness when admitted, the laboratory director should be consulted.

The requisition, in addition to the identifying information mentioned, should also include the following:

1. Diagnosis (Preferably this should indicate why transfusion is considered necessary.)
2. Transfusion history
3. Date of last transfusion
4. Obstetric history
5. Test(s) required
6. Number and type of blood products required
7. Time and date of intended transfusion

The requisition should be signed by the individual who initiated the request for blood, preferably the physician in charge of the case.

Before the crossmatch procedure is performed the following steps are necessary:

1. Review the records of previous transfusions. If the patient has been previously tested, check the recorded group and type and note any irregular red cell antibodies that may have been previously identified.
2. Perform ABO grouping, Rh typing and red cell antibody screening. Be sure that the results obtained correlate with previous records.
3. Perform ABO grouping, Rh typing and red cell antibody screening on the chosen unit(s) of blood. (*Note*: Antibody screening need not be repeated if it has been performed by the collecting laboratory).

The One-Tube Crossmatch Procedure

1. Place four to six drops of the recipient's serum in an appropriately labeled 10 × 75 mm or 12 × 75 mm test tube.
2. Add one drop of a 2 to 5 per cent saline suspension of red cells from the donor. Mix.
3. Incubate at room temperature for 15 to 30 minutes.
4. Centrifuge at 3400 rpm for 15 seconds.
5. Examine for hemolysis and for agglutination with an optical aid (see under the heading Reading and Interpretation).
6. Record result.
7. *Optional:* add two or three drops of 22 to 30 per cent bovine albumin.
8. Mix well.
9. Incubate at 37° C for 15 to 30 minutes.
10. Centrifuge at 3400 rpm for 15 seconds immediately upon removal from the incubator.
11. Examine for hemolysis and for agglutination with an optical aid (see under the heading Reading and Interpretation).
12. Record results.

13. Wash the red cells three or four times in large volumes of normal saline. Decant as completely as possible after each wash.
14. Add one to two drops of antiglobulin serum.
15. Mix well.
16. Centrifuge at 3400 rpm for 15 seconds.
17. Examine for agglutination using an optical aid.
18. Record results.
19. *Optional:* Add one drop of known sensitized red cells to all negative tests. Centrifuge and examine for agglutination; record results. If no agglutination is seen, the antiglobulin phase must be repeated.

The unit of blood can be considered safe for transfusion purposes if no hemolysis or agglutination is seen in any phase. It is extremely important not to ignore hemolysis, since this may indicate the presence of an antibody capable of binding complement and therefore of causing intravascular destruction of red cells.

Cold agglutinins may cause difficulty in the saline phase of this procedure. The two-tube crossmatch may resolve this difficulty.

The Two-Tube Crossmatch Procedure

1. Place two drops of the recipient's serum in each of two appropriately labeled 10 × 75 mm or 12 × 75 mm test tubes.
2. Add one drop of a 2 to 5 per cent saline suspension of red cells from the donor to each tube.
3. Incubate the first tube at room temperature for 15 to 30 minutes.
4. *Optional:* add 2 to 3 drops of 22 to 30 per cent bovine albumin to the second tube and mix. Incubate the second tube at 37° C for 15 to 30 minutes.
5. Centrifuge both tubes at 3400 rpm for 15 seconds. This should be done as soon as the second tube is removed from the incubator.
6. Examine each tube for hemolysis and for agglutination with an optical aid (see under the heading Reading and Interpretation).
7. Record results and discard the first tube.
8. Wash the red cells in the second tube three or four times in large amounts of normal saline. Decant as completely as possible after each wash.
9. Add one to two drops of antiglobulin serum.
10. Mix well.
11. Centrifuge at 3400 rpm for 15 seconds.
12. Examine for agglutination using an optical aid.
13. Record results.
14. *Optional:* Add one drop of known sensitized red cells to all negative tests. Centrifuge and examine for agglutination; record results. If no agglutination is seen, the antiglobulin phase must be repeated.

Reading and Interpretation

As soon as centrifugation is complete, the contents of the tube(s) should be examined for hemolysis. The appearance of free hemoglobin that was not present in the original sample must be interpreted as a positive reaction. Hemolysis can easily be observed against a white light or white background.

Technique for Resuspending the Cell Button
1. Hold the test tube at a sharp angle in such a way that the fluid, moving across the cell button, assists in dislodging the red cells.
2. Shake the tube *very gently* until all the red cells have been dislodged from the wall of the tube.
3. Tilt the tube back and forth to obtain an even suspension of cells or agglutinates.

Precautions
1. Never read more than one tube at a time.
2. Take care not to overshake or undershake. Overshaking can break up fragile agglutinates. Undershaking may give the appearance of a positive reaction.
3. Use a consistent light source with an optical aid.
4. Check all negative reactions microscopically. A microscope can also be useful in distinguishing rouleaux formation (Chapter 24) from true agglutination.

All reactions should be graded as described in Chapter 2 of this text.

Interpretation
The crossmatch should be considered compatible only if no agglutination or hemolysis is seen in any phase of the test. If incompatibility is seen in an early phase of the crossmatch, the testing should be completed to provide information as to the temperature and media when these reactions occur, variability of these reactions and in some cases the approximate percentage of compatible donors. This information will assist in choosing the correct conditions for identification of the antibody or antibodies (see Chapter 22).

Notes on the Crossmatch Procedure

1. A clotted specimen (one taken into a tube without anticoagulant) should always be used for crossmatching. It should contain fresh, not inactivated, serum less than 48 hours old. Do not attempt to crossmatch with a specimen containing anticoagulant, since the action of

fibrinogen in the plasma may cause spontaneous fibrin clots to form that may interfere with the test. Note also that anticoagulants are *anti-complementary*, which may prevent the detection of certain complement-binding antibodies. In the clotted specimen, a good firm clot should be formed before crossmatching is undertaken. Centrifugation of the specimen will help in this respect.

2. In performing ABO grouping on the patient, bear in mind the causes of anomalous results — in particular, leukemia, hypogammaglobulinemia (see Chapter 3).

3. Check the donor units macroscopically. Clots in the unit that could be due to inadequate mixing of anticoagulant when the unit was collected, while serologically insignificant, can often cause clogging of the administration set.

4. Since autoantibodies are a common source of difficulty in routine crossmatching, an *autocontrol* should be set up in parallel with the crossmatch through all phases. This autocontrol consists of the addition of the recipient's red cells to his or her own red cells.

5. When a series of transfusions are to be given over a period of several days, a new sample of the recipient's blood, obtained within 48 hours of the next scheduled transfusion, should be used to ensure that antibodies that may appear in the recipient's circulation in response to blood previously transfused will be detected. If there is an interval of 48 hours between transfusions, donor blood previously crossmatched must be *recrossmatched* with a new recipient specimen before transfusion.

6. Hemolyzed recipient samples should not be used, since they may mask hemolysis of donor red cells.

7. Red cells suspended in serum should not be used if the serum contains autoagglutinins, cold agglutinins or abnormal proteins, which cause rouleaux formation (Chapter 24).

The Emergency Crossmatch

In certain instances, blood may be required more rapidly than the standard crossmatch will allow. In cases such as these, the patient's physician must weigh the risk of transfusing uncrossmatched or incompletely crossmatched blood against the consequences of waiting for routine crossmatch tests to be completed.

The following is recommended:

1. Requests for compatibility tests labeled "stat" or "emergency" must take precedence over all other work in the laboratory.

2. The attending physician should indicate the urgent nature of the situation, and, if un-crossmatched or incompletely crossmatched blood is required, should be made aware of the inherent risks involved.

3. Group-specific and type-specific blood should be given whenever possible.

4. Begin the routine crossmatch and continue even if the blood is released. The use of low ionic-strength solution as a suspending medium will allow the safe reduction of incubation time.

5. If incompatibility is detected in any phase of the crossmatch, immediately notify the patient's physician and the blood bank physician.

MASSIVE TRANSFUSION

The rapid infusion of blood in amounts approaching or exceeding the recipient's total blood volume is known as massive transfusion. If such a transfusion is planned, a specimen of blood should be obtained well in advance and ABO, Rh, antibody detection and identification tests should be performed. (*Note:* If hypothermia is to be used, special care must be taken in the identification of antibodies detected at room temperature.) Ensure that sufficient serum less than 48 hours "old" is available for crossmatching. While interdonor compatibility testing is not required, donor units containing irregular antibodies should not be used. If additional units are required within a 48-hour period, the immediate pretransfusion sample may be used. At any time after that, a new sample must be obtained from the patient.

It should be noted that an antibody present in the original specimen may·be weak or undetectable in subsequent post-transfusion specimens because of the dilution effect of massive transfusion. It is essential that blood lacking the corresponding antigen be selected for transfusion by typing the units with commercial (reagent) antiserum before crossmatching.

If large amounts of citrated blood are given, signs of *citrate toxicity* are likely to develop when the blood is transfused at a rate of 1 liter in 10 minutes. These toxic effects can be minimized by giving calcium (e.g., 10 ml of 10 per cent calcium gluconate for every liter of citrated blood). When even higher rates of transfusion are used, larger amounts of calcium should be given (see Firt and Hejhal, 1957).

The problem of acidosis as a result of massive transfusion of ACD blood appears not to be of practical importance — at least not in healthy young subjects — because the base deficiency is rapidly corrected *in vivo*. When CPD rather than ACD is used, the problem of acidosis after massive transfusion is negligible.

CROSSMATCHING OF PATIENTS WITH COAGULATION ABNORMALITIES

Blood samples from patients with coagulation abnormalities may not be fully clotted when serum and cells are separated, which may result in the formation of a fibrin "web" and trapping of the red cells when the serum is incubated with donor red cells. This problem can often be solved by the addition of thrombin (50 units/ml) to the serum. Care should be taken not to add excess thrombin, since this may cause the nonspecific agglutination of all donor red cells. As an alternative, the addition of glass beads to the serum with subsequent gentle agitation will often aid in clot formation.

If anticoagulated specimens are used, the donor red cells must be well washed to ensure that there is no carryover of fibrinogen. The addition of one drop of protamine sulfate to samples of blood from *heparinized patients* will promote clotting but may also cause rouleaux, and in excess may also prolong clotting.

CROSSMATCHING OF PATIENTS AFTER INFUSION OF SYNTHETIC PLASMA EXPANDERS

When plasma expanders such as some dextrans or other large molecular weight plasma substitutes are used, crossmatching may be complicated by rouleaux formation. In cases such as these, the saline replacement technique can be used for crossmatching (see Chapter 23), and antiglobulin testing should be performed *without* the addition of high-protein media.

THE ISSUING OF BLOOD

When all crossmatching tests have been completed and the blood is found to be compatible, blood may be issued for transfusion. Before issue from the laboratory, however, all clerical details must be checked to ensure *absolute correlation* of information. The expiration date and appearance of the blood must also be checked just before the release of the unit.

The final identification of the recipient is the responsibility of the transfusionist.

The blood specimen from the recipient and a donor sample must be sealed or stoppered and retained at 2° C to 6° C for at least seven days following transfusion. The serum should be separated from the clot and stored at −20° C for the same period of time. After transfusion is complete, the empty blood bag should be returned to the blood bank within 24 hours, and should be retained at 2° C to 6° C for at least one week.

Blood should not be issued (or reissued) from the blood bank if it has been out of the refrigerator for more than 30 minutes.

TYPICAL EXAMINATION QUESTIONS

Select the phrase, sentence or symbol that completes the statement or answers the question. More than one answer may be correct in each case. Answers are given in the back of this book.

1. The so-called "minor" crossmatch is performed using
   (a) saline room temperature tests only
   (b) the antiglobulin test only
   (c) the patient's serum and the donor's red cells
   (d) the patient's red cells and the donor's serum
   (Introduction)

2. Saline techniques are designed to detect
   (a) IgM antibodies
   (b) IgG antibodies
   (c) IgA antibodies
   (d) major ABO grouping errors
   (Saline Techniques)

3. Albumin autoagglutinating factor is due to an antibody
   (a) directed against bovine albumin

   (b) directed against sodium caprylate
   (c) directed against fatty acid salts
   (d) none of the above
   (Albumin Techniques)

4. Enzyme techniques have the following limitations in routine crossmatching
   (a) they are insensitive
   (b) they are unable to detect certain antibodies in the MNSs and Duffy blood group systems
   (c) they detect a high incidence of "nonspecific" agglutinins
   (d) certain enzymes may become inactive if they are improperly stored
   (Enzyme Techniques)

5. The role of anti-complement in the antiglobulin reagent is to
   (a) detect complement-binding, clinically significant antibodies that may be missed by pure anti-IgG
   (b) enhance the reactions of complement-binding antibodies

(c) detect IgM antibodies, which invariably bind complement yet may elute off the red cells with increase in temperature, leaving complement components alone on the red cells

(d) none of the above

(Role of Anti-Complement in the Antiglobulin Reaction)

6. The indirect antiglobulin test is used to detect red cells that have been sensitized
   (a) *in vitro*
   (b) after elution tests have been performed
   (c) *in vivo*
   (d) with any IgM antibody
   (e) *in vitro* or *in vivo*

   (The Indirect Antiglobulin Test)

7. Under standard conditions, a positive antiglobulin test will be obtained when the test red cells are coated with
   (a) 10 to 20 antibody molecules per cell
   (b) 100 to 500 antibody molecules per cell
   (c) 1000 to 5000 antibody molecules per cell
   (d) 20 to 50 antibody molecules per cell

   (Discussion of the Various Phases of the Antiglobulin Test)

8. The optimum serum:red cell ratio for antibody detection that is within the realm of practical application has been reported to be
   (a) 80:1
   (b) 10:1
   (c) 500:1
   (d) 1:1

   (The Effect of the Serum:Red Cell Ratio)

9. A patient with septicemia
   (a) may have a false positive antiglobulin test
   (b) may have a false negative antiglobulin test
   (c) may have T-activated red cells
   (d) all of the above

   (Sources of Error)

10. Patients of group A with anti-HI(Anti-O) in their sera that is not inhibited by H substance should receive blood of group
    (a) A_2
    (b) O
    (c) A_2B
    (d) A_1

    (Selection of Blood for Transfusion — Routine Situations)

11. A unit of blood may be considered safe for transfusion purposes when the crossmatch tests

(a) show no agglutination or hemolysis in the antiglobulin test only

(b) show hemolysis but no agglutination in any of the tubes

(c) show incompatibility in every tube in all phases

(d) are free of hemolysis and agglutination in every tube in all phases

(Reading and Interpretation)

12. Blood may not be reissued from the blood bank if it has been out of the refrigerator for more than
    (a) 120 minutes
    (b) 5 minutes
    (c) 30 minutes
    (d) 6 hours

    (The Issuing of Blood)

ANSWER TRUE OR FALSE

13. Saline techniques are adequate as a sole test for compatibility.

    (Saline Technique)

14. The serologic characteristics of IgG anti-IgG and IgM anti-IgG are identical.

    (Preparation of Antiglobulin Reagent)

15. The enzyme-antiglobulin test is reported to be particularly suitable for the detection of anti-Jk^a.

    (Use of Enzyme-Treated Cells in the Antiglobulin Test)

16. Antiglobulin reagent should be added to the red cells in the antiglobulin test *immediately* following the completion of washing.

    (Discussion of the Various Phases of the Antiglobulin Test — Washing Phase)

17. Insufficient incubation time may result in a false positive antiglobulin test.

    (Sources of Error)

18. Crossmatch-compatible Rh-negative blood may be given to an Rh-positive recipient if Rh-positive blood is unavailable.

    (Selection of Blood for Transfusion)

19. When large amounts of citrated blood are given to a particular recipient, the problem of citrate toxicity can be minimized by the administration of calcium gluconate.

    (Massive Transfusion)

20. A positive direct antiglobulin test indicates *in vitro* cell sensitization.

    (The Direct Antiglobulin Test)

GENERAL REFERENCES

1. Issitt, P. D. and Issitt, C. H.: Applied Blood Group Serology, 2nd Ed. Spectra Biologicals, Oxnard, California, 1975. *(The student will find this book particularly useful in its discussion of the antiglobulin test.)*

2. Mollison, P. L.: Blood Transfusion in Clinical Medicine. 6th Ed. Blackwell Scientific Publications, Oxford, 1979. *(Excellent coverage of the subjects covered in this chapter.)*

3. Standards for Blood Banks and Transfusion Services, 8th Ed. American Association of Blood Banks, Washington, D.C., 1976.

4. Technical Manual of the American Association of Blood Banks, 7th Edition, AABB, Washington, D.C., 1977.

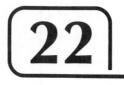

ANTIBODY IDENTIFICATION AND TITRATION

OBJECTIVES — ANTIBODY IDENTIFICATION AND TITRATION

The student will know, understand and be prepared to explain:

1. Methods of antibody detection using screening cells
2. Methods of antibody identification, specifically to include:
   (a) The use of red cell panels
   (b) The recognition of potentially useful information
   (c) Preliminary tests
      (1) Saline (room temperature and 15° C) panel, including choice of cells
      (2) Albumin (immediate spin, 37° C and antiglobulin test)
      (3) Enzyme-enhanced antiglobulin test
      (4) Antiglobulin test

3. The interpretation of results with respect to:
   (a) A single, specific antibody
   (b) A mixture of antibodies
   (c) Autoantibodies
4. The alternative techniques that can be used in antibody identification, specifically to include:
   (a) Absorption
   (b) Elution
   (c) Inhibition
   (d) Enhancement technique
   (e) Thiol reduction
   (f) Dissociation of bound IgG from red cells
5. Titration

Introduction

The detection of incompatibility in antibody detection (screening) tests or crossmatching presents a choice of two courses of action for the technologist: (1) to identify the antibody(ies) and select blood that lacks the corresponding antigen(s) for crossmatching and (2) to perform crossmatching using several other donor units in an attempt to find units that fail to react with the recipient serum. These units are then regarded as compatible and issued for transfusion.

The second course of action is much less desirable than the first and should be used only in cases of extreme emergency in which the provision of blood is the first priority. In following the first course of action (identification of the antibody or antibodies) a careful, planned methodology will reduce the waste of valuable serum and aid in the final solution to the problem.

Before starting an antibody identification procedure it is important to *complete the crossmatch*, in spite of the fact that the units may not

be used for transfusion, because knowledge of the *phases* at which incompatibility occurs can aid in solving the problem. In addition to this, it is often wise to repeat the crossmatch with the same donor(s) using a fresh specimen of blood from the patient. For reasons not yet understood, this often results in a compatible crossmatch. The incompatibility could have been the result of poor specimen procurement or contamination of the original specimen.

It should not be immediately presumed that incompatibility is due to the presence of antibody. Many different factors may cause red cell agglutination, such as overcentrifugation or contamination of serum or apparatus (see Chapter 21).

The identification of antibodies is rapidly becoming a complex and highly specialized field. The account given in this chapter is aimed at the routine laboratory worker, who will, no doubt, seek the advice of more experienced personnel when meeting a problem. As such, it covers only the most common types of reactions incurred. The interested student requiring more detailed coverage is referred to the list of general references at the end of this chapter.

THE DETECTION OF ANTIBODY

Commercial panels for antibody identification are usually accompanied by at least two separate "screening cells" for the detection of antibodies. These red cells (group O) contain as many common antigens as possible. Pooled reagent screening cells are *not* recommended for the detection of antibodies in patients, since weak antibodies may not be detected because all of the cells will probably not possess the same antigenic determinants.

Antibody detection red cells will, in most cases, not detect antibodies to low-frequency antigens because these antigens will probably not be found on detection cells. Antibodies of this type will therefore be detected only when an antibody identification procedure is performed because of the presence of *another* antibody in the serum, or when a crossmatch is found to be incompatible or if a newborn presents with or develops jaundice after delivery.

Antibody-detection (screening) cells should be set up in parallel with crossmatching procedures through all phases and with all other laboratory procedures in which it is important to detect the presence of irregular antibodies, such as in pre- and postnatal investigations. The screening cells' protocol is provided with the cells and should be closely examined whenever an irregular antibody is detected. It may, in some cases, serve as an aid in identification of the antibody.

An example of a typical screening cell protocol is given in Table 22–1.

ANTIBODY IDENTIFICATION

Panels

Antibody identification is performed using a "cell panel." These are commercially prepared, though they may be made up by the individual laboratory. They consist of a number of cells from different donors (usually eight to ten) of group O that have been carefully selected and tested for the presence or absence of most of the common antigens. Institutions that prefer to prepare their own panels can fully phenotype individuals on staff and bleed them regularly, or freeze large donations from these individuals in glycerol or liquid nitrogen.

Panels are commonly phenotyped for the following red cell antigens: D, C, E, c, e, f, C^w, V, K, k, Kp^a, Kp^b, Js^a, Js^b, Fy^a, Fy^b, Jk^a, Jk^b, Xg^a, Le^a, Le^b, S, s, M, N, P_1, Lu^a, Lu^b. Additional low-frequency and high-frequency antigens for which the cells have been typed and found to be all negative or all positive respectively are usually noted separately on the protocol. Any special typing that has been found is usually listed in line with the other reactions of the cell (shown in Table 22–2). Certain antigens (especially P_1) that show variation of antigenic strength are also so marked on most panel protocols.

An example of a typical "panel sheet" (or "protocol") is given in Table 22–2.

In general, a useful cell panel will include some red cells that possess as many as possible of the common antigenic determinants and some that lack these. The cells are chosen in such a manner that a distinct pattern of reactions is available for the easy identification of most "single" antibodies and of many "multiple" antibodies.

Special cells (those either possessing a low-frequency antigen or lacking a high-frequency antigen) can be stored frozen for future complicated identifications rather than being used in routine situations. In this way, laboratories can develop a library of unusual red cell specimens.

Commercial panel cells are usually suspended in modified Alsever's solution to a 3 to 6 per cent concentration and should be stored at 2 to 6° C when not in use. Care should be taken to avoid contamination of the cells with bacteria or with blood or serum. The dating period of the panel (date of expiration) should be respected. Toward the end of the dating period, the reactivity of some of the more labile antigens may be slightly diminished.

As with the crossmatch, no particular rules govern the performance of antibody identification. A routine format is usually set by each laboratory, which should, in general, duplicate the type of testing used in the crossmatch procedure. In difficult cases, additional tests (or techniques) often assist in reaching a conclusion, as do confirmation and exclusion panels.

The following procedure is offered for those students who are not exposed to practical investigation formats while in training.

Reviewing Potentially Useful Information

Before beginning an investigation, it is useful to review the following information:

Table 22–1   A TYPICAL "SCREENING CELLS" PROTOCOL

Donor No.	Genotype	D	C	E	c	e	f	C^w	K	k	Fy^a	Fy^b	Jk^a	Jk^b	Xg^a	Le^a	Le^b	S	s	M	N	P_1	Lu^a
1	$R_1{}^wR_1$	+	+	0	0	+	0	+	0	+	+	+	+	+	+	0	+	+	+	+	+	+	0
2	R_2r	+	0	+	+	+	+	0	+	+	0	+	0	+	+	+	0	+	+	+	0	+	0

Table 22–2   A TYPICAL PANEL SHEET OR PROTOCOL

Donor (Cell) No.	Rh/Hr Genotype	Rh/Hr							Kell		Duffy		Kidd		X-linked	Lewis		MNSs				P	Lutheran		Special Antigen Typing
		D	C	E	c	e	f	C^w	K	k	Fy^a	Fy^b	Jk^a	Jk^b	Xg^a	Le^a	Le^b	S	s	M	N	P_1	Lu^a	Lu^b	
1	R_1R_1	+	+	0	0	+	0	0	0	+	0	+	+	0	0	0	+	0	+	+	0	0	0	+	
2	$R_1{}^wR_1$	+	+	0	0	+	0	+	0	+	0	+	+	0	0	0	+	0	+	+	+	$+^s$	0	+	Bg(a+)
3	R_2R_2	+	0	+	+	0	0	0	0	+	0	+	0	+	+	0	0	+	0	0	+	+	0	+	Kp(a+)
4	R_0r	+	0	0	+	+	+	0	0	+	+	0	+	0	+	0	+	0	0	0	+	$+^s$	0	+	Sd(a+)
5	$r'r$	0	+	0	+	+	+	0	0	+	0	+	0	+	+	0	0	+	+	+	+	0	+	+	
6	$r''r$	0	0	+	+	+	+	0	+	+	0	0	+	+	+	0	+	0	+	+	+	+	0	+	Bg(a+),Wr(a+)
7	rr	0	0	0	+	+	+	0	0	+	+	0	+	0	0	+	0	0	+	+	+	$+^s$	0	+	
8	rr	0	0	0	+	+	+	0	+	+	+	0	0	+	+	0	+	0	+	+	+	+	0	+	Mg+,Co(b+)

1. Results of previous testing
2. History of transfusion or pregnancy
3. Diagnosis
4. Drug therapy (including Rh immune globulin)
5. Results of tests for whatever red cell antigens may appear to be pertinent (preferably performed on a pretransfusion specimen).

With respect to the results of previous testing, the following data may be particularly useful:

1. Effect of temperature
2. Effect of the suspending medium
3. Effect of enzyme treatment
4. Frequency of positive reactions with the red cells of random donors
5. Strength of positive reactions
6. Presence of hemolysis
7. Whether the antibodies appear to detect dosage

Preliminary Tests

Perform ABO forward and reverse grouping using anti-A, anti-B, Anti-A$_1$B, A$_1$ red cells and A$_2$ red cells (if indicated). If the patient is group A, perform A subtyping using anti-A$_1$. Also perform Rh phenotyping and a direct antiglobulin test.

These preliminary tests may provide the following information:

1. If the ABO reverse grouping shows irregular agglutination, a saline (IgM) antibody could be present.
2. If the patient belongs to a subgroup of A, anti-A$_1$ may be present. (This will be revealed in ABO reverse grouping if A$_1$ and A$_2$ red cells are used.)
3. If the direct antiglobulin test is positive, an autoagglutinin could be present. Note that a positive direct antiglobulin test is not *necessarily* indicative of autoagglutinins and may be caused by several other factors (see The Direct Antiglobulin Test, Chapter 21). (See also Chapter 15.)

Saline (Room Temperature) Panel

Purpose

To identify cold-reacting (IgM) alloagglutinins (e.g., −M−N, −Le^a, Le^b, −Lu^b) and autoagglutinins (e.g., −I, −IH, −H)

Selection of Cells

1. *If the patient is group O:* panel cells, patient's own cells for the autocontrol, two group O cord cells (one Rh+, one Rh−).

2. *If the patient is group A:* panel cells, patient's own cells for the autocontrol, one group A$_1$ (adult), one group A$_2$ (adult), two group O (cord) cells (one Rh+, one Rh−), one group A (cord) cells.

3. *If the patient is group B:* panel cells, patient's own cells for the autocontrol, one group B (adult), two group O (cord) cells (one Rh+, one Rh−), one group B (cord) cells.

4. *If the patient is group AB:* panel cells, patient's own cells for the autocontrol, one group A$_1$ (adult), one group A$_2$ (adult), one group B (adult), two group O (cord) cells (one Rh+, one Rh−), one group A (cord), one group B (cord).

Method

1. Set up the appropriate number of 10 × 75 mm test tubes required, based on the group requirements just outlined. Be sure that tubes are clearly labeled.
2. Add two drops of the patient's serum to each tube.
3. Add one drop of a washed (3 to 5 per cent) saline suspension of the appropriate red cells to each tube.
4. Incubate at room temperature for 30 to 60 minutes. *Note:* cold agglutinins are usually enhanced in their reactions by lowering the temperature to 15 to 18° C. This can be achieved by incubating the tubes in a pan of cold tap water to which a few ice cubes have been added.
5. Shake gently and read macroscopically. Record results.
6. Centrifuge at 3400 rpm (Serofuge) for 15 seconds. *Note:* This will usually be unnecessary if incubation has been for 60 minutes.
7. Shake gently and read macroscopically. Negative readings should be checked microscopically.
8. Grade all positive reactions (see Chapter 2) and record all results.

Note: If the 15 to 18° C temperature has been used, it should be maintained while reading. This can be achieved by eliminating the centrifugation step and reading each tube directly from the water bath.

Albumin (Immediate Spin, 37° C, Antiglobulin Test)

Purpose

To detect warm-reacting (IgG and complement binding IgG and IgM) alloantibodies and autoantibodies.

Note: This technique may be set up at the same time or during the incubation as the saline (room temperature) test.

Selection of Cells

All groups: panel cells and patient's own cells for the autocontrol.

Method (Eight-Cell Panel)

1. Set up nine 10 × 75 mm tubes in a test tube rack.
2. Label the tubes A1 to A8 and "autocontrol," respectively.
3. Place four to six drops of the patient's serum in each tube.
4. Add one drop of each appropriate panel cell to tubes A1 to A8.
5. Add one drop of a washed 3 to 5 per cent saline suspension of red cells from the patient to the "autocontrol."
6. Add 2 to 3 drops of 22 to 30 per cent bovine albumin to each tube.
7. Mix the contents of each tube well.
8. Centrifuge immediately at 3400 rpm (Serofuge) for 15 seconds.
9. Read macroscopically and record results. Results should be carefully graded.
10. After reading, mix the contents of each tube well.
11. Incubate all tubes at 37° C for 15 to 30 minutes in heat blocks or in a water bath.
12. Centrifuge immediately after incubation at 3400 rpm for 15 seconds.
13. Read macroscopically and record results. Results should be carefully graded.
14. After reading, mix the contents of each tube well.
15. Wash three times in large volumes of normal saline. Decant each wash as completely as possible.
16. Add one to two drops of antiglobulin reagent to each tube.
17. Mix well.
18. Centrifuge at 3400 rpm for 15 seconds.
19. Read macroscopically and record results. Negative reactions should be checked microscopically. Results should be carefully graded.
20. Interpret results as outlined below.

Enzyme-Enhanced Antiglobulin Test

Purpose

A back-up test for the detection of warm-reacting (IgG or complement-binding) alloantibodies and autoantibodies. This technique serves to enhance the reactions of certain Rh, Lewis, and Kidd antibodies.

Note: This technique may be set up in parallel with or during the incubation of the albumin-enhanced antiglobulin test.

Selection of Cells

All groups: panel cells, patient's own cells for the autocontrol.

Method (Eight-Cell Panel)

1. Enzyme-treat the panel cells and the patient's own cells as described in Chapter 23, depending on the enzyme of choice. Prepare a 3 to 5 per cent saline suspension of these cells.
2. Set up nine 10 × 75 mm tubes in a test tube rack.
3. Label the tubes EA1 to EA8 and "autocontrol," respectively.
4. Add two to four drops of the patient's serum to each tube.
5. Add one drop of the appropriate enzyme-treated panel cells to tubes EA1 to EA8.
6. Add one drop of a 3 to 5 per cent suspension of enzyme-treated patient's own cells to the autocontrol.
7. Incubate all tubes at 37° C for 15 to 30 minutes in heat blocks or in a water bath.
8. Centrifuge all tubes at 3400 rpm for 15 seconds.
9. Read macroscopically and record results. Results should be carefully graded.
10. Wash all cells three times in large volumes of normal saline. Decant each wash as completely as possible.
11. Add one to two drops of antiglobulin reagent to each tube.
12. Mix well.
13. Centrifuge at 3400 rpm for 15 seconds.
14. Read macroscopically and record results. Negative reactions should be checked microscopically. Results should be carefully graded.

INTERPRETATION OF RESULTS

In establishing the identity of an antibody, it is good practice to use a process of basic elimination, based on the *temperature(s)* at which the reactions occur, the *technique(s)* that give reactions and the *frequency* of the positive results obtained. For example, an antibody reacting strongly at 37° C and not at all at room temperature allows, in the majority of cases, for many cold-reacting antibodies (e.g., anti-P_1, anti-M, anti-N, anti-Le[a]) to be discounted. An antibody reacting with several donor units in the antiglobulin test would probably discount many antibodies directed against low-frequency antigens, unless they occur as part of an antibody mixture.

There are several clues to antibody identity provided by a routine work-up, and with experience, a technologist should be able to recognize these clues and use them to the best advantage. For example, an antibody reacting with approximately one in ten donor units *could* be anti-K, based on frequency statistics; an antibody that causes the hemolysis of the panel cells *could* be Lewis antibody. Knowing the racial origin of the patient is also often helpful, based on the frequency and specificity differences of particular antigens (or antibodies) within that race. In addition, a patient who has never been transfused or pregnant will probably possess a "non-red-cell-immune" (naturally occurring) antibody. This should be interpreted with caution because of the general unreliability of information regarding the transfusion and obstetric history of many patients.

In difficult interpretations, the possibility that the original tests are inaccurate should not be discounted. A set of results that defies identification can often be resolved by a fresh start with a new specimen from the patient.

The establishment of specificity of an antibody is often an arduous task. In this discussion, an attempt will be made to examine the most common possibilities and to present guidelines, through examples, toward accurate and reliable results.

The Single, Specific Antibody

Once the results of an investigation procedure are known and recorded, an attempt should be made to establish a *pattern of reactions* in accordance with those given on the panel sheet (see Example 1).

The test results in Example 1 exactly duplicate the reactions on the panel sheet for the Fy^a antigen. The antibody, therefore, reacts with all Fy^a-positive red cells and fails to react with all Fy^a-negative red cells. The specificity of the antibody therefore appears to be anti-Fy^a. The patient's red cells, tested with known (commercial) anti-Fy^a, show that the Fy^a antigen is not present (see Special Phenotype, Example 1). Note the negative reactions obtained in the enzyme antiglobulin test, which offers a further clue to identity (see Chapter 7).

It is important to realize that the results of the tests do not prove that anti-Fy^a is the only antibody present. All other possibilities must be excluded. For instance, in Example 1, anti-K or anti-Lu^a or both could be "masked" by the reaction. In addition, if the reactive cells possess any "special" antigens, the corresponding antibodies could also be present. The panel

given is the same as that given in Table 22–2, and by referring to that table, it can be seen that cell No. 6 is Wr (a+) and cell No. 8 is Mg+ and Co(b+). (*Note:* although cell No. 6 is also Bg(a+), the presence of this antibody can be discounted because cell No. 2, also Bg(a+), has failed to react.) The presence of anti-Lu^a in the sample is unlikely, because that antibody tends to react at low temperatures and the saline (RT) test shows no evidence of its presence. Anti-K, anti-Co^b, anti-Mg and anti-Wr^a may, of course, be present; however, this is unlikely, because one would expect some evidence of their presence in the enzyme antiglobulin test. Moreover, reactions are of constant strength, which also suggests the presence of a single antibody.

In order to prove or disprove the presence of these antibodies, so-called "exclusion" cells can be used, which lack the antigen corresponding to the primary antibody detected (in this case, anti-Fy^a) yet possess the antigens corresponding to the suspect antibodies. In this case, the following exclusion cells will be required:

1. Fy(a−), Lu(a+), Wr(a−), Mg−, K−, Co (b−) (To prove or disprove the presence of anti-Lu^a)

2. Fy(a−) Lu(a−), Wr(a+), Mg−, K−, Co(b−) (To prove or disprove the presence of anti-Wr^a)

3. Fy(a−), Lu(a−), Wr(a−), Mg+, K−, Co(b−) (To prove or disprove the presence of anti-Mg)

4. Fy(a−), Lu(a−), Wr(a−), Mg−, K+, Co(b+) (To prove or disprove the presence of anti-K)

5. Fy(a−), Lu(a−), Wr(a−), Mg−, K−, Co(b+) (To prove or disprove the presence of anti-Co^b)

If these cells are not available, an attempt can be made to *absorb* the anti-Fy^a from the patient's serum with Fy(a+), Lu(a−), Wr(a−) Mg−, K−, Co(b−) red cells, following which the investigation can be repeated using the absorbed serum. If no reaction is seen with the absorbed serum or if all "exclusion" cells give negative reactions, it can be concluded with some confidence that the serum contains specific anti-Fy^a.

DIFFICULT CASES

In some cases a specific set of reactions are observed that *do not* duplicate a pattern of reactions on the panel sheet. If this problem is encountered, several possibilities should be investigated.

PANEL SHEET

Example 1

Cell No.	D	C	E	c	e	f	Cw	K	k	Fya	Fyb	Jka	Jkb	Xga	Lea	Leb	S	s	M	N	P1	Lua	Lub
1	+	+	0	0	+	0	0	0	+	0	+	+	0	0	+	0	0	+	+	0	0	0	+
2	+	+	0	0	+	0	+	0	+	0	+	+	0	+	0	+	0	+	+	+	+s	0	+
3	+	0	+	+	0	0	0	0	+	0	+	0	+	+	0	0	+	0	+	0	+s	0	+
4	+	0	0	+	+	+	0	0	+	0	+	+	0	+	0	+	0	0	0	+	+s	0	+
5	0	+	0	0	+	0	0	+	+	+	0	+	+	+	+	0	+	+	+	+	0	+	+
6	0	0	+	+	+	+	0	0	+	+	0	0	+	+	0	0	0	+	+	+	+	0	+
7	0	0	0	+	+	+	0	+	0	+	+	0	+	0	+	0	0	+	+	+	+s	0	+
8	0	0	0	+	+	+	0	0	+	0	0	+	+	+	+	0	+	+	+	+	+	+	0

TEST RESULTS

ABO ___O___ $Rh_o(D)$ ___Positive___

Rh phenotype ___$CDe(R_1R_1)$___

Direct antiglobulin test ___Negative___

Specific phenotype ___Fy(a − b+)___

Cell No.	Saline (RT)	Albumin (IS)	Albumin 37° C	Albumin (AHG)	Enzyme (AHG)
1	0	0	0	0	0
2	0	0	0	0	0
3	0	0	0	0	0
4	0	0	0	0	0
5	0	2+	3+	3+	0
6	0	2+	3+	3+	0
7	0	2+	3+	3+	0
8	0	2+	3+	3+	0
Auto-control	0	0	0	0	0

SPECIFICITY ___Anti-Fya (See text)___

Example 2

PANEL SHEET

Cell No.	D	C	E	c	e	f	Cʷ	K	k	Fyᵃ	Fyᵇ	Jkᵃ	Jkᵇ	Xgᵃ	Leᵃ	Leᵇ	S	s	M	N	P₁	Luᵃ	Luᵇ
1	+	+	0	0	+	0	0	0	+	0	+	+	0	0	+	0	0	+	+	0	0	0	+
2	+	+	0	0	+	0	+	0	+	0	+	+	0	+	0	+	0	+	+	+	+ˢ	0	+
3	+	0	+	+	0	0	0	0	+	0	+	0	+	+	0	0	+	0	+	0	+	0	+
4	+	0	0	+	+	+	0	0	+	0	+	+	0	+	0	+	0	0	0	+	+ˢ	0	+
5	0	+	0	0	+	0	0	+	+	+	0	+	+	+	0	0	+	+	+	+	0	+	+
6	0	0	+	+	+	+	0	0	+	+	0	0	+	+	+	0	0	+	+	+	+	0	+
7	0	0	0	+	+	+	0	+	0	+	+	0	+	0	0	+	0	+	+	+	+ˢ	0	+
8	0	0	0	+	+	+	0	0	+	+	0	+	+	+	+	0	+	+	+	+	+	+	0

TEST RESULTS

ABO ___O___ Rhₒ(D) ___Negative___

Rh phenotype ___cde(rr)___

Direct antiglobulin test ___Negative___

Specific phenotype ___M − N+___

Cell No.	Saline (RT)	Albumin (IS)	Albumin 37° C	Albumin (AHG)	Enzyme (AHG)
1	3+	0	0	0	0
2	0	0	0	0	0
3	3+	0	0	0	0
4	0	0	0	0	0
5	0	0	0	0	0
6	0	0	0	0	0
7	0	0	0	0	0
8	0	0	0	0	0
Auto-control	0	0	0	0	0

SPECIFICITY ___Anti-M (showing "dosage")___

PANEL SHEET

Example 3

Cell No.	D	C	E	c	e	f	Cw	K	k	Fya	Fyb	Jka	Jkb	Xga	Lea	Leb	S	s	M	N	P1	Lua	Lub
1	+	+	0	0	+	0	0	0	+	0	+	+	0	0	+	0	0	+	+	0	0	0	+
2	+	+	0	0	+	0	+	0	+	0	+	+	0	+	0	+	0	+	+	+	+s	0	+
3	+	0	+	+	0	0	0	0	+	0	+	0	+	+	0	0	+	0	+	0	0	0	+
4	+	0	0	+	+	+	0	0	+	0	+	+	0	+	0	+	0	0	0	+	+s	0	+
5	0	+	0	0	+	0	0	+	+	+	0	+	+	+	0	0	+	+	+	+	0	+	+
6	0	0	+	+	+	+	0	0	+	+	0	0	+	+	+	0	0	+	+	+	+	0	+
7	0	0	0	+	+	+	0	+	0	+	+	0	+	0	0	+	0	+	+	+	+s	0	+
8	0	0	0	+	+	+	0	0	+	0	0	+	+	+	+	0	+	+	+	+	+	+	0

TEST RESULTS

ABO ___A___ Rho(D) ___Positive___

Rh phenotype ___CDe(R1R1)___

Direct antiglobulin test ___Negative___

Specific phenotype ___P1-negative___

Cell No.	Saline (RT)	Albumin (IS)	Albumin (AHG)	Albumin 37° C	Albumin (AHG)	Enzyme (AHG)
1	0	0	0	0	0	0
2	2+	0	0	0	0	0
3	0	0	0	0	0	0
4	2+	0	0	0	0	0
5	0	0	0	0	0	0
6	0	0	0	0	0	0
7	2+	0	0	0	0	0
8	0	0	0	0	0	0
Auto-control	0	0	0	0	0	0

SPECIFICITY Anti-P1 (reacting with cells possessing strong P1 antigen only)

1. *A mixture of antibodies.*

2. *Dosage effect.* Certain antibodies show reactions with red cells possessing the corresponding antigen in *double dose* only (i.e., when the causative gene is present in the homozygous state). Also, some antibodies react more strongly with "homozygous" than with "heterozygous" cells. Example 2 shows an anti-M antibody reacting in this fashion. Homozygous *MM* cells (possessing the M antigen in double dose) are reacting, whereas heterozygous *MN* cells (possessing the M antigen in single dose) are not.

3. *Variation in antigenic strength.* Certain antigens (e.g., P_1, Le^a, Le^b, Vel, Chido) have great variation of strength from one individual to another. Example 3 shows an anti-P_1 reacting in this fashion: only P_1+^s (strong) cells show reaction — other P_1+ red cells fail to react.

4. *Weak antibody.* Establishing the specificity of an antibody is difficult unless the reactions obtained are in the 1+ range or stronger. Weak antibodies will often cause confusion and may defy accurate identification. Such antibodies may increase in strength in certain circumstances, either because the antibody, when tested, is in the process of development, or because of continued stimulation such as in pregnancy. It is worth testing a later sample in these cases before reaching a conclusion regarding specificity.

5. *Contamination.* Apparent specificity may result from contamination of panel cells or patient's serum. This can be considered possible if only one cell on a panel shows a positive result. If the patient's serum is contaminated, all panel cells will probably give positive reactions. That particular cell should be examined against various other sera that are known *not* to contain irregular antibodies to determine if it is reacting nonspecifically with all sera.

6. *An antibody not represented by an antigen on the panel cells in use.* A rare antibody not represented by an antigen on the particular panel cells in use may be the cause of the problem. This can sometimes be established with the use of a different panel that has been more extensively phenotyped, if available. In cases in which specificity cannot be established, the patient's specimen may be referred to another laboratory specializing in this sort of investigation and that would therefore possess large and comprehensive exclusion panels.

7. *A new antigen-antibody system.* This is an exciting but rather remote possibility. The establishment of a new blood group system is a complicated research project and as such is beyond the scope of this book.

A Mixture of Antibodies

The identification of antibody "mixtures" often constitutes a difficult and complex serologic undertaking. Yet the occurrence of such mixtures is not uncommon, since individuals who produce antibodies to one antigenic stimulus quite often readily produce others.

The suggestion that a mixture of antibodies is present in a serum sample may be indicated by any or all of several situations.

1. *A varying distribution of positive and negative reactions at different temperatures.* This phenomenon indicates a possible mixture of warm and cold-reacting antibodies (Example 4). In Example 4, both anti-K and anti-P_1 are detectable — the anti-K reacting only in the indirect antiglobulin test and the anti-P_1 reacting only in the saline (room temperature) test.

This type of mixture is often relatively simple to identify, provided that there is no carry-over of reactions through a wide thermal range. For instance, in the example given, both anti-K and anti-P_1 could show reactions in both the saline (room temperature) and the antiglobulin techniques. Confirmation of results, if this was the case, could be achieved by confining the room temperature tests to red cell samples that are K-negative. The same basic rule applies if the anti-P_1 is active at 37° C.

2. *A varying distribution of positive and negative results in different techniques.* Certain antibodies react preferentially in certain techniques; for example, anti-Fy^a, which reacts in the indirect antiglobulin technique, yet fails to react with enzyme-treated red cells. The presence of a second antibody reactive in enzyme techniques or in saline (room temperature) techniques would not be influenced by the reaction of the anti-Fy^a. Any such mixture is usually simple to identify, even if both antibodies react within the same thermal range (see Example 5).

3. *Varying strengths of reactions in the same technique in which "dosage" is not evident.* A serum containing anti-M and anti-Lu^a, for example, cannot be differentiated by using different techniques or temperatures, since both are *cold agglutinins* and commonly react in saline at or below room temperature. In cases such as this, noting the antigens on the red cells (if any) that *fail to react* can aid in the identification of the components of the mixture (that is,

PANEL SHEET

Example 4

Cell No.	D	C	E	c	e	f	Cw	K	k	Fya	Fyb	Jka	Jkb	Xga	Lea	Leb	S	s	M	N	P1	Lua	Lub
1	+	+	0	0	+	0	0	0	+	0	+	+	0	0	+	0	0	+	+	0	0	0	+
2	+	+	0	0	+	0	+	0	+	0	+	+	0	+	0	+	0	+	+	+	+s	0	+
3	+	0	+	+	0	0	0	0	+	0	+	0	+	+	0	0	+	0	+	0	+	0	+
4	+	0	0	0	+	+	0	0	+	0	+	+	0	+	0	+	0	0	0	+	+s	0	+
5	0	+	0	+	+	0	0	+	+	+	0	+	+	+	0	0	+	+	+	+	0	+	+
6	0	0	+	+	+	+	0	0	0	+	0	0	+	+	+	0	0	+	+	+	+	0	+
7	0	0	0	+	+	+	0	+	+	+	+	0	+	0	0	+	0	+	+	+	+s	0	+
8	0	0	0	+	+	+	0	0	+	+	0	+	+	+	+	0	+	+	+	+	+	+	0

TEST RESULTS

ABO __B__   Rho(D) __Negative__

Rh phenotype __cde(rr)__

Direct antiglobulin test __Negative__

Specific phenotype __K−, P1−__

Cell No.	Saline (RT)	Albumin (IS)	Albumin 37° C	Albumin (AHG)	Enzyme (AHG)
1	0	0	0	0	0
2	3+	0	0	0	0
3	1+	0	0	0	0
4	3+	0	0	0	0
5	0	0	1+	3+	2+
6	1+	0	0	0	0
7	3+	0	1+	3+	2+
8	1+	0	0	0	0
Auto-control	0	0	0	0	0

SPECIFICITY __Anti-P1 + Anti-K__

PANEL SHEET

Example 5

Cell No.	D	C	E	c	e	f	Cw	K	k	Fya	Fyb	Jka	Jkb	Xga	Lea	Leb	S	s	M	N	P1	Lua	Lub
1	+	+	0	0	+	0	0	0	+	0	+	+	0	0	+	0	0	+	+	0	0	0	+
2	+	+	0	0	+	0	+	0	+	0	+	+	0	+	0	+	0	+	+	+	+s	0	+
3	+	0	+	+	0	0	0	0	+	0	+	0	+	+	0	0	+	0	+	0	+	0	+
4	+	0	0	+	+	+	0	0	+	0	+	+	0	+	0	+	0	0	0	+	+s	0	+
5	0	+	0	0	+	0	0	+	+	+	0	+	+	+	0	0	+	+	+	+	0	+	+
6	0	0	+	+	+	+	0	0	+	+	0	0	+	+	+	0	0	+	+	+	+	0	+
7	0	0	0	+	+	+	0	+	0	+	+	0	+	0	0	+	0	+	+	+	+s	0	+
8	0	0	0	+	+	+	0	0	+	+	0	+	+	+	+	0	+	+	+	+	+	+	0

TEST RESULTS

ABO   __A__ $Rh_o(D)$ __Positive__

Rh phenotype   __cDEe(R_2r)__

Direct antiglobulin test   __Negative__

Specific phenotype   __Fy(a −), C −__

Cell No.	Saline (RT)	Albumin (IS)	Albumin 37° C	Albumin (AHG)	Enzyme (AHG)
1	0	0	0	0	4+
2	0	0	0	0	4+
3	0	0	0	0	0
4	0	0	0	0	0
5	0	0	0	4+	4+
6	0	0	0	4+	0
7	0	0	0	4+	0
8	0	0	0	4+	0
Auto-control	0	0	0	0	0

SPECIFICITY   __Anti-Fya + Anti-C (enzyme only)__

Example 6

PANEL SHEET

Cell No.	D	C	E	c	e	f	C^w	K	k	Fy^a	Fy^b	Jk^a	Jk^b	Xg^a	Le^a	Le^b	S	s	M	N	P_1	Lu^a	Lu^b
1	+	+	0	0	+	0	0	0	+	0	+	+	0	0	+	0	0	+	+	0	0	0	+
2	+	+	0	0	+	0	+	0	+	0	+	+	0	+	0	+	0	+	+	+	+^s	0	+
3	+	0	+	+	0	0	0	0	+	0	+	0	+	+	0	0	+	0	+	0	+	0	+
4	+	0	0	0	+	+	0	0	+	0	0	+	0	+	0	+	0	0	0	+	+^s	0	+
5	0	+	0	0	+	0	0	0	+	0	0	+	+	+	0	0	0	+	+	+	0	+	+
6	0	0	+	+	+	+	0	+	+	+	+	0	+	0	0	+	0	+	+	+	+	0	+
7	0	0	0	+	+	+	0	+	0	+	0	0	+	+	+	0	0	+	+	+	+^s	0	+
8	0	0	0	+	+	+	0	0	+	+	0	+	+	+	+	0	+	+	+	+	+	+	0

TEST RESULTS

ABO ___O___ Rh_o(D) ___Negative___

Rh phenotype ___cde(rr)___

Direct antiglobulin test ___Negative___

Specific phenotype ___Lu(a−), M−___

Cell No.	Saline (RT)	Albumin (IS)	Albumin 37° C	Albumin (AHG)	Enzyme (AHG)
1	2+	0	0	0	0
2	1+	0	0	0	0
3	2+	0	0	0	0
4	(0)	0	0	0	0
5	(4+)	0	0	0	0
6	1+	0	0	0	0
7	1+	0	0	0	0
8	(4+)	0	0	0	0
Auto-control	0	0	0	0	0

Lu(a−), M−   Lu(a+), M+

SPECIFICITY ___Anti-M + Anti-Lu^a___

cells that are N-negative and Lu^a-negative) (see Example 6). Note that in Example 6 the only cells showing a negative reaction with the patient's serum are Lu(a−) and M−.

The same basic principle applies to mixtures of more than two antibodies, though in these cases, additional panels may be necessary. Isolating the cells that give the *strongest* reaction can also often give a clue to the identity of the antibodies present. In Example 6, cells No. 5 and No. 8 give 4+ reactions, whereas all other positive reactions are 2+. Cells No. 5 and No. 8 are positive for both Lu^a and M.

Identification of Difficult Mixtures

Complicated mixtures of antibodies can sometimes be identified with the use of titration, absorption and elution. These techniques are discussed later in this chapter.

1. *Titration.* Before titration methods are used as an aid in the identification of antibodies in a mixture, the possibility of dosage must first be ruled out, since this phenomenon can obviously cause titration variation. If dosage effect has been excluded, the titration of serum containing antibodies with various selected red cells can provide a clue to antibody specificity, because the components of a mixture are unlikely to react at equal strengths. In these cases, however, it is important that the particular specificity be *suspected*, since titration with random red cells will often be time-consuming and wasteful of the patient's serum. Titration is also used in the identification of HTLA antibodies (see later discussion).

2. *Absorption.* Absorption of an antibody in the serum under test may result in total separation of the components of the mixture. In cases such as these, all other possible combinations should be excluded before specificity is assigned.

3. *Elution.* If the red cells have absorbed antibody, elution often makes possible the separation of one antibody from a mixture of two or more. The major drawback of this type of elution is that often antibodies may be eluted and recovered together, particularly if they belong to the same blood group system.

AUTOANTIBODIES

Autoantibodies represent one of the most common and harassing problems encountered in blood banking. Whereas alloantibodies are characterized by the fact that they are produced by individuals whose red cells lack the corresponding antigen, autoantibodies are formed *in spite* of the existence of the corresponding antigen on the individual's red cells. Mention of autoantibodies has been made in Chapter 15 (Autoimmune Hemolytic Anemia); these may be attributed to certain disease states or to drug therapy.

Cold autoantibodies can react through a wide thermal range, though they are most commonly encountered in the saline phase at or below room temperature; that is, as "cold" agglutinins. Characteristically, these antibodies increase in strength as the temperature of the test is lowered. In some instances, however, the reactions may still be evident at 37° C owing to complement activity. (The problem can usually be solved with the use of the "Prewarming Technique," discussed later.) Since autoantibodies can be clinically significant if they are reactive over a wide thermal range, tests for such antibodies should always be performed through the temperature range 4 to 37° C.

Cold agglutinins most often have anti-I, anti-H or anti-IH specificity. In these cases all (adult) panel cells will give positive reactions. The identity of these antibodies can usually be established through the reactions of the patient's serum with his or her own red cells and with the selected A_1A_2, B adult and O cord cells as described in the saline (room temperature) technique. The method of interpreting these results is given in Table 22–3. An aid in the differentiation of anti-H and anti-IH is the fact that anti-H is inhibited (neutralized) by H secretor saliva, whereas anti-IH is not. It should also be noted that great variation of reaction strength may occur in the definition of anti-H, anti-I or anti-IH.

Note that even when specificity is established as anti-I, anti-H or anti-IH, it is possible that another antibody is being "masked" by the reaction. For this reason, the anti-I, anti-H or anti-IH should be absorbed with the patient's own red cells and the absorbed serum retested for the presence of antibodies.

For the most part, cold agglutinins appear to have no clinical significance in transfusion therapy. Reactions at 37° C (warm autoantibodies), however, may well cause the *in vivo* destruction of red cells (see Autoimmune Hemolytic Anemia, Chapter 15). Whenever possible, incompatible transfusions in these cases should be avoided.

Certain high-titered cold agglutinins react at temperatures above 22° C but usually show a negative direct antiglobulin test. Occasionally, reactions occur through the temperature range

Table 22–3 IDENTIFICATION OF ANTI-I, ANTI-H AND ANTI-IH

	Panel	Auto-control	0 (Adult)	A₁ (Adult)	A₂ (Adult)	B (Adult)	0 (Cord)	A (Cord)	B (Cord)
Anti-H									
1 Patient group A	4+	Neg (Mi)	4+	1+	3+	0	4+	2+	0
2 Patient group B	4+	Neg (Mi)	4+	0	0	1+	4+	0	1+
3 Patient group AB	4+	Neg (Mi)	4+	1+	3+	1+	4+	2+	1+
Anti-I (all groups)	4+*	3+†	4+	4+	4+	4+	Neg‡	Neg‡	Neg‡
Anti-IH									
1 Patient group A	4+	1+ or neg	4+	2+	4+	0	1+	Wk (Mi)	Wk (Mi)
2 Patient group B	4+	1+ or neg	4+	0	0	2+	1+	Wk (Mi)	Wk (Mi)
3 Patient group AB	4+ₚ	1+ or neg	4+	1+	3+	2+	1+	Wk (Mi)	Wk (Mi)

*Variation of antigen strength may cause varying reactions in the panel.

†This reaction may be weaker than 3+ in some cases and even negative. This is caused by the fact that the antigen receptors are "blocked" with antibody, and none is available to proceed to the second stage of agglutination.

‡With a powerful anti-I, these reactions may be positive, and dilution or titration may be necessary to demonstrate weaker reactions with cord cells than with adult cells.

0 = Test not performed.

4° C to 37° C. This can be caused by the action of complement, which binds quickly to the red cells at low temperatures and remains bound to the red cells as the temperature of the test is raised, even though the causative IgM antibody elutes from the cells with increase in temperature. This is sometimes referred to as complement "carry-over."

In order to demonstrate that reactions seen at 37° C are due to the activation of complement in this way, the following *prewarming technique* is recommended. Blood from the patient is collected into a *warm* (37° C) container, transported to the laboratory immersed in warm water and transferred directly into a heated centrifuge. All reagents used in the test (including saline) are "prewarmed" to 37° C and this temperature is maintained *throughout the test*. Performing the test in this way will not permit the binding of the cold antibody to the red cells — and therefore complement will also not be bound. If it is necessary to harvest serum from a sample of blood that has been allowed to clot at room temperature or lower, the sample should be warmed at 37° C for at least one hour before the serum is separated.

Other Autoantibodies

The agglutination of all panel cells as well as the patient's own cells in bovine albumin or when enzyme-treated cells are used may be caused by *albumin autoagglutinating factor* (Chapter 19) or by *enzyme autoagglutinating factor*, respectively. With respect to enzyme autoagglutinating factor, specificity can occasionally be established (most often anti-I). However, many examples have no apparent specificity. Like albumin-autoagglutinating factor, the phenomenon appears to have no clinical significance.

Moreover, certain sera give the appearance of agglutination without apparent specificity or cause. The reason for this is not clear.

Positive Reactions With all Panel Cells — Autocontrol Negative

This type of reaction can be caused by any of five situations:

1. *A mixture of antibodies.* Resolution of the problem may require additional cells that are more fully phenotyped or a more comprehensive red cell panel.

2. *An antibody corresponding to an antigen of high frequency.* If the reaction occurs in the cold, anti-I, anti-H or anti-IH may again be suspected and tested for as just described. Other high-frequency (public) antigens include K2(k), K4(Kpᵇ), Vel, and Luᵇ. If the corresponding antisera is available, the patient's cells may be tested for the presence or absence of these

Example 7

	Patient's Serum
Ch(a−)	1+
Rg(a−)	1+
Cs(a−)	1+
Yk(a−)	0
Gy(a−)	1+
Hy(a−)	1+
Kn(a−)	1+
McC^a(−)	1+
JMH(−)	1+
Yt(a−)	1+

SPECIFICITY Anti-Yk^a

antigens. This could provide a valuable clue to the identity of the antibody. Alternatively, a panel of cells that lack certain high-frequency antigens can be tested against the patient's serum. Anti-Le^a and anti-Le^b occurring together can also cause the phenomenon if no Le(a−b−) cells are present on the panel.

3. *An antibody that reacts preferentially with group O cells.* An example is anti-H.

4. *Anti-Sd^a.* If the reactions are extremely weak in saline at room temperature, giving a "mixed-field" appearance when observed microscopically, anti-Sd^a may be suspected. This is a relatively common antibody. Anti-Sd^a shows different strengths of reaction with different cells, but the difference tends to be in the *number* of agglutinates, rather than in their *size*. The agglutination is quite distinctive and, once seen, will never be forgotten or mistaken for something else. The individual agglutinates look almost spherical, which is unusual, and will stand up to washing in saline. Suspect sera should be incubated at 16° C, washed three times in saline, then placed on a slide and reincubated in a moist chamber (*Note:* a 20 per cent saline cell suspension should be used.) The slides may be read after 30 minutes.

5. *A high titer–low avidity (HTLA) antibody.* Antibodies that fall into this category include Ch^a(Chido), Rg^a(Rogers), Cs^{a}Cost/Sterling), Yk^a(York), Gy^a(Gregory), Hy(Holly), Kn^a(Knops), McC^a(McCoy), JMH(JM Hagen) and Yt^a(Cartwright). Since all of these antigens occur with high frequency, weak positive reactions are usually seen with all cells (excluding the patient's own cells) in the indirect antiglobulin test with weakened or negative reactions with enzyme-treated cells. Suspect sera can be titrated using the panel cells that give the strongest reaction. If a high titration score results, the

antibody can usually be identified using a panel of cells that are negative for these antigens, if available (see Example 7). Since Ch^a and Rg^a substances are present in the serum of individuals possessing these antigens, neutralization (inhibition) tests can be useful in the identification of these antibodies (see Crookston, 1975).

Negative Reactions With all Panel Cells — Autocontrol Positive

This sort of reaction will be seen when all free antibody in the patient's serum has been taken up by his own cells. The phenomenon can also involve drug-related antibodies. Identification involves the elution of the antibody from the patient's cells, followed by routine antibody identification procedures using the eluate.

Negative Reactions Throughout

This type of finding may, of course, suggest the absence of irregular antibodies in the patient's serum. The following possibilities, however, should first be considered:

1. Faulty or poorly selected technique
2. Antibody inactivation or neutralization
3. An antibody not directed against group O red cells (e.g. anti-A$_1$)
4. Inactivated anti-complement activity in the antiglobulin reagent used.
5. An antibody directed against a low-frequency antigen not represented on the panel

In cases such as these, the serum should be retested by the method with which the antibody was first detected, and a fresh specimen of blood should be collected from the patient for repeat testing. A more comprehensive cell panel should be used, if available, and a fresh bottle of antiglobulin reagent (see under the heading Alternative Techniques in Antibody Identification).

ALTERNATIVE TECHNIQUES IN ANTIBODY IDENTIFICATION

In cases in which the identity of an antibody or antibodies in a patient's serum cannot be established using the techniques described, certain alternative procedures can be used, chosen according to the type of problem encountered. These procedures will be briefly described, with emphasis on their application to antibody identification. Specific techniques and a brief discussion of their other applications are given in Chapter 23 of this text.

Absorption. In antibody identification, absorption can be used for the removal of cold or warm autoantibody activity to permit the evaluation of a coexisting ("masked") alloantibody, or for the separation of mixed antibodies in serum or eluate. It should be noted that if the patient has been transfused within the previous two to three months, the procedure should be used with caution, since alloantibody may be removed in addition to autoantibody.

Elution. In antibody identification, elution can be used for the following purposes:

1. To identify the antibody on an infant's red cells in hemolytic disease of the newborn.

2. To identify the antibody producing a positive direct antiglobulin test in acquired hemolytic anemia or in suspected transfusion reactions.

3. To produce a small amount of useful single-antibody preparations after the separation of a mixture of antibodies by absorption.

4. To remove antibody from the patient's red cells so that they can be used for autoabsorption, or to render them suitable for further testing.

5. To demonstrate that cells have adsorbed on antibody and therefore that they possess the corresponding antigen.

Inhibition (Neutralization). Inhibition (neutralization) techniques can be useful as a means of identifying certain antibodies (such as Sd[a], Ch[a], and Rg[a]) and for the removal of certain antibodies from the serum, enabling the identification of coexisting antibodies. The procedure is, of course, limited by the fact that it can be used only when the appropriate blood group substance *exists*. In practice, therefore, the procedure is limited to work involving the following antibodies: anti-A, anti-B (substances obtainable from human secretor saliva, cyst fluids, animal blood), anti-P[1] (substance from hydatid cyst fluid), anti-Le[a], anti-Le[b] (substances from human secretor saliva, acacia), anti-Ch[a], anti-Rg[a] (substances from human serum), anti-Sd[a] (substance from human urine) and anti-I (substance from human milk).

Enhancement Techniques. In antibody identification, weak antibodies, or those that may not be demonstrable by routine techniques, can often be enhanced in their reactions by using alternative suspending media such as

enzymes and low ionic-strength solution. Enhancement is also achieved by concentration of the serum (see The Concentration of Serum-Containing Antibody, Chapter 23) or in the case of anti-M by modification of the pH of the suspending medium (see Chapter 23).

Thiol Reduction of IgM Antibodies (2-ME, Dithiothreitol). The technique of splitting I9S IgM molecules into 7S subunits using 2-mercaptoethanol or dithiothreitol can be used in antibody identification to inactivate an IgM antibody in a mixture of IgG and IgM antibodies.

Dissociation of Bound IgG From the Red Cells (ZZAP). A reagent known as ZZAP, containing 0.1 per cent papain and 0.1M dithiothreitol, has been reported to dissociate IgG from red blood cells (Branch and Petz, 1980). The reagent has no effect on Rh and Kidd antigens, but destroys Duffy, MNS and Kell antigens. In antibody identification, this could prove useful in cases involving multiple alloantibodies. ZZAP is also useful in cell typing of patients with a positive direct antiglobulin test owing to IgG sensitization.

TITRATION

Titration can be defined as a semiquantitative means of measuring the amount of antibody in a serum. A titer, therefore, refers to the strength of an antibody, measured by determining the greatest dilution of antibody-containing serum that will produce a detectable reaction with a standard volume of red cells possessing the corresponding antigen.

Titration is most often used to demonstrate an increase in the strength of a maternal antibody during pregnancy as an indication of the possible severity of hemolytic disease of the newborn. However, it is most useful when comparing a particular serum against several cell samples to clarify differences in strength between alloactive and autoactive antibodies in a serum as, for example, between cord and adult red cells in the identification of anti-I, or in the search for "least incompatible" units when crossmatching difficulties are encountered.

In fact, the results of a titration offer only a very approximate indication of antibody strength, since only the amount of antibody *actually* taken up by the red cells is estimated — free antibody (that which is not taken up by the cells) is not taken into account.

Techniques for single titration and for master dilution are given in Chapter 23.

TYPICAL EXAMINATION QUESTIONS

Select the phrase, sentence or symbol that completes the statement or answers the question. More than one answer may be acceptable in each case. Answers are given in the back of this book.

1. Antibody detection cells will, in most cases, not detect antibodies to
   (a) high-frequency antigens
   (b) low-frequency antigens
   (c) enzyme-reactive antibodies
   (d) saline-reactive antibodies
   (The Detection of Antibody)

2. When not in use, panel cells should be stored at
   (a) room temperature
   (b) 2 to 6° C
   (c) 37° C
   (d) frozen
   (Panels)

3. Anti-A$_1$ in a patient's serum will be revealed with the use of
   (a) panel cells
   (b) *Dolichos biflorus* lectin
   (c) absorbed anti-A$_1$
   (d) A$_1$ and A$_2$ red cells
   (Preliminary Tests)

4. If a pattern of reactions is observed in the investigation of an antibody that does not duplicate a pattern of reactions on the panel sheet, which of the following could be the cause?
   (a) contamination
   (b) a mixture of antibodies
   (c) a new antigen-antibody system
   (d) none of the above
   (The Single, Specific Antibody)

5. If positive reactions are obtained with a serum specimen against all panel cells, but not with the patient's own red cells, the cause could be
   (a) a mixture of antibodies
   (b) an antibody to an antigen of low frequency

   (c) anti-Jk^a
   (d) anti-Kn^a
   (Positive Reactions With all Panel Cells — Autocontrol Negative)

6. Which of the following HTLA antibodies can be identified using neutralization (inhibition) techniques?
   (a) anti-Kn^a
   (b) anti-Ch^a
   (c) anti-JMH
   (d) anti-Rg^a
   (Positive Reactions With all Panel Cells — Autocontrol Negative)

7. Weak antibodies can often be enhanced in their reactions by using
   (a) enzymes
   (b) saline
   (c) 2-ME
   (d) serum concentration techniques
   (Enhancement Techniques)

ANSWER TRUE OR FALSE

8. Titration gives a precise indication of antibody strength.
   (Titration)

9. Elution techniques can be used in the identification of antibody on an infant's red cells in hemolytic disease of the newborn.
   (Elution)

10. If negative reactions are obtained with an eight-cell panel when tested with a particular serum, this proves that no antibody is present in the serum.
    (Negative Reactions Throughout)

11. Autoantibodies only react at or below room temperature.
    (Autoantibodies)

12. Antibody detection cells are of blood group O.
    (The Detection of Antibody)

GENERAL REFERENCES

1. Issitt, P. D. and Issitt, C. H.: Applied Blood Group Serology, 2nd Ed. Spectra Biologicals, 1975. *(Chapter 23 of this text is devoted to antibody detection and identification and crossmatching. The discussion is comprehensive, brief, easy to understand.)*

2. Mollison, P. L.: Blood Transfusion in Clinical Medicine. 6th Ed. Blackwell Scientific Publications, Oxford, 1979. *(Concise yet thorough coverage of antibody identification and titration. Extremely useful.)*

3. Standards for Blood Banks and Transfusion Services, 8th Ed. American Association of Blood Banks, Washington, D.C., 1976.

4. Technical Manual of the American Association of Blood Banks, 7th Ed. American Association of Blood Banks, Washington, D.C., 1977.

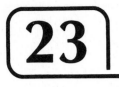

TECHNIQUES

Introduction

Knowledge of specific techniques is generally not an essential requirement for students of immunohematology. Techniques are included here to provide a reference for students in their practical training and to initiate the newcomer into the essential art of following a new procedure from a text without assistance. The application of these tests is largely the choice of each individual laboratory. Each will establish a priority, or place a particular importance on or favor one technique over another. For this reason, it must be stressed that the inclusion of a particular technique here does not in any way suggest that this is the only or for that matter the best technique available for the purpose.

The theory behind each test is not presented in this section, although the purpose and applications of each are. The student is advised to refer to the applicable chapter in doubtful cases. When using commercial antisera, it is always advised that the method recommended in the direction insert with the product be used, since this represents the technique in which the particular product has been found to give best results.

SECTION 1 ALBUMIN TECHNIQUES

Technique 1.1: Albumin Layering Technique

Purpose
For the detection of IgG antibodies, especially anti-Rh, that may be undetectable by other methods.

Method
1. **To a tube containing a dry button of red cells, add two drops of the test serum.**
2. **Mix well and incubate at 37° C for 15 to 30 minutes.**
3. **Centrifuge at 3400 rpm (Serofuge) for 15 seconds.**

4. **Without disturbing the red cell button, allow two drops of 30 per cent bovine albumin to run down the inside of the tube. Because the specific gravity of the albumin is greater than that of the cell-serum mixture, the albumin will settle as a layer on the top of the cell button.**
5. **Without mixing, return the tube to 37° C incubation for a further 15 minutes.**
6. **Shake gently to resuspend the red cells or pipette the button of red cells, spread on a slide and read microscopically.**
7. **Read tests and record results.** *Note:* **If reading is macroscopic, an optical aid should be used.**

REFERENCE

Case, J. *Vox Sang,* 4:403, 1959.

SECTION 2 ENZYME TECHNIQUES

Note: The preparation of the various stock enzyme solutions is given under the heading Preparations, Section 14.

Technique 2.1: Two-Stage Trypsin Technique

Purpose
For antibody detection or identification or both.

Method
1. **Wash the donor's red cells three times in saline to remove the "trypsin inhibitor" present in normal serum.**
2. **Add four volumes (e.g., four drops) of diluted buffered trypsin stock solution to one volume (e.g., one drop) of packed red cells.**
3. **Mix well.**
4. **Incubate in a water bath or in heat blocks at 37° C for 30 minutes.**
5. **Wash the red cells once in saline and make up to a final 5 per cent suspension in saline.**

6. Warm the patient's serum to 37° C for five minutes.
7. Add equal volumes of patient's warmed serum to the trypsinized red cells, which have been kept warm at 37° C.
8. Incubate in a water bath or in heat blocks at 37° C for one hour.
9. Shake gently and examine macroscopically for agglutination.
10. Record results.

Technique 2.2: One-Stage Ficin Technique

Purpose

For antibody detection or identification or both.

Method

1. To one drop of a 4 to 6 per cent saline suspension of washed red cells, add one drop of the test serum.
2. Mix well.
3. Add one drop of 1 per cent ficin stock solution.
4. Incubate at room temperature for 15 to 60 minutes, or at 37° C for 15 to 60 minutes.
5. Centrifuge at 3400 rpm (Serofuge) for 15 seconds (or for one minute at 500 rcf). *Care must be taken to avoid overcentrifugation.*
6. Shake gently and examine for macroscopic agglutination.
7. Record results.

Technique 2.3: Two-Stage Ficin Technique

Purpose

For antibody detection or identification or both.

Method

1. Dilute the 1 per cent ficin solution to an 0.1 per cent or 0.05 per cent solution by mixing, respectively, one volume of the 1 per cent ficin with 9 volumes or 19 volumes of pH 7:3 buffered saline.
2. To one volume of washed, packed red cells, add one volume of 0.1 per cent or 0.05 per cent ficin solution.
3. Incubate at 37° C for 10 to 15 minutes.
4. Wash the red cells three times in isotonic saline.
5. Resuspend the pre-treated red cells to a 4 to 6 per cent suspension.
6. Mix one drop of ficinized red cell suspension with two drops of the serum under test.

7. Incubate at 37° C for 15 to 30 minutes in a water bath or in heat blocks.
8. Observe macroscopically for agglutination.
9. Record results.

Technique 2.4: One-Stage Papain Technique

Purpose

For antibody detection or identification or both.

Method

1. To one drop of a 4 to 6 per cent suspension of washed red cells add one drop of the test serum.
2. Mix well.
3. Add one drop of one per cent activated papain stock solution.
4. Incubate at room temperature for 15 to 60 minutes or at 37° C for 15 to 30 minutes in a water bath or in heat blocks.
5. Centrifuge at 3400 rpm (Serofuge) for 15 seconds or for one minute at 500 rcf. *Care must be taken to avoid overcentrifugation.*
6. Shake gently and examine for macroscopic agglutination.
7. Record results.

Technique 2.5: Two-Stage Papain Technique

Purpose

For antibody detection or identification or both.

Method

1. Pipette 0.1 ml of thrice-washed, packed red cells (and the patient's red cells as a control) into labeled tubes.
2. Add 0.2 ml of papain working solution to each of the tubes.
3. Incubate in a water bath or in heat blocks at 37° C for 30 minutes, agitating frequently.
4. Wash the red cells three times with phosphate-buffered saline (pH 7.4). (Preparation of phosphate buffered saline is outlined in Technique 14.3.)
5. Dilute to 2 to 5 per cent suspension in isotonic saline.
6. Place two drops of the patient's serum in a labeled test tube.
7. Add one drop of papainized patient's red cells to two drops of patient's serum in a tube labeled "control."
8. Mix well.
9. Incubate in a water bath or in heat blocks at 37° C for 15 to 30 minutes.

10. Examine macroscopically for agglutination or hemolysis using an optical aid.
11. Record results.
12. If no reaction occurs, this technique may be immediately followed with the antiglobulin technique.

Technique 2.6: One-Stage Bromelin Technique

A suggested method for this technique is given in Chapter 21 of this text, page 266.

Technique 2.7: Two-Stage Bromelin Technique

Purpose
For antibody detection or identification or both.

Method
1. Add one volume (e.g., one drop) of a washed, 5 per cent saline suspension of the donor's red cells to one volume (e.g., one drop) of stock bromelin solution.
2. Incubate in a water bath or in heat blocks at 37° C for 10 minutes.
3. Wash once in saline and make up to a final 5 per cent saline suspension.
4. Add one drop of the bromelinized red cells to one drop of the patient's serum.
5. Incubate in a water bath or in heat blocks at 37° C for 15 minutes.
6. Centrifuge at 3400 rpm (Serofuge) for 15 seconds.
7. Shake gently and examine macroscopically for agglutination or hemolysis.
8. Record results.

SECTION 3 CROSSMATCH TECHNIQUES

Technique 3.1: Prewarmed Antiglobulin Technique

Purpose
To prevent the attachment of cold antibodies to red blood cells, and the production of incompatible reactions in the antiglobulin phase caused by complement binding to the red cells.

Method
1. Warm a 2 to 5 per cent saline suspension of washed donor red cells in a properly labeled tube at 37° C for 10 to 15 minutes.

2. Warm two drops of the patient's serum separately in a labeled tube at 37° C for 10 to 15 minutes.
3. Add one drop of prewarmed red cell suspension to the prewarmed serum without removing the tubes from the water bath or heat blocks.
4. Mix well.
5. Incubate at 37° C for 30 minutes.
6. During incubation, warm a bottle of saline to 45° C, then let stand in a water bath at 37° C.
7. After incubation, wash the red cells three to four times with the warm saline, decanting as completely as possible after each wash.
8. Add two drops of antiglobulin reagent. Antiglobulin reagent should be at room temperature.
9. Mix well.
10. Centrifuge at 3400 rpm (Serofuge) for 15 seconds and examine for agglutination, using an optical aid.
11. Add one drop of known sensitized red cells to all negative tests (control). Centrifuge and examine for agglutination using an optical aid. If negative reactions are seen after this step, the test results are invalid.
12. Record results.

REFERENCE

Technical Manual, American Association of Blood Banks, 1977.

Technique 3.2: Saline Replacement Technique

Purpose
To disperse rouleaux formation.

Method
1. After incubation and resuspension of the red cells, re-spin the serum-cell mixture.
2. Remove the serum.
3. Replace the serum with an equal volume of saline (two drops).
4. Mix well.
5. Spin the saline-cell mixture at 3400 rpm (Serofuge) for 15 seconds.
6. Resuspend the saline-cell mixture and observe for agglutination. Rouleaux formation will disperse but true agglutination will remain.

REFERENCE

Technical Manual, American Association of Blood Banks, 1977.

Technique 3.3: Crossmatching in the Presence of Strong Rouleaux: Titration Technique

Purpose

To determine compatibility in the presence of strong rouleaux formation.

Method

1. Place two drops of patient serum in each of two sets of five labeled tubes.
2. Add saline to each set as follows:
   Tube 1: None
   Tube 2: One drop
   Tube 3: Two drops
   Tube 4: Three drops
   Tube 5: Four drops
3. To one set of tubes add one drop of 2 to 5 per cent suspension of donor cells. To the other set of tubes add one drop of 2 to 5 per cent suspension of patient's washed red cells.
4. Mix well.
5. Complete the compatibility test and compare the result of the two sets of tubes. Compatibility is indicated if the set of tests with the donor cells is negative at the same or lower tube number than the corresponding tube with recipient red cells.

Technique 3.4: "In Vivo" Crossmatch Procedure

Purpose

To determine the survival of transfused red cells in an alloimmunized recipient.

Equipment Required

10 cc sterile vacutainer tubes (yellow stoppered)
Medical injection sites for blood bags
^{51}Cr, sterile for injection (approximately 100 μCi/ml)
Disposable syringes (10 cc, 5 cc, 1 cc)
Needles (18 gauge and 25 gauge)
Sterile saline for injection (20 ml bottles)
Volumetric pipettes (2 ml)
Counting vials
Saponifier
Purple-stoppered vacutainer tubes (7 cc)
Blood collection equipment
Capillary pipettes and centrifuge for hematocrit determination
Alcohol swabs, sterile gauze, plastic absorbant paper, disposable gloves
Radioactive waste container
Centrifuge
Gamma counter

Preparation

The work area is prepared by covering the tabletop with plastic-lined absorbent paper. Proper radioactive waste containers must be available. Sterile techniques must be observed and special care must be taken not to cross-contaminate blood samples. Each sample is processed independently. Disposable gloves, which are kept free of contamination, must be worn by the technologist throughout the procedure. Autopipettes are used whenever volumetric samples are measured.

Generally, the most incompatible unit is used so that any significant drop in erythrocyte survival can be measured.

Method

1. Label the tubes, syringes and counting vials for each blood sample. Mix the donor red cells and insert a medical injection site. Swab the external surface of the site with alcohol.
2. Draw 10 cc red blood cell volume into the syringe labeled "draw syringe" with an 18-gauge needle.
3. Empty 7 cc of red blood cells into the sterile (yellow-stoppered) vacutainer tube and determine the hematocrit. *Note:* When the risk of *in vivo* incompatibility seems great, 1 to 3 cc of red blood cells should be used.
4. Add 10 to 15 μCi ^{51}Cr to the red blood cell concentrate. Mix well and incubate at room temperature for 30 minutes. *Note:* The smaller the volume of ^{51}Cr required, the better. Smaller volumes of chromium disappear rapidly in the circulation, should additional *in vivo* crossmatches be required later.
5. Draw approximately 4 cc of sterile saline into the first wash syringe with an 18-gauge needle, and deliver into the sterile tube. Mix well and centrifuge at 2400 rpm for five minutes (Dupont Sorvall GLC–2).
6. Draw off the supernatant with the same syringe as in step 5, and discard into the radioactive waste container.
7. Repeat step 5 with a second wash syringe.
8. Draw off the supernatant with the same syringe as in step 7 and deliver into a saline wash tube (wash control).
9. Draw approximately 4 cc of sterile saline into the ^{51}Cr red blood cell syringe with an 18-gauge needle and deliver into the sterile tube to complete 11 cc.
10. Mix well and draw accurately 8 cc of labeled red blood cells into the ^{51}Cr labeled red cells.
11. Determine the hematocrit of the ^{51}Cr labeled red cells.
12. Mix and draw 2 cc of labeled red cells with a volumetric pipette and deliver into a counting

vial labeled "^{51}Cr RBC." Add 2 drops of saponifier and cap tightly.

13. Within two or three hours of preparation, inject the labeled red cells into the recipient. First, enter the vein with a 21-gauge butterfly needle attached to a saline syringe containing 5 cc of sterile saline. After making sure that the needle is in the vein, switch to the ^{51}Cr labeled red cells through the injection syringe and inject. Note the time and measure the amount infused very accurately.

14. To ensure maximal delivery of the labeled red cells, wash the IV butterfly line with saline from the saline syringe.

15. Samples of blood are taken from the recipient at 3, 10, 20, 30, 60 minutes, at 2 hours, 4 hours and 24 hours from the opposite arm, then serveral times during the next four weeks to determine the survival curve. Blood is collected into EDTA tubes and the hematocrit determined; 2 ml are drawn with a volumetric pipette into the counting vials. Two drops of saponifier are added and the vials tightly capped and labeled.

16. Count all vials with a gamma counter and determine counts per minute per milliliter, subtracting the background. Obtain counts per minute per milliliter by dividing the above by the hematocrit. Correct the ^{51}Cr decay if counts are not done all on the same day. Plot the semilog paper counts per minute per milliliter of red cells along the ordinate (log) and time along the abscissa (linear). Draw best fit curve. Note shape of curve and determine T½.

Interpretation

Except when the destruction is very rapid, the three-minute sample will contain approximately 100 per cent of the injected red cells. If substantial numbers of the red cells are cleared by the liver, the concentration of the surviving cells will be substantially lower in the 10-minute sample. When the destruction occurs predominantly in the spleen, there will be little fall in the concentration of surviving red cells at 10 minutes, with a substantial fall at the end of 60 minutes. The radioactivity in the red cells and the plasma of the 10- and 60-minute samples should be counted separately, because if there is intravascular hemolysis, a substantial amount of ^{51}Cr will be released into the plasma. Because ^{51}Cr is cleared from the plasma relatively slowly, one may obtain a false notion about the pattern of destruction if only whole blood samples are counted. (*Note:* This technique is taken from the *Technical Manual of the American Association of Blood Banks,* 1977.)

SECTION 4 THIOL REDUCTION TECHNIQUES

Technique 4.1: Inactivation of IgM Antibodies by 2-Mercaptoethanol

Purpose

To separate multiple cold and warm antibodies for the purpose of identification or to determine the immunoglobulin nature of the antibody. The latter application may be particularly useful in predicting whether an antibody is likely to cause hemolytic disease of the newborn.

Reagents Required

1. Phosphate buffer pH 7.4, prepared as follows:
   (a) Dissolve 9.47 g anhydrous Na_2HPO_4 in 1000 ml distilled water.
   (b) Dissolve 9.08 g crystalline KH_2PO_4 in 1000 ml distilled water.
   (c) Mix 80.8 ml of Na_2HPO_4 solution with 19.2 ml KH_2PO_4 solution at room temperature.
2. 0.2 M 2-Mercaptoethanol, prepared by adding 100 ml phosphate buffer, pH 7.4 to 1.56 ml 2-mercaptoethanol. *Note:* This solution should not be stored for more than one month at 4° C.
3. Buffered saline.
4. 0.2 M iodoacetamide, prepared by dissolving 0.37 g iodoacetamide in 100 ml buffered saline, pH 7.4.

Method

1. Mix 1 ml of 2-mercaptoethanol with 1 ml of the test serum.
2. Incubate at 37° C for 15 minutes with a control consisting of equal volumes of isotonic saline and test serum.
3. Add 1 ml iodoacetamide to the test serum and control (or dialyze overnight (16 hours) against phosphate-buffered saline).
4. Test both mixtures against appropriate red cells by saline technique (immediate spin and room temperature), convert to high-protein test (albumin), read after immediate spin, then again after 30 minutes at 37° C and convert to the antiglobulin technique.
5. If indicated, titer both mixtures by serial dilution in isotonic saline (see Titration Techniques, Section 7) and test against appropriate red cells by standard procedures to measure the effectiveness of inactivation.

Interpretation

If no reactivity is noted in the control, this indicates dilution of the antibody and invalidates the results. If no reactivity is noted in the test but reactivity is noted in the control mixture, this indicates that only IgM antibodies are present. Reactivity in the text mixture only in the indirect antiglobulin test and reactivity in the control mixture indicates that IgG antibodies are present. If reactivity is noted in the same phases of both the test and control tubes, titration studies should be performed. A fourfold reduction of activity (two-tube difference in titer) when compared to the control indicates the presence of an IgM antibody. No reduction of activity indicates that only IgG antibody is reacting, or that the 2-mercaptoethanol is not working properly.

Notes

2-Mercaptoethanol has a noxious odor and should therefore be used under a hood. Most recent investigations show 2-mercaptoethanol to be more effective than dithiothreitol for this purpose (see Technique 4.2); however, a few very potent antibodies still may not be inactivated even with prolonged incubation. The addition of iodoacetamide is necessary to prevent false positives. If the added dilution caused by the iodoacetamide is undesirable, the 2-mercaptoethanol serum mixture may be dialyzed overnight (16 hours) against phosphate buffered saline, as described.

REFERENCE

Special Serological Techniques Useful in Problem Solving, AABB Technical Workshop, October, 1976.

Technique 4.2: Inactivation of IgM Antibodies by Dithiothreitol

Purpose

To separate multiple cold and warm antibodies for the purpose of identification or to determine the immunoglobulin nature of the antibody. The latter application may be particularly useful in predicting whether an antibody is likely to cause hemolytic disease of the newborn.

Reagents Required

1. 0.01M Dithiothreitol, prepared by dissolving 0.77 g DTT in isotonic saline to a volume of 500 ml. *Note:* The DTT solution is stable at −20° C for up to six months but is not stable at 4° C.

Method

1. **Mix equal volumes of DTT solution and test serum.**
2. **Incubate at 37° C for 30 minutes with a control consisting of equal volumes of isotonic saline and test serum.**
3. **Test both mixtures against appropriate red cells**

by saline techniques (immediate spin and room temperature), convert to high-protein test (immediate spin and 37° C), then carry to antiglobulin test.
4. **If indicated, titer both mixtures by serial dilutions in isotonic saline (see Technique 7.1 and 7.2, Section 7) and test against appropriate red cells by standard procedures to measure the effectiveness of inactivation.**

Interpretation

If no reactivity is noted in the control, this indicates the dilution of the antibody and invalidates the results. No activity in the test but reactivity in the control mixture indicates that only IgM antibodies are present. Reactivity in the test mixture only in the indirect antiglobulin test and reactivity in the control mixture indicates that IgG antibodies are present.

If reactivity is noted in the same phase in both the test and control tubes, titration studies should be performed. A fourfold reduction of activity (two-tube difference in titer) when compared to the control indicates the presence of IgM antibodies. No reduction of activity indicates that only IgG antibody is reacting or that the DTT is not working properly.

Notes

DTT is not as odorous as 2-mercaptoethanol and provides a more rapid test. However, it may not be as effective as 2-mercaptoethanol against more potent antibodies.

REFERENCE

Special Serological Techniques Useful in Problem Solving, AABB Technical Workshop, October, 1976.

SECTION 5 ABSORPTION TECHNIQUES

Technique 5.1: Cold Autoabsorption Technique

Purpose

This technique is indicated when antibody reactivity is seen at room temperature with screening cells and with the patient's autocontrol. If the patient has been transfused recently, however, it should be noted that this technique may also remove alloantibodies in addition to autoantibody.

Note: For better absorption results, fresh blood samples should be obtained. *Serum For Absorptions:* Clotted specimen drawn and immediately placed in an ice bath; allow clot formation under refrigerated conditions; remove serum from clot maintaining iced conditions. *Cells For Absorptions:* Anticoagulated specimen drawn and immediately placed in 37° C environment. Allow cells to settle by gravity. Remove plasma; wash remaining cells three times with warm (37° C) saline.

Method 1 Using Untreated Red Cells
1. Wash the red cells three times in isotonic saline. (This can be omitted if specimens have been collected as just described.)
2. Completely remove the supernatant saline after the last wash.
3. Add one volume of undiluted serum to one volume of washed packed red cells.
4. Mix and incubate in an ice bath or refrigerator for 30 to 60 minutes. Mix frequently during incubation for maximum absorption.
5. Centrifuge and immediately harvest serum.
6. Test the absorbed serum against autologous cells to ensure that absorption is complete. If absorbed serum is still reactive with the auto-control, absorption is not complete and should be repeated with a fresh aliquot of washed packed red cells.

Method 2 Using Enzyme-Treated Red Cells
1. Add one volume of enzyme solution to one volume of washed, packed autologous red cells.
2. Mix and incubate at 37° C for 15 minutes.
3. Wash red cells several times. Mix cells by inversion on each saline wash to ensure complete removal of the enzyme solution.
4. To one volume of washed, packed enzyme-treated red cells, add one volume of patient's serum.
5. Mix and incubate in an ice bath or refrigerator for 15 to 60 minutes. Mix frequently during incubation for maximum absorption.
6. Centrifuge and immediately harvest serum.
7. Test absorbed serum against autologous cells to ensure that absorption is complete. If autologous control is still positive, the procedure should be repeated.

REFERENCE

Technical Manual, American Association of Blood Banks, 1981.

Technique 5.2: Warm Autoabsorption Technique

Purpose
This technique is indicated when antibody reactivity is seen at 37° C with screening cells and with the patient's autocontrol. This procedure

should be used with caution if the patient has been transfused in the last 2 to 3 months.

Method
1. Collect a sample of the patient's red cells in anticoagulant.
2. Wash a volume of the patient's red cells six times with warm (45° C) normal saline. *Note:* The volume of packed red cells should be at least twice the volume of serum to be tested.
3. Suspend the washed patient's red cells in saline at 1:1 ratio. Divide the sample into two aliquots of equal volume.
4. Elute the cells gently into equal volumes of saline at 56° C for 3 to 4 minutes, mixing constantly (or at 44° C for 60 minutes if red cells are very fragile). *Note:* The eluate may be reserved for tests to define specificity of the autoantibody, but this should not replace testing an eluate prepared by ether or digitonin techniques.
5. Wash each sample four times in warm saline.
6. Spin and remove excess saline.
7. Add one half to one volume of Bromelase to each volume of packed red cells.
8. Incubate at 37° C for 30 minutes.
9. Wash three or four times with saline to remove enzyme and decant the last wash as completely as possible to minimize serum dilution.
10. Add an equal volume of patient's serum to one aliquot of the enzyme-treated red cells.
11. Incubate at 37° C for 30 to 60 minutes, mixing occasionally.
12. Centrifuge immediately and recover serum.
13. Add the once-absorbed serum to the second aliquot of Bromelase-treated red cells.
14. Repeat steps 11 and 12.
15. Test serum for antibody reactivity by performing either an antibody screen, a panel, or a compatibility test.
16. If the autoantibody reactivity has not been completely removed, the procedure should be repeated.

REFERENCES

Technical Manual, American Association of Blood Banks, 1981.
Morel, P. A., Bergen, M. O., and Frank, B. S.: AABB Poster Session. 31st Annual Meeting, AABB, New Orleans, 1978.

Technique 5.3: Allo-Absorption Technique

Purpose
To remove an "unwanted" antibody from serum for the purpose of antibody identification, or to prepare reagent antisera.

Method

1. Wash a large volume of the red cells to be used in the absorption three times in normal saline. These cells must possess the antigen corresponding to the antibody that is to be absorbed and should lack the antigen corresponding to the antibody, if any, that is not to be absorbed (i.e., to remain in the serum).
2. After the final wash, centrifuge the cells so that they are tightly packed and remove as much of the saline from the cells as possible.
3. Add a volume of serum equal to the volume of the absorbing cells.
4. Incubate at the optimal temperature at which the antibody to be absorbed will react for 30 to 60 minutes.
5. Test the serum to ensure that the absorption is complete. If not, repeat the procedure using another aliquot of packed red cells. Always test to ensure that the antibody, if any, that is to remain in the serum is sufficiently reactive before continuing with repeat absorptions.

SECTION 6 ELUTION TECHNIQUES

Technique 6.1: Digitonin Elution Technique

Purpose

To recover antibody from sensitized red cells for the purpose of identification, or in order to accurately phenotype the red cells.

Reagents Required

1. Digitonin – 5 mg/ml in saline (stable at 4° C).
2. Glycine buffer– 0.1 M pH 3.0, prepared by mixing 3.754 gm glycine with 500 ml of distilled water. Correct pH by adding about 34 drops 12N HCl.
3. Phosphate buffer – 0.8 M pH 8.2, prepared as follows:
   Add 113.57 gm Na_2HPO_4 to 1 liter of distilled water
   Add 108.87 gm KH_2PO_4 to 1 liter of distilled water
   Final solution: Add 0.35 ml KH_2PO_4 solution to 9.65 ml Na_2HPO_4 solution (stable at 4° C).

Method

1. Warm the phosphate buffer to room temperature.
2. Wash 1 ml of red cells from which the eluate is to be prepared six times in large volumes of normal saline. Carefully aspirate the supernatant saline between washes. Note: Do *not* decant by pouring off the saline.
3. After the last wash, remove as much saline as possible.

Note: Save an aliquot of the last wash saline from the area nearest to the cells to test for residual antibody. To two drops of this saline, add one drop of antiglobulin serum and one drop of Coombs control cells (sensitized red cells). Spin and read. A negative result indicates, in most cases, neutralization of the antiglobulin serum and that all residual antibody was not removed. *Alternatively,* test the final wash saline in parallel with the eluate. There should be no antibody activity in the saline.

4. Add 9 ml of normal saline to the washed packed red cells.
5. Seal the test tube, and mix by inversion. Add 0.5 ml digitonin solution.
6. Invert several times until a clear hemolysate is visable.
7. Centrifuge for 3 to 5 minutes at 3400 rpm (Serofuge).
8. Remove and discard the supernatant.
9. Wash the cell stroma four times with normal saline or until the stroma appears snow white. *Note:* Other elution methods may be applied to the white stroma.
10. Add 2 ml glycine buffer.
11. Invert for one minute and centrifuge for five minutes at 3400 rpm. Save the supernatant; this is the eluate.
12. Add 0.2 ml phosphate buffer to the supernatant (eluate).
13. Mix and centrifuge for two minutes (3400 rpm) to remove any precipitate. The supernatant is the final eluate.
14. Test the eluate following the normal testing procedure for the demonstration of antiglobulin-reactive antibodies.

REFERENCE

Special Serological Techniques Useful in Problem Solving, AABB, 1976.

Technique 6.2: Acid Elution Technique

Purpose

To recover antibody from sensitized red cells for the purpose of identification, or in order to phenotype the red cells accurately.

Reagents Required

1. Glycine-HCl buffer pH 3.0, prepared by mixing 7.507 g glycine and 5.844 g NaCl and bringing to one liter with deionized water. Adjust the pH to 3.0 with 0.1N HCl.
2. Tris (hydroxymethyl) aminomethane — 0.5 M pH 10.5.

Method

1. Chill normal saline and glycine buffer.
2. Wash the red cells from which the eluate is to be prepared six times in large volumes of normal saline. Save an aliquot of the last wash saline from the area nearest the cells and test for residual antibody as described in Technique 6.1.
3. To the washed packed red cells, add an equal volume of chilled (4° C) saline.
4. To the chilled 50 per cent saline cell suspension, add an equal volume of chilled glycine buffer.
5. Incubate the mixture in an ice bath for one minute with gentle agitation.
6. Centrifuge for two minutes at 3400 rpm (Serofuge).
7. Remove the supernatant eluate and place in a labeled tube.
8. Adjust the pH to 7.0 by adding 0.2 ml Tris per ml of supernatant.
9. Centrifuge to remove any precipitate.
10. If the eluate is to be frozen, add 10 mg/ml bovine albumin (one drop of 30 per cent albumin per ml of eluate).
11. To test the eluate, follow normal testing procedure for the demonstration of anti-globulin-reactive antibodies.

REFERENCE

Revig, O.P. and Hannestad, K.: Vox Sang. 32:280, 1977.

Technique 6.3: Ether Elution Method (Rubin)

Purpose

To recover antibody from sensitized red cells for the purpose of identification, or in order to accurately phenotype the red cells.

Method

1. Wash the red cells from which the eluate is to be prepared six times in large volumes of normal saline. Carefully aspirate the supernatant saline between washes. (*Note:* Do not decant by pouring off the saline.)
2. After the final wash, remove as much saline as possible. Save an aliquot of the last wash saline from the area nearest the red cells and test for residual antibody as described in Technique 6.1.
3. To the washed packed red cells add an equal volume of saline and mix well.
4. To the total volume of red cells plus saline add an equal volume of reagent grade diethyl ether.

5. Stopper. Mix by inversion for one minute. Carefully remove stopper to release the volatile ether. (*Note:* A more potent eluate can be prepared after this step by incubating the tube at 37° C for 30 minutes.)
6. Centrifuge at 3400 rpm (Serofuge) for 10 minutes.
7. Three layers will be visible, the top layer representing clear ether, the middle layer representing red cell stroma and the bottom layer representing hemoglobin-stained eluate.
8. Aspirate the eluate.
9. Incubate the eluate at 37° C for 15 minutes to drive off the residual ether.
10. The eluate is now ready for testing or freezing.
11. To test the eluate follow normal testing procedures for the demonstration of anti-globulin-reactive antibodies.

REFERENCE

Rubin, H.J.: J. Clin. Pathol. 16:70, 1963.

Technique 6.4: Xylene Elution Technique

Purpose

To recover antibody from sensitized red cells for the purpose of identification, or in order to phenotype the red cells accurately.

Method

1. Wash the red cells from which the eluate is to be prepared six times in large volumes of normal saline. Save an aliquot of the last wash saline from the area nearest to the cells and test for residual antibody as described in Technique 6.1.
2. To the washed, packed red cells, add an equal volume of normal saline and mix well.
3. To the 50 per cent saline-cell suspension, add two volumes of reagent grade xylene. Stopper and mix well by repeated inversion.
4. Incubate for 10 minutes at 56° C, agitating occasionally.
5. Remove the stopper and centrifuge for 5 minutes at 3400 rpm (Serofuge).
6. Remove and discard the top two layers (xylene and red cell stroma, respectively).
7. Test for eluate (bottom layer) according to normal testing procedures.

REFERENCE

Chan-Shu, S.A. and Blair, O.: Transfusion 19 (2):182–185, 1979.

Technique 6.5: Lui Easy Freeze Elution Technique

Purpose

To recover antibody from sensitized red cells for the purpose of identification, or in order to phenotype the red cells accurately. This technique seems well suited to situations in which a small volume of eluate only is required or in which only a small volume of cells has been obtained. This applies well to diagnosing hemolytic disease of the newborn due to ABO incompatibility.

Method

1. Wash 0.5 ml of the antibody-coated red cells six times using 10 ml of normal saline per wash.
2. After the sixth wash and centrifugation, remove and discard all the supernatant saline except for the 0.5 ml directly over the red cells. This portion is removed and tested for "free" antibody. If positive, additional washes are needed; if negative, proceed to the next step.
3. Place eight drops of washed packed red cells and two drops of normal saline (or two drops of bovine albumin) in a 10 or 12 × 75 mm test tube.
4. Stopper and rotate the tube so that the red cells coat the inside of the tube.
5. Place the tube on its side in a −6° C to 30° C freezer until frozen (a minimum of ten minutes). (*Note:* No deterioration of the antibody has been noted when the red cells are stored at this stage for several weeks.)
6. Thaw the red cells rapidly under running tap water.
7. Remove the stopper and centrifuge the tube for two minutes at 3400 rpm (Serofuge).
8. Transfer the supernatant (eluate) to a small clean test tube and test the eluate with appropriate cells by the indirect antiglobulin test.

REFERENCE

Eicher, C. J. South Central Association of Blood Banks, Vol. 19, Fall 1976.

SECTION 7 TITRATION TECHNIQUES

Technique 7.1: Titration

Purpose

A semiquantitative means of measuring the amount of antibody in a given serum.

Discussion

Ideally, when several serums are compared by titration, red cells from the same donor, freshly drawn and prepared, should be used each time. If commercially prepared reagent red cells are used, the same genotype should be employed consistently. If the antibody is diluted with saline, the red blood cells should be suspended in saline. If a high-protein medium is used for dilution, the red cells should be suspended in albumin or serum.

Meticulous pipetting technique is necessary for meaningful titration results. Mouth pipetting is not permitted. Semiautomatic pipettes are recommended. A clean pipette tip should be used for each dilution.

Results should be read macroscopically. The prozone phenomenon may produce weaker reactions in the first one or two tubes than in the higher dilutions, so the entire series of tubes should be evaluated, starting with the most dilute and ending with the most concentrated sample.

Optimal incubation time, temperature and centrifugation condition should be determined in preliminary evaluation of the antibody. Once determined, these should be used consistently.

If serums are to be compared, the titrations should be done at the same time. With prenatal specimens, successive samples should be stored frozen for comparison with subsequent specimens. Each specimen should be tested along with the immediately preceding sample. *Note:* Only a titer change of two tubes or more is significant.

Method 1 Single Titration Technique

1. Label a row of tubes according to the serum dilution, usually 1:1 through 1:512.
2. Deliver 0.1 ml of saline into the bottom of all tubes except the first.
3. Add 0.1 ml of serum to tubes 1 and 2 (dilutions 1:1 and 1:2).
4. With a clean pipette, mix the contents of tube 2 several times, then transfer 0.1 ml of the mixture to tube 3 (1:4 dilution).
5. Continue same technique through all dilutions. Remove 0.1 ml from the 512 tube and discard or save for use in further dilutions, if required.
6. Add 0.1 ml of a saline suspension of appropriate red cells to each tube.
7. Incubate in the appropriate manner according to the antibody being tested.
8. Centrifuge (3400 rpm for 15 seconds).
9. Gently dislodge the red cell button and observe macroscopically for agglutination, starting with the 512 tube. Record results. Express the end point as saline titer.
10. All unagglutinated or weakly agglutinated specimens are then washed three or four times for the antiglobulin test, if this is desired. Express this end point as the antiglobulin titer.

Method 2 Master Titration Technique

When a diluted serum is to be studied for reactivity against several red blood cell specimens, the dilutions are kept constant by preparing a master dilution. The method is the same as that described for the single titration, except that larger volumes of serum and diluent are used. The diluted serum for each tube in each titration series can now be transferred from the corresponding master tube. Even if one cell is to be used, a large-volume dilution may be easier than the 0.1 ml technique.

REFERENCE

Technical Manual, American Association of Blood Banks, 1977.

SECTION 8 EVALUATION AND QUALITY CONTROL TECHNIQUES

Technique 8.1: Avidity Test for Anti-A and Anti-B Reagents

Purpose

To establish the avidity of blood grouping reagents used in routine laboratory work.

Method

1. Prepare a 40 per cent saline suspension of washed red cells of the appropriate group (i.e., A cells for anti-A, B cells for anti-B).
2. Use a wax pencil to draw a 25-mm circle on a slide or tile.
3. Place one drop of the red cell suspension in the center of this area and near it, one drop of the grouping serum to be tested.
4. Mix rapidly over the 25-mm area and accurately time with a stopwatch the interval between mixing and the beginning of agglutination.
5. Rotate the tile (or slide) from side to side intermittently from the first mixing of cells and serum. *Do not use an Rh-view box for reading.*
6. The beginning of agglutination is the end point. The aggregates must be distinct on macroscopic observation.
7. Some of the aggregates or clumps formed must be 1 mm^2 in surface area or larger before two minutes have elapsed.

REFERENCE

Technical Manual, American Association of Blood Banks, 1977.

Technique 8.2 Testing for Anticomplement Activity in Antiglobulin Serum

Purpose

To determine the amount of anticomplement activity in antiglobulin serum.

Method 1 Using Red Cells Sensitized With C3b and C4b (Using A "Nonagglutinating" Anti-Lewis)

1. To nine volumes of anti-Lewis antiserum, add one volume of neutral EDTA (4.45 per cent K_2H_2 EDTA + 0.3 per cent NaOH).
2. Add one volume of 50 per cent suspension of washed Lewis-positive red cells.
3. Incubate at 37° C for 30 to 60 minutes.
4. Wash four times.
5. To the button of red cells, add five volumes of fresh normal serum as a source of complement.
6. Reincubate at 37° C for 15 minutes.
7. Wash four times.
8. Resuspend to 2 to 5 per cent in saline and perform the antiglobulin test using the antiglobulin serum under investigation.

Method 2 Using Red Cells Sensitized With C3b and C4b (Using Anti-I)

1. Dilute anti-I in fresh normal serum (select a dilution that gives approximately 2+ agglutination).
2. Add one tenth volume of 50 per cent washed red cells.
3. Incubate at 20 to 25° C for 30 minutes.
4. Incubate at 37° C for approximately 15 minutes (to allow agglutination to disperse).
5. Wash the red cells four times at 37° C.
6. Resuspend to 2 to 5 per cent in saline and perform the antiglobulin test using the antiglobulin serum under investigation. *Note:* The degree of complement sensitization can be varied by altering the amount of antibody sensitization (e.g., using dilutions of strong anti-Lewis or anti-I).

Method 3 Using Red Cells Sensitized With C4b (But Not With C3b)

1. Add 10 ml of 10 per cent sucrose in water to a 16 × 100 mm EDTA vacutainer tube, containing 12 or 15 mg K EDTA.
2. Add 1 ml of whole blood, which can be fresh or ACD or CPD blood, that has been stored at 4° C for less than three weeks.
3. Incubate at 37° C for 15 minutes.
4. Wash four times.
5. Resuspend to 2 to 5 per cent in saline and perform the antiglobulin test using the antiglobulin serum under investigation.

REFERENCE

Technical Manual, American Association of Blood Banks, 1977.

SECTION 9 INHIBITION TECHNIQUES

Technique 9.1: Sd^a Neutralization Test

Purpose

To neutralize the Sd^a antibody in serum, enabling identification.

Method

1. Add one drop of Sd^a-positive urine (first morning urine is preferable, if available) to three drops of serum from the patient under test.
2. As a control, add one drop of saline to three drops of serum from the patient under test to a separate tube.
3. Incubate both tubes at room temperature for 15 minutes.
4. The anti-Sd^a should now be completely removed from the serum, which can be used for identification of other antibodies. If the test is used for the identification of anti-Sd^a, test the neutralized serum with Sd(a+) and Sd(a−) red cells by the technique through which the antibody was first found to react. If no antibody activity is noted with the neutralized serum, the antibody is identified as anti-Sd^a.

Technique 9.2: Anti-P$_1$ Neutralization with Hydatid Cyst Fluid

Purpose

To neutralize anti-P$_1$ for purposes of identification or to identify additional antibodies in the same serum complicated by the presence of anti-P$_1$.

Method

1. Set up and label two sets of four tubes — the first four to be used as the "test" and the second four to be used as the "control."
2. Add two drops of serum (containing anti-P$_1$, or suspected of containing anti-P$_1$) to all tubes.
3. To the first set of four tubes, add one drop of hydatid cyst fluid. To the second set of tubes, add one drop of saline.
4. Incubate both sets of four tubes at room temperature for ten minutes.
5. Add red cells as follows:
   (a) To the first tube in each set add red cells of phenotype P$_1$+, Le(a+b−), I+(weak).
   (b) To the second tube in each set add red cells of phenotype P$_1$+, Le(a−b+), I+(strong).
   (c) To the third tube in each set add red cells of phenotype P$_1$ (strong), Le(a−b−), I+.
   (d) To the fourth tube in each set add red cells of phenotype P$_1$−, Le(a−b+), I+.

Note: The red cells used should be washed and brought to a 5 per cent saline suspension.

6. Centrifuge all tubes for 15 seconds (3400 rpm).
7. Read and record results.
8. Incubate all tubes at room temperature for 15 minutes.
9. Centrifuge for 15 seconds (3400 rpm).
10. Read and record results.
11. Incubate all tubes at 5° C for 15 minutes.
12. Centrifuge for 15 seconds (3400 rpm).
13. Read and record results.

Interpretation

Inhibition of the antibody in the "test" tubes at any temperature with no inhibition at the same temperature in the "control" tube indicates anti-P$_1$ specificity. The neutralized serum can now be used for the identification of other antibodies if necessary.

Technique 9.3: Anti-I Neutralization With Human Milk

Purpose

To neutralize anti-I antibodies in order to determine if that antibody is masking other clinically important antibodies and as a possible aid to identification.

Method

1. Set up and label three test tubes.
2. Add two drops of the serum from the patient under test to each tube.
3. Add one drop of human milk to tubes 1 and 2.
4. Add one drop of saline to tube 3 (this is the dilution control).
5. Mix and incubate all tubes at room temperature for 15 minutes.
6. Add red cells as follows:
   (a) One drop adult I+ red cells to tube 1
   (b) One drop cord cells to tube 2
   (c) One drop adult I+ red cells to tube 3
7. Incubate all tubes at room temperature for 30 minutes.
8. Centrifuge all tubes at 3400 rpm for 15 seconds.
9. Read and record results.

Interpretation

Inhibition of the anti-I tubes 1 and 2 with no inhibition in tube 3 indicates the presence of anti-I. The resulting neutralized serum may now be used for the identification of other antibodies.

Technique 9.4: Neutralization of Lewis Antibodies With Human Lewis Blood Group Substances

Purpose

To aid in the identification of Lewis blood group antibodies or to assure the absence of an underlying antibody in the same serum.

Method

1. Set up and label three test tubes.
2. To the first two tubes, add a sufficient quantity of serum to allow for antibody identification or detection or both. To the third tube add two drops of serum as a control.
3. To the first tube, add Lewis blood group substance (human; available from commercial sources) in the ratio of one part of substance to five parts of serum.
4. To the second tube, add saline in the ratio of one part of saline to five parts of serum.
5. Mix the contents of each tube carefully and thoroughly.
6. Allow the tubes to stand at room temperature for 5 minutes.
7. Mix thoroughly.
8. Test each substance-treated and saline-diluted serum specimen with Le(a+) or Le(b+) red cells or both.
9. Read and record results.

Interpretation

If the substance-treated serum does not react with Le(a+) or Le(b+) red cells or both that are agglutinated by the saline-diluted serum, the presence of antibody or antibodies to antigens of the Lewis system is confirmed. The resultant neutralized serum can now be used for the identification of other underlying antibodies if indicated.

SECTION 10 TECHNIQUES IN HEMOLYTIC DISEASE OF THE NEWBORN

Technique 10.1: Plasma Microbilirubin Estimation On Infants

Method

1. Obtain a heparinized specimen from the baby and centrifuge at 3400 rpm for five minutes. Remove the plasma into a dry 12 × 100 mm tube.
2. Measure 3.0 ml of buffered saline into a 13 × 100 mm disposable test tube.

3. Add 100 lambda of the baby's plasma to the buffered saline, using an Oxford Sampler pipette.
4. Mix well on a vortex mixer and transfer to a cuvette.
5. Set the spectrophotometer at 0 per cent transmittance with the cuvette well darkened.
6. Using a cuvette of buffered saline as the blank, set the spectrophotometer at an optical density of 450 mμ.
7. Read the optical density value for the test.
8. Using the same blank, set the spectrophotometer to "0" optical density at 540 mμ.
9. Read the optical density value for the test.
10. Subtract the reading obtained at 540 mμ from the reading obtained at 450 mμ and determine the bilirubin value from the calibration curve.

Technique 10.2: Acid Elution Method for Detection of Fetal Cells In Maternal Circulation (Kleihauer Technique)

Method

1. Maternal fresh whole blood mixed with anticoagulant is spread on ordinary films or glass slides and allowed to air-dry for not longer than one hour.
2. Fix the films in 80 per cent ethanol for five minutes.
3. Rinse with tap water and dry.
4. Prepare a buffer solution containing 26.6 ml 0.2 M anhydrous Na_2HPO_4 and 73.4 ml 0.1 M citric acid. The final pH should be 3.3.
5. Warm the buffer to 37° C and place the slides vertically into it.
6. Move the slides up and down from time to time.
7. Elution is complete in 5 to 15 minutes.
8. Wash the slides in tap water and stain with acid hematoxylin for three minutes, then with eosin (0.3 per cent solution in water) for 30 seconds.

Interpretation

Adult hemoglobin is soluble at pH 3.3, but fetal hemoglobin is not. Fetal cells stand out as dark cells in a field of ghosts.

SECTION 11   AMNIOTIC FLUID TECHNIQUES

Technique 11.1: Amniocentesis

Purpose

To give an indication of the severity of hemolytic disease of the fetus (in utero) and thereby to provide a therapeutic guide to the timing of delivery of erythroblastotic infants.

Method

1. Collect an ample volume of amniotic fluid. Keep the specimen away from light (wrap aluminum foil around sample tube). Note that exposure to light will invalidate readings.
2. Centrifuge the amniotic fluid at 3000 rpm for 10 minutes.
3. Filter through Whatman No. 42 filter paper using millipore apparatus.
4. If the specimen is turbid, dilute with distilled water until optical density (OD) readings can be obtained. Diagnostic curves are based on deviations of the optical density from the normal linear curve and not on absolute values.
5. Place 2.5 ml water in one cuvette for the "Blank."
6. Place 2.5 ml amniotic fluid in the other cuvette for the "test."
7. Take OD readings of the amniotic fluid against water at the following wavelengths: 700, 650, 550, 500, 480, 470, 460, 450, 440, 430, 420, 415, 410, 400, 390, 380, 370, 365, 360 and 350. (Use the tungsten lamp for all readings.)

   Note: Be sure to zero the blank with the slit control and that the absorbance scale is at zero each time the wavelength is changed.

Calculations

1. Using semilog paper, plot OD readings obtained against the wavelength settings used. Use vertical axis for OD and horizontal axis for nm. Start the 700 nm at the lower left corner of the paper at the same point as the zero OD.
2. Draw a straight line from the 550-nm plot to the 365-nm plot on the graph paper.
3. To determine the rise in OD at 450 nm: read the OD reading at 450 nm where the drawn straight line crosses it. Subtract this value from the plotted value at 450 nm.
4. A hemoglobin peak at 415 nm may add to the absorption at 450 nm. This error can be corrected by subtracting 5 per cent of the specific rise in OD at 415 nm for the rise in OD at 450 nm.

   The normal values will be dependent on gestation time. A rise in OD of 0.1 or greater at any time is indicative of disease.

REFERENCE

Technical Manual, American Association of Blood Banks, 1977.

Technique 11.2: Spectrophotometric Analysis of Amniotic Fluid Using a Recording Spectrophotometer

Purpose

To give an indication of the severity of hemolytic disease of the fetus (in utero) and thereby to provide a therapeutic guide to the timing of delivery of erythroblastotic infants.

Method

1. Immediately following aspiration, the amniotic fluid is placed in an amber glass bottle or test tube wrapped in aluminum foil to protect it from light.
2. Centrifuge the fluid at 2000 rpm for five minutes (700 g) to sediment the red cells and other particulate debris.
3. Filter through No. 40 Whatman filter paper or through 3μ membrane filter. This must be done in an area protected from sunlight.
4. Using an automatic continuous-recording spectrophotometer with a 1-cm cuvette filled with distilled water, set the pen of the recorder at zero optical density on the chart paper.
5. Remove the sample cuvette and drain the water from it as completely as possible. Fill the cuvette with the clarified amniotic fluid and return it to the instrument.
6. Scan the clear amniotic fluid from 350 nm to 700 nm using distilled water as a reference.
7. Tear off the chart paper and draw a straight line from 375 nm to 525 nm along the amniotic fluid curve to approximate a normal curve (Fig. 23–1).
8. Measure the optical density difference at 450 nm (ΔOD 450) from the top of the bilirubin peak to the straight line drawn to simulate the base (Fig. 23–1).

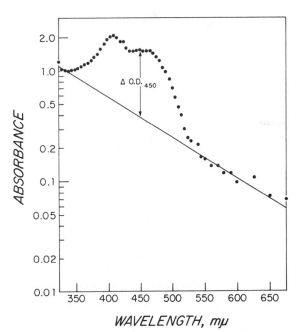

Figure 23–1 Visible absorption spectrums of amniotic fluid. Log absorbance plotted against wavelength. The tangent drawn to each curve corrects for background absorbance. (From AABB Technical Manual, American Association of Blood Banks, Washington, D.C., 1977, p. 342.)

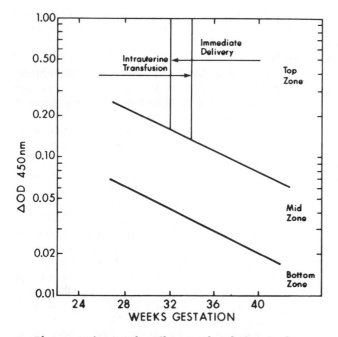

Figure 23–2 The Liley graph. (*AABB Technical Manual*, American Association of Blood Banks, Washington, D.C., 1977, p. 343.)

9. Place a point on the Liley graph relating to the ΔOD 450 logarithmic scale on the vertical axis and the weeks of gestation on the horizontal axis (Fig. 23–2).

Notes

1. Amniotic fluid may be held for analysis for up to 24 hours at room temperature if protected from light.
2. Samples may be preserved in the frozen state with little or no change in the ΔOD 450.
3. The presence of trace amounts of hemoglobin in the amniotic fluid will cause an absorbance peak at 415 nm. If this peak is large, it may override and obscure the bilirubin peak at 450 nm, making interpretation impossible. This problem can be minimized by the centrifugation of the fluid immediately following collection.

REFERENCE

Technical Manual, American Association of Blood Banks, 1977. See also Chapter 16 of this text for additional references and discussion.

SECTION 12   TECHNIQUES IN AUTOIMMUNE HEMOLYTIC ANEMIA

Technique 12.1: Detection of Antibodies to Penicillin and Cephalothin

Method

1. Prepare penicillin-treated red cells as follows:
   (a) Group O red cells (preferably fresh) are washed three times in saline.
   (b) To 1 ml of packed, washed red cells add 1×10^6 units (approximately 600 mg) of K-benzyl penicillin G dissolved in 15 ml of 0.1 M barbital buffer pH 9.5 to 10.0.
   (c) Incubate for one hour at room temperature with gentle mixing.
   (d) Wash the cells three times in saline. Slight hemolysis may occur during incubation and a small "clot" may form in the red cells, which can be removed with applicator sticks before washing cells. Once prepared, the cells may be kept in ACD at 4° C for up to one week; they do deteriorate slowly during this time, but not significantly.
2. Prepare cephalothin-treated red cells as follows:
   (a) Group O red cells (preferably fresh) are washed three times in saline.
   (b) To 1 ml of washed packed red cells, add 400 mg cephalothin dissolved in 10 ml of pH 9.5 to 10.0 buffered saline; i.e., one part pH 9.5 to 10.0 barbital buffer plus nine parts normal saline.
   (c) Incubate at 37° C for two hours with gentle mixing.
   (d) Wash the red cells three times in saline.
3. Perform the following tests on the patient's serum and eluate:
   (a) If the results of the direct antiglobulin test are positive, prepare an eluate by a standard method.
   (b) The eluate and the patient's serum should be tested against normal group O red cells and the same cells treated with penicillin. Usually, serial dilutions of the patient's serum are tested.

(c) Two volumes of eluate or serum dilutions should be incubated with one volume of 2 to 5 per cent suspension of penicillin-treated and untreated group O red cells in saline.

(d) Incubate at room temperature for 15 minutes. Centrifuge and inspect for agglutination.

(e) Wash the red cells four times in saline.

(f) Add antiglobulin serum to the button of washed red cells. Centrifuge and inspect for agglutination.

Interpretation

IgM penicillin antibodies will agglutinate saline-suspended penicillin-treated red cells but not the same cells untreated. IgG penicillin antibodies will react by the indirect antiglobulin test against penicillin-treated red cells but not against the same red cells untreated.

If indirect antiglobulin tests are used to detect cephalothin antibodies, it must be remembered that cephalothin-treated red cells can absorb proteins nonimmunologically. Therefore, all normal sera will give a positive result in indirect antiglobulin tests if incubated with cephalothin-treated red cells for a long enough period of time. The reaction does not usually occur once the normal protein is diluted out to more than 1:20. The amount of protein present in red cell eluates does not seem to be enough to give nonspecific results, so a positive result usually indicates the presence of antibody to cephalothin or a cross-reacting penicillin antibody.

REFERENCES

Spath, P., Garratty, G., Petz, L. D.: J. Immunol. 107:854, 1971.

Technical Manual, American Association of Blood Banks, 1977.

SECTION 13 HB$_s$Ag TECHNIQUES

Technique 13.1: Radioimmunoassay for the Detection of HB$_s$Ag

Method

The technique described is that intended for use with the Austria 11-125 kit provided by Abbott Laboratories, North Chicago, IL.

Materials. The kit contains:
1. Beads, coated with hepatitis B surface antigen (guinea pig)
2. Vials (10 ml each) of anti-HB$_s$ ^{125}I (human), approximately 7 microcuries per vial. Preservative: 0.1 per cent sodium azide

3. Vial (5 ml) of negative control (nonreactive for HB$_s$Ag). Preservative: 0.1 per cent sodium azide
4. Vial (3 ml) of positive control (positive for HB$_s$Ag). Preservative: 0.1 per cent sodium azide
5. Four reaction trays (20 wells each), 8 sealers and 80 tube identification inserts
6. Counting tubes (8 cartons, 20 tubes each) properly positioned for transfer of beads from reaction trays

Additional materials needed (not provided with the kit):
1. Precision pipettes or similar equivalent to deliver 0.2 ml
2. Device for delivery of rinse solution such as Cornwall syringe, Filamatic or equivalent
3. An aspiration device for washing coated beads, such as a cannula or aspirator tip and a vacuum source and trap for retaining the aspirate
4. A well-type gamma scintillation detector capable of efficiently counting ^{125}I
5. Gently circulating water bath, capable of maintaining temperature at 45° C ± 1° C
6. Austria confirmatory neutralization test kit (Note: All Austria 11-125 reactive samples must be confirmed with the test procedure provided with this kit.)

Collection and Preparation of Specimens

1. **Only serum and recalcified plasmas can be tested. Collect blood specimens and separate the serum from the sample. Plasma can be tested only after conversion to serum.**
2. **If specimens are to be stored, they should be refrigerated at 2 to 8° C or frozen. If specimens are to be shipped, they should be frozen.**

Procedure. Seven negative and three positive controls should be assayed with each run of unknowns. Be sure that reaction trays containing controls and reaction trays of unknowns are subjected to the same process and incubation times. Use a clean pipette or disposable tip for each transfer to avoid cross-contamination.

1. **Adjust the temperature of the water bath to 45° C.**
2. **Remove the cap from the clear plastic tube that contains antibody-coated beads. Hold the bead dispenser directly over the top of the reaction tray incubation well and push down with the index finger to release one bead into a well for each sample to be tested.**
3. **Using precision pipettes, add 0.2 ml of serum and positive and negative controls to the bottom of their respective wells. Make sure that the antibody-coated bead is completely surrounded by serum. Tap the reaction tray to**

release any air bubbles that may be trapped in the serum sample.

4. Apply a cover sealer to each tray and incubate the trays in the 45° C water bath for two hours.

5. At the end of two hours, remove the trays from the water bath. Remove the cover sealer and discard. Using a semiautomated aspiration and rinsing system, aspirate the serum; rinse each well and bead with a total of 5 ml distilled or deionized water. Repeat this wash procedure one additional time.

   Note: A manual system of washing the wells and beads may also be used. Using disposable pipettes or cannulas and a Cornwall syringe delivery system, or equivalent, and a vacuum source, rinse each well and bead with extreme care not to overflow the reaction well but assuring that the bead is totally immersed throughout the wash procedure. Place the pipette or cannula, attached to the vacuum source, into the bottom of the well next to the bead and simultaneously add slowly, with the Cornwall syringe, 5 ml of distilled or deionized water.

6. With precision pipettes, add 0.2 ml of ^{125}I-anti-HB_s (human) to the bottom of each reaction well. Make sure that the antibody-coated bead is completely surrounded by the labeled antibody solution. Tap the tray to release any air bubbles that may be trapped in the solution.

7. Apply a new cover sealer to each tray and incubate the trays in the 45° C water bath for one hour.

8. At the end of one hour, remove the trays from the water bath. Remove the cover sealer, aspirate the antibody solution from each well and rinse the well and antibody-coated bead it contains with a total of 5 ml of distilled or deionized water, as in step 5.

9. Transfer the beads from the reaction wells to properly identified counting tubes; align the inverted rack of oriented counting tubes over the reaction tray, press the tubes tightly over the wells and then invert the tray and tubes together so that beads fall into properly labeled tubes.

10. Place the counting tubes in a suitable well-type gamma scintillation counter and determine the count rate. The position of the bead at the bottom of the counting tube is not important. Although it is not critical that the counting be done immediately, it should be performed as soon as practicable. All control samples and unknowns must be counted together.

Interpretation: The presence or absence of HB_sAg is determined by relating net counts per minute of the unknown sample to net counts per minute of the negative control mean times the factor 2.1. Unknown samples whose net count rate is higher than the mean cutoff value established with the negative control are to be considered positive with respect to HB_sAg.

The mean value for the positive control samples should be at least five times the negative control mean. If not, the technique may be suspect and the run should be repeated.

Note: For gamma counters that do not automatically subtract machine background, the gross counts may be used if the cutoff value for the negative control is calculated as described below.

Calculation of the Negative Control Mean

Example:

Negative Control Sample Number	Net Count Rate Per Minute
1	380
2	400
3	410
4	375
5	350
6	390
7	400
	Total 2705

$$\frac{\text{Total net cpm}}{7} = \frac{2705}{7} = \frac{386 \text{ net cpm}}{\text{(mean)}}$$

Elimination of Aberrant Values

Method. Discard those individual values in the negative control samples that fall outside the range of 0.5 to 1.5 times the mean.
Example:

$0.5 \times 386 = 193$ and $1.5 \times 386 = 579$
Range = 193 cpm to 579 cpm

Note: In this example, no negative control sample is rejected as aberrant. The negative control mean therefore need not be revised. Typically, all negative control values should fall within the range of 0.5 to 1.5 times the control mean. If more than one value is consistently found outside this range, technique problems should be suspected.

Calculation of the Cutoff Value
1. Multiple the net negative control mean, 386 cpm, by the factor 2.1.
2. The calculated cutoff value is then 811 cpm.

3. Unknowns whose net count rate is higher than the cutoff value should be considered positive with respect to HB_sAg.

Note: Many gamma counters have no capacity for automatically subtracting background. In this case, as an alternative to subtracting instrument background manually from each sample, uncorrected sample counts per minute can be compared with a cutoff modified as follows:

$$\text{(Negative control mean} - \text{Background)} \times$$
$$2.1 + \text{Background} = \text{Cutoff}$$

Example:

Gross negative control mean = 436 cpm
Instrument background = 50 cpm
Cutoff = $(436 - 50) \times 2.1 + 50 = 861$

Samples with gross count rates greater than 861 are to be considered reactive with respect to HB_sAg.

Calculation of Positive Control to Negative Control Ratio

1. Divide the positive control mean value by the negative control mean value after correcting for background:

$$\frac{\text{Net positive control mean}}{\text{Net negative control mean}} = \text{P/N ratio}$$

2. This ratio should be at least 5, or the technique may be suspect and the run should be repeated.
Example:

Net positive control mean value = 5906 cpm
Net negative control mean value = 386 cpm
P/N Ratio = $5906 \div 386 = 15.3$

Technique is acceptable, and data should be considered valid.

Limitations of the Procedure

Nonrepeatable Positives. Some positive results may test nonreactive on repeat. This phenomenon is highly dependent on the technique used in running the test. The most common sources of such nonrepeatable positives are (1) inadequate rinsing of the bead and (2) cross-contamination of nonreactive samples caused by transfer of residual droplets of high-titer, antigen-containing sera on the pipetting device.

Nonspecific False Positives. The nonspecific false positives resulting from cross-reactions with guinea pig serum are essentially eliminated by using ^{125}I-anti-HB_s of human origin; however, all sensitive immune systems have a potential for false positives, and before notifying a patient or donor that he may be a carrier of HB_sAg, positive results must be confirmed as follows:

Repeatability. Further testing of the sample in question will verify whether it is repeatedly positive. In making an evaluation of data, consideration should be given to the actual test values obtained. The value 2.1 times the negative control mean is used as the cutoff for single determinations. This value has been selected in order to decrease the total number of nonrepeatable positives.

If repeat testing shows the sample to be less than 2.1 times the negative control mean, the original result may be classified as a nonrepeatable positive. If repeats are above the cutoff value, the sample should be presumed reactive for HB_sAg. Such results are contingent on determination of the specificity of the repeatable positives.

Specificity. Specificity analysis must be performed prior to informing a donor that he is a HB_sAg carrier. A suitable method must be used for confirmation of screening procedure on all reactive specimens. A repeatable reactive specimen, confirmed by neutralization with human antiserum, must be considered HB_sAg-positive.

SECTION 14   PREPARATIONS

Technique 14.1: Preparation of Bromelin Stock Solution

Method
1. **Add 0.5 per cent bromelin stock solution (by weight) to nine parts of saline and one part phosphate solution.**
2. **The pH should be 5.5.**
3. **Add sodium azide in a final concentration of 0.1 per cent.**
4. **Storage at 4° C or at −20° C.**
   Note: The solution of 0.5 per cent EDTA will stabilize the solution for about 12 hours at room temperature.

Technique 14.2: Preparation of Ficin Stock Solution

Method
1. **Prepare a Hendry's buffer solution as follows:**
   (a) **Add 2.34 g $NaH_2PO_4 2H_2O$ to 100 ml of distilled water.**

(b) Add 1.63 g NaHPO$_4$ to 100 ml of distilled water.
(c) Add 19 ml of the NaH$_2$PO$_4$2H$_2$O solution to 81 ml of the Na$_2$HPO$_4$ solution.

2. Dissolve 250 mg of crude ficin in 25 ml of the Hendry's buffer.

Technique 14.3: Preparation of Trypsin Stock Solution

Method

1. Dissolve 0.1 g of pure crystalline trypsin in 10 ml of N/$_{20}$HCl. (This is a stock solution and can be stored at 4° C until ready for use.)
2. As required, dilute the above solution with 0.1 M phosphate buffer 1 in 10 v/v. (The buffer is of pH 7.7 and is prepared by mixing one part of M/$_{15}$ KH$_2$PO$_4$ with nine parts of M/$_{15}$ NaHPO$_4$·2H$_2$O. Eight grams of sodium chloride are added to each liter.)

Technique 14.4: Preparation of Papain Stock Solution

Method 1: Papain-EDTA

1. To one volume of 0.2 M acetate buffer (pH 5.8) add nine volumes of saline.
2. To 495 ml of this buffered saline add 5 g of papain powder and 5 ml of a 50 g per liter aqueous solution of K$_2$EDTA · 2H$_2$O.
3. Stopper the container and shake vigorously for ten minutes.
4. Store at 4° C overnight.
5. Shake well and centrifuge at 1200 g for ten minutes.
6. Filter through Whatman No. 1 paper at 4° C.
7. Dispense into small portions and store at −25° C. The pH of the final product should be 5.3 to 5.5.

Method 2: Papain-Cystine

1. Add 450 ml of saline to 50 ml of 0.2 M acetate buffer.
2. To 470 ml of this buffered saline add 5 ml of a 50 g per 1 solution of K$_2$EDTA·2H$_2$O and 5 g of papain powder.
3. Stopper the container and shake vigorously for ten minutes.
4. Centrifuge at 1200 g for ten minutes.
5. Filter through Whatman No. 1 paper.
6. Add freshly prepared, neutralized L-cystine to a final concentration of 0.025 m.
7. Dissolve 2.0 g of L-cystine hydrochloride in 12.5 ml of distilled water and add sufficient 1.0 N NaOH to bring the pH of the solution to 6.9 to 7.1 (approximately 10 to 12 ml will be required).

8. Add all of the neutralized solution to the papain solution.
9. Incubate at 37° C for 60 minutes.
10. Check the pH, which should be 5.5 to 5.7.
11. Dispense into small portions and store at −25° C.

Technique 14.5: Preparation of Low Ionic-Strength Solution

Method

1. Dissolve 18 g Glycine in approximately 500 ml of distilled water.
2. Add 1.0 M NaOH drop-wise, with stirring, until the pH reaches 6.7. (Approximately 0.35 ml of 1.0 M NaOH will be needed.)
3. Add 20 ml phosphate buffer, 0.15 M at pH 6.7. (Made by mixing approximately equal volumes of 0.15 M Na$_2$HPO$_4$ and 0.15 M NaH$_2$PO$_4$.)
4. Add 1.79 g NaCl dissolved in approximately 100 ml distilled water.
5. Make up to one liter with distilled water. The conductivity of the final solution should be 3.7 mmho/cm at 23° C.

REFERENCE

Moore, H. C., and Mollison, P. L.: Transfusion 16:291, 1976.

Technique 14.6: Preparation of Isotonic Saline

Method

1. Dissolve 8.5 g sodium chloride in one liter of distilled water.
2. Shake well and use immediately. Do not store.
   Note: Saline should be buffered because the pH of distilled water varies enormously. This can be achieved by the addition of 8.6 g of hemagglutination buffer to each liter of saline prepared.

Technique 14.7: Preparation of ACD Solution

Method

1. Measure out 2.2 g of trisodium citrate (dihydrate).
2. Measure out 0.8 g citric acid (monohydrate).
3. Measure out 2.5 g dextrose.
4. Place all three in a suitable beaker and add distilled water to make 100 ml.

Technique 14.8: Preparation of CPD Solution

Method

1. Measure out and combine:

(a) 26.30 g trisodium citrate (dihydrate)

(b) 3.27 g citric acid (monohydrate)

(c) 2.22 g sodium dihydrogen phosphate (monohydrate)

(d) 25.50 g dextrose

2. Add distilled water to make 1 liter.

SECTION 15 RED CELL FREEZING TECHNIQUES

Technique 15.1: Freezing of Red Cells in Liquid Nitrogen

Red cells for storage in liquid nitrogen should be collected in either EDTA, CPD or ACD. The cells should not be more than two days old when they are frozen if antigens are to store well. Immediately before freezing, the blood should be mixed with half its volume of 40 per cent sucrose in buffered saline, added slowly and mixed well.

Method

1. Two-inch plastic tubing and a transfusion "taking" set needle are fitted to a siliconed 50-ml syringe.

2. The syringe is suspended over a 2-liter beaker (lined with absorbent cotton batton on sides and bottom).

3. The beaker is filled with liquid nitrogen, and the syringe is filled with blood (prepared as above).

4. The blood is dropped into the liquid nitrogen from the syringe, which is fitted with a clip to ensure uniform drops that do not coalesce on entering the liquid nitrogen.

5. The pellets of frozen blood are transferred with a cooled spoon to cardboard boxes filled with liquid nitrogen, then placed in a liquid nitrogen container.

Recovery of Red Cells Frozen in Liquid Nitrogen

To recover red cells frozen in liquid nitrogen, simply remove the pellets from the liquid nitrogen container and place them in 1 per cent NaCl at 45° C. Agitate the solution. The pellets will melt quickly and are washed in isotonic saline until the supernatant fluid shows no hemolysis.

Technique 15.2: Freezing of Red Cells in Glycerol

Method

1. A buffered citrate-glycerol solution is prepared by adding 19.4 g tripotassium citrate (monohydrate), 3.1 g sodium dihydrogen phosphate (dihydrate) and 2.8 g disodium hydrogen phosphate (anhydrous) to 600 ml of distilled water. Then 400 ml of glycerol is added to 600 ml of buffer citrate. The final pH is 6.9 to 7.0.

2. Pack the red cells to be frozen and remove *all* of the supernatant plasma.

3. Note the volume of packed cells and measure out an equal volume of buffered citrate-glycerol.

4. Add the buffered citrate-glycerol to the cells in small quantities, mixing constantly. The addition should take at least five minutes, depending on the quantity of cells to be frozen.

5. Divide the cells into small portions and freeze at −30° C. The proportion of glycerol must be altered for temperatures lower than −30° C. P. L. Mollison gives details of this in Blood Transfusion in Clinical Medicine, 4th edition, p. 726.

Recovery of Glycerolyzed Red Cells by Dialysis

Thaw the frozen cells. Pour the thawed cells into a length(s) of dialysis tubing in a saline bath for 30 to 60 minutes.* Remove the cells from the dialysis tubing into conveniently sized tubes and wash in saline until the supernatant is free of hemolysis.

Note: P. L. Mollison, in Blood Transfusion in Clinical Medicine, 6th edition, 1979, suggests the use of citrate-phosphate solution rather than saline for dialysis, and after dialysis, giving the cells a single wash in citrate-phosphate before washing in saline. The method of preparation of the citrate-phosphate solution is provided in the above mentioned publication on page 726.

SECTION 16 OTHER TECHNIQUES

Technique 16.1: Addition of Complement to "Old" Serum

Purpose

To demonstrate certain antigen-antibody reactions that require the presence of complement, and that therefore would not be demonstrated in "old" serum.

Method 1

1. Add one volume of fresh serum to three volumes of "old" serum. (If Lewis antibodies are suspected, use fresh serum from Le(a+b−) donors, or use Method 2.) Note: Different ratios of fresh serum to "old" serum can be used although the initial strength of the antibody should be considered when large amounts of fresh serum are added.

---

*Constant stirring of the saline with a magnetic stirrer improves the efficiency of this step.

Method 2

1. Prepare a solution containing 4.0 gm dipotassium EDTA and 0.3 gm NaOH in 100 ml of distilled water. The final pH should be between 7.0 and 7.4.
2. To 1 ml of antibody-containing serum add 0.1 ml EDTA solution (final concentration 4 mg per 1 ml serum).
3. To a dry button of red cells add four drops of the EDTA-treated serum and mix well.
4. Incubate at 37° C for at least 15 minutes.
5. Wash the red cells three times in saline.
6. After the last wash, drain off all the saline.
7. To each tube add two drops of fresh, compatible serum as a source of complement.
8. Incubate at 37° C for 15 minutes.
9. Wash as in steps 5 and 6.
10. To each dry button of washed cells, add two drops of antiglobulin serum and mix well.
11. Centrifuge.
12. Read and record results. Negative reactions may be read microscopically.

REFERENCES

Polly, M. J. and Mollison, P. L.: Transfusion 1:9, 1961.
Technical Manual, American Association of Blood Banks, 1977.

Technique 16.2: Donath-Landsteiner Technique (Qualitative)

Purpose

A diagnostic test for paroxysmal cold hemoglobinuria.

Method 1: Direct Test

1. Warm two dry tubes to 37° C.
2. Take 10 ml of venous blood from the individual under test and divide the blood immediately between the two dry, warmed tubes.
3. Leave one tube at 37° C; place the other at 0° C in crushed ice for 30 minutes. Then, without disturbing the clot, transfer the cold tube to the water bath at 37° C for one hour.

Interpretation

If the test is positive, the tube which was placed at 0° C will show gross hemolysis, while the tube kept at 37° C throughout the test will show no trace of free hemoglobin.

Method 2: Indirect Test

1. Separate the serum from the clot at 37° C. (Note that the sample of blood should not have been allowed to cool.)

2. Add nine drops of serum from the individual under test to one drop of washed packed red cells (group O) in tube 1.
3. To the second tube add equal parts of serum from the individual under test, fresh normal serum to act as a source of complement and washed packed red cells (group O).
4. Place the first tube and the second tube at 0° C on crushed ice for 30 minutes. Negative controls are provided by keeping a duplicate of tubes 1 and 2 at 37° C throughout the test. Transfer the tubes at 0° C to the water bath (37° C) for one hour.
5. Examine for hemolysis.

Interpretation

A positive test shows hemolysis in tubes 1 and 2 (or in 2 only, if the patient is deficient in complement). No hemolysis should be observed in the negative controls.

Technique 16.3: Donath-Landsteiner Technique (Quantitative)

Method

1. Make serial doubling dilutions of the patient's serum in fresh normal AB serum.
2. Add an equal volume of a washed 2 per cent suspension of group O red cells to each tube.
3. Immerse the tubes in crushed ice at 0° C for 30 minutes, then transfer them to a 37° C water bath for one hour.
4. Centrifuge and examine each tube for the degree of hemolysis. Read according to the following scale:
   - 4+ = complete hemolysis
   - 3+ = deep red supernatant
   - 2+ = red supernatant
   - 1+ = pale pink supernatant
   - ± = weak hemolysis

Interpretation

The hemolytic titer is the reciprocal of the highest dilution giving a ± reaction.

Technique 16.4: VDRL Screening Test

Purpose

To examine the plasma of blood donations for evidence of venereal disease.

Method

1. Prepare a buffered saline by dissolving 0.093 g of $Na_2HPO_4 \cdot 12H_2O$, 0.170 g of KH_2PO_4 and 10.0 g of NaCl in 1 liter of distilled water. Add

0.5 ml of formaldehyde. The final pH of the mixture is 6.0 ± 0.1.

2. Prepare the antigen emulsion by adding 0.5 ml of the antigen (commercially prepared) to 0.4 ml of buffered saline. Rotate the solution *while adding the antigen* and for a further ten seconds to ensure good mixing. Then add 4.1 ml of buffered saline, stopper the container and shake vigorously for a further ten seconds. (This prepared emulsion can be stored at 4° C until needed.)

3. The sera to be tested are inactivated for 30 minutes at 56° C.

4. Place 0.05 ml of the serum under test into a well on a slide and add one drop of antigen emulsion. Known positive and negative sera must be run as controls.

5. Rotate the slide for four minutes on a mechanical rotator.

6. Read macroscopically.

Interpretation

A positive reaction is a clumping of emulsified particles. Large and medium clumps are read as a definite positive; an even distribution of small clumps is read as a weak positive; no clumping is read as a negative. If a sample is found to be positive, it should be exposed to further testing before results are given. Usually these are performed by large research laboratories and are beyond the scope of this book.

Technique 16.5: pH Modified Serum Testing

Purpose

To demonstrate certain naturally occurring antibodies that react optimally at a lower pH than normal.

Method

1. Acidify serum by adding one volume of 0.1N HCl to four volumes serum. Mix and test acidified serum with nitrazine paper to make sure that the pH is near 6.5.

2. Let the test serum and dilution control remain at room temperature for 15 minutes.

3. Test against the same panel of cells as were used for testing unmodified serum.

4. To each tube add two drops of acidified serum and one drop of the appropriate cells. Mix.

5. Centrifuge for 15 seconds at 1000 rpm. Read and record.

6. Incubate for 30 minutes at room temperature.

7. Centrifuge for 15 seconds at 1000 rpm. Read and record.

8. Incubate for 30 minutes at 5° C.

9, Centrifuge for 15 seconds at 1000 rpm. Read and record.

Note: A dilution control should be run to be sure the antibody activity is not diluted. This control consists of one volume of isotonic saline in four volumes of serum.

REACTIONS THAT MAY MISLEAD IN THE EXAMINATION OF AGGLUTINATION TESTS

OBJECTIVES—REACTIONS THAT MAY MISLEAD IN THE EXAMINATION OF AGGLUTINATION TESTS

The student shall know, understand and be prepared to explain:

1. Rouleaux formation
2. Panagglutination
3. Polyagglutination, to include:
   (a) T-activation
   (b) Tk-activation
   (c) Tn-activation
   (d) VA polyagglutination
4. Albumin-autoagglutinating factor
5. Enzyme-autoagglutinating factor
6. Antigen on stored red cells
7. Antigen on red cells freshly washed in saline
8. Wharton's jelly
9. Prozone phenomenon
10. Colloidal silica

ROULEAUX FORMATION

Appearance. *Rouleaux formation* is a form of pseudoagglutination in which the red cells give the appearance of "stacks of coins" (Fig. 24–1). When it is heavy, rouleaux formation may be difficult to distinguish from true agglutination, especially when the cells do not all adhere together in neat piles but tend to form large clumps. Conversely, weak agglutination in colloid media can closely resemble rouleaux formation, such as in the titration of partly neutralized immune anti-A sera against A cells in a medium of serum.

Most samples of human serum, when diluted with an equal volume of saline, will not cause rouleaux formation — a fact of value in distinguishing rouleaux formation from true agglutination. Note, however, that this dilution process will also destroy weak agglutination. Other substances that have an inhibitory effect on rouleaux formation, such as glycine (Koop and Bullitt, 1945) and sodium salicylate (Ino-

kuchi, 1950), are of little practical value, since the concentrations needed to inhibit rouleaux formation also interfere with agglutination (Mollison, 1956). Adding a few drops of saline to the reaction and then mixing will usually break up rouleaux. Saline is added *after* and not *before* the reaction; if it is added before, the antibody will be diluted before it has time to react. If added after the reaction, the antibody reaction is complete and will not be affected by dilution.

Causes. Rouleaux formation is seen if red cells are allowed to sediment in their own plasma. The rate of sedimentation depends on the degree of this tendency to aggregate; therefore, rapid, intense rouleaux formation is seen in individuals with a high sedimentation rate.

Rouleaux formation is also often encountered in certain disease states involving high levels of immunoglobulin — notably myelomatosis and macroglobulinemia. It is also often seen in patients with serum protein abnormalities.

320

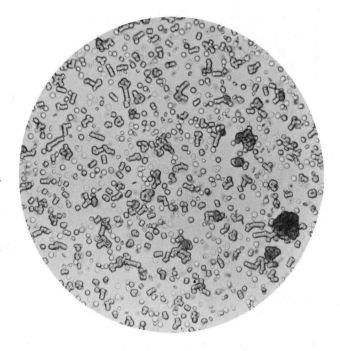

Figure 24–1   Rouleaux formation.

Certain synthetic plasma expanders can also produce rouleaux formation. Dextran, for example, when the dextran molecules exceed a certain size, can be causative (Bull *et al*, 1949). It has been suggested that a monolayer of large dextran molecules serves to increase the distance between the red cells so that there is weaker electrical repulsion. This monolayer also provides a large absorption area on the red cell surface, which provides a bridging force (Chien and Kung-Ming, 1973).

Fibrinogen (in plasma samples) has a great influence on rouleaux formation; this is yet another indication for the use of serum rather than plasma in blood grouping. Fibrinogen therapy also induces strong rouleaux formation in the recipient.

PANAGGLUTINATION

Definition. *Panagglutination* is the spontaneous agglutination of all red cells irrespective of blood group by a given serum. The phenomenon is also known as "bacteriogenic agglutination" and as the "Heubener-Thomsen phenomenon." All red cells are agglutinated — often even the red cells from the individual from whom the serum was derived.

Causes. Panagglutination is frequently a result of bacterial action and does not usually occur when blood and sera are fresh and sterile. The bacterial contaminant in the given *serum* may expose a latent receptor on the red cells known as T (see later discussion under Polyag-

glutination). This receptor then reacts with the anti-T in the given serum, causing agglutination of the red cells. Bacteriogenic agglutination of this kind can also occur in certain patients with sepsis whose red cells have become polyagglutinable.

POLYAGGLUTINATION

Strictly speaking, "polyagglutinability" means that a sample of *red cells* is agglutinated by many samples of human serum. There are several circumstances in which red cells become agglutinable due to the *exposure* of antigens that form part of the structure of the normal cell membrane, but that are usually "hidden." Those that occur *in vivo* and sometimes *in vitro* include the exposure of the T, Tk, Tn and VA antigens. Since antibodies for these four antigens are found in almost all samples of normal adult serum, the conditions are often described as polyagglutinability.

T-Activation

A latent receptor, T, contained in all human red cells, can be activated by various strains of bacteria or by enzymes derived from them. Red cells that are T-activated are agglutinated by most samples of serum from adults because the antibody, anti-T, is normally present in these sera.

T-activation may occur *in vitro*, as evidenced by the original observations of Hübener (1925), Thomsen (1927) and Friedenreich (1930), who found that suspensions of red cells might become agglutinable by ABO-compatible serum after standing at room temperature for many hours and that this agglutination was associated with infection of the suspension with certain enzyme-producing bacteria (such as corynebacteria) or with infection *in vivo*, where it usually occurs as a transient phenomenon. This has also been observed in apparently healthy subjects (see Henningsen, 1948; Reepmaker, 1952).

The characteristics of the reactions of T-activated red cells are as follows:

1. The cells are agglutinated by the sera of a proportion of adults, but are not agglutinated by most sera from newborn infants.

2. The reactions are strongest at room temperature and may be very weak or absent at 37° C.

3. Although the agglutinates may be large, many "free" red cells are normally present.

4. The reactions are strongest with fresh serum. Sometimes no reaction will be seen with serum that has been stored frozen (Stratton, 1954; Hendry and Simmons, 1955; Chorpenning and Hayes, 1959).

5. T-activated red cells react better with sera containing anti-A than with those that do not (Race and Sanger, 1975).

6. T-activated red cells fail to agglutinate with their own serum (the titer of anti-T being low due presumably to absorption by exposed T). The red cells give a negative direct antiglobulin reaction. At 37° C they are not sensitized to an antiglobulin serum by human sera, which agglutinate them at room temperature.

Other Notes about T-Activation

In general, T-activated red cells can be ABO grouped without difficulty using commercial anti-A and anti-B reagents, probably because the anti-T has been "diluted out." If problems are encountered, however, tests can be carried out strictly at 37° C, where anti-T is unlikely to interfere.

The titer of anti-T varies considerably in samples of serum from different adults. The agglutinins are not present in the serum of newborn infants but are present at the age of six months; they are quite distinct from normal cold agglutinins. Anti-T can be removed from human serum by absorption with T-activated cells. An anti-T lectin can be extracted from the peanut, *Arachis hypogaea* (Bird, 1964).

Leukocytes and platelets can also become

Table 24–1 THE REACTIONS OF DIFFERENT KINDS OF POLYAGGLUTINABLE RED CELLS*

	Arachis Hypogaea	*Dolichos Biflorus*†	*Salvia Sclaera*	*Polybrene*
T	+	0	0	0
Tk	+	0	0	+
Tn	0	+	+	+

*Modified from Bird, 1977.
†Test used only with group 0 or group B red cells.

T-activated, although this does not impair platelet function (Hysell *et al*, 1976).

Most patients with T-activated red cells do not have an associated hemolytic process, although a few such cases have been described (van Loghem, 1965; Moores *et al*, 1975; Rickard *et al*, 1969). Severe hemolytic transfusion reaction has been reported as a result of the transfusion of normal plasma containing anti-T to an infant with polyagglutinable red cells (van Loghem *et al*, 1955; Poon, Saunders and Wakelin, cited by Mollison, 1979).

T-activated red cells are deficient in sialic acid, and therefore have a reduced negative charge. For this reason, T-activated red cells are not agglutinated by polybrene, whereas normal red cells are. This can be useful in the identification of the reactions observed with polyagglutinable red cells in determining the cause (see Table 24–1).

A method of testing red cells with polybrene, taken from Issitt and Issitt (1975), is as follows:

1. Prepare a stock solution by dissolving polybrene in normal saline to a final concentration of 40 g/l. (This stock solution is stored in a plastic container at room temperature.)

2. Prepare a "working" solution containing 1 mg polybrene per ml. by diluting the stock solution 1 in 40 in saline.

3. To one drop of the working solution, add one drop of a 5 per cent suspension of red cells in a small test tube. (Normal red cells are used as a control.)

4. A positive reaction (agglutination) of the normal cells but not of the test cells indicates that the test cells are deficient in sialic acid.

Tk-Activation

Polyagglutinability of red cells due to Tk-activation is similar to T-activation in that it is a transient phenomenon associated with infection and in that the red cells are agglutinated by the lectin from peanuts. Unlike T-activated red cells, however, Tk-activated cells have normal amounts of sialic acid, as evidenced by the fact that they are agglutinated by polybrene (Bird and Wingham, 1972). This fact is used in the differentiation of the two forms of polyagglutination (see Table 24–1). Inglis *et al* (1975a, 1975b) reported that Tk activation is associated with *Bacteroides fragilis*.

Tn-Activation

Polyagglutinability due to Tn-activation differs from that due to the antigen T not only serologically but also in being *persistent* and not transient; it is *not* associated with gross infection, but rather with hematologic disorders such as acquired hemolytic anemia, leukopenia and thrombocytopenia — and may also be found in people described as always healthy. A case of probable Tn-activation *in utero* has recently been described (Wilson *et al*, 1980). The condition was first described by Moreau *et al* (1957, 1959) and the antigen was named Tn because it first appeared that the polyagglutinability observed resembled that due to T-activation. These similarities included the fact that anti-Tn, like anti-T, is present in all normal adult sera and absent from most samples of cord serum — and also that Tn red cells, like T-activated cells, are deficient in sialic acid and therefore, unlike normal red cells, are not aggregated by polybrene (Bird *et al*, 1971).

In Tn polyagglutination, only 50 per cent of the red cells may be polyagglutinable and it is therefore also known as "persistent mixed-field polyagglutination" (Myllylä *et al*, 1971). The condition is thought to be due to somatic mutation in stem cells (Bird *et al*, 1971, 1976). Tn red cells have deficiency of galactose and of alkali-labile sialic acid (Dahr *et al*, 1975). The Tn antigen is thought to be a cryptic determinant from the alkali-labile tetrasaccharide that has been isolated from human red cell glycopeptide (Dahr *et al*, 1974).

Treatment of Tn cells with papain abolishes their polyagglutinability; the effect of trypsin and ficin is not clearcut, and neuraminidase has no effect (Myllylä *et al*, 1971; Gunson *et al*, 1970). Tn cells, when injected into a normal volunteer, were noted to have a considerably shortened survival, although these same cells in the patient's own circulation were found to survive normally (Myllylä *et al*, 1971). When normal cells are transfused to a subject with Tn polyagglutination, the transfused cells survived normally and did not become Tn-positive (Hayes *et al*, 1970).

Tn red cells are agglutinated by an extract of *Dolichos biflorus* seeds (Gunson *et al*, 1970) and by snail anti-A and show a certain affinity for human anti-A (Myllylä *et al*, 1971). The Tn reaction with human anti-A and with *Dolichos biflorus* is inhibited by N-acetyl-galactosamine, which suggests that this substance may be an important determinant of Tn specificity (Bird *et al*, 1971; Myllylä *et al*, 1971).

Seed extracts are useful in distinguishing Tn from T (see Table 24–1), particularly the extract from *Salvia sclaera* (Bird and Wingham, 1973), which must be diluted to avoid nonspecific activity, but then reacts strongly with Tn cells and not at all with T-activated cells.

VA Polyagglutination

Graninger et al (1977a, 1977b) described a case of this abnormality that was associated with hemolytic anemia; the polyagglutinability was "persistent." The patient's red cells were weakly agglutinated with almost all adult sera, but only up to a temperature of 18° C. There was a depression of H receptors on the red cells and a slight (3.8 per cent) reduction in sialic acid. However, the red cells were agglutinated by polybrene because the deficiency in red cell sialic acid must exceed about 12 per cent before cells fail to be agglutinated by polybrene in a tube test (Steane, cited by Mollison, 1979). Interestingly, when the cells were treated with Anti-A$_{HP}$ (Helix somatin) and studied by immunofluorescence, a stippled appearance was observed.

ALBUMIN-AUTOAGGLUTINATING FACTOR

This factor is discussed in Chapter 19.

ENZYME-AUTOAGGLUTINATING FACTOR

Agglutinins specific for trypsin-treated, papain-treated, bromelin-treated, neuraminidase-treated and periodate-treated red cells can all be found in normal serum (Mellbye, 1969). The agglutinin for trypsin-treated red cells is the only one found in cord serum and the only one whose reactions are reversed by the addition of histidine, a factor "reversor" that occurs in normal serum after heating to 60° C for two hours. A warm hemolysin for papain-treated red cells has been found in 0.1 per cent of sera from normal subjects. This antibody does not affect the survival of red cells *in vivo* (Bell *et al*, 1973). Agglutinins reacting with bromelin-treated red cells were found in 2 per cent of normal donors by Randazzo *et al*, (1973).

In 1965, Heistö *et al* found that the serum of 94 out of 961 normal donors would hemolyse the subject's own trypsinized red cells. The hemolysin (which was shown to be inherited) was shown not to be inhibited by trypsin itself, and was twice as common in women as in men.

ANTIGEN ON STORED RED CELLS

Brendemoen (1952) described a cold agglutinin that reacted only with stored red cells. The red cells become agglutinable by this antibody after 4 to 7 days' storage at room temperature or 2 days at 37° C or 30 minutes at 56° C.

Further examples, all in patients with clinical evidence of hemolytic anemia, were described by Jenkins and Marsh (1961); Stratton *et al* (1960); and Ozer and Chaplin (1963). Another patient in whom there was no definite evidence of hemolytic anemia was described by Beaumont *et al* (1976).

Little is known about the agglutinin or its antigen, although there is no evidence to suggest that the development of the antigen on stored red cells is related to loss of sialic acid from the cells.

ANTIGEN ON RED CELLS FRESHLY WASHED IN SALINE

A panagglutinin that acts on a subject's own red cells and on other red cells only if they have been freshly washed in saline was described by Freiesleben and Jensen (1959). The agglutinin reacted best at 4° C, less well at room temperature and not at all at 37° C and reacted with stored as well as fresh cells, provided that they were freshly washed.

It was later discovered by Allan *et al* (1972), in reporting four further cases, that:

1. The reactions became negative after standing at room temperature for periods between five minutes and four hours.

2. The reactions were maximal after three saline washes.

3. The red cells did not become agglutinable after being washed in ACD or Alsever's solution.

4. The activity could be absorbed onto red cells and eluted from them.

Davey *et al* (1976) reported a further example in which it was found that the patient's plasma caused both agglutination and the binding of complement to all red cells that had been freshly washed in saline. When either donor red

cells or the patient's own cells were labeled with ^{51}Cr and then washed in saline and injected into the patient's circulation, more than 50 per cent were destroyed within one hour.

The change in the red cell membrane induced by saline washing that renders the red cells agglutinable has yet to be explained.

WHARTON'S JELLY

Wharton's jelly is usually present in cord samples that have been collected by cutting the umbilical cord and allowing the blood to drain into a collection tube. Samples contaminated with Wharton's jelly may agglutinate spontaneously (Wiener, 1943). If a sample is believed to be contaminated with Wharton's jelly, three to five saline washes will usually eliminate the reaction. If Wharton's jelly contamination is a common problem, it is best to advise the delivery room to collect cord blood samples from the umbilical vein rather than allowing the blood to drain from the cord into the collection tube. This will eliminate the problem.

PROZONE PHENOMENON

This is a phenomenon observed at times in titration of antibodies in which the antibody apparently reacts more strongly when the serum is diluted than when it is undiluted (Table 24–2). The phenomenon has often been attributed to the lack of optimal proportions between antigen and antibody, although according to Wiener (1970), it may actually occur in one of two ways:

1. It may be due to the use of fresh serum containing complement. This can be proved by inactivating the serum and re-titrating, whereupon the prozone disappears.

2. It may be due to the presence of both IgM (agglutinating) and IgG (blocking) antibodies in the same serum. This prozone will disappear if the tests are carried out in a high-viscosity medium (e.g., human AB serum, bovine albumin) in place of saline.

A prozone phenomenon is occasionally seen in the antiglobulin technique as a result of

Table 24–2 PROZONE PHENOMENON

Dilutions of Serum								
1/1	1/2	1/4	1/8	1/16	1/32	1/64	1/128	1/256
–	–	–	–	1+	2+	2+	1+	–

partial neutralization of the antiglobulin reagent.

COLLOIDAL SILICA

When solutions are stored in glass bottles (particularly if the solution is alkaline, such as trisodium citrate), they may become contaminated with colloidal silica, which may bring about nonspecific agglutination of red cells or lysis of red cells if complement is present. Colloidal silica may also coat red cells without agglutinating them, and such red cells may then agglutinate if suspected in serum.

Undiluted serum inhibits the agglutination caused by silica; however, if diluted serum is used, silica may cause false positive results when tests are performed on glass slides, when stirred with a glass rod or when mixed with another glass slide (Stratton and Renton, 1955). When stirring red cell suspensions on glass slides, a wooden stick should be used as this should avoid any problem that might otherwise arise from silica.

OTHERS

There are many other substances that cause red cells to agglutinate nonspecifically; e.g., multivalent metallic ions such as Cr^{3+}, tannic acid and $CrCl_3$ (chromic chloride). This nonspecific absorption of proteins or other antigens by tannic acid or $CrCl_3$ has been used in the technique of "passive hemagglutination" using subagglutinating doses for the detection of anti-Gm, anti-IgA and (in a slight modification) in testing plasma for the presence of the HBs antigen (see Gold and Fudenberg, 1967).

TYPICAL EXAMINATION QUESTIONS

Choose the phrase, sentence or symbol that completes the statement or answers the question. More than one answer may be correct in each case. Answers are given in the back of this book.

1. Rouleaux formation is encountered frequently when testing specimens from patients suffering from
   (a) myelomatosis
   (b) macroglobulinemia
   (c) serum protein abnormalities
   (d) leukemia
   (Rouleaux Formation)
2. Panagglutination
   (a) is the spontaneous agglutination of all red cells by a given serum
   (b) is the spontaneous agglutination of all sera by given red cells
   (c) is also known as bacteriogenic agglutination
   (d) all of the above
   (Panagglutination)
3. Anti-T
   (a) is present in 20 to 40 per cent of all adult sera
   (b) can be extracted from the peanut *Arachis hypogaea*
   (c) is present in most samples of serum from adults and newborn infants
   (d) none of the above
   (Polyagglutination)
4. Tn red cells
   (a) are agglutinated by an extract of *Dolichos biflorus* seeds
   (b) when treated with papain are not polyagglutinable

   (c) react strongly with an extract from *Salvia sclaera*
   (d) are agglutinated by snail anti-A
   (Tn Activation)
5. A warm hemolysin for papain-treated red cells has been found in:
   (a) 1 per cent of normal subjects
   (b) 2 per cent of normal subjects
   (c) 0.1 per cent of normal subjects
   (d) 1.5 per cent of normal subjects
   (Enzyme-Autoagglutinating Factor)
6. A "prozone" is
   (a) an area of the laboratory reserved for experienced workers
   (b) the delay before a transfusion reaction occurs
   (c) an antibody elution technique
   (d) none of the above
   (Prozone Phenomenon)

ANSWER TRUE OR FALSE

7. Sodium salicylate has an inhibitory effect on rouleaux formation
   (Rouleaux Formation)
8. The reaction of anti-T with T-activated red cells is strongest at 37° C and may be weak or absent at room temperature.
   (T-activation)
9. Leukocytes and platelets can become T-activated.
   (Other Notes About T-Activations)
10. The development of the antigen on *stored* red cells is related to loss of sialic acid from the cells. *(Antigen on Stored Red Cells)*

GENERAL REFERENCES

1. Erskine, A. G. and Socha, W. W.: The Principles and Practice of Blood Grouping. 2nd Ed. C. V. Mosby Company, St. Louis, 1978. *(Valuable general discussion of all areas covered in this chapter.)*

2. Mollison, P. L.: Blood Transfusion in Clinical Medicine. 6th Ed. Blackwell Scientific Publications, Oxford, 1979.

ADVERSE REACTION TO TRANSFUSION

OBJECTIVES — ADVERSE REACTION TO TRANSFUSION

The student shall know, understand and be prepared to explain:
1. Febrile transfusion reactions
2. Allergic transfusion reactions
3. Hemolytic transfusion reactions
4. Delayed hemolytic transfusion reactions
5. Bacteriogenic reactions
6. Circulatory overload
7. The transmission of disease, specifically to include:
   (a) Post-transfusion viral hepatitis
   (b) Malaria
   (c) Syphilis
8. Alloimmunization
9. Investigation of adverse reaction to transfusion

Introduction

Any unfavorable response by a patient that occurs as a result of the transfusion of blood or blood products may be classified as adverse reaction to transfusion. These are usually referred to in the laboratory as transfusion reactions, although the term is not strictly correct, because a transfusion "reaction" can be either favorable or unfavorable.

Not all adverse transfusion reactions are caused by incompatibility of the blood in terms of antigens and antibodies — in fact, this represents a relatively small percentage of all adverse reactions. In a study by R. H. Walker (cited by Mollison, 1979), adverse reactions were recorded in 6.6 per cent of recipients, of which the majority were febrile (55 per cent). There was shivering without recorded fever in 14 per cent; allergic reactions (mainly urticaria) constituted 20 per cent; 6 per cent developed serum hepatitis; 4 per cent had a hemolytic reaction and 1 per cent had circulatory overload.

The account of the various types of adverse transfusion reactions given here is not intended as an in-depth coverage of the subject. The interested reader is referred to Mollison (1979)

(see General References at the end of this chapter) for such coverage.

FEBRILE REACTIONS

A febrile transfusion reaction is one in which the patient develops fever and chills during or after the transfusion of blood or blood products, but has none of the other more serious signs of adverse transfusion reaction. The rise in temperature may be due to leukocyte antibodies, platelet antibodies or pyrogens.

Leukocyte Antibodies. Brittingham and Chaplin (1957) clearly showed the role of leukocytes in causing adverse transfusion reactions in patients with leukocyte antibodies. They transfused five patients who had a history of severe febrile reactions following blood transfusion and whose serum contained leukoagglutinins with two extracts of blood from the same donor — one containing more than 90 per cent of the buffy coat and the other containing less than 10 per cent of the buffy coat. The transfusion of the unit containing 90 per cent of the buffy coat resulted in severe febrile reactions, characterized by flushing within five minutes of the start of the transfusion, with a feeling of warmth, presumably due to complement activation. This was followed, one hour later, by chills, severe hypotension with cyanosis, increased respiratory rate, fibrinolysis and fever. The transfusion of the unit containing less than 10 per cent of the buffy coat, on the other hand, caused no reaction.

Subsequent complementary observations were made by Payne (1957), who found leukoagglutinins in 32 out of 49 patients with a history of febrile reactions. Perkins *et al* (1961) reported that the degree of temperature elevation was related to the number of incompatible leukocytes transfused.

Platelet Antibodies. The role of platelets in causing adverse transfusion reaction is difficult to assess, since platelet suspensions are always contaminated to some extent with leukocytes and also since platelet alloantibodies are usually associated with leukocyte antibodies. There is, however, no doubt that the destruction of platelets by alloantibodies may cause adverse reactions, as was evidenced by Aster and Jandl (1964). They transfused $P_1^{B_1}$-negative recipients with P_1-positive platelets and, a day or two later, with serum containing anti-$P_1^{B_1}$. Three out of four of these patients developed frontal headache after 30 minutes and rigors (which lasted 15 to 30 minutes) after 45 to 50 minutes followed by fever.

Marchal *et al* (1960) and Cooper *et al* (1975) described cases in which severe febrile reactions were almost certainly caused by incompatible platelets, but may have been partly caused by contamination with transfused leukocytes.

Pyrogens. Certain solutions and chemical substances (e.g., citrate, sodium chloride) may be contaminated with bacterial polysaccharides known as *pyrogens* (i.e., foreign substances including waste products of bacterial growth). When pyrogenic substances are transfused, a febrile reaction occurs, characterized by increased blood pressure, chills, fever, nausea, headache and back pain.

Pyrogenic reactions can be virtually eliminated by the use of plastic infusion sets and blood bags, provided that care is taken in the preparation of solutions to avoid contamination.

Methods of Avoiding or Suppressing Febrile Reactions

Crossmatching. In giving leukocyte transfusions, the donor leukocytes should be crossmatched against the recipient's serum. This is partly to avoid reactions but is also considered necessary because incompatible antibodies inhibit the bactericidal power of granulocytes (Goldstein *et al*, 1971).

Use of Leukocyte-Poor Blood. Perkins *et al* (1966) concluded that the least number of leukocytes that would produce an adverse reaction in a recipient with leukoagglutinins varied from 0.25×10^9 to more than 2.5×10^9. In preparing leukocyte-poor blood for transfusion to these patients, therefore, the aim should be to remove at least 90 per cent of the leukocytes. A discussion of leukocyte-poor blood and a method of preparation is found in Chapter 18.

Microfiltration. Wenz *et al* (1979) studied 45 patients with a history of febrile reaction due to leukoagglutinins by transfusing these patients with a total of 212 units of centrifuged, microaggregate-filtered red cells. The microaggregate filter used had a standard pore size of 40 microns. This size was found to reduce the total white cell mass by 60 per cent and virtually eliminated granulocytes in the majority of units. The mean postfiltration white blood cell count was $8 \pm 3.7 \times 10^8$ per unit, which is below the mean value for leukocyte-induced febrile reactions observed by Perkins *et al* (1966). The frequency of febrile reactions in these patients was decreased by 95 per cent.

Drugs. Smith (1940) and Altschule and Freidberg (1945) showed that pyrogenic reactions could be modified by the previous administration of antipyretic drugs. Dare and Mogey 1945) found that one gram of aspirin administered at the onset of shivering had the same effect. Jandl and Tomlinson (1958) reported that one gram of aspirin given one hour before transfusion was also effective. Leverenz *et al* (1975) found that administration of more than 50 mg of prednisolone a day prevented febrile transfusion reactions, as did 50 mg of cortisone given orally every 6 hours for up to 48 hours before transfusion (Jandl and Tomlinson, 1958).

Antihistamines, on the other hand, do not appear to prevent febrile reactions (see Wilhelm *et al*, 1955; Hobsley, 1958).

Others. The severity of febrile transfusion reactions can probably be mitigated by warming the patient (see Altschule and Freidberg, 1945). A moderate *rate* of transfusion can also be of significance in reducing the severity of febrile reactions (see Grant and Reeve, 1951).

ALLERGIC REACTIONS

The most common type of allergic reaction is one in which wheals develop on the body (urticaria) during or following transfusion. A severe allergic (or anaphylactic-type) reaction in which the patient has flushing of the skin, dyspnea and hypotension is rare — the incidence has been given as 1 per 20,000 transfusions (Bjerrum and Jersild, 1971). Milder allergic reactions (sometimes described as "anaphylactoid") characterized by urticaria have been reported to have an incidence of approximately 3 per cent (Stephen *et al*, 1955). Many of these are of little importance, since often the wheals do not itch and are almost certain to be overlooked unless they occur on an exposed part of the body. In general, however, if mild urticaria is noted, the transfusion should be discontinued.

Probably the commonest cause of severe anaphylactic reactions following transfusion is the interaction between transfused IgA and class-specific anti-IgA in the recipient's plasma (for full discussion see Mollison, 1979, pp. 626–629). The relative importance of other antigens and antibodies known to be or suspected of being associated with milder (anaphylactoid) reactions is little understood. These include IgG-anti-IgG (see Barandun *et al*, 1962), IgM-anti-IgM (Ropars *et al*, 1973), human albumin (Ring and Messmer, 1977), atopens (Maunsell, 1944), hypersensitivity to passively acquired antibodies (see Ramirez, 1919), passively acquired penicillin antibody (McGinnis and Goldfinger, 1971) and sensitivity to nickel (Stoddart, 1960).

It has been shown that antihistamines such as diphenhydramine (Benadryl) are effective in reducing the incidence of allergic reactions. These should be given by mouth or, if necessary, by injection to patients with a history of previous allergic manifestations, one hour before transfusion and a further 50 mg after the start of transfusion. If an allergic response develops in a patient who has not been given antihistamines prophylactically, 25 mg of diphenhydramine or 10 mg of chlorpheniramine may be given intravenously. This prophylaxis refers primarily to the suppression of urticarial reactions. If a severe allergic reaction occurs, epinephrine should be given.

Alternatively, patients who are known to have severe allergic reactions may be given steroids prophylactically (Fox *et al*, 1958) or may be transfused with washed red cells or platelets (Silvergleid *et al*, 1977).

HEMOLYTIC TRANSFUSION REACTIONS

Introduction

A hemolytic transfusion reaction refers to the destruction of red cells following and as a result of the transfusion of incompatible blood. In addition, hemolytic transfusion reactions may be caused by the following:

1. Transfusion of red cells damaged by exposure to 5 per cent dextrose
2. Injection of water into the circulation
3. Transfusion of hemolyzed blood
4. Transfusion of overheated blood
5. Transfusion of frozen blood
6. Transfusion of infected blood
7. Transfusion of blood under great pressure

Fairley (1940) suggested the recognition of two types of red cell destruction — *intravascular* and *extravascular*. Intravascular destruction refers to the rupture of red cells within the blood stream, with consequent liberation of hemoglobin into the plasma. Extravascular destruction refers to the removal of red cells from the blood stream by the cells of the reticuloendothelial system.

Hemolytic Transfusion Reactions Involving Intravascular Red Cell Destruction

The most common cause of intravascular red cell destruction is the transfusion of incompatible red cells to a patient whose plasma contains an antibody directed against an antigen on the transfused red cells, which is capable of causing rapid activation of complement (e.g., anti-A or anti-B). In such cases, the complement activation sequence proceeds from the EAC1 to the EAC9 stage causing the hemolysis of the transfused cells at, or near to, the site of infusion.

The signs of intravascular red cell destruction include flushing, a feeling of apprehension, fever, chills, burning sensation at the site of infusion, nausea, vomiting, feeling of chest restriction, back pain and shock (often severe and life threatening). If the reaction is not checked through discontinuing the transfusion, hemoglobinemia, hemoglobinuria, hypotension, disseminated intravascular coagulation, acute renal failure and death can result.

The type of reaction described is most likely to be caused by antibodies of the ABO blood group system, which are rapidly lytic *in vitro*. Antibodies that are slowly lytic *in vitro* (e.g., Lewis antibodies) may also cause intravascular red cell destruction, but the incidence of this is low, presumably due to the fact that the cells are cleared by the reticuloendothelial system before they have had time to be lysed.

Oddly, the most common cause of hemolytic transfusion reaction involving intravascular red cell destruction is the administration of the wrong blood to the recipient owing to inadequate patient identification, clerical error, and so forth.

Hemolytic Transfusion Reactions Involving Extravascular Red Cell Destruction

Antibodies that are nonhemolytic *in vitro* bring about destruction of red cells that is predominantly *extravascular* (outside of the blood vessels) but that is characteristically accompanied by some degree of hemoglobinemia. In such cases, the antibody attaches to the corresponding antigen on the red cells, rendering them susceptible to destruction by tissue bound macrophages, as follows: the macrophages can be considered in this instance as cells that attempt to remove the protein (IgG or C3) from the red cell. In the process of tearing off the protein, however, irreversible damage is caused to the red cells, which may become fragmented or deformed or may become spheroidal, probably as a result of the removal of part of the red cell membrane by the macrophages in their attempt to remove the abnormal protein. When red cells become fragmented, deformed or spheroidal, their membrane area is reduced but their internal content is not altered; they therefore become inflexible and rigid, and as such are not able to pass through the microcapillaries in the liver and spleen. The red cells are thus trapped in these organs and removed from the circulation.

The signs of extravascular red cell destruction are similar to those seen in reactions involving intravascular destruction, although they are generally less severe. Fever and chills are most common, although these may not occur until some time after the transfusion is over. Jaundice is also seen in many patients after transfusion. The hemoglobinemia that is fairly commonly seen is thought to be caused by the damage to the red cells as a result of contact with macrophages.

Extravascular red cell destruction is commonly caused by Rh antibodies but can also be caused by other IgG, nonagglutinating, noncomplement-binding forms of antibodies directed against antigens such as K, k, S, Fy[a].

OTHER CAUSES OF HEMOLYTIC TRANSFUSION REACTION

Hemolytic transfusion reactions, as mentioned, can be caused by a number of factors besides red cell incompatibility.

Exposure to 5 Per Cent Dextrose. Patients receiving transfusions of whole blood passed through a bottle containing 5 per cent dextrose in 0.225 per cent saline have been reported to have hemolytic transfusion reactions (Ebaugh *et al*, 1958, cited by DeCesare *et al*, 1964). Although it may appear obvious that the mechanism was simply cell-swelling on exposure to hypertonic solution followed by rupture on return to the circulation, studies by DeCesare *et al* (1964) revealed that cells swollen to 155 per cent of their normal volume survived normally. These same workers also reported that red cells exposed to a solution containing 5 per cent dextrose and 0.9 per cent saline survived normally after reinjection into the circulation. They concluded that glucose was not responsible for the effects they had observed. Jones *et al* (1962) also showed that loss of red cells did not always follow immediately on reinjection into the circulation of red cells exposed to 5 per cent dextrose in 0.225 per cent saline, as would be expected if the effects were due solely to the fact that in glucose solutions the cells became hypertonic and subsequently ruptured by osmotic lysis after exposure to normal plasma. It was therefore concluded that exposure of red cells to 5 per cent glucose not only makes them hypertonic but also produces some kind of damage that has yet to be explained.

Injection of Water into the Circulation. Red cells are damaged by the intravenous injection of water into the circulation of a human adult. In two patients described by J. Wallace (cited by Mollison, 1979) who were accidentally given 1.5 to 2 liters of distilled water by rapid intravenous injection during the Second World War, rigors, hemoglobinuria and persistent hypotension developed and both patients became oliguric and died.

Transfusion of Hemolyzed Blood. Hemoglobinemia as a result of the injection of free hemoglobin into the circulation may be misinterpreted as a sign of intravascular hemolysis. Free hemoglobin may be injected in the following circumstances:

Overheating. At a temperature of 50° C or higher, red cells hemolyze. This can occur if blood is warmed prior to infusion in a vessel containing hot water — and for this reason, blood should *not* be warmed before transfusion. If there is thought to be a good justification for warming blood, the temperature of the water used for this purpose must be carefully monitored to ensure that it does not exceed body temperature.

Freezing. If blood freezes in an unregulated refrigerator, it may be severely hemolyzed when it is subsequently thawed. Blood that has been hemolyzed in this way has a purple appearance, which should provide a warning.

Infection. Blood becomes grossly hemolyzed when contaminated with certain bacteria, with hemoglobinuria produced if such blood is transfused. Of course, this effect is relatively insignificant compared to the toxic effects of bacteria.

Injection Under Pressure. Red cells may rupture as a result of being forced through a needle with considerable pressure (see example cited by Macdonald and Berg, 1959).

Transfusion of Blood Containing Antibody. Adverse transfusion reaction can occur when antibody transfused in the donor's plasma is directed against an antigen on the recipient's red cells. This type of reaction is virtually never serious, since the antibody is subject to dilution in the recipient's plasma and since the antibody is rapidly used up because of the gross excess of antigen. One consideration of this type of incompatibility is the transfusion of group O blood to group A, B or AB recipients, in whom the amount of antibody passively transferred increases with each unit given. In such cases, the cumulative effects of many transfusions may eventually lead to red cell destruction. It should also be noted that the transfusion of group O blood having hemolytic anti-A and anti-B (i.e., hemolysin positive) can cause rapid red cell destruction and even death.

DELAYED HEMOLYTIC TRANSFUSION REACTION

On some occasions when incompatible blood has been transfused, a weak antibody in the recipient may be incapable of causing rapid, immediate red cell destruction, but the transfusion may provoke an anamnestic (secondary) immune response. The antibody concentration increases a few days after transfusion, causing rapid destruction on the transfused red cells at that time. In most cases the patient has been primarily immunized by previous transfusion, although sometimes the only previous stimulus has been a pregnancy. Generally, the antibody is too weak to be detected in routine crossmatch tests but becomes detectable about three to seven days after transfusion.

Howard (1973), in reviewing 21 published papers, found that of the 43 antibodies found to cause delayed hemolytic transfusion reaction, 19 were within the Rh system and 14 were within the Kidd system. The remaining 10 had various other specificities, and in 38 per cent of the cases more than one antibody was detected.

Sixty-nine per cent of the reactions occurred in women.

Clinically, there are no signs of red cell destruction at the time of transfusion and for a variable number of days afterward. At this time there is a rapid fall in hemoglobin concentration and a rise in serum bilirubin that may reach levels at which the patient becomes clinically jaundiced. This jaundice most commonly is seen on days five to seven after transfusion (Pinkerton *et al*, 1959; Stuckey *et al*, 1964; Joseph *et al*, 1964; Day *et al*, 1965; Rauner and Tanaka, 1967; Morgan *et al*, 1967). However, this may occur as late as 10 days after transfusion (Croucher *et al*, 1967). In some cases, hemoglobinuria may occur, after an average interval of 7.9 days (Mollison, 1979, averaging the results of 15 reported cases). Renal failure associated with delayed hemolytic transfusion reaction is very rare. On the other hand, spherocytosis is often noted in blood films taken from patients during a delayed hemolytic reaction, and may be the first indication that red cell destruction is occurring.

BACTERIOGENIC REACTIONS

Adverse transfusion reactions may be caused by bacteria that may contaminate solutions or equipment before sterilization. The solutions or equipment, after sterilization, then remain contaminated with heat-stable bacterial *products*. Alternatively, bacteria may survive sterilization or may contaminate solutions after they have been properly sterilized. Or they may gain entrance to the blood container during venisection. These reactions may be due to pyrogens, to contamination at the time of blood collection, or to flaws in the blood container.

Contamination at the Time of Blood Collection. When a normal donation of blood is mixed with a relatively small volume of citrate, any organisms present are usually killed so that the blood is normally sterile (Spooner, 1942). In examining 1700 samples of fresh bank blood (stored at 4° C for only 24 hours) Braude *et al* (1952) found that 2.2 per cent of the samples were contaminated. With a longer period of storage, most of these contaminants would probably have died, however, because they were mostly staphylococci presumably growing preferentially at 37° C (Mollison, 1979).

Flaws in the Blood Container. Blood may become contamined due to very small cracks in glass bottles or pinhole lesions in plastic bags, which allow organisms to gain entrance into the container.

Transfusion reactions due to contamination can be severe, dramatic and often fatal. The reaction is characterized by the rapid onset of chills, high fever, vomiting, diarrhea, marked hypotension and often acute renal tubular necrosis. Gram-negative organisms capable of proliferation at refrigerator storage temperatures are most often implicated.

In order to minimize the risk of infection of blood, the following precautions should be strictly observed:

1. Blood should be maintained at refrigerator temperature at all times during storage.

2. The container should not be opened or punctured to obtain a sample.

3. The recommended storage time must not be exceeded.

4. Components prepared by "open" procedures must be used within 24 hours.

5. Blood should be examined routinely for unusual color or the presence of hemolysis, both of which may suggest bacterial contamination.

CIRCULATORY OVERLOAD

This type of transfusion reaction may result from the transfusion of a patient with a normal blood volume, but a reduced red cell volume. In simple terms, the total circulatory volume becomes too great for the pumping action of the heart and may precipitate congestive heart failure manifested by coughing, cyanosis and difficulty in breathing. Patients with normal blood volumes (who are therefore susceptible to circulatory overload) should be transfused with packed red blood cells at a rate no faster than 1 ml per kilogram of body weight per hour (Marriott and Kekwick, 1940).

TRANSMISSION OF DISEASE

Post-Transfusion Viral Hepatitis

The occasional occurrence of post-transfusion hepatitis remains a serious consequence of blood transfusion. Many blood components such as plasma, platelets, cryoprecipitate (factor VIII concentrate), factor IX concentrate and fibrinogen are capable of transmitting hepatitis — the risk being proportional to the number of donors whose blood is used to prepare the component. On the other hand, some components (albumin, plasma protein fraction and immunoglobulin preparations) can be regarded as "safe" derivatives, since hepatitis virus is usually inactivated or removed during preparation.

Tests for the hepatitis B surface antigen (HBsAg) have allowed detection of most carriers of hepatitis B virus, yet it has become clear that much work and research is still required before post-transfusion hepatitis is completely prevented. Hepatitis A virus, the agent of *infective* hepatitis, seems to be a relatively uncommon cause of post-transfusion hepatitis; in fact, most of the cases of hepatitis now seen following transfusion with blood screened for HBsAg by certain routine techniques (i.e., radioimmunoassay or reversed passive hemagglutination) is not caused by either hepatitis A or hepatitis B virus (Alter *et al*, 1975).

Antigens and Antibodies Associated with Hepatitis B Virus

An antigen, originally called Australia antigen, was first recognized in the serum of an Australian aborigine by Blumberg *et al* (1965) and was thought to have an association with acute leukemia. The association of the antigen with hepatitis was realized three years later by Prince (1968) and by Blumberg *et al* (1968). The complete hepatitis B virus consists of a 27 nm nucleocapsid DNA-containing core surrounded by an outer lipoprotein coat, and is known as the *Dane particle*, which has a diameter of 42 nm (Fig. 25–1). The "Australia antigen" is now known to be unassembled viral coat, or surface antigen, and is termed HS_sAg^* (hepatitis B surface antigen). The core carries an independent antigen known as HB_cAg (hepatitis B core antigen). The antibodies to the surface antigen and to the core antigen are known as anti-HB_s and anti-HB_c, respectively. A soluble antigen

---

*Terminology is that of WHO, 1977.

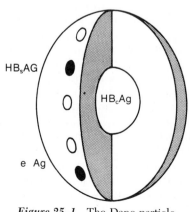

Figure 25–1 The Dane particle.

(which is also particle associated) known as HB_eAg is found only in some sera containing HB_sAg— its presence appears to be related to the degree of infectivity of the serum. It appears that there is a correlation between HB_eAg, DNA polymerase (which, with double-stranded DNA, makes up the core), Dane particle count and infectivity (Tong *et al*, 1977; Hindman *et al*, 1976). Anti-HB_c occurs in a majority of sera containing HB_sAg from voluntary blood donors and can be detected, as can HB_cAg, by radioimmunoassay.

Transmission by Transfusion

The incidence of HB_sAg among voluntary blood donors in the United States and Canada is about 0.1 per cent (Wallace *et al*, 1972; Cherubin and Prince, 1971). Among paid donors, however, the incidence of positives is about ten times greater (Walsh *et al*, 1970; Cherubin and Prince, 1971). This may be due to the fact that the practice of paying donors tends to attract a proportion of undesirable donors such as alcoholics or drug addicts, in whom the risk of hepatitis B is high. The commercial blood donor also is less likely to give an accurate history of his present and past health.

Because there is currently no known, completely effective method for detecting the infectivity of all blood products capable of transmitting hepatitis, the disease remains a lethal complication of blood transfusion. Murray (1955) and Drake *et al* (1952) found that minimum infective dose of plasma from a carrier (given by subcutaneous or intravenous injection) that could transmit the disease was 1×10^{-6} ml. and 4×10^{-5} respectively. Of the tests available for the detection of HB_sAg, radioimmunoassay is the most sensitive (see Chapter 23 for details of this technique).

Other Notes on the Hepatitis Viruses

Incubation Period. In post-transfusion hepatitis due to hepatitis B virus, the incubation period was taken as 60 to 180 days by the World Health Organization (1973). It is now thought that cases with an incubation period of more than 120 days are rare. The incubation period of non-A, non-B post-transfusion hepatitis has been reported to be 51 days (14 to 105 days) by Feinstone *et al* (1975) and 56 days (37 to 75 days) by Prince (1975). In the occasional case due to virus A, the incubation period is about 30

days (Purcell *et al*, 1975; Hollinger *et al*, 1977).

Effect of Heat on Hepatitis B Virus. Although human serum albumin when heated to 60° C for 10 hours is usually incapable of transmitting hepatitis B virus, serum (and possibly plasma protein solution) when subjected to the same conditions might still be capable of transmitting the virus, especially when heavily contaminated.

MALARIA

Malaria, when transmitted by transfusion, is occasionally fatal. Malaria parasites of all species can remain viable in stored blood for at least a week (Hutton and Shute, 1939) and sometimes, although rarely, for up to two weeks (Bruce-Chwatt, 1974). The requirements of the AABB with respect to donors who may transmit malaria are outlined in Chapter 17. The indirect fluorescent antibody test for the detection of occult malaria infection may prove useful if possible carriers have to be used as donors of whole blood. Prophylactic treatment of donors or recipients of blood or both with chloroquine also appears to be effective in preventing the transmission of malaria.

Malaria can be transmitted by transfusion of fresh plasma, presumably because the product contains a few intact red cells (Lozner and Newhouser, 1943; see also Dike, 1970). Frozen or dried plasma, however, has never been known to transmit malaria.

SYPHILIS

Blood that is fresh (i.e., less than four days old) can transmit syphilis to the recipient. Citrated blood stored at 2 to 6° C for more than four days, however, is unlikely to transmit syphilis, and can be considered virtually safe from this point of view, since the causative spirochetes are unable to survive these conditions. Few cases of post-transfusion syphilis are seen nowadays as a result both of refrigeration of blood before administration and of routine testing of all blood donations.

OTHER DISEASES

Other diseases that may be transmitted by transfusion include cytomegalovirus infection (see Diosi *et al*, 1969; Perham *et al*, 1971; see also Mollison, 1979), infectious mononucleosis (Solem and Jörgensen, 1969; Turner *et al*, 1972) brucellosis (Wood, 1955), Chagas' disease (Rohwedder, 1969), trypanosomiasis and leishmaniasis (see Wolfe, 1974).

ALLOIMMUNIZATION

The transfusion of blood products always entails exposure to foreign antigens, which may result in alloimmunization to red blood cell, leukocyte and platelet antigens lacking in the patient. The probability of stimulating one or more antibodies to red cell antigens after one blood transfusion has been estimated to be about 1 per cent (Giblett, 1961).

INVESTIGATION OF ADVERSE REACTION TO TRANSFUSION

Suggested Procedure

When notification of an adverse reaction is received, the following procedure is recommended.
1. Check all relevant paperwork — the number of units transfused, the identity of the patient, the crossmatching results, records of previous transfusions, and so forth. Ensure that the transfusion was without fault through any clerical error.
2. The following specimens are required:
    (a) Pre-reaction blood specimen from the recipient
    (b) Post-reaction blood specimen from the recipient (anticoagulated and clot tubes)
    (c) Blood from the integral donor tubing or container implicated in the reaction

    (d) Post-transfusion urine (spun specimen)
3. Perform the following procedures:
    (a) Examine for visible hemolysis in all specimens. In the case of the post-reaction blood specimen from the patient, use the anticoagulated tube, because it is less likely to show spurious *in vitro* hemolysis and can be more rapidly evaluated (centrifuge and observe).
    (b) Repeat the ABO typing on specimens a, b and c.
    (c) Repeat the Rh typing on specimens a, b and c.
    (d) Perform a direct antiglobulin test on specimens a and b.
    (e) Repeat the crossmatch (major and minor) and the antibody screening using specimens a, b and c.
    (f) If irregular antibodies are detected, identify the antibodies. If antibodies are detected in the post-reaction blood specimen from the recipient (b) and not in the pre-reaction blood specimen (a), verify the presence of the implicated red cell antigen in the donor specimen (c) and the lack of this antigen on the recipient's red cells (specimen a).
    (g) Perform a bacteriologic smear and culture on specimen c.
4. In addition to these tests, the following optional procedures may prove to be informative.
    (a) Haptoglobin (specimens a and b)
    (b) Methemalbumin (specimens a and b)
    (c) Bilirubin (specimen b)
    (d) Creatinine
    (e) Direct antiglobulin test (specimen c)
    (f) Tests for leukocyte and platelet antibodies (specimens a and b)
    (g) Tests for antibodies to IgA (specimens a and b)

TYPICAL EXAMINATION QUESTIONS

Choose the phrase, sentence or symbol that answers the question or completes the statement. More than one answer may be correct in each case. Answers are given in the back of this book.

1. Febrile transfusion reactions may be due to
    (a) leukocyte antibodies in the recipient
    (b) platelet antibodies in the recipient
    (c) pyrogens in solutions or chemical substances
    (d) all of the above
    (Febrile Reactions)

2. The incidence of allergic transfusion reactions can be reduced by
    (a) administration of anti-histamines
    (b) prophylactic administration of steroids
    (c) use of washed red cells
    (d) transfusion of heated blood
    (Allergic Reactions)
3. Intravascular red cell destruction may be caused by antibodies of the
    (a) Rh blood group system
    (b) ABO blood group system
    (c) Duffy blood group system

(d) Kell blood group system
   (*Hemolytic Transfusion Reactions Involving*
        Intravascular Red Cell Destruction)
4. Bacteriogenic transfusion reactions may be caused by
   (a) pyrogens
   (b) contamination at time of blood collection
   (c) contamination of blood after transfusion
   (d) flaws (cracks) in the blood container
                    (*Bacteriogenic Reactions*)
5. Which of the following diseases is not transmitted by transfusion?
   (a) malaria
   (b) leukemia
   (c) syphilis
   (d) infectious mononucleosis
                    (*Transmission of Disease*)
6. Which of the following types of adverse transfusion reaction is most commonly encountered in modern blood tranfusion practice?
   (a) allergic

(b) pyrogenic
(c) febrile
(d) hemolytic

                    (*Introduction*)

Answer True or False

7. Extravascular red cell destruction is commonly caused by Rh antibodies.
   Hemolytic Transfusion Reactions Involving
        Extravascular Red Cell Destruction
8. Delayed hemolytic transfusion reaction occurs more commonly in women than in men.
   Delayed Hemolytic Transfusion Reaction
9. The incidence of HB_sAg among voluntary blood donors in the United States is 1 per cent.
   (*Post-Transfusion Viral Hepatitis-Transmission*
        by Transfusion)
10. Malaria can be transmitted by transfusion of frozen plasma.
                    (*Malaria*)

GENERAL REFERENCES

Many related texts contain information regarding adverse reaction to transfusion. Mollison (1979) is undoubtedly the most comprehensive. The texts that have proven most useful in the preparation of this chapter include:

1. Bryant, N. J.: Laboratory Immunology and Serology. W. B. Saunders Co. Phila., 1978. (*Information re syphilis and hepatitis.*)
2. Issitt, P. D. and Issitt, C. H.: Applied Blood Group Serology. 2nd Ed. Spectra Biologicals, 1975. (*Comprehensive discussion on intravascular and extravascular red cell destruction. Chapter 24 is devoted to transfusion reactions.*)
3. Mollison, P. L.: Blood Transfusion in Clinical Medicine. 6th Ed. Blackwell Scientific Publications, Oxford, 1979.
4. Technical Manual of the American Association of Blood Banks, 7th Edition, AABB, Washington, 1977.

LITERATURE REFERENCES

Abbal, M.: Les substances inhibitrices des anti-I et anti-I des liquides biologiques humains et animaux. Thesis, Université Paul Sabatier, Toulouse, 1971.

Abelson, N. M., and Rawson, A. J.: Studies of blood group antibodies, V. Fractionation of examples of anti-B, anti-A,B, anti-M, anti-P, anti-JA^a, anti-Le^a, anti-D, anti-CD, anti-K, anti-Fy^a and anti-Good. Transfusion 1:116, 1961.

Abraham, G. N., Petz. L. D., and Fudenberg, H. H.: Immunohematological cross-allergenicity between penicillin and cephalothin in humans. Clin. Exp. Immunol. 3:343, 1968.

Abramson, N. and Schur, P. H.: The IgG subclasses of red cell antibodies and relationship to monocyte binding. Blood 40:500, 1972.

Adams, J., Broviac, M., Brooks, W., Johnson, N. R. and Issitt, P. D.: An antibody, in the serum of a Wr(a+) individual, reacting with an antigen of very high frequency. Transfusion 11:290, 1971.

Adinolfi, A., Mollison, P. L., Polley, M. J. and Rose, J. M.: γA-blood group antibodies. J. Exp. Med. 123:951, 1966.

Adinolfi, M., Polley, M. J., Hunter, D. A. and Mollison, P. L.: Classification of blood group antibodies as β_2M or gamma globulin. Immunology 5:566, 1962.

Agote, L.: Nuevo procedimiento para la transfusion de la sangre. Ann. Inst. Modelo. Clin. Med. (Buenos Aires, November 1–3), 1915.

Ahn, Y. S.: Platelet transfusions in clinical medicine. Adv. Intern. Med. 20:379, 1975.

Ahrons, S.: HL-A antibodies: influence on the human fetus. Tissue Antigens 1:129, 1971.

Akerblom, O.: Evaluation of frozen blood preserved as ACD-adenine blood prior to freezing. International Working Conference on the Freeze-preservation of Blood. Office of Naval Research, Washington, D.C., 1967.

Akerblom, O., De Verdier, C.-H., Finnson, M., Garby, L., L., Högman, C. F. and Johansson, S. G. O.: Further studies on the effect of adenine in blood preservation. Transfusion 7:1, 1967.

Albrey, J. A., Vincent, E. E. R., Hutchinson, J., Marsh, W. L., Allen, F. H., Jr., Gavin, J., and Sanger, R.: A new antibody, anti-Fy3, in the Duffy blood group system. Vox Sang. 20:29, 1971.

Allan, C. J., Lawrence, R. D., Shih, S. C., Williamson, K. R., Sweatt, M. A. and Taswell, H. F.: Agglutination of erythrocytes freshly washed with saline solution. Four saline-autoagglutinating sera. Transfusion 12:306, 1972.

Allen, F. H.: Selection of blood for exchange transfusion in erythroblastosis fetalis. Proc. 11th Congr. Int. Soc. Blood Trans., Sydney, 1968, p. 241

Allen, F. H., and Lewis, S. J.: Kp^a (Penney), a new antigen in the Kell blood group system. Vox Sang. 2:81–87, 1957.

Allen, F. H. Marsh, W. L., Jensen, L. and Fink, J.: Anti-IP: another antibody defining a product of interaction be-tween the genes of the I and P blood group systems. Vox Sang. 27:442–446, 1974.

Allen, F. H. Jr., Issitt, P., Degnant, T., Jackson, V., Reinart, J., Knowlin, R. and Adelbane, M.: Further observations on the Matuhasi-Ogata phenomenon. Vox Sang. 16:47, 1969.

Allen, F. H., Jr., Madden, H. J. and King, R. W.: The MN gene MU, which produces M and U but no N, S or s. Vox Sang. 8:549–556, 1963.

Allen, F. H., Krabbe Sissel, M. R. and Corcoran P. A.: A new phenotype (McLeod) in the Kell blood-group system. Vox Sang. 6:555–560, 1961.

Allen, F. H., Jr., Corcoran, P. A. and Ellis, F. R.: Some new observations on the MN system. Vox Sang. 5:224, 1960.

Allen, F. H., Corcoran, P. A., Kenton, H. B. and Breare, N.: M^g, a new blood group antigen in the MNS system. Vox Sang. 3:81–91, 1958.

Allen, F. H., Jr., Diamond, L. K. and Niedziela, B.: A new blood-group antigen. Nature 167:482, 1951.

Allgood, J. W. and Chaplin, H.: Idiopathic acquired autoimmune hemolytic anemia: a review of 47 cases treated from 1955 through 1965. Am. J. Med. 43:254, 1967.

Alter, A. A. and Rosenfield, R. E.: The nature of some subtypes of A. Blood 23:605, 1964.

Alter, A. A., Gelb, A. G., Chown, B., Rosenfield, R. E. and Cleghorn, T. E.: Gonzales (Go^a), a new blood group character. Transfusion 7:88–91, 1967.

Alter, A. A., Gelb, A. G. and Lee, St. L.: Hemolytic disease of the newborn caused by a new antibody (anti-Go^a). Proc. 9th Congr. Int. Soc. Blood Trans., Mexico, 1962, 341–343, 1964.

Alter, H. J., Purcell, R. H., Holland, P. V., Feinstone, S. M., Morrow, A. G. and Moritsugu, Y.: Clinical and serological analysis of transfusion-associated hepatitis. Lancet ii:838, 1975.

Altschule, M. D. and Freidberg, A. S.: Circulation and respiration in fever. Medicine 24:403, 1945.

Ambrus, M. and Bajtai, G.: A case of an IgG-type cold agglutinin disease. Hematologia 3:225, 1969.

Ames, A. C. and Lloyd, R. S.: A scheme for the antenatal prediction of ABO hemolytic disease of the newborn. Vox Sang. 9:712, 1964.

Amiel, J. F.: Study of the leukocyte phenotypes in Hodgkin's disease. In Curtoni, E. S., Mattiuz, P. L., and Tosi, R. M. (eds): Histocompatibility Testing 1967. Munksgaard, Copenhagen, 1967, pp. 79–81.

Amos, D. B.: Genetics of the HLA system in the biology and function of the major histocompatibility complex. AABB, November 1980, presented at 33rd Annual Meeting, AABB.

Andersen, J.: Modifying influence of the secretor gene on the development of the ABH substance. A contribution of the conception of the Lewis group system. Vox Sang. 3:251–261, 1958.

Andersen, J. and Munk-Andersen, G.: Cited by Kissmeyer-Nielsen, F. (1965). 1957.

Anderson, C., Hunter, J., Zipursky, A., Lewis, M. and Chown, B.: Antibody defining a new blood group antigen, Bu[a]. Transfusion 3:30–33, 1963.

Anderson, L. D., Race G. J. and Owen, M.: Presence of anti-D antibody in an Rh (D)-positive person. Am. J. Clin. Pathol. 30:228–229, 1958.

André R. and Salmon, C.: Étude sérologique comparée de neuf exemples non apparentés de groupe sanguin "A faible." Rev. Hémat. 12:668, 1957.

Andresen, P. H.: Relations between the ABO, secretor/nonsecretor, and Lewis systems with particular reference to the Lewis system. Am. J. Hum. Genet. 13:396–412, 1961.

Andresen, P. H.: Blood group with characteristic phenotypical aspects. Acta Path. Microbiol. Scand. 25:616–618, 1948.

Andresen, P. H.: The blood group system L. A new blood group L$_2$. A case of epistasy within the blood groups. Acta Path. Microbiol. Scand. 25:728–731, 1948.

Andresen, P. H. and Jordal, K.: An incomplete agglutinin related to the L-(Lewis) system. Acta Path. Microbiol. Scand. 26:636–638, 1949.

Angevine, C. D., Andersen, B. R. and Barnett, E. V.: A cold agglutinin of the IgA class. J. Immunol. 96:578, 1966.

Anonymous: Successful case of transfusion. Lancet i:431, 1828.

Applethwaite, F. Ginsberg, V., Cerena, J., Cunningham, C. A. and Gavin, J.: A very frequent red cell antigen, At[a]. Vox Sang. 13:444, 1967.

Arcara, P. C., O'Connor, M. A., and Dimmette, R. M.: A family with three Jk(a–b–) members. Transfusion 9:282, 1969.

Arcilla, M. B. and Sturgeon, P.: Le[a], the spurned antigen of the Lewis blood group system. Vox Sang. 26:425–438, 1974.

Argall, C. I., Ball, J. M. and Trentelman, E.: Presence of anti-D antibody in the serum of a D[u] patient. J. Lab. Clin. Med. 41:895–898, 1953.

Ascari, W. Q., Jolly, P. C., and Thomas, P. A.: Autologous blood transfusion in pulmonary surgery. Transfusion 8:111, 1968.

Ashurst, D. E., Bedford, D. and Coombs, R. R. A.: Examination of the human platelets for the ABO, MN, Rh, Tj[a], Lutheran and Lewis systems of antigens by means of mixed erythrocyte-platelet agglutination. Vox Sang. 1:235, 1956.

Aster, R. H. and Jandl, J. H.: Platelet sequestration in man. II. Immunological and clinical studies. J. Clin. Invest. 43:856, 1964.

Aster, R. H., Becker, G. A. and Filip, D. J.: Studies to improve methods of short-term platelet preservation. Transfusion 16:4, 1976.

Ayland, J., Horton, M. A., Tippet, P. and Waters, A. H.: Complement binding anti-D made in a D[u] variant woman. Vox Sang. 34:40, 1978.

Bach, F. H.: Immunogenetics of the major histocompatibility complex in mouse and man. In The Biology and Function of the Major Histocompatibility Complex. AABB, November 1980.

Badakere, S. S. Bhatia, H. M., Sharma, R. S. and Bharucha, Z.: Anti-Fy[b] (Duffy) as a cause of transfusion reaction. Ind. J. Med. Sci. 24:565–568, 1970.

Baer, H. Naylor, I., Gibbel, N. and Rosenfield, R. E.: The production of precipitating antibody in chickens to a substance present in the fluids of nonsecretors of blood groups A, B and O. J. Immunol. 82:183–189, 1959.

Baldini, M., Costea, N. and Dameshek, W.: The viability of stored human platelets. Blood 16:1669, 1960.

Ballas, S. K. and Sherwood, W. C.: Rapid in vivo destruction of Yt(a+) erythrocytes in a recipient with anti-Yt[a]. Transfusion 17:65, 1977.

Barandun, S., Kistler, P., Jeunet, F. and Isliker, H.: Intravenous administration of human Y-globulin. Vox Sang. 7:157, 1962.

Barnes, A. E., Sarasti, H., Mavioglu, H., and Jensen, W. N.: The detection and quantification of Rh(D) antigen sites on human leukocytes. Blood 22:690, 1963.

Bauer, D. C. and Stavitsky, A. B.: On the different molecular forms of antibody synthesized by rabbits during the early response to a single injection of protein and cellular antigens. Proc. Natl. Acad. Sci. USA 47:1667, 1961.

Beattie, K. M., Ferguson, S. J., Burnie, K. L., Barr, R. M., Urbaniak, S. T., and Atherton, P. J.: Chloramphenicol antibody causing interference in antibody detection and identification tests. Transfusion 16:174, 1976.

Beattie, K. M. and Zuelzer, W. W.: The frequency and properties of pH-dependent anti-M. Transfusion 5:322, 1965.

Beaumont, J. L., Lorenzelli, L., Delplanque, B., Zittoun, R., and Homberg, J. C.: A new serum lipoprotein-associated erythrocyte antigen which reacts with monoclonal IgM. The stored human red blood cell SHRBC antigen. Vox Sang. 30:36, 1976.

Beck, M. L., Hicklin, B. and Pierce, S. R.: Unexpected limitations in the use of commercial antiglobulin reagents. Transfusion 16:71, 1976a.

Beck, M. L., Edwards, R. L., Pierce, S. R., Hicklin, B. L. and Bayer, W. L.: Serologic activity of the fatty acid dependent antibodies in albumin-free systems. Transfusion 16:434, 1976b.

Beck, M. L., Butch, S. H., Armstrong, W. D. and Oberman, H. A.: An autoantibody with U-specificity in a patient with myasthenia gravis. Transfusion 12:280–283, 1972.

Beck, M. L., Dixon, J., Lawson, N. S. and Oberman, H. A.: Anti-C as a naturally occurring antibody. Transfusion 8:387, 1969.

Behzad, O., Lee, C. L., Gavin, J. and Marsh, W. L.: A new anti-erythrocyte antibody in the Duffy system: anti-Fy4. Vox Sang. 24:337–342, 1973.

Bell, C. A., Zwicker, H. and Nevius, D. B.: Nonspecific warm hemolysis of papain-treated cells: serologic characterization and transfusion risk. Transfusion 13:207, 1973.

Benesch, R., and Benesch, R. E.: The effect of organic phosphates from the human erythrocyte on the allosteric properties of hemoglobin. Biochem. Biophys. Res. Commun. 26:162, 1967.

Bergstrom, H., Nilsson, L. A., Nilsson, L. and Ryttinger, L.: Demonstration of Rh antigens in a 38-day-old fetus. Am. J. Obstet. Gynecol. 99:130, 1967.

Bernstein, F.: Ergebnisse einer biostatischen zusammenfassenden Betrachtung über die erblichen Blutstrukturen des Menschen. Klin. Wschr 3:1495, 1924. (Translated and published by the Blood Transfusion Division, U.S. Army Medical Research Laboratory, Fort Knox, Kentucky 40121.)

Bernstein, F.: Zusammenfassende Betrachtungen über die erblichen Blutstrukturen des Menschen. Z. f. indukt, Abstamm. u. Vererblehre, 37:237, 1925. (Translated and published by the Blood Transfusion Division, U.S. Army Medical Research Laboratory, Fort Knox, Kentucky 40121.)

Bertrams, J., Kuwert, E. and Noll K.: Leukocyten-Isoantikörper. III. Identifizierung und Charakterisierung monospezifischer HL-A-Antiseren zur Histokompatibilitätstestung. Z. Med. Mikrobiol. U. Immunol. 156:132–148, 1971.

Bettigole, R., Harris, J. P., Tegoli, J. and Issitt P. D.: Rapid *in vivo* destruction of Yt(a+) red cells in a patient with anti-Yt^a. Vox Sang. 14:143–146, 1968.

Beutler, E.: The maintenance of red cell function during liquid storage. *In* Schmidt, P. J. (ed.): Progress in Transfusion and Transplantation. Washington, D.C., American Association of Blood Banks, 1972, pp. 285–297.

Bhatia, H. M., Sanghvi, L. D., Bhide, Y. G., and Jhala, H. I.: Anti-II in two siblings in an Indian family. J. Ind. Med. Assoc., 25:545–548, 1955.

Bhende, Y. M. Despande, C. K., Bhatia, H. M., Sanger, R., Race, R. R., Morgan, W. T. J. and Watkins, W. M.: A "new" blood-group character related to the ABO system. Lancet i:903, 1952.

Bier, O. G., Leyton, G., Mayer, M. M. and Heidelberger, M.: A comparison of human and guinea-pig complements and their component fractions. J. Exp. Med. 81:445, 1945.

Billingham, R. E., Brent, L. and Medawar, P. B.: "Active acquired tolerance" of foreign cells. Nature 172:603, 1953.

Bird, G. W. G.: Erythrocyte polyagglutination. *In* Greenwalt, T. and Steane, E. (eds): CRC Handbook Series in Clinical Laboratory Science Section D: Blood Banks. Vol. 1, p. 443. CRC Press, Inc., Cleveland, 1977.

Bird, G. W. G.: Anti-T in peanuts. Vox Sang. 9:748–749, 1964.

Bird, G. W. G.: Haemagglutinins in seeds. Br. Med. Bull. 15:165–168, 1959.

Bird, G. W. G.: Erythrocyte agglutinins from plants. PhD thesis, London, 1958.

Bird, G. W. G.: Seed agglutinins and the T receptor. J. Pathol. Bacteriol. 68:289–291, 1954.

Bird, G. W. G.: Observations on haemagglutinin "linkage" in relation to isoagglutinins and auto-agglutinins. Br. J. Exp. Pathol., 34:131–137, 1953.

Bird, G. W. G.: Relationship of the blood sub-groups A₁, A₂ and A₁B, A₂B to haemagglutinins present in the seeds of *Dolichos biflorus*. Nature 170:674, 1952.

Bird, G. W. G.: Anti-A hemagglutinins in seeds. J. Immunol. 69:319–320, 1952.

Bird, G. W. G.: Specific agglutinating activity for human red blood corpuscles in extracts of *Dolichos biflorus*. Curr. Sci. 20:298–299, 1951.

Bird, G. W. G. and Wingham, J.: Anti-N antibodies in renal dialysis patients. Lancet i, 1218, 1977.

Bird, G. W. G. and Wingham, J.: Tk: a new form of red cell polyagglutination. Br. J. Haemat. 23:759, 1972.

Bird, G. W. G. and Wingham, J.: Seed agglutinin for rapid identification of Tn-polyagglutination (Letter). Lancet i:677, 1973.

Bird, G. W. G. and Wingham, J.: Changes in specificity of erythrocyte autoagglutinins. Vox Sang. 22:364, 1972.

Bird, G. W. G., *et al*:Erythrocyte membrane modification in malignant disease of myeloid and lymphoreticular tissues. I. Tn-polyagglutination in acute myelocytic leukaemia. Br. J. Haematol. 33:289, 1976.

Bird, G. W. G., Shinton, N. K. and Wingham, J.: Persistent mixed-field polyagglutination. Br. J. Haematol. 21:443, 1971.

Biro, C. E. and Garcia, G.: The antigenicity of aggregated and aggregate-free human gamma-globulin for rabbits. Immunology 8:411, 1965.

Bitter-Suermann, D., Dierich, M., Köning, W. and Hadding, U.: Bypass-activation of the complement system starting with C3. Immunology 23:267, 1972.

Bjerrum, O. J. and Jersild, C.: Class-specific anti-IgA associated with severe anaphylactic transfusion reactions in a patient with pernicious anemia. Vox Sang. 21:411, 1971.

Bjorum, A. and Kemp, T.: Untersuchungen über den Empfindlichkeitsgrad der Blutkörperchen gegenüber Isoag-glutininen im Kindesalter. Acta Pathol. Microbiol. Scand. 6:218–234, 1929.

Blajchman, M. A., Hui, Y. T., Jones, T. E. and Luke, K. H.: Familial autoimmune hemolytic anemia with autoantibody demonstrating U specificity. Program. AABB Meeting, 1971, p. 82.

Blum, L., Pillemer, L. and Lepow, I. H.: The properdin system and immunity XIII. Assay and properties of a heat-labile serum factor (factor B) in the properdin system. Z. Immunitaetsforsch. 118:349, 1959.

Blumberg, B. S., Sutnick, A. I. and London, W. T.: Hepatitis and leukemia: their relation to Australia antigen. Bull. N.Y. Acad. Med. 44:1566, 1968.

Blumberg, B. S., Alter, H. J. and Visnich, S.: A new antigen in leukemia sera. JAMA 191:541, 1965.

Blumenthal, G. and Pettenkofer, H. J.: Über das neuentdeckte anti-Duffy^b (Fy^b). Z. Immun. Forsch. 109:267, 1952.

Blundell, J.: Experiments on the transfusion of blood by the syringe. Medicochir. Trans. 9:56, 1818.

Bokisch, V. A., Müller-Eberhard, H. J. and Cochrane, C. G.: Isolation of a fragment (C3a) of the third component of human complement containing anaphylatoxin and chemotactic activity and description of an anaphylatoxin inactivator of human serum. J. Exp. Med. 129:1109, 1969.

Boorman, K. E., and Lincoln, P.J.: A suggestion as to the place of r^G and r^M on the Rh system. Ann. Hum. Genet. 26:51, 1962.

Boorman, K. E., Dodd, B. E. and Lincoln, P. J.: Blood Group serology: Theory, Techniques, Practical Applications. 5th Ed. Churchill Livingstone, 1977.

Booth, P. B.: Anti-N^A. An antibody subdividing Melanesian N. Vox Sang. 21:522–530, 1971.

Booth, P. B.: Anti-I^{T}P$_1$: an antibody showing a further association between the I and P blood group systems. Vox Sang. 19:85–90, 1970.

Booth, P. B. and MacGregor A.: The incidence of cold autohemagglutinins in Melanesian children and adults. Vox Sang. 11:720–723, 1966.

Booth, P. B., Plaut, G., James, J. D., Ikin, E. W., Moores, P., Sanger, R. and Race, R. R.: Blood chimerism in a pair of twins. Br. Med. J. i:1456, 1957.

Bornsteins, S. and Israel, M.: Agglutinogens in fetal erythrocytes. Proc. Soc. Exp. Biol. N.Y. 49:718–720, 1942.

Borsos, T. and Rapp, H. J.: Hemolysin titration based on fixation of the activated first component of complement: evidence that one molecule of hemolysin suffices to sensitize an erythrocyte. J. Immunol. 95:559, 1965.

Bouguerra-Jacquet, A., Reviron J., Salmon, D. and Salmon, C.: Un exemple de chromosome cis A₁B. Etude thermodynamique de l'antigene B induit. Nouw. Ref. Franç. Hémotol. 9:329, 1969.

Bove, J. R., Allen, F. H., Chiewsilp, P., Marsh, W. L. and Cleghorn, T. E.: Anti-Lu4: a new antibody related to the Lutheran blood group system. Vox Sang. 21:302–310, 1971.

Bove, J. R., Johnson, M., Francis, B. J., Hatcher, D. E., and Gelb, A. G.: Anti-K² defining a new antigenic determinant. Program, 18th Ann. Meeting, AABB, Florida, 1965, p. 60.

Bowley, C. C. and Dunsford, I.: The agglutinin anti-M associated with pregnancy. Br. Med. J. ii:681, 1949.

Bowman, H. S.: Red cell preservation in citrate-phosphate-dextrose and in acid-citrate-dextrose. Transfusion 3:364–367, 1963.

Bowman, H. S., Marsh, W. L., Schumacher, H. R., Owen, R. and Reihard: Auto anti-N immunohemolytic anemia in infectious mononucleosis. Am. J. Clin. Pathol. 61:465, 1974.

Bowman, J. M., Chown, B., Lewis, M. and Pollack, J.: Rh

immunization during pregnancy; antenatal prophylaxis. Can. Med. Assoc. J. 118:623, 1978.

Boyd, W. C.: Blood groups. Tabulae Biologicae 17:113, 1939.

Boyd, W. C. and Shapleigh, E.: Separation of individuals of any blood group into secretors and nonsecretors by use of a plant agglutinin (lectin). Blood 9:1195–1198, 1954.

Boyd, W. C. and Reguera, R. M.: Hemagglutinating substances for human cells in various plants. J. Immunol. 62:333–339, 1949.

Boyd, W. C., Everhart, D. L. and McMaster, M.H.: The anti-N lectin of Bauhinia purpura. J. Immunol. 81:414, 1958.

Brain, P.: Subgroups of A in the South African Bantu. Vox Sang. 11:686–698, 1966.

Branch, D. R. and Petz, L. D.: A new reagent having multiple applications in immunohematology. Proc. 33rd Ann Meeting, AABB, Washington, 1980.

Brendemoen, O. J.: A cold agglutinin specifically active against stored red cells. Acta Pathol. Microbiol. Scand. 31:574, 1952.

Brendemoen, O. J.: Studies of agglutination and inhibition in two Lewis antibodies. J. Lab. Clin. Med. 34:538–542, 1949.

Brent, L. and Medawar, P. B.: Tolerance and autoimmune phenomena. Symposia at VIIth International Congress for Microbiology. Tunevall, J. (ed): Recent progress in Microbiology. Blackwell Scientific Publications, Oxford, 1958.

Brewerton, D. A., Caffrey, M., Hart, F. D., James, D. C. O., Nicholls, A. and Sturrock, R. D.: Ankylosing spondylitis and HL-A27. Lancet i:904–907, 1973.

Brittingham, T. E. and Chaplin, H., Jr.: Febrile transfusion reactions caused by sensitivity to donor leukocytes and platelets. JAMA 165:819, 1957.

Broman B., Heiken, A. Tippett, A. and Giles, C. M.: The D (C) (e) gene complex revealed in the Swedish population. Vox Sang. 8:588–593, 1963.

Brown, D. L. and Cooper, A. G.: The *in vivo* metabolism of radioiodinated cold agglutinins of anti-I specificity. Clin. Sci. 38:175, 1970.

Brown, P. C., Glynn, L. E., and Holborow, E. J.: Lewis[a] substance in saliva. A qualitative difference between secretors and nonsecretors. Vox Sang. 4:1–12, 1959.

Bruce-Chwatt, L. J.: Transfusion malaria. Bull. WHO 50:337, 1974.

Bryant, N. J.: Disputed Paternity: The Value and Application of Blood Tests. Brian C. Decker, New York, 1980.

Bryant, N. J.: Laboratory Immunology and Serology. W. B. Saunders Co., 1979.

Bryant, N. J. Shanahan, L. S. and Sutton, D. M. C.: A rapid tube technique for fetal cell typing. Transfusion 19:190, 1979.

Bryson, M. J., Gabert, H. A., and Stenchever, M. A.: Amniotic fluid lecithin/sphingomyelin ratio as an assessment of fetal pulmonary maturity. Am. J. Obstet. Gynecol. 114:208, 1972.

Buchanan, D. I. and Afaganis, A.: The Bennett-Goodspeed-Sturgeon or "Donna" red cell antigen and antibody. Vox Sang. 8:213–218, 1963.

Bukowski, R. M., Hewlett, J. S., Harris, J. W., Hoffman, G. C., Battle, J. D., Jr., Silverblatt, E. and Yang, I.-Y.: Exchange transfusions in the treatment of thrombotic thrombocytopenic purpura. Semin. Hematol. 13:219, 1976.

Bull, J. P., Ricketts, C., Squire, J. R., Maycock, W.D'A, Spooner, S. J. L., Mollison, P. L. and Paterson, J. C. S.: Dextran as a plasma substitute. Lancet i:134, 1949b.

Burkart, P., Rosenfield, R. E., Hsu, T. C. S., Wong, K. Y., Nusbacker, J., Shaikh, S. H. and Kochwa, S.: Instrumented PVP-augmented antiglobulin tests. I. Detection of allogeneic antibodies coating otherwise normal erythrocytes. Vox Sang. 26:289, 1974.

Burki, U., Degnan, T. J. and Rosenfield, R. E.: Stillbirth due to anti-U. Vox Sang. 9:209–211, 1964.

Burnet, F. M. and Fenner, F.: The Production of Antibodies, 2nd Ed. Macmillan, 1949.

Burnie, K.: Ii antigens and antibodies. Can. J. Med. Technol. 35:5–26, 1973.

Burton, M. S. and Mollison, P. L.: Effect of IgM and IgG iso-antibody on red cell clearance. Immunology 14:861, 1968.

Bush, M. Sabo, B., Stroup, M. and Masouredis, S. P.: Red Cell D antigen sites and titration scores in a family with weak and normal D^u phenotypes inherited from a homozygous D^u mother. Transfusion 14:433, 1974.

Buskard, N. A., Varghese, Z. and Willis, M. R.: Correction of hypocalcaemic symptoms during plasma exchange. Lancet ii:344, 1976.

Callender, S. T. and Race, R. R.: A serological and genetical study of multiple antibodies formed in response to blood transfusion by a patient with lupus erythematosus diffusus. Ann. Eugen. 13:102–117, 1946.

Callender, S., Race, R. R. and Paykoc, Z. V.: Hypersensitivity to transfused blood. Br. Med. J. ii:83, 1945.

Cameron, C., Dunsford, I., Sickles, G. R., Cahan, A., Sanger, R. and Race, R. R.: Acquisition of a B-like antigen by red blood cells. Br. Med. J. ii,29:1959.

Cameron, G. L. and Staveley, J. M.: Blood Group P substance in hydatid cyst fluids. Nature, 179:147–148, 1957.

Cameron, J. W. and Diamond, L. K.: Chemical, clinical and immunological studies on the products of human plasma fractionation XXIX. Serum albumin as a diluent for Rh typing reagents. J. Clin. Invest. 24:793, 1945.

Capra, J. D., Dowling, P., Cooks, S. and Kunkel, H. G.: An incomplete cold-reactive γG antibody with i specificity in infectious mononucleosis. Vox Sang. 16:10–17, 1969.

Carr, J. B., de Quesada, A. M., and Shires, D. L.: Decreased incidence of transfusion hepatitis after exclusive transfusion with reconstitued frozen erythrocytes. Ann. Intern. Med. 78:693, 1973.

Case, J.: The albumin layering method for D typing. Vox Sang. 4:403, 1959.

Caspersson, T., Zechs, L., Johansson, C. and Modest, E. J.: Identification of human chromosomes by DNA-binding fluorescent agents. Chromosoma 30:215, 1970.

Cazal, P. and LaLaurie, M.: Recherches sur quelques phytoagglutinines spécifiques des groups sanguins ABO. Acta Hematol. 8:73–80, 1952.

Cazal, P., Monis, M. and Bizot, M.: Les antigènes cad et aleurs rapports avec les antigènes A. Rev. Franç. Transf. 14:321–334, 1971.

Cazal, P., Monis M., Caubel, J. and Brives, J.: Polyagglutinabilité héréditaire dominante: antigène privé (Cad) correspondant à un anticorps public et à une lectine de *Dolichos biflorus*. Rev. Franç. Transf. 11:209–221, 1968.

Celano, M. J. and Levine, P.: Anti-LW specificity in autoimmune acquired hemolytic anemia. Transfusion 7:265, 1967.

Celano, M. J., Levine, P. and Lange, S.: Studies on eluates from Rhesus and human A red cells. Vox Sang. 2:375, 1957.

Ceppellini, R.: Physiological genetics of human factors. Ciba Found. Symp. on Biochemistry of Human Genetics, Churchill, London, 242, 1959.

Ceppellini, R.: Nuova interpretazione sulla genetica dei carratteri Lewis eritrocitarie salivali derivante dall'analist di 87 famiglie. Ric. Sci. Mem. (Suppl) 25:3–9 (in offprint), 1955.

Ceppellini, R.: On the genetics of secretor and Lewis characters: a family study. Proc. 5th Congr. Int. Soc. Blood Transf., Paris, 1955, pp. 207–211.

Ceppellini, R. and Siniscalco, M.,: Una nuova ipotesi genetica per il sistema Lewis secretore e suoi riflessi nei riguardi di alcune evidence di linkage con altri loc. Revista dell' Istituto Sieroterapico Italiano 30:431–445, 1955.

Ceppellini, R., Dunn, L. C. and Turri M.: An interaction between alleles at the Rh locus in man which weakens the reactivity of the Rh_0 factor (D^u). Proc. Nat. Acad. Sci., USA, 41:283–288, 1955.

Chalmers, J. N. M. and Lawler, S. D.: Data on linkage in man: elliptocytosis and blood groups. I. Families 1 and 2. Ann. Eugen. 17:267–271, 1953.

Chanutin, A.: The effect of the addition of adenine and nucleosides at the beginning of storage on the concentrations of phosphates of human erythrocytes during storage in acid-citrate-dextrose and citrate-phosphate-dextrose. Transfusion 7:120, 1967.

Chanutin, A., and Curnish, R. B.: Effect of organic and inorganic phosphates on the oxygen equilibrium of human erythrocytes. Arch. Biochem. Biophys. 121:96, 1967.

Chaplin, H., Jr., Crawford, H. A. L., Cutbush, M. and Mollison, P. L.: Post-transfusion survival of red cells stored at −20° C. Lancet i:852, 1954.

Cherubin, C. E. and Prince, A. M.: Serum hepatitis specific antigen (SH) in commercial and volunteer sources of blood. Transfusion 11:25, 1971.

Chien, S. and Kung-Ming, J.: Ultrastructural basis of the mechanism of Rouleaux formation. Microvasc. Res. 5:155, 1973.

Chien, S., Simchon, S., Abbott, R. E., and Jan, K. M.: Surface absorption of dextrans on human red cell membrane. J. Coll. Interf. Sci. 62:461, 1977.

Chorpenning, F. W. and Hayes, J. C.: Occurrence of the Thomsen-Friedenreich phenomenon *in vivo*. Vox Sang. 4:210, 1959.

Chown, B.: XIIIth John G. Gibson II Lecture Published by Columbia Presbyterian Medical Center College of Physicians and Surgeons, New York, 1964.

Chown, B.: On a search for rhesus antibodies in very young fetuses. Arch. Dis. Childh. 30:237, 1955.

Chown, B., and Lewis, M.: The occurrence of an Rh hemagglutinin of specificity anti-C^w in the absence of known stimulation: suggestions as to cause. Vox Sang. (O.S.) 4:41–45, 1954.

Chown, B., Lewis, M., Kaita, H. and Lowen B.: An unlinked modifier of Rh blood groups: effects when heterozygous and when homozygous. Am. J. Hum. Genet. 24:623–637, 1972.

Chown, B., Lewis, M., Kaita, H., Hahn, D., Schackelton, K. and Shepeard, W. L.: On the antigen Go^a and the Rh system. Vox Sang. 15:264–271, 1968.

Chown, B., Lewis, M. and Kaita, H.: The Duffy blood group system in Caucasians: evidence for a new allele. Am. J. Hum. Genet. 17:384–389, 1965.

Chown, B., Lewis, M., Kaita, H. and Philipps, S.: The Rh antigen D^W (Wiel). Transfusion 4:169–172, 1964.

Chown, B., Lewis, M. and Kaita, H.: The Bennett-Goodspeed antigen or antigens. Vox Sang. 8:281–288, 1963.

Chown, B., Lewis, M. and Kaita, H.: A "new" Rh antigen and antibody. Transfusion 2:150–154, 1962.

Chown, B., Lewis, M. and Kaita, H.: A "new" Kell blood group phenotype. Nature 180:711, 1957.

Clark, D., Pincus, L., Hubbell, D., Oliphant, M. and Davey, F.: HLA-A2 antigens associated with chronic lung disease in neonates. Proc. 33rd Ann. Meeting, AABB, Washington, DC, November, 1980.

Cleghorn, T. E.: The frequency of the Wr^a, By and M^g blood group antigens in blood donors in the South of England. Vox Sang. 5:556–560, 1960.

Cohen, D. W., Garratty, G., Morel, P. and Petz, L. D.: Autoimmune hemolytic anemia associated with IgG auto anti-N. Transfusion 19:329, 1979.

Cohen, S. and Freeman, T.: Metabolic heterogeneity of human γ-globulin. Biochem. J. 76:475, 1960.

Colledge, K. I., Pezzulich, M. and Marsh, W. L., Anti-Fy5, an antibody disclosing a probable association between the Rhesus and Duffy blood group genes. Vox Sang. 24:193, 1973.

Constandoulakis, M. and Kay, H. E. M.: A and B antigens of the human fetal erythrocyte. Br. J. Hematol. 8:57–63, 1962.

Constantoulis, N. C., Paidoussis, M. and Dunsford, I.: A naturally occurring anti-S agglutinin. Vox Sang. (O.S.) 5:143, 1955.

Contreras, M. and Tippett, P.: The Lu(a−b−) syndrome and an apparent upset of P_1 inheritance. Vox Sang. 27:369–371, 1934.

Contreras, M., Stebbing, B., Blessing, M. and Gavin, J.: The Rh antigen Evans. Vox Sang 34:208, 1978.

Cook, I. A., Polley, M. J. and Mollison, P. L.: A second example of anti-Xg^a. Lancet i:857–859, 1963.

Coombs, H. I., Ikin, E. W., Mourant, A. E. and Plaut, G.: Agglutinin anti-S in human serum. Brit. Med. J. i:109, 1951.

Coombs, R. R. A. and Race, R. R.: Further observations on the "incomplete" or "blocking" Rh antibody. Nature 156:233, 1945.

Coombs, R. R. A., Bedford, D. and Rouillard, L. M.: A and B blood-group antigens on human epidermal cells demonstrated by mixed agglutination. Lancet i:461–463, 1956.

Coombs, R. R. A., Mourant, A. E. and Race, R. R.: *In vivo* isosensitization of red cells in babies with hemolytic disease. Lancet i:264, 1946.

Coombs, R. R. A., Mourant, A. E. and Race, R. R.: A new test for the detection of weak and 'incomplete' Rh agglutinins. Br. J. Exp. Path. 26:255, 1945.

Cooper, A. G. and Brown, M. C.: Serum i antigen: a new human blood-group glycoprotein. Biochem. Biophys. Res. Commun. 55:297–304, 1973.

Cooper, A. G., Hoffbrand, A. V. and Worlledge, S. M.: Increased agglutinability by anti-i of red cells in sideroblastic and megaloblastic anemia. Br. J. Hemat. 15:381–387, 1968.

Cooper, R. A.: Abnormalities of cell-membrane fluidity in the pathogenesis of disease. N. Engl. J. Med. 297:371, 1977.

Cooper, M. R., Heise, E., Richards, F., Kaufmann, J. and Spurr, C. L.: A prospective study of histocompatible leucocyte and platelet transfusions during chemotherapeutic induction of acute myelobastic leukaemia, In Leucocytes: Separation, Collection and Transfusion. Goldman, J. M. and Lowenthal, R. M. (eds): Academic Press, New York, 1975.

Cornwall, S., Wright, J. and Moore, B. P. L.: Further examples of the antigen Mur (Murrell), a rare blood group associated with the MNSs system. Vox Sang 14:295–298, 1968.

Costea, N., Yakulis, V. J. and Heller, P.: Inhibition of cold agglutinins (anti-I) by *M. pneumoniae* antigens. Proc. Soc. Exp. Biol. 139:476, 1972.

Crawford, M. N., Tippett, P. and Sanger, R.: Antigens Au^a, i and P_1 of cells of the dominant type of Lu(a−b−), Vox Sang. 26:283–287, 1974.

Crawford, M. N., Greenwalt, T. J., Sasaki, T., Tippett, P., Sanger, R. and Race, R. R.: The phenotype Lu(a−b−) together with unconventional Kidd groups in one family. Transfusion 1:228–232, 1961.

Cregut, R., Lewin, D., Lacomme, M. and Michot, O.: Un cas d'anasarque foetoplacentaire par iso-immunisation contre un antigène 'privé.' Rev. Franç. Transf. 11:139–143, 1968.

Crome, P. and Moffatt, B.: IgM lymphocytotoxic antibodies following multiple transfusion. Vox Sang. 21:11, 1971.

Crookston, J. H.: Hemolytic anemia with IgG and IgM autoantibodies and alloantibodies. Arch. Intern. Med. 135:1314, 1975.

Crookston, J. H., Crookston, M. C., Burnie, K L., Francome, W. H., Dacie, J. V., Davis, J. A. and Lewis, S. M.: Hereditary erythroblastic multinuclearity associated with a positive acidified-serum test: a type of congenital dyserythropoietic anemia. Br. J. Hemat. 17:11, 1969a.

Crookston, J. H., Crookston, M. C. and Rosse, W. F.: Red cell membrane abnormalities in hereditary erythroblastic multinuclearity (Abstract). Blood 34:844, 1969b.

Crookston, M. C., Tilley, C. A., and Crookston, J. H.: Human blood chimera with seeming breakdown of immune tolerance. Lancet ii:1110–1112, 1970.

Crosby, W. H.: Trends in blood transfusion. Ann. N.Y. Acad. Sci. 115:399, 1964.

Crosby, W. H., and Stefanini, M.: Pathogenesis of the plasma transfusion reaction with especial reference to the blood coagulation system. J. Lab. Clin. Med. 40:374, 1952.

Cross, D. E., Whittier, F. C., Schimke, R. N., Greiner, R. F., Foxworth, J. A., O'Kell, R. T.: A crossover in the HL-A system traced through three generations. Tissue Antigens 6:265, 1975.

Crossland, J. D., Pepper, M. D., Giles, C. M. and Ikin, E. W.: A British family possessing two variants of the MNSs blood group system, M^v and a new class within the Miltenberger complex. Vox Sang. 18:407–413, 1970.

Croucher, B. E. E., Crookston, M. C. and Crookston, J. H.: Delayed transfusion reactions simulating auto-immune hemolytic anemia. Vox Sang. 12:32, 1967.

Cruz, W. O. and Junqueira, P. C.: Resistance of reticulocytes and young erythrocytes to the action of specific hemolytic serum. Blood 7:602, 1952.

Curtain, C. C.: Anti-I agglutinins in non-human sera. Vox Sang. 16:161–171, 1969.

Curtain, C. C., Baumgarten, A., Gorman, J., Kidson, C., Champness, L., Rodriguez, R. and Gajdusek, D. C.: Cold hemagglutinins: unusual incidence in Melanesian populations. Br. J. Hemat. 11:471–479, 1965.

Cutbush, M. and Mollison, P. L.: Relation between characteristics of blood-group antibodies in vitro and associated patterns of red cell destruction in vivo. Br. J. Hemat. 4:115, 1958.

Cutbush, M. and Chanarin, I.: The expected blood-group antibody, anti-Lu^b. Nature 178:855–856, 1956.

Cutbush, M., Giblett, E. R. and Mollison, P. L.: Demonstration of the phenotype Le(a+b+) in infants and in adults. Br. J. Hemat. 2:210, 1956.

Cutbush, M., Mollison, P. L. and Parkin, D. M.: A new human blood group. Nature 165:188, 1950.

Dacie, J. V.: Autoimmune hemolytic anemia. Arch. Intern. Med. 135:1293, 1975.

Dacie, J. V.: The Hemolytic Anaemias, Congenital and Acquired, 2nd ed. Part II — The Auto-Immune Hemolytic Anemias. Churchill, London, 1962.

Dacie, J. V.: Transfusion of saline-washed red cells in nocturnal hemoglobinuria. Clin. Sci. 7:65, 1948.

Dacie, J. V. and Worlledge, S. M.: Auto-immune hemolytic anemias. Progr. Hematol. 6:82, 1969.

Dacie, J. V. and Cutbush, M.: Specificity of autoantibodies in acquired hemolytic anemia. J. Clin. Pathol. 7:18, 1954.

Dacie, J. V., Crookston, J. H. and Christenson, W. N.: "Incomplete" cold antibodies: role of complement in sensitization to antiglobulin serum by potentially hemolytic antibodies. Br. J. Hematol. 3:77, 1957.

Dacie, J. V., and Firth, D.: Blood transfusion in nocturnal hemoglobinuria. Brit. Med. J. i:626, 1943.

Dahr, W., Uhlenbruck, G., Gunson, H. H. and Hart, M. Van Der: Studies on glycoproteins and glycopeptides from Tn-polyagglutinable erythrocytes. Vox Sang. 28:249, 1975.

Dahr, W., Uhlenbruck, G. and Knott, H.: Immunochemical aspects of the MNSs blood group system. J. Immunogenet. 2:87, 1975.

Dahr, W., Uhlenbruck, G., and Bird, G. W. G.: Cryptic A-like receptor sites in human erythrocyte glycoproteins: proposed nature of Tn-antigen. Vox Sang. 27:29, 1974.

Dair, P.: Über im Menschenserum natürlich vorkommendes anti-M Agglutinin. Klin. Wschr. 20:1273, 1941.

Dalmasso, A. P. and Müller-Eberhard, H. J.: Physiochemical characteristics of the third and fourth component of complement after dissociation from complement-cell complexes. Immunology 13:293, 1967.

Dare, J. G. and Mogey, G. A.: Rabbit responses to human threshold doses of a bacterial pyrogen. J. Pharm. Pharmacol. 6:325, 1954.

Darnborough, J.: Further observations on the Verweyst blood group antigen and antibodies. Vox Sang. 2:362, 1957.

Darnborough, J. Dunsford, I. and Wallace, J. A.: The En^a antigen and antibody. A genetical modification of human red cells affecting their blood grouping reactions. Vox Sang. 17:241–255, 1969.

Darnborough, J., Firth, R., Giles, C. M., Goldsmith, K. L. G. and Crawford, M. N.: A "new" antibody anti-Lu^aLu^b and two further examples of the genotype Lu(a−b−). Nature 198:796, 1963.

Daussett, J.: Iso-leuco-anticorps. Acta Hematol. 20:156–166, 1958.

Daussett, J.: Leuco-agglutinins IV. Leuco-agglutinins and blood transfusion. Vox Sang. 4:190, 1954.

Dausset, J. and Colombani, J.: The serology and the prognosis of 128 cases of autoimmune hemolytic anemia. Blood 14:1280, 1959.

Dausset, J. and Nenna, A.: Présence d'une leucoagglutinine dans le sérum d'un cas d'agranulocytose chronique. C. R. Soc. Biol. 146:1539, 1952.

Dausset, J., Moullec, J., and Bernard, J.: Acquired hemolytic anemia with polyagglutinability of red blood cells due to a new factor present in normal human serum (anti-Tn). Blood 14:1079–1093, 1959.

Dausset, J., Colombani, J., Jean, R. G., Caulorte, P. and Lelong, M.: Sur un cas d'anémie hémolytique aigüe de l'enfant avec présence d'une hémolysine immunologique et d'un pouvoir anticomplémentaire du sérum. Sang. 28:351, 1957.

Davey, M. G.: Antenatal administration of anti-Rh: Australia 1969–1975. Proceedings of Symposium on Rh Antibody Mediated Immunosuppression, Ortho Research Institute, Raritan, N. J., 1976.

Davey, M. G., Campbell, A. L. and James, J.: Some consequences of hyperimmunization to the rhesus (D) blood group antigen in man (Abstract). Proc. Austr. Soc. Immunol., Adelaide, December 1969.

Davey, R. J., O'Gara, C. and McGinniss, M. H.: An unusual agglutination phenomenon of saline-washed red cells. Commun. AABB, San Francisco, 1976.

Davidsohn, I.: Reflections on the past, present and future of blood transfusion. In Heustis, D. W., Bove, J. R. and Busch, S.: Practical Blood Transfusion. Little, Brown and Co., 1969.

Davidsohn, I., Ni Louisa, Y. and Steiskal, R.: Tissue isoantigens A, B and H in carcinoma of the pancreas. Cancer Res. 31:1244–1250, 1971.

Davidsohn, I., Ni Louisa, Y. and Steiskal, R.: Tissue isoantigens A, B and H in carcinoma of the stomach. Arch. Pathol. 92:456–464, 1971.

Davidsohn, I., Kovarik, S. and Ni Louisa, Y.: Isoantigens A, B and H in benign and malignant lesions of the cervix. Arch. Pathol. 37:306–314. 1969.

Davidsohn, I., Kovarik, S. and Lee, C. L.: A, B and O substances in gastrointestinal carcinoma. Arch. Pathol. 31:381–390, 1966.

Davidsohn, I., Stern, K., Strauser, E. R. and Spurrier, W.: Be^a, a new "private" blood factor. Blood 8:747–754, 1953.

Dawson, R. B., Jr.: The control of hemoglobin function in blood stored for transfusion purposes. In Proceedings, International Symposium on Blood Oxygenation, University of Cincinnati, 1969. In Blood Oxygenation. Plenum Press. 1970, pp 231–242.

Dawson, R. B., Kocholaty, W. F., Camp, R., Crater, D., Ellis, T. J., Spurlock, W., Billings, T. A. and Ledford, E. B.: Hemoglobin function in stored blood. XIII. A citrate-adenine preservative with optimal pH to maintain red cell 2,3-DPG (function) and ATP (viability). Haematologia 9:49, 1975.

Day, D., Perkins, H. A. and Sams, B.: The minus minus phenotype in the Kidd system. Transfusion 5:315, 1965.

De Boissezon J.-F., Marty, Y., Ducos, J. and Abbal, M.: Presence constante d'une substance inhibitrice de l'anticorps anti-i dans le serum humain normal. C. R. Acad. Sci. 271:1448–1451, 1970.

Decastello, A. V. and Sturli, A.: Iso-agglutinins in the serum of healthy and sick persons. Munchen. Med. Wschr. 26:1090, 1902.

De Cesare, W. R., Bove, J. R. and Ebaugh, F. G., Jr.: The mechanism of the effect of iso- and hyperosmolar dextrose-saline solutions on in vivo survival of human erythrocytes. Transfusion 4:237, 1964.

Degnan, T. J. and Rosenfield, R. E.: Hemolytic transfusion reaction associated with poorly detectable anti-Jk^a. Transfusion 5:245–247, 1965.

Denatale, A., Cahan, A., Jack, J. A., Race, R. R. and Sanger, R. V.: A "new" Rh antigen, common in Negroes, rare in white people. JAMA 159:247–250, 1955.

Dennis, H. G. and Konugres, A. A.: Comparative studies of the effectiveness of complement obtained from different species in the alpha hemolysis test on human sera. J. Med. Lab. Technol. 16:284, 1959.

Denys, J. B.: Philos. Trans. 2 (No 27):489, 1667.

Dern, R. J.: Double label studies of the poststorage viability of erythrocytes in trauma patients. In Modern Problems of Blood Preservation. Spielmann, W. and Seidl, S. (eds). Gustav Fischer, 1970.

Dern, R. J., Wiorkowski, J. J. and Matsuda, T.: Studies on the preservation of human blood. V. The effect of mixing anticoagulated blood during storage on the poststorage erythrocyte survival. J. Lab. Clin. Med. 75:37, 1970.

Dern, R. J., Brewer, G. J. and Wiorkowski, J. J.: Studies on the preservation of human blood. II. The relationship of erythrocyte adenosine triphosphate levels and other in vitro measures to red cell storageability. J. Lab. Clin. Med. 69:968, 1967.

DeVerdier, C.-H, Finnson, M., Garby L., Högman, C. F. Johansson, S. G. O. and Akerblom, O.: Experience of blood preservation in ACD adenine solution. Proc. 10th Congr. Europ. Soc. Haemat., Strasburg, 1965.

De Verdier, C.-H., Högman, C., Garby, L. and Killander, J.: Storage of human red blood cells. II. The effect of pH and of the addition of adenine. Acta Physiol. Scand. 60:141, 1964a.

De Verdier, C.-H., Garby, L., Hjelm, M., Högman, C. and Eriksson, A.: Adenine in blood preservation: posttransfusion viability and biochemical changes. Transfusion 4:337, 1964b.

DeWit, D. C. and Van Gastel, C.: Red cell age and susceptibility to immune hemolysis. Scand. J. Hematol. 6:373, 1969.

Diamond, L. K.: Erythroblastosis fetalis or hemolytic disease of the newborn. Proc. Roy. Soc. Med. 40:546, 1947.

Diamond, L. K. and Allen, F. H.: Rh and other blood groups. N. Engl. J. Med. 241:867, 1949.

Diamond, L. K. and Denton, R. L.: Rh agglutination in various media with particular reference to the value of albumin. J. Lab. Clin. Med. 30:821, 1945.

Dike, A. E.: Two cases of transfusion malaria. Lancet ii:72, 1970.

Diosi, P., Moldovan, E. and Tomescu, N.: Latent cytomegalovirus infection in blood donors. Br. Med. J. iv:660, 1969.

Dobson, A. and Ikin, E. W.: The ABO blood groups in the United Kingdom: Frequencies based on a very large sample. J. Pathol. Bacteriol. 58:221, 1946.

Dodd, B. E.: Linked anti-A and anti-B antibodies from group O sera. Br. J. Exp. Pathol., 33:1–18, 1952.

Doinel, C., Ropars, C. and Salmon, C.: Quantitative and thermodynamic measurements on I and i antigens of human red blood cells. Immunology 30:289, 1976.

Donahue, R. P., Bias, W. B., Renwick, J. H., and McKusick, V. A.: Probable assignment of the Duffy blood group locus to chromosome 1 in man. Proc. Natl. Acad. Sci. USA, 61:949, 1968.

Dorfmeier H., Hart, M. V. D., Nijenhuis, L. E. and Loghem, J. J. Van: A "new" blood group antigen of rare occurrence (Ot). Proc. 7th Congr. Int. Soc. Blood Transf., 608–610, 1959.

Dorner, I. M., Parker, C. W. and Chaplin, H., Jr.: Autoagglutinin developing in a patient with acute renal failure. Characterization of the autoagglutinin and its relation to transfusion therapy. Br. J. Hemat. 14:383, 1968.

Drachmann, O. and Brogaard, H. K.: Hemolytic disease of the newborn due to anti-s. Scand. J. Hematol. 6:93–98, 1969.

Drake, M. E., Hampil, B., Pennell, R. B., Spizizen, J., Henle, W. and Stokes, J.: Effect of nitrogen mustard on virus of serum hepatitis in whole blood. Proc. Soc. Exp. Biol. 80:310, 1952.

Dube, V. E., House, R. F., Jr., Moulds, J. and Polesky, H. F.: Hemolytic anemia caused by auto anti-N. Am. J. Clin. Pathol. 63:828, 1975.

Dungern, E. V. and Hirszfeld, L.: Über gruppenspezifische Strukturen des Blutes III. Z. Immun. Forsch, 8:526, 1911. (Translated and published by the Blood Transfusion Division, U.S. Army Medical Research Laboratory, Fort Knox, Kentucky, 40121.)

Dungern, E. v. and Hirszfeld, L.: Ueber Vererbung gruppenspezifischer Strukturen des Blutes. Strukturen des Blutes. (Z. Immun Forsch, 6, 284, 1910. See translation by G. P. Pohlmann: Transfusion 2:70, 1962.)

Dunsford, I.: A new Rh antibody — anti-CE. Proc. 8th Congr. Europ. Soc. Hemat., Vienna, 1961.

Dunsford, I.: A critical review of the ABO subgroups. Proc. 6th Congr. Int. Soc. Blood Transf., Rome, p. 687, 1959.

Dunsford, I.: The Wright blood groups system. Vox Sang. 4:160, 1954.

Dunsford, I., Bowley, C. C., Hutchinson, A. M., Thompson, J. S., Sanger, R., and Race, R. R.: A human blood-group chimera. Br. Med. J. ii:81, 1953.

Dunsford, I., Ikin, E. W. and Mourant, A. E.: A human blood group gene intermediate between M and N. Nature 172:688–689, 1953.

Dupont, B.: Mechanisms for HLA and disease associations. In The Biology and Function of the Major Histocompatibility Complex. AABB, 1980.

Dybkjear, E.: Anti-E antibodies disclosed in the period 1960–1966. Vox Sang. 13:446, 1967.

Dybkjear, E.: Enzyme methods for the demonstration of

incomplete antibodies. Proc. 10th Congr. Int. Soc. Blood Transfus., Stockholm, 1964.

Dybkjear, E., Lylloff, K. and Tippett, P.: Weak Lu9 antigen in one Lu:−6 member of a family. Vox Sang. 26:94–96, 1974.

Dzierzkowa-Borodej, W., Meinhard, W. Nestorowicz, S. and Pirog, J.: Successful elution of anti-A and certain anti-H reagents from two "Bombay" (O$_h$) blood samples and investigation of isoagglutinins in their sera. Arch. Immunol. Ther. Exp. 20:841–849, 1972.

Dzierzkowa-Borodej, W., Seyfried, H., Nichols, M., Reid, M., and Marsh, W. L.: The recognition of water-soluble I blood group substance. Vox Sang. 18:222–234, 1970.

Eaton, B. R., Morton, J. A., Pickles, M. M. and White, K. E.: A new antibody, anti-Yt^a, characterizing a blood group of high incidence. Br. J. Hematol., 2:333–341, 1956.

Economidous, J., Hughes-Jones, N. C., and Gardner, B.: Quantitative measurements concerning A and B antigen sites. Vox Sang. 12:321, 1967.

Edelman, G. M.: Antibody structure and molecular immunology. In Immunoglobulins. Kochwa, S. and Kunkel, H. G. (eds). Ann. N.Y. Acad. Sci. 190:5, 1971.

Edwards, J. H., Allen, F. H., Glenn, K. P., Lamm, L. U. and Robson, E. B.: The linkage relationships of HL-A. In Histocompatibility Testing, Munksgaard, Copenhagen, 745–751, 1973.

Edwards, R. G., Ferguson, L. C. and Coombs, R. R. A.: Blood group antigens on human spermatozoa. J. Reprod. Fertil. 7:153–161, 1964.

Elliot, M., Bossom, E., Dupuy, M. E., and Masouredis, S. P.: Effect of ionic strength on the serologic behavior of red cell isoantibodies. Vox Sang. 9:396, 1964.

Ellisor, S. S., Reid, M. E., and Shoemaker, M. M.: Autoabsorption of anti-Chido using C4 coated red cells. Proc. 33rd Ann. Meeting, AABB, Washington, 1980.

Engelfriet, C. P., Beckers, D., Von Dem Borne, A., Reynierse, E. and Van Loghem, J. J.: Hemolysins probably recognizing the antigen p. Vox Sang. 23:176–181, 1971.

Engelfriet, C. P., Pondman, K. W., Wolters, G., Von Dem Borne, A., Beckers, D., Misset-Groenveld, G. and Van Loghem, J. J.: Autoimmune hemolytic anaemia. III. Preparation and examination of specific antisera against complement components and products and their use in serological studies. Clin. Exp. Immunol. 6:721, 1970.

Epstein, A. A. and Ottenberg, R.: Simple method of performing serum reactions. Proc. N.Y. Path. Soc. 8:117, 1908.

Epstein, W. V.: Specificity of macroglobulin antibody synthesized by the normal human fetus. Science 148:1591, 1965.

Erskine, A. G.: The Principles and Practice of Blood Grouping. C. V. Mosby Co., 1973.

Escolar, J. and Mueller-Eckhardt, C.: Untersuchungen zur Identifizierung HL-A-spezifischer Antiseren für die Gewebetypisierung. Dtsch. Med. Wschr. 96:58–62, 1971.

Evans, R. S., Turner, E. and Bingham, M.: Studies with radio-iodinated cold agglutinins of 10 patients. Am. J. Med. 38:378, 1965.

Eyster, M. E., and Jenkins, D. E.: γG erythrocyte autoantibodies: comparison of in vivo complement coating and in vitro "Rh" specificity. J. Immunol. 105:221, 1970.

Factor IX complex and hepatitis: FDA Drug Bulletin 6:22, 1976.

Fairley, N. H.: The fate of extracorpuscular circulating hemoglobin. Br. Med. J. ii: 213, 1940.

Feinstone, S. M., Kapikian, A. Z., Purcell, R. H., Alter, H. J. and Holland, P. V.: Transfusion-associated hepatitis not due to viral hepatitis type A or B. N. Engl. J. Med. 292:767, 1975.

Feizi, T. Kabat, E. A., Vicari, G., Anderson, B. and Marsh, W. L.: Immunochemical studies on blood groups. XLVII. The I antigen complex-precursors in the A, B, H, Le^a and Le^b blood group system — hemagglutination-inhibition studies. J. Exp. Med. 133:39–52, 1971a.

Feizi, T., Kabat, E. A., Vicari, G., Anderson, B. and Marsh, W. L.: Immunochemical studies on blood groups. XLIX. The I antigen complex: specificity differences among anti-I sera revealed by quantitative precipitin studies; partial structure of the I determinant specific for one anti-I serum. J. Immunol. 106:1578–1592, 1971b.

Feller, C. W., Shenker, L., Scott, E. P. and Marsh, W. L.: An anti-Diego^b (Di^b) antibody occurring during pregnancy. Transfusion 10:279–280, 1970.

Fellous, M., Gerbal, A., Tessier, C., Frézal, J., Dausset, J. and Salmon, C.: Studies on the biosynethic pathway of human erythrocyte antigens using somatic cells in culture. Vox Sang. 26:518–536, 1974.

Fellous, M., Tessier, C., Gerbal, A., Salmon, C., Frézal, J. and Dausset, J.: Genetic dissection of P biosynthesis pathway. Bull. Europ. Soc. Hum. Genet., Nov., 1972.

Ferguson, S. J., Boyce, F., and Blajchman, M. A.: Anti-Yt^b in pregnancy. Transfusion 19:581–582, 1979.

Figur, A. M. and Rosenfield, R. E.: The cross-reaction of anti-N with type M erythrocytes. Vox Sang. 10:169, 1965.

Filitti-Wurmser, S., Jacquot-Armand, Y., Aubel-Lesure, G. and Wurmser, R.: Physicochemical study of human isohemagglutination. Ann. Eugen. 18:183–302, 1954.

Finn, R.: In Report of the Liverpool Medical Institution. Lancet i:526, 1960.

Finn, R., Clarke, C. A., Donohoe, W. T. A., McConnell, R. B., Sheppard, P. M., Lehane, D. and Kulke, W.: Experimental studies on the prevention of Rh hemolytic disease. Br. Med. J. i:1486, 1961.

Firt, P., and Hejhal, L.: Treatment of severe haemorrhage. Lancet ii:1132, 1957.

Fischer, W. and Hahn, F.: Ueber auffallende Schwäche der gruppenspezifischen Reaktions-Fähigkeit bei einem Erwachsenen. Z. Immun. Forsch. 84:177, 1935.

Fisher, N.: Unpublished observations. Cited by Race and Sanger, 1975.

Fisher R. A.: Cited by Race R. R. An "incomplete" antibody in human serum. Nature 153:771–772, 1944.

Fisk, R. T., and Foord, A. G.: Observations on the Rh agglutinogen of human blood. Am. J. Clin. Pathol. 12:545, 1942.

Fletcher, J. L. and Zmijewski, C. M.: The first example of auto-anti-M and its consequences in pregnancy. Int. Arch. Allerg. 37:586, 1970.

Flückiger, P., Ricci, C. and Usteri, C.: Zur Frage der Blutgruppenspezifität von Autoantikörpern. Acta Hematol. 13:53, 1955.

Folkerd, E. J., Ellory, J. C. and Hughes-Jones, N. C.: A molecular size determination of Rh (D) antigen by radiation inactivation. Immunochemistry 14:529, 1977.

Formaggio, T. G.: Development and secretion of the blood group factor O in the newborn. Proc. Soc. Exp. Biol. N.Y. 76:554–556, 1951.

Forre, Ø., Gaarder, P. I. and Natvig, J. B.: V$_H$ subgroup restriction in human erythrocyte antibodies: studies of anti-A, anti-B and anti-Duffy antibodies. Scand. J. Immunol. 6:149, 1977.

Fox, C. L., Jr., Einbinder, J. M. and Nelson, C. T.: Comparative inhibition of anaphylaxis in mice by steroids, tranquilizers and other drugs. Am. J. Physiol. 192:241, 1958.

Frame, M., Mollison, P. L. and Terry, W. D.: Anti-Rh activity of human gamma G4 proteins. Nature 225:641, 1970.

Francis, B. J. and Hatcher, D. E.: MN blood types. The S−s−U+ and the M₁ phenotypes. Vox Sang. 11:213–216, 1966.

Franklin, E. C. and Kunkel, H. G.: Comparative levels of high molecular weight (19S) gamma globulin in maternal and umbilical cord sera. J. Lab. Clin. Med. 52:724, 1958.

Freda, V. J., Gorman, J. G. and Pollack, W.: Rh factor: prevention of immunization and clinical trial on mothers. Science 151:828, 1966.

Freedman, J. and Newlands, M.: Autoimmune hemolytic anemia with the unusual combination of both IgM and IgG autoantibodies. Vox Sang. 32:61, 1977.

Freedman, J., Newlands, M. and Johnson, C. A.: Warm IgM anti-I^T causing autoimmune hemolytic anemia. Vox Sang. 32:135, 1977.

Freiesleben, E. and Jensen, K. G.: An antibody specific for washed red cells. Commun. 7th Congr. Europ. Soc. Hemat., London, Abstract 330, 1959.

Friedenreich, V.: The Thomsen Hemagglutination Phenomenon. Levin and Munksgaard, 1930.

Fudenberg, H. H., Drews, G., and Nisonoff, A.: Serologic studies with proteolytic antibody fragments and "hybrid" antibodies. Vox Sang. 9:14, 1964.

Fudenberg, H. H., Kunkel, H. G. and Franklin, E. C.: High molecular weight antibodies. Acta Hematol. Fasc. 10:522, 1959.

Furuhata, T., Kitahama, M. and Nozawa, T.: A family study of the so-called blood group chimera. Proc. Imp. Acad. Japan 35:55–57, 1959.

Furuhjelm, U., Nevanlinna, H. R., Nurkka, R., Gavin, J. and Sanger, R.: Evidence that the antigen Ul^a is controlled from Kell complex locus. Vox Sang. 16:496–499, 1969.

Furuhjelm, U., Myllylä, G., Nevanlinna, H. R., Nordling, S., Pirkola, A., Gavin, J., Gooch, A., Sanger, R. and Tippett, P.: The red cell phenotype En (a−) and anti-En^a: serological and physicochemical aspects. Vox Sang. 17:256–278, 1969.

Furuhjelm, U., Nevanlinna, H. R., Nurkka, R., Gavin, J, Tippett, P., Gooch, A. and Sanger, R.: The blood group antigen Ul^a (Karhula). Vox Sang. 15:118–124, 1968.

Gammelgaard, A.: Om Sjaeldne, Svage A-receptorer (A₃, A₄, A₅ og A$_x$), Hos Mennesket, Nyt Nordisk Forlag, Copenhagen. (English translation published in 1964 by Walter Reed Army Institute of Medical Research, Washington, D.C., 1942.)

Gandini, E., Sacchi, R., Reali, G., Veratti, M. A., and Menini, C.: A case of Lewis negative "Bombay" blood type. Vox Sang. 15:142–146, 1968.

Gardas, A.: Studies on the I Blood group–active sites on macroglycolipids from human erythrocytes. Europ. J. Biochem. 68:185, 1976.

Garratty, G. and Petz, L. D.: The significance of red cell bound complement components in development of standards and quality assurance for the anti-complement components of antiglobulin sera. Transfusion 16:297, 1976.

Garratty, G., Petz, L. D. and Hoops, J. K.: The correlation of cold agglutinin titrations in saline and albumin with hemolytic anemia. Br. J. Hematol. 35:587, 1977.

Garratty, G., Petz, L. D., Wallerstein, R. O. and Fudenberg, H. H.: Autoimmune hemolytic anemia in Hodgkin's disease associated with anti-I^T. Transfusion 14:226, 1974.

Garratty, G., Petz, L. D., Brodsky, I. and Fudenberg, H. H.: An IgA high-titer cold agglutinin with an unusual blood group specificity within the Pr complex. Vox Sang. 25:32, 1973.

Garratty, G., Haffleigh, B., Dalziel, J. and Petz, L. D.: An IgG anti-I^T detected in a Caucasian American. Transfusion 12:325, 1972.

Garretta, M., Müller, A. and Gener, J.: Détermination du facteur D^u sur Groupamatic. Étude comparée avec les techniques manuelles. Bilan sur 203,240 examens. Rev. Franç. Trans. 17:211, 1974.

Garrison, F. H.: An Introduction to the History of Medicine, 3rd Ed. W. B. Saunders Co., 1924.

Gartler, S. M., Waxman, S. H. and Giblett, E.: An XX/XY human hermaphrodite resulting from double fertilization. Proc. Nat. Acad. Sci. USA 48:332, 1962.

Gavin, J., Daniels, G. L., Yamaguchi, H., Okubo, Y., and Seno, T.: The red cell antigen once called Levay is the antigen Kp^c of the Kell system. Vox Sang. 36:31–33, 1979.

Geiger, J. and Wiener, A. S.: An Rh₀ positive mother with serum containing potent Rh antibodies, apparently of specificity anti-Rh₀, causing erythroblastosis fetalis. Proc. 6th Congr. Int. Soc. Blood Transf., 36–40, 1958.

Gerbal, A., Ropars, C., Gerbal, R., Cartron, J. P., Maslet, C. and Salmon, C.: Acquired B antigen disappearance by in vitro acetylation associated with A₁ activity restoration. Vox Sang. 31:64, 1976.

Gerbal, A., Maslet, C. and Salmon, C.: Immunological aspects of the acquired B antigen. Vox Sang. 28:398, 1975.

Gerbal, A., Lavallée, R., Ropars, C., Doinel, C., Lacombe, M. and Salmon C.: Sensibilisation des hématies d'un nouveau-né par un auto-anticorps anti-i d'origine maternelle de nature IgG. Nouv. Rev. Franç. Hematol., 11:689–700, 1971.

Gerlough, T. D.: Some immunological, physical and chemical properties of purified human gamma-globulin solution stored for prolonged periods at approximately 4° C. Vox Sang. 3:67, 1958.

Gershowitz, H.: An unusual human anti-N serum. Proc. 2nd Int. Congr. Hum. Genet., Rome 1962, pp. 833–835, 1964.

Gershowitz, H. and Fried K.: Anti-M^v, a new antibody of the MNS blood group system. I. M^v, a new inherited variant of the M gene. Am. J. Hum. Genet. 18:264–281, 1966.

Giblett, E. R.: A critique of the theoretical hazard of inter-vs. intra-racial transfusion. Transfusion 1:233, 1961.

Giblett, E. R. and Crookston, M. C.: Agglutinability of red cells by anti-i in patients with thalassemia major and other hematological disorders. Nature 201:1138–1139, 1964.

Giblett, E. R. and Chase, J.: Js^a, a "new" red cell antigen found in Negroes; evidence for an eleventh blood group system. Br. J. Hematol., 5:319–326, 1959.

Giblett, E., Chase, J. and Crealock, F. W.: Hemolytic disease of the newborn resulting from anti-s antibody. Am. J. Clin. Pathol., 29:254–256, 1958.

Gibson, J. G., Gregory, C. B. and Button, L. N.: Citrate-phosphate-dextrose solution for preservation of human blood. Transfusion 1:280, 1961.

Gibson, J. G., Rees, S. B., McManus, T. J. and Scheitlin, W. A.: A citrate-phosphate-dextrose solution for the preservation of human blood. Am. J. Clin. Pathol. 28:569, 1957.

Giles, C. M.: Serologically difficult red cell antibodies, with special reference to Chido and Rodgers blood groups. In Human Blood Groups. J. F. Mohn et al (eds). S. Karger, 1977.

Giles, C. M.: Survey of uses for ficin in blood group serology. Vox Sang. 5:467, 1960.

Giles, C. M. and Howell, P.: An antibody in the serum of an MN patient which reacts with M₁ antigen. Vox Sang. 27:43–51, 1974.

Giles, C. M. and Skov, F.: The CDe rhesus gene complex; some considerations revealed by a study of a Danish family with an antigen of the rhesus gene complex

(C)D(e) defined by a "new" antibody. Vox Sang. 20:328–334, 1971.

Giles, C. M. and Metaxas, M. N.: Identification of the predicted blood group antibody anti-Yt^b. Nature 202:1122–1123, 1964.

Giles, C. M., Crossland, J. D., Haggas, W. K. and Longster, G.: An Rh gene complex which results in a "new" antigen detectable by a specific antibody, anti-Rh33. Vox Sang. 21:289–301, 1971.

Giles, C. M., Bevan, B. and Hughes, R. M.: A family showing independent segregation of Bu^a and Yt^b. Vox Sang. 18:265–266, 1970.

Giles, C. M., Darnborough, J., Aspinall, P. and Fletton, M. W.: Identification of the first example of anti-Co^b. Br. J. Hemat. 19:267–269, 1970.

Giles, C. M., Metaxas-Bühler, M., Romanski, Y. and Metaxas, M. N.: Studies on the Yt blood group system. Vox Sang., 13:171–180, 1967.

Giles, C. M., Huth, M. C., Wilson, T. E., Lewis, H. B. M. and Grove, G. E. B.: Three examples of a new antibody anti-Cs^a, which reacts with 98% of red cell samples. Vox Sang. 10:405–415, 1965.

Giles, C. M., Mourant, A. E. and Atabuddin, A.-H.: A Lewis-negative "Bombay" blood. Vox Sang. 8:269–272, 1963.

Gilliland, B. C., Baxter, E., and Evans, R. S.: Red cell antibodies in acquired hemolytic anemia with negative antiglobulin serum tests. N. Engl. J. Med. 285:252, 1971.

Gilliland, B. C., Leddy, J. P., and Vaughan, J. H.: The detection of cell-bound antibody on complement-coated human red cells. J. Clin. Invest. 49:898, 1970.

Gillund, T. D., Howard, P. L., and Isham, B.: A serum agglutinating human red cells exposed to EDTA. Vox Sang. 23:369, 1972.

Gleichmann, H. and Breininger, J.: Over 95% sensitization against allogeneic leukocytes following single massive blood transfusion. Vox Sang. 28:66, 1975.

Glynn, A. A., Glynn, L. E., and Holborow, E. J.: The secretor status of rheumatic fever patients. Lancet ii:759–762, 1956.

Göbel, U., Drescher, K. H., Pöttgen, W. and Lehr, H. J.: A second example of anti-Yt^a with rapid in vivo destruction of Yt(a+) red cells. Vox Sang. 27:171–175, 1974.

Gold, E. and Dunsford, I.: An A$_1$ antigen with abnormal serological properties. Vox Sang. 5:574–578, 1960.

Gold, E. R. and Fudenberg, H. H.: Chromic chloride: a coupling reagent for passive hemagglutination reactions. J. Immunol. 99:859, 1967.

Gold, E. R., Gillespie, E. M., and Tovey, G. H.: A serum containing 8 antibodies. Vox Sang. 6:157–163, 1961.

Golde, D. W., McGinnis, M. H. and Holland, P. V.: Mechanism of the albumin agglutination phenomenon. Vox Sang. 16:465, 1969.

Goldman, J. M., Lowenthal, R. M., Buskard, N. A., Spiers, A. S. D., Th'Ng, K. H. and Park, D. S.: Chronic granulocytic leukemia — selective removal of immature granulocytic cells by leukapheresis. Series Hematologica 8:28, 1975.

Goldsmith, K. L. G.: The effect of bovine serum albumin on red cell agglutination. In Enhancement of Serological Reactions. Proceedings of Symposium published by Biotest Folex Ltd., 1974.

Goldsmith, K. L. G., Albrey, J., Brunnelhuis, H. G. J., Gunson, H. H., Ikin, E. W., Kerwick, R. A., Metaxas, M., Moore, B. P. L., Yasuda, J., and Phillips, T. T. B.: A study performed on batches of serum albumin used as diluents in Rh testing. Br. J. Hemat. 32:215, 1976.

Goldsmith, K. L. G., Jones, J. M. and Kekwick, R. A.: The effects of polymers on the efficiency of bovine serum albumin used as a diluent in the detection of incomplete Rh antibodies. Proc. 12th Congr. Int. Soc. Blood Transf.,

Moscow, 1969. Bibl. Haemat. No. 38, part 1, Karger, 1971.

Goldstein, E. I.: Investigation of the inheritance of the U factors: emphasis on dosage studies of S and s and studies with anti-U^A and U^B. Master of Science Thesis, University of Cincinnati, 1966.

Goldstein, I. M., Eyre, H. J., Terasaki, P. I., Henderson, E. S. and Graw, R. G., Jr.: Leukocyte transfusions: role of leukocyte alloantibodies in determining transfusion response. Transfusion 11:19, 1971.

Gonzenbach, R., Hässig, A. and Rosin, S.: Über posttransfusionelle Bildung von Anti-Lutheran-Antikörpern. Die Häufigkeit des Lutheran-Antigens Lu^a in de Bevölkerung Nord-, West- und Mitteleuropas. Blut 1:272–274, 1955.

Goodall, H. B., Hendry, D. W. W., Lawler, S. D. and Stephen, S. A.: Data on linkage in man: elliptocytosis and blood groups. III. Family 4. Ann. Eugen. 18:325–327, 1954.

Goodall, H. B., Hendry, D. W. W., Lawler, S. D. and Stephen, S. A.: Data on linkage in man: elliptocytosis and blood groups. II. Family 3. Ann. Eugen. 17:272–278, 1953.

Goodman, H. S. and Masaitis, L.: Analysis of the isoimmune response to leukocytes. I. Maternal cytotoxic leukocyte isoantibodies formed during the first pregnancy. Vox Sang. 16:97, 1967.

Götze, O. and Müller-Eberhard, H. J.: The alternative pathway of complement activation. Advances in Immunology 24:1, 1976.

Gower, D. B. and Davidson, W. M.: The mechanism of immune hemolysis. I. The relationship of the rate of destruction of red cells to their age, following the administration to rabbits of an immune hemolysin. Br. J. Hematol. 9:132, 1963.

Gralnick, H. R. and McGinniss, M. H.: Immune cross-reactivity of penicillin and cephalothin. Nature 215:1026, 1967.

Gralnick, H. R., McGinniss, M. H., Elton, W. and McCurdy, P.: Hemolytic anemia associated with cephalothin. JAMA 217:1193, 1971.

Gralnick, H. R., Wright, L. D. and McGinniss, M. H.: Coombs' positive reactions associated with sodium cephalothin therapy. JAMA 199:725, 1967.

Graninger, W., Ramesis, H., Fischer, K., Poschmann, A., Bird, G. W. G., Wingham, J. and Neumann, E.: "VA," a new type of erythrocyte polyagglutination characterized by depressed H receptors and associated with hemolytic anemia. I. Serological and hematological observations. Vox Sang. 32:195, 1977.

Graninger, W., Poschmann, A., Fischer, K., Schedl-Giovannoni, I., Hörandner, H. and Klaushofer, K.: "VA," a new type of erythrocyte polyagglutination characterized by depressed H receptors and associated with hemolytic anemia. II. Observations by immunofluorescence, electron microscopy, cell electrophoresis and biochemistry. Vox Sang. 32:201, 1977.

Grant, R. T. and Reeve, E. B.: Observations on the general effects of injury in man, with special reference to wound shock. Spec. Rep. Ser. Med. Res. Coun. No. 277, 1951.

Graw, R. G., Jr.: Leukocyte transfusion therapy — past, present and future. In Goldman, J. M. and Lowenthal, R. M. (eds): Leukocytes: Separation, Collection and Transfusion. Academic Press, 1975.

Graw, R. G., Jr., Herzig, G., Perry, S. and Henderson, E. S.: Normal granulocyte transfusion. Treatment of septicemia due to gram-negative bacteria. N. Engl. J. Med. 287:367, 1972.

Gray, D. F.: Immunology. American Elsevier Publishing Co., 1970.

Gray, M. P.: A human serum factor agglutinating human red cells exposed to lactose. Vox Sang. 9:608, 1964.

Green, F. A.: Phospholipid requirement of Rh antigenic activity. J. Biol. Chem. 243:5519, 1968.

Green, F. A.: Erythrocyte membrane sulfhydryl groups and Rh antigen activity. Immunochemistry 4:247, 1967.

Green, H., Barrow, P. and Goldberg, B.: Effects of antibody and complement on permeability control in ascites tumor cells and erythrocytes. J. Exp. Med. 110:699, 1959.

Green, N. M.: Electron microscopy of the immunoglobulins. Advanc. Immunol. II:1, 1969.

Greenbury, C. L., Moore, D. H. and Nunn, L. A. C.: Reaction of 7S and 19S components of immune rabbit antisera with human group A and AB cells. Immunology 6:421, 1963.

Greendyke, R. M. and Chorpenning, F. W.: Normal survival of incompatible red cells in the presence of anti-Lu^a. Transfusion 2:52–57, 1962.

Greendyke, R. M., Banzhaf, J. C. and LaFerla, J. J.: Determination of Rh blood group of fetuses in abortions by suction curettage. Transfusion 16:267, 1976.

Greenwalt, T. J. and Sasaki, T.: The Lutheran blood groups: a second example of anti-Lu^b and three further examples of anti-Lu^a. Blood 12:998–1003, 1957.

Greenwalt, T. J. and Sanger, R.: The Rh antigen E^w. Br. J. Hematol. 1:52–54, 1955.

Greenwalt, T. J., Sasaki, T. and Steane, E. A.: The Lutheran blood groups: a progress report with observations on the development of the antigens and characteristics of the antibodies. Transfusion 7:189–200, 1967.

Greenwalt, T. J., Walker, R. H., Argall, C. I., Steane, E. A., Can, R. T. and Sasaki, T. T.: Js^b of the Sutter blood group system. Proc. 9th Congr. Int. Soc. Blood Transf., Mexico, 1962.

Greenwalt, T. J., Sasaki, T. and Gajewski, M.: Further examples of haemolytic disease of the newborn due to anti-Duffy (anti-Fy^a). Vox Sang. 4:138, 1959.

Greenwalt, T. J., Sasaki, T., Sanger, R. Sneath, J. and Race, R. R.: An allele of the S(s) blood group genes. Proc. Nat. Acad. Sci. USA 40:1126–1129, 1954.

Grubb, R.: Observations on the human group system Lewis. Acta Pathol. Microbiol. Scand. 28:61–81, 1951.

Grubb, R.: Dextran as a medium for the demonstration of incomplete anti-Rh agglutinins. J. Clin. Pathol. 2:223, 1949.

Grubb, R.: Correlation between Lewis blood group and secretor character in man. Nature 162:933, 1948.

Grumet, F. C.: HLA and disease associations. Transplant. Proc. 9:1839–1844, 1977.

Grundbacher, F. J.: Changes in the human A antigen of erythrocytes with the individual's age. Nature 204:192–194, 1964.

Guévin, R. M., Taliano, V. and Waldmann, O.: The Côté serum, an antibody defining a new variant in the Kell system. 24th Annual Meeting, AABB, p. 100, 1971.

Gundolf, F.: Anti-A₁Le^b in serum of a person of a blood group A₁h. Vox Sang. 25:411–419, 1973.

Gunson, H. H. and Phillips, P. K.: An inhibitor to erythrocyte agglutination in bovine albumin preparation. Vox Sang. 28:207, 1975.

Gunson, H. H. and Donohue, W. L.: Multiple examples of the blood genotype C^wD−/C^wD− in a Canadian family. Vox Sang. 2:320, 1957.

Gunson, H. H., Stratton, F. and Cooper, D. G.: Primary immunization of Rh-negative volunteers. Br. Med. J. i:593, 1970a.

Gunson, H. H., Stratton, F. and Mullard, G. W.: An example of polyagglutinability due to the Tn antigen. Br. J. Hematol. 18:309, 1970b.

Gurevitch, J. and Nelken, D.: Elution of isoagglutinins absorbed by platelets. Nature 175:822, 1955.

Gurevitch, J. and Nelken, D.: ABO groups in blood platelets. J. Lab. Clin. Med. 44:562–570, 1954.

Gurevitch, J. and Nelken, D.: ABO blood groups in blood platelets. Nature 173:356, 1954.

Gurner, B. W. and Coombs, R. R. A.: Examination of human leukocytes for the ABO, MN, Rh, Tj^a, Lutheran and Lewis systems of antigens by means of mixed erythrocyte-leukocyte agglutination. Vox Sang. 3:13, 1958.

Haber, G. and Rosenfield, R. E.: Ficin-treated red cells for hemagglutination studies. P. H. Andresen — Papers in Dedication of his 60th Birthday. Munksgaard, 1957.

Habibi, B., Tippett, P., Lebesnerais, M. and Salmon, C.: Protease inactivation of the red cell antigen Xg^a. Vox Sang. 36:367–368, 1979.

Habibi, B., Fouillade, M. T., Duedari, N., Issitt, P. D., Tippett, P. and Salmon, C.: The antigen Duclos: a new high frequency red cell antigen related to Rh and U. Vox Sang. 34:302, 1978.

Hamaguchi, H. and Cleve, H., Solubilization of human erythrocyte membrane glycoproteins and separation of the MN glycoprotein from a glycoprotein with I, S, and A activity. Biochem. Biophys. Acta 278:271, 1972.

Hamerton, J. L.: Chromosomes in medicine. Little Club Clinics in Developmental Medicine, No. 5. William Heinemann Ltd., London, 1962.

Hammer, C. H., Nicholson, A. and Mayer, M. M.: On the mechanism of cytolysis by complement: evidence on insertion of C5b and C7 subunits of the C5b,6,7 complex into phospholipid bilayers of erythrocyte membranes. Proc. Nat. Acad. Sci. USA 72:5076, 1975.

Hamstra, R. D. and Block, M. H.: Erythropoiesis in response to blood loss in man. J. Appl. Physiol. 27:503, 1969.

Haradin, A. R., Weed, R. I. and Reed, C. F.: Changes in physical properties of stored erythrocytes: relationship to survival in vivo. Transfusion 9:229, 1969.

Harboe, M., Müller-Eberhard, H. J., Fudenberg, H., Polley, M. J. and Mollison, P. L.: Identification of the components of complement participating in the antiglobulin reaction. Immunology 6:412, 1963.

Harris, J. P., Tegoli, J., Swanson, J., Fisher, N., Gavin, J. and Noades, J.: A nebulous antibody responsible for crossmatching difficulties. Vox Sang. 12:140, 1967.

Harrison, J.: The "naturally occurring" anti-E. Vox Sang. 19:123, 1970.

Hart, M. Van der, Szaloky, A. and Van Loghem, J. J.: A "new" antibody associated with the Kell blood group system. Vox Sang. 15:456–458, 1968.

Hart, M. Van der, Moes, M., Veer Marga, V. D. and Van Loghem, J. J.: Ho and Lan — two new blood group antigens. Paper read at the VIIIth Europ. Cong. Hemat., 1961.

Hayashida, Y. and Watanabe, A.: A case of a blood group p Taiwanese woman delivered of an infant with hemolytic disease of the newborn. Jpn. J. Legal Med. 22:10, 1968.

Haynes, C. R. and Chaplin, H., Jr.: The role of macromolecular components in anti-γ, α, μ, κ, λ, C₃ and C₄ antiglobin sera. Br. J. Hematol. 21:277, 1971a.

Haynes, C. R. and Chaplin, H., Jr.: An enhancing effect of albumin on the determination of cold hemagglutinins. Vox Sang. 20:46, 1971b.

Haynes, C. R., Dorner, I., Leonard, G. L., Arrowsmith, W. R. and Chaplin, H., Jr.: Persistent polyagglutinability in vivo unrelated to T-antigen activation. Transfusion 10:43, 1970.

Heidelberger, M. and Mayer, M. M.: Quantitative studies on complement. Advanc. Enzymol. 8:71, 1948.

Heiken, A.: Observations on the blood group receptor P1

and its development in children. Hereditas 56:83–98, 1966.

Heistö, H., Guévin, R.-M., Taliano, V., Mann, J., Macilroy, M., Marsh, W. L., Tippet, P. and Gavin, J.: Three further antigen-antibody specificities associated with the Kell blood group system. Vox Sang. 24:179–180, 1973.

Heistö, H., Van Der Hart, M., Madsen, G., Moes, M., Noades, J., Pickles, M. M., Race, R. R., Sanger, R. and Swanson, J.: Three examples of a new red cell antibody, anti-Co^a. Vox Sang. 12:18–24, 1967.

Heistö, H., Harboe, M. and Godal, H. C.: Warm hemolysins active against trypsinized red cells: occurrence, inheritance, and clinical significance. Proc. 10th Congr. Int. Soc. Blood Transfus., Stockholm, 1965.

Hektoen, L.: Isoagglutination of human corpuscles. J. Infect. Dis. 4:297, 1907a.

Hektoen, L.: Isoagglutination of human corpuscles with respect to demonstration of opsonic index and to transfusion of blood. JAMA 48:1739, 1907b.

Hendry, P. I. A. and Simmons, R. T.: An example of polyagglutinable erythrocytes, and reference to panagglutination, polyagglutination and autoagglutination as possible sources of error in blood grouping. Med. J. Aust. i:720, 1955.

Henningsen, K.: OM Blodtypesystemet, P.M.D. Thesis. Dansk Videnskabs Forlag A/S, Copenhagen, 1952.

Henningsen, K.: On the heredity of blood factor P. Acta Pathol. Microbiol. Scand. 26:769–785, 1949.

Henningsen, K.: Investigations on the blood factor P. Acta Pathol. Microbiol. Scand. 26:639–654, 1949.

Henningsen, K.: A case of polyagglutinable human red cells. Acta Pathol. Microbiol. Scand. 26:339, 1949.

Herst, R. and Shepherd, F. A. (eds): Clinical Guide to Transfusion. The Canadian Red Cross Society, Toronto, 1980.

Hindman, S. H., Gravelle, C. R., Murphy, B. L., Bradley, D. W., Budge, W. R. and Maynard, J. E.: "e" antigen, Dane particles, and serum DNA polymerase activity in HBs Ag carriers. Ann. Intern. Med. 85:458, 1976.

Hinz, C. C. and Boyer, J. T.: Dysgammaglobulinemia in the adult manifested as autoimmune hemolytic anemia. N. Engl. J. Med. 269:1329, 1963.

Hirsch, W., Moores, P., Sanger, R. and Race, R. R.: Notes on some reactions of human anti-M and anti-N sera. Br. J. Hematol. 3:134, 1957.

Hirszfeld, L. and Hirszfeld, H.: Serological differences between the blood of different races. The result of research on the Macedonian front. Lancet ii:675, 1919.

Hobbs, J. R., Byrom, N., Elliott, P., Oon, C.-J and Retsas, S.: Cell separators in cancer immunotherapy. Exp. Hemat. 5:Suppl. 1, p. 95, 1977.

Hobsley, M.: Chlorpheniramine maleate in prophylaxis of pyrexial reactions during blood transfusions. Lancet i:497, 1958.

Högman, C. F., Akerblom, O., Arturson, G., De Verdier, C.-H., Kreuger, A. and Westman, M.: Experience with new preservatives: summary of the experiences in Sweden. In Greenwalt, T. J. and Jamieson, G. A. The Human Red Cell in vitro. Grune and Stratton, 1974.

Holburn, A. M., and Masters, C. A.: The radioimmunoassay of serum and salivary blood group A and Le glycoproteins. Br. J. Hematol. 28:157–167, 1974.

Holländer, L.: Das Lutheran-Blutgruppensystem. Die Häufigkeit des Lutheran-Antigens in der Bevölkerung Basels. Schweiz. Med. Wschr. 85:10–11, 1955.

Holländer, L.: Study of the erythrocyte survival time in a case of acquired hemolytic anaemia. Vox Sang. 4:164, 1954.

Hollinger, F. B., Dreesman, G. R., Fields, H. and Melnick, J. L.: HB$_c$Ag, anti-HB$_c$ and DNA polymerase activity in transfused recipients followed prospectively. Am. J. Med. Sci. 270:343, 1975.

Holman, C. A.: A new rare human blood-group antigen (Wr^a). Lancet ii:119, 1953.

Holman, C. A. and Karnicki, J.: Intrauterine transfusion for haemolytic disease of the newborn. Br. Med. J. ii:594, 1964.

Høstrup, H.: A and B blood group substances in the serum of the newborn infant and the fetus. Vox Sang. 8:557–566, 1963.

Høstrup, H.: A and B blood group substances in the serum of normal subjects. Vox Sang. 7:704–721, 1962.

Howard, A., and Pelc, S. R.: Synthesis of deoxyribonucleic acid in normal and irradiated cells and its relation to chromosome breakage. Heredity 6, Suppl. 261, 1953.

Howard, P. L.: Delayed hemolytic transfusion reactions. Ann. Clin. Lab. Sci. 3:13, 1973.

Howell, E. D. and Perkins, H. A.: Anti-N-like antibodies in the sera of patients undergoing chronic hemodialysis. Vox Sang. 23:291, 1972.

Hrubiško, M., Čalkovská, Z., Mergancová, O. and Gallová, K.: Beobachtungen über Varianten des Blutgruppensystems ABO. I. Studien der Variante A$_m$. Blut 13:137–142, 1966.

Hrubiško, M., Čalkovská, Z., Mergancová, O. and Gallová, K.: Beobachtungen über Varianten des Blutgruppensystems ABO. II. Beitrag zur Erblichkeit der A$_m$ Variante. Blut 13:232–239, 1966.

Hubbard, A. L. and Cohn, Z. A.: The enzymatic iodination of the red cell membrane. J. Cell. Biol. 55:390, 1972.

Hübener, G.: Untersuchungen über Isoagglutination, mit besonderer Berücksichtigung scheinbarer Abweichungen vom Gruppenschema. Z. Immun.-Forsch. 45:223, 1925.

Huestis, D. W., White, R. F., Price, M. J. and Inman, M.: Use of hydroxyethyl starch to improve granulocyte collection in the Latham blood processor. Transfusion 15:559, 1975.

Huestis, D. W., Busch, S., Hanson, M. L. and Gurney, C. W.: A second example of the antibody anti-Js^b of the Sutter blood group system. Transfusion 3:260–262, 1963.

Hughes-Jones, N. C.: Nature of the reaction between antigen and antibody. Br. Med. Bull. 19:171, 1963.

Hughes-Jones, N. C. and Gardner, B.: The Kell system: studies with radioactively labelled anti-K. Vox Sang. 21:154, 1971.

Hughes-Jones, N. C., Gardner, B. and Lincoln, P.: Observations of the number of available cDc and E antigen sites on red cells. Vox Sang. 21:210, 1971.

Hughes-Jones, N. C., Gardner, B., and Telford, R.: The effect of pH and ionic strength on the reaction between anti-D and erythrocytes. Immunology 7:72, 1964.

Hughes-Jones, N. C., Polley, M. J., Telford, R., Gardner, B. and Kleinshmidt, G.: Optimal conditions for detecting blood group antibodies by the antiglobulin test. Vox Sang 9:385, 1964.

Hughes-Jones, N. C., Gardner, B. and Telford, R.: Studies on the reaction between the blood group antibody anti-D and erythrocytes. Biochem. J. 88:435, 1963.

Hughes-Jones, N. C., Mollison, P. L. and Robinson, M. A.: Factors affecting the viability of erythrocytes stored in the frozen state. Proc. R. Soc. 147:476, 1957.

Humphrey, A. and Morel, P.: Evidence that anti-Jk3 is not cross-reacting anti-Jk^a Jk^b. Transfusion 16:242, 1976.

Humphrey, J. H. and Dourmashkin, R. R.: Electron microscope studies of immune cell lysis. In Ciba. Found. Symp. Complement, J. A. Churchill, 1965.

Huprikar, S. V. and Springer, G. F.: Structural aspects of blood-group M and N specificity. In Blood and tissue antigens. Aminoff, D. (ed.) Academic Press, 1970.

Hurd, J. K., Jacox, R. F., Swisher, S. N., Cleghorn, T. E., Carlin, S. and Allen, F. H., Jr.: S$_2$, a new phenotype in the MN blood group system. Vox Sang. 9:487–491, 1964.

Hutton, E. L. and Shute, P. G.: The risk of transmitting malaria by blood transfusion. J. Trop. Med. Hyg. 42:309, 1939.

Hysell, J. K., Hysell, J. W., Nichols, M. E., Leonardi, R. G. and Marsh, W. L.: *In vivo* and *in vitro* activation of T-antigen receptors on leukocytes and platelets. Vox Sang. 31:9, 1976.

Ikin, E. W.: The production of anti-M^g in rabbits. Vox Sang. 11:217–218, 1966.

Ikin, E. W., Kay, H. E. M., Playfair, J. H. L. and Mourant, A. E.: P_1 antigen in the human foetus. Nature 192:883, 1961.

Ikin, E. W., Mourant, A. E., Pettenkofer, H. J. and Blumenthal, G.: Discovery of the expected hemagglutinin, anti-Fy^b. Nature 168:1077, 1951.

Inglis, G., Bird, G. W. G., Mitchell, A. A. B., Miline, G. R. and Wingham, J.: Erythrocyte polyagglutination showing properties of both T and Tk, probably induced by *Bacteroides fragilis* infection. Vox Sang. 28:314, 1975a.

Inglis, G., Bird, G. W. G., Mitchell, A. A. B., Miline, G. R. and Wingham J.: Effect of *Bacteroides fragilis* on the human erythrocyte membrane: pathogenesis of Tk polyagglutination. J. Clin. Pathol. 28:964, 1975b.

Inokuchi, K.: Agglomerating action of sodium alginate on red blood cells. Mem. Fac. Sci. Kyüshü Univ. Ser. C, Chem, I. 109, 167, 1950.

International Society of Blood Transfusion. International Committee for Standardization in Hematology. Working Party on the Standardization of Antiglobulin. Reagents of the Expert Panel of Serology. Vox Sang. 38:178–179, 1980.

Iseki, S., Masaki, S. and Shibasaki, K.: Studies on Lewis blood group system. I. Le^a blood group factor. Proc. Imp. Acad. Japan 33:492–497, 1957.

Ishimori, T. and Hasekura, H.: A Japanese with no detectable Rh blood group antigens due to silent Rh alleles or deleted chromosomes. Transfusion 7:84–87, 1967.

Ishimori, T. and Hasekura, H.: A case of a Japanese blood with no detectable Rh blood group antigen. Proc. Jpn. Acad. 42:658–660, 1966.

Ishizaka, T., Tada, T. and Ishizaka, K.: Fixation of C′ and C′Ia by rabbit gamma-G and gamma-M-antibodies with particulate and soluble antigens. J. Immunol. 100:1145, 1968.

Ishizaka, T., Ishizaka, K., Salmon, S. and Fudenberg, H.: Biologic activity of aggregated gammaglobulin. VIII. Aggregated immunoglobulins of different classes. J. Immunol. 99:82, 1967.

Ishizaka, K., Ishizaka, T., Lee, E. H. and Fudenberg, H. H.: Immunochemical properties of human gamma-A isohemagglutinin. I. Comparisons with gamma-G and gamma-M-globulin antibodies. J. Immunol. 95:197, 1965.

Issitt, P. D., Pavone, B. G., and Shapiro, M.: Anti-Rh 39-A "new" specific Rh system antibody. Transfusion 19:389, 1979.

Issitt, P. D., Pavone, B. G., Goldfinger, D., Zwicker, J., Issitt, C. H., Tessel, J. A., Kroovand, S. W. and Bell, C. A.: Anti-Wr^b, and other autoantibodies responsible for positive direct antiglobulin tests in 150 individuals. Br. J. Hematol. 34:5, 1976.

Issitt, C. H., Duckett, J. B., Osborne, B. M., Gut, J. B. and Beasley, J.: Another example of an antibody reacting optimally with p red cells. Br. J. Hematol. 34:19, 1976.

Issitt, P. D., Pavone, B. G. and Goldfinger, D.: The Phenotype En(a−), Wr(a−b−). Commun. 14th Congr. Int. Soc. Blood. Transfus., Helsinki, 1975.

Issitt, P. D., Issitt, C. H., and Wilkinson, S. L.: Evaluation of commercial antiglobulin sera over a two-year period. Part

II. Anti-IgG and Anti-IgM levels and undesirable contaminating antibodies. Transfusion 14:103, 1974.

Issitt, P. D., Issitt, C. H., Moulds, J. and Berman, H. J.: Some observations on the T, Tn and Sd^a antigens and the antibodies that define them. Transfusion 12:217, 1972.

Issitt, P. D., Tegoli, J., Jackson, V., Sanders, C. W. and Allen, F. H.: Anti-JP_1: antibodies that show an association between the I and P blood group systems. Vox Sang. 14:1–8, 1968.

Issitt, P. D., Haber, J. M. and Allen, F. H., Jr.: Sj, a new antigen in the MN system, and further studies on TM. Vox Sang. 15:1–14, 1968.

Issitt, P. D., Tegoli, J., Jackson, V., Sanders, C. W. and Allen, F. H.: Anti-IP_1: antibodies that show an association between the I and P blood group systems. Vox Sang 14:1–8, 1968.

Issitt, P. D., Haber, J. M. and Allen, F. H., Jr.: Anti-Tm, an antibody defining a new antigenic determinant within the MN bloodgroup system. Vox Sang. 10:742–743, 1965.

Ito, K., Mukomoto, Y. and Konishi, H.: An example of "naturally-occurring" anti-Js^a (K6) in a Japanese female. Vox Sang. 37:350, 1979.

Jack, J. A., Tippett, P., Noades, J., Sanger, R. and Race, R. R.: M_1, a subdivision of the human blood-group antigen M. Nature 186:642, 1960.

Jackson, D. P., Krevans, J. R. and Conley, C. L.: Mechanism of the thrombocytopenia that follows multiple whole blood transfusion. Trans. Assoc. Am. Physicians 69:155, 1956.

Jakobowicz, R., Williams, L. and Silberman, F.: Immunization of Rh negative volunteers by repeated injections of very small amounts of Rh positive blood. Vox Sang. 23:376, 1972.

Jakobowicz, R., Bryce, L. M. and Simmons, R. T.: The occurrence of unusual positive Coombs reactions and M factors in the blood of a mother and her first baby. Nature 165:158, 1950.

Jakobowicz, R., Bryce, L. M. and Simmons, R. T.: The occurrence of unusual positive Coombs reactions and M variants in the blood of a mother and her first child. Med. J. Austral. 2:945–948, 1949.

James, J., Stiles, P., Boyce, F. and Wright, J.: The HL-A type of Rg(a−) individuals. Vox Sang. 30:214, 1976.

Jandl, J. H. and Tomlinson, A. S.: The destruction of red cells by antibodies in man. II. Pyrogenic, leukocytic and dermal responses to immune hemolysis. J. Clin. Invest. 37:1202, 1958.

Jansky, I.: Hematologic studies in psychotics. Klinky Sbornik, No. 2, 1906.

Jeannet, M., Schapira, M., and Magnin, C.: Mise en évidence d'anticorps lymphocytotoxiques dirigés contre les antigènes A et B et contre des antigènes d'histocompatibilité non-HL-A. Schweiz. Med. Wschr. 104:152, 1974.

Jeannet, M., Bodmer, J. G., Bodmer, W. F., and Schapira, M.: Lymphocytotoxic sera associated with the ABO and Lewis red cell blood groups. Histocompatibility Testing. Munksgaard, 1972.

Jeannet, M., Metaxas-Bühler, M. and Tobler, R.: Anomalie héréditaire de la membrane érythrocytaire avec test de Coombs direct positif et modification de l'antigène de groupe N. Vox Sang. 9:52–55, 1964.

Jeannet, M., Metaxas-Bühler, M. and Tobler, R.: Anomalie héréditaire de la membrane érythrocytaire avec tests de Coombs positif et modification de l'antigène de groupe N. Schweiz. Med. Wschr. 93:1508–1509, 1963.

Jenkins, W. J. and Marsh, W. L.: Unpublished observations. (Cited by Race and Sanger, 1975).

Jenkins, W. J., Marsh, W. L. and Gold, E. R.: Reciprocal

relationship of antigens "I" and "i" in health and disease. Nature 205:813, 1965.

Jenkins, W. J., Koster, H. G., Marsh, W. L. and Carter, R. L.: Infectious mononucleosis: an unsuspected source of anti-i. Br. J. Hematol. 11:480–483, 1965.

Jenkins, W. J., Marsh, W. L., Noades, J., Tippet, P., Sanger, R. and Race, R. R.: The I antigen and antibody. Vox Sang. 5:97–106, 1960.

Jensen, K. G. and Freiesleben, E.: Inherited positive Coombs' reaction connected with a weak N-receptor (N_2). Vox Sang. 7:696–703, 1962.

Jerry, L. M., Kunkel, H. G. and Grey, H. M.: Absence of disulphide bonds linking the heavy and light chains: a property of a genetic variant of gamma A_2 globulins. Proc. Nat. Acad. Sci. USA 65:557, 1970.

Jones, A. R., Steinberg, A. G., Allen, F. H., Jr., Diamond, L. K. and Kriete, B.: Observations on the new Rh agglutinin anti-f. Blood 9:117, 1954.

Jones, J. M., Kekwick, R. A. and Goldsmith, K. L. G.: Influence of polymers on the efficacy of serum albumin as a potentiator of "incomplete" Rh agglutinins. Nature 224:510, 1969.

Jones, J. H., Kilpatrick, G. S. and Franks, E. H.: Red cell aggregation in dextrose solutions. J. Clin. Pathol. 15:161, 1962.

Jordal, K.: The Lewis blood groups in children. Acta Pathol. Microbiol. Scand. 39:399–406, 1956.

Joseph, J. I. J., Awer, E., Laulicht, M. and Scudder, J.: Delayed hemolytic transfusion reaction due to appearance of multiple antibodies following transfusion of apparently compatible blood. Transfusion 4:367, 1964.

Joshi, S. R. and Bhatia, H. M.: A new red cell phenotype I-i-: Red cells lacking both I and i antigens. Vox Sang. 36:34–38, 1979.

Judson, G., Jones, A., Kellogg, R., Buckner, D., Eisel, R., Perry, S. and Greenough, W.: Closed continuous-flow centrifuge. Nature 217:816, 1968.

Juel, E.: Anti-A agglutinins in sera from A_2B individuals. Acta Pathol. Microbiol. Scand. 46:91–95, 1959.

Kaita, H., Lewis, M., Chown, B. and Gard, E.: A further example of the Kell blood group phenotype K−, k−, Kp(a−b−). Nature 183:1586, 1959.

Kattlove, H. E. and Alexander, B.: The effect of cold on platelets. I. Cold-induced platelet aggregation. Blood 38:39, 1971.

Kaufman, B. and Masouredis, S. P.: Effect of formalin and periodic acid on red cell Rh_v(D) antigen. J. Immunol. 91:233, 1963.

Keith, P., Corcoran, P. A., Caspersen, K. and Allen, F. H.: A new antibody; anti-Rh [27] (cE) in the Rh blood group system. Vox Sang. 10:528–535, 1965.

Keleman, J., Hedlund, W., Orlin, J. B., Berkmen, E. M., and Munsat, T. L.: Failure of partial plasma exchange (PPE) and immunosuppression to effect the course of lower motor neuron disease. Proc. 33rd Ann. Meeting, AABB, Washington, D.C., 1980.

Kemp, T.: Über den Empfindlichkeitsgrad der Blutkörperchen gegenüber Isohämagglutininen im Fötattleben und im Kindesalter beim Menschen. Acta Path. Microbiol. Scand. 7:146–156, 1930.

Kerde, C., Brunk, R., Fünfhausen, G. and Prokop, O.: Über die Herstellung von anti-Lewis-Seren an Capra Hircus L. Z. ImmunForsch. 119:462–468, 1960.

Kerde, C., Fünfhausen, G., Brunk, R. E., and Brunk, R. U.: Über die Gewinnung von hochwertigen Anti-P-Immunseren durch Immunisierung mit Echinkokken-zystenflüssigkeit. Z. ImmunForsch. 119:216–224, 1960.

Kerr, R. O., Dalmasso, A. P. and Kaplan, M. E.: Erythrocyte-bound C_5 and C_6 in autoimmune hemolytic anemia. J. Immunol. 107:1209, 1971.

Kim, B. K., Tanque, L. and Baldini, M. G.: Storage of human platelets by freezing. Vox Sang. 30:401, 1976.

Kindler, M.: Ein weiteres Beispiel einer schwachen A-Eigenschaft (A_m). Blut 4:373–377, 1958.

Kirkman, N. N.: Further evidence for a racial difference in frequency of ABO hemolytic disease. J. Pediatr. 90:717, 1977.

Kissmeyer-Nielsen, F.: Irregular blood group antibodies in 200,000 individuals. Scand. J. Hemat. 2:331, 1965.

Kissmeyer-Nielsen, F.: A further example of anti-Lu^b as a cause of mild hemolytic disease of the newborn. Vox Sang. 5:532–537, 1960.

Kissmeyer-Nielsen, F. and Kristensen, T.: An overview of the HLA system: clinical aspects. Transplant. Proc. 9:1789–1794, 1977.

Kissmeyer-Nielsen, F. and Thorsby, E.: Human transplantation antigens. Transplant. Rev. 4, 1970.

Kissmeyer-Nielsen, F., and Kjerbye E.: Lymphocytotoxic microtechnique. Purification of lymphocytes by flotation. Histocompatibility testing 1967. Munksgaard, 1967.

Kissmeyer-Nielsen, F. and Gavin, J.: Unpublished observations. 1967 Cited by Lao and Sanger, 1975.

Kitahama, M.: Chimera and mosaic in blood group. J. Jpn. Soc. Blood Transf. 5:210–212, 1959.

Kochwa, S., Rosenfield, R. E., Tallal, L. and Wasserman, L. R.: Isoagglutinins associated with erythroblastosis. J. Clin. Invest. 40:874, 1961.

Konugres, A. A. and Winter, N. M.: Sul, a new blood group antigen in the MN system. Vox Sang. 12:221–224, 1967.

Konugres, A. A., Brown, L. S. and Corcoran, P. A.: Anti-M^A, and the phenotype M^aN, of the MN blood-group system (A new finding). Vox Sang. 11:189–193, 1966.

Konugres, A. A., Huberlie, M. M., Swanson, J. and Matson, G. A.: The production of anti-Mt^a in rabbits. Vox Sang. 8:632–633, 1963.

Koop, C. E. and Bullitt, L.: The effect of gelatin infusion on the subsequent typing and cross-matching of the blood with a method of eliminating the phenomenon of pseudoagglutination. Am. J. Med. Sci. 219:28, 1945.

Kornstad, L., Ryttinger, L. and Högman, C.: Two sera containing probably naturally occurring anti-C^w, one of them also containing a naturally occurring anti-Wr^a. Vox Sang. 5:330–334, 1960.

Kortekangas, A. E., Kaarsalo, E., Melartin, L., Tippett, P., Gavin, J., Noades, J., Sanger, R. and Race, R. R.: The red cell antigen P^k and its relationship to the P system: the evidence of three more P^k families. Vox Sang. 10:385–404, 1965.

Kortekangas, A. E., Noades, J., Tippett, P., Sanger, R. and Race, R. R.: A second family with the red cell antigen P^k. Vox Sang. 4:337–349, 1959.

Kourilsky, F. M., Dausset, J., Feingold, N., et al.: Leukocyte groups and acute leukemia. J. Natl. Cancer Inst. 41:81, 1968.

Kreuger, A.: Adenine metabolism during and after exchange transfusions in newborn infants with CPD-adenine blood. Transfusion 16:249, 1976.

Kunkel, H. G. and Prendegast, R. A.: Subgroups of gamma-A immune globulins. Proc. Soc. Exp. Biol. Med. 122:910, 1966.

Kunkel, H. G., and Rockey, J. H.: β_2A and other immunoglobulins in isolated anti-A antibodies. Proc. Soc. Exp. Biol. 113:278, 1963.

Lalezari, P.: Discussion. In Histocompatibility Testing, Terasaki, P. I., (ed.) p. 307. Munksgaard, 1970.

Lalezari, P. and Murphy, G. B.: Cold reacting leukocyte agglutinins and their significance. In Histocompatibility

Testing. Curtoni, E. S., Mattiuz, P. L. and Tosi, R. M. (eds). p. 421. Munksgaard, 1967.

Landois, L.: Blood Transfusion. Leipzig, 1875.

Landsteiner, K.: Über Agglutinationserscheinungen normalen menschlichen Blutes, Wien. Klin. Wschr. 14:1132, 1901. (Translated and published by the Blood Transfusion Division, U.S. Army Medical Research Laboratory, Fort Knox, Kentucky, 40121.)

Landsteiner, K.: Zur Kenntnis der antifermentativen, lytischen und agglutinierenden Wirkungen des Blutsvums und der Lymph. Zbl. Bakt., 27:357, 1900. (Translated and published by the Blood Transfusion Division, U.S. Army Medical Research Laboratory, Fort Knox, Kentucky 40121.)

Landsteiner, K. and Wiener, A. S.: An agglutinable factor in human blood recognizable by immune sera for Rhesus blood. Proc. Soc. Exp. Biol. 43:223, 1940.

Landsteiner, K. and Levine, P.: The differentiation of a type of human blood by means of normal animal serum. J. Immunol. 20:179–185, 1931.

Landsteiner, K. and Levine, P.: On the inheritance and racial distribution of agglutinable properties of human blood. J. Immunol. 18:87–94, 1930.

Landsteiner, K. and Levine, P.: On the racial distribution of some agglutinable structures of human blood. J. Immunol. 16:123–131, 1929.

Landsteiner, K. and Levine, P.: Further observations on individual differences of human blood. Proc. Soc. Exp. Biol. 24:941–942, 1927.

Landsteiner, K. and Levine, P.: A new agglutinable factor differentiating individual human bloods. Proc. Soc. Exp. Biol. 24:600–602, 1927.

Landsteiner, K. and Witt, D.: Observation on the human blood groups. J. Immunol. 11:221–247, 1926.

Landsteiner, K., Strutton, W. R. and Chase, M. W.: An agglutination reaction observed with some human bloods, chiefly among Negroes. J. Immunol. 27:469–472, 1934.

Lanset, S., Ropartz, C., Rousseau, P.-Y., Guerbet, Y. and Salmon, C.: Une famille comportant les phénotypes Bombay: O_h^{AB} et O_h^B. Transfusion (Paris) 9:255–263, 1966.

Lau, F. O. and Rosse, W. F.: The reactivity of red blood cell membrane glycophorin with "cold-reacting" antibodies. Clin. Immunol. Immunopath. 4:1, 1975.

Lawler, S. D. and Shatwell, H. S.: Are Rh antigens restricted to red cells? Vox Sang. 7:488, 1962.

Lawler, S. D. and Marshall, R.: Lewis and secretor characters in infancy. Vox Sang 6:541–544, 1961.

Lawler, S. D. and Marshall, R.: Significance of the presence of Lewis substances in serum during infancy. Nature 190:1020, 1961.

Lawler, S. D. and Sandler, M.: Data on linkage in man: elliptocytosis and blood groups. IV. Families 5, 6 and 7. Ann. Eugen. 18:328–334, 1954.

Lawson, N. W., Ochsner, J. L., Mills, N. L., and Leonard, G. L.: The use of hemodilution and fresh autologous blood in open heart surgery. Anesth. Analg. 53:672, 1974.

Layrisse, Z. and Layrisse, M.: High incidence cold autoagglutinins of anti-I^T specificity in Yanomama Indians of Venezuela. Vox Sang 14:369–382, 1968.

Layrisse, M. and Arends, T.: The Diego blood factor in Chinese and Japanese. Nature 177, 1083–1084, 1956.

Layrisse, M., Layrisse, Z., Garcia, E., Wilbert, J. and Parra, R. J.: New Rh phenotype Dcce^{i}e^{i}f found in a Chibcha Indian tribe. Nature 191:503–504, 1961.

Layrisse, M., Layrisse, Z. Garcia, E. and Parra, J.: Genetic studies of the new Rh chromosome Dce^{i}f(Rh$_o$^{i}) found in a Chibcha tribe. Vox Sang. 6: 710–719, 1961.

Layrisse, M., Arends, T. and Dominguez Sisco, R.: Nuevo grupo sanguineo encontrado en descendientes de Indios. Acta Medica Venezolana 3:132–138, 1955.

Leddy, J. P. and Bakemeier, R. F.: A relationship of direct Coombs test pattern to autoantibody specificity in acquired hemolytic anemia. Proc. Soc. Exp. Biol. 125:808, 1967.

Leddy, J. P., Bakemeier, R. F. and Vaughan, J. H.: Fixation of complement components to autoantibodies eluted from human RBC (abstract). J. Clin. Invest. 44:1066, 1965.

Lee, L. S. N., Ying, K. L., and Bowen, P., Position of the Duffy locus on chromosome 1 in relation to breakpoints for structural rearrangements. Am. J. Hum. Genet. 26:93, 1974.

Leikola, J. and Pasanen, V. J.: Influence of antigen receptor density on agglutination of red blood cells. Int. Arch. Allergy 39:352, 1970.

Lepow, I. H., Naff, G. B. and Pensky, J.: Mechanisms of activation of C'1 and inhibition of C' esterase. In Ciba Foundation Symposium, Complement, p. 74. Churchill, 1965.

Levene, C., Sela, R., Rudolphson, Y., Nathan, A., Karplus, M. and Dvilansky, A.: Hemolytic disease of the newborn due to anti-PP$_1$P^k (anti-Tj^a). Transfusion 17:569, 1977.

Leverenz, S., Ihle, R. and Frick, G.: HL-A-System und Transfusionstreaktionen. 2. Mitteilung. Dtsch. Ges.-Wesen. 30:1688, 1975.

Leverenz, S., Ihle, R. and Frick, G.: HL-A-System und Transfusionstreaktionin. I. Mitteilung. Dtsch. Ges.-Wesen. 29:1546, 1974.

Levine, P. and Celano, M.: The antigenicity of Lewis (Le^a) substance in saliva coated onto tanned red cells. Vox Sang. 5:53–61, 1960.

Levine, P. and Celano, M. J.: Antigenicity of P substance in Echinococcus cyst fluid coated onto tanned rabbit cells. Fed. Proc. 18, 1959.

Levine, P. and Koch, E. A.: The rare human isoagglutinin anti-Tj^a and habitual abortion. Science 120:239–241, 1954.

Levine, P. and Katzin, E. M.: Pathogenesis of erythroblastosis fetalis; absence of the Rh factor from saliva. Proc. Soc. Exp. Biol. 48:126, 1941.

Levine, P. and Stetson, R.: An unusual case of intra-group agglutination. JAMA 113:126–127, 1939.

Levine, P., Celano, M. J., Falkowski, F., Chambers, J., Hunter, O. B. and English, C. T.: A second example of ---/--- or Rh$_{null}$ blood. Transfusion, 5:492–500, 1965.

Levine, P., Chambers, J. W., Celano, M. J., Falkowski, F., Hunter, O. B. and English, C. T.: A second example of ---/--- or Rh$_{null}$ blood. Proc. 10th Congr. Int. Soc. Blood Transf., Stockholm 1964, 350–356, 1965.

Levine, P., Celano, M. J., Falkowski, F., Chambers, J., Hunter, O. B. and English, C. T.: A second example of ---/--- blood, or Rh$_{null}$. Nature 204:892, 1964.

Levine, P., Celano, M. J. and Falkowski, F.: The specificity antibody in paroxysmal cold hemoglobinuria (PCH). Transfusion 3:278–280, 1963.

Levine, P., Rosenfield, R. E. and White, J.: The first example of the Rh phenotype r^{G}r^G. Am. J. Hum. Genet. 13:299–305, 1961.

Levine, P., Celano, M., Fenichel, R. and Singher, H.: A "D"-like antigen in Rhesus red blood cells and in Rh-positive and Rh-negative red cells. Science 133:332–333, 1961.

Levine, P., Celano, M., Fenichel, R., Pollack, W. and Singher, H.: A "D-like" antigen in rhesus monkey, human Rh positive and human Rh negative red blood cells. J. Immunol. 87:747–752, 1961.

Levine, P., Celano, M. and Staveley, J. M.: The antigenicity of P substance in Echinococcus cyst fluid coated onto tanned red cells. Vox. Sang. 3:434–438, 1958.

Levine, P., Celano, M., Lange, S. and Berliner, V.: On anti-M in horse sera. Vox Sang. 2:433, 1957.

Levine, P., Sneath, J. S., Robinson, E. A., and Huntingdon, P. W.: A second example of anti-Fy^b. Blood 10:941, 1955.

Levine, P., Ferraro, L. R. and Koch, E.: Hemolytic disease of the newborn due to anti-S. Blood 7:1030, 1952.

Levine P., Bobbitt O. B., Waller, R. K. and Kuhmichel, A.: Isoimmunization by a new blood factor in tumor cells. Proc. Soc. Exp. Biol. 77:402–405, 1951.

Levine, P., Kuhmichel, A. B., Wigod, M. and Koch, E.: A new blood factor, s, allelic to S. Proc. Soc. Exp. Biol. 78:218–220, 1951.

Levine, P., Backer, M., Wigod, M. and Ponder, R.: A new human hereditary blood property (Cellano) present in 99.8% of all bloods. Science 109:464–466, 1949.

Levine, P., Burnham, L., Katzin, E. M. and Vogel, P.: The role of isoimmunization in the pathogenesis of erythroblastosis fetalis. Am. J. Obstet. Gynecol. 42:925–937, 1941.

Levine, P., Katzin, E. M. and Burnham, L.: Isoimmunization in pregnancy, its possible bearing on the etiology of erythroblastosis fetalis. JAMA 116:825–827, 1941.

Levine, P., Vogel, P., Katzin, E. M. and Burnham, L.: Pathogenesis of erythroblastosis fetalis: statistical evidence. Science 94:371–372, 1941.

Lewis, M., Kaita, H. and Chown, B.: Scianna blood group system. Vox Sang. 27:261–264, 1974.

Lewis, M., Kaita, H. and Chown, B.: The Duffy blood group system in Caucasians. A further population sample. Vox Sang. 23:523–527, 1972.

Lewis, M., Chown, B., Kaita, H., Hahn, D., Kangelos, M., Shepeard, W. L. and Shackelton, K.: Blood group antigen Go^a and the Rh system. Transfusion 7:440–441, 1967.

Lewis, M., MacPherson, C. R. and Gayton, J.: The Rh complex R$_1$^{wD} (CD^{w}e). Can. J. Genet. Cytol. 7:259–261, 1965.

Lewis, M., Chown, B., Schmidt, R. P. and Griffitts, J. J.: A possible relationship between the blood group antigens Sm and Bu^a. Am. J. Hum. Genet. 16:254–255, 1964.

Lewis, M., Kaita, H., Duncan, D. and Chown, B.: Failure to find hypothetic K^a (KKp^a) of the Kell blood group system. Vox Sang. 5:565–567, 1960.

Lewis, M., Ayukawa, H., Chown, B. and Levine, P.: The blood group antigen Diego in North American Indians and in Japanese. Nature 177:1084, 1956.

Lewis, S. M., Grammaticos, P. and Dacie, J. V.: Lysis by anti-I in dyserythropoietic anemias: role of increased uptake of antibody. Br. J. Haematol. 18:465, 1970.

Lewisohn, R.: Blood transfusion by the citrate method. Surg. Gynecol. Obstet. 21:37, 1915.

Liley, A. W.: Intrauterine transfusion of fetus in hemolytic disease. Br. Med. J. ii: 1107, 1963.

Liley, A. W.: Liquor amnii analysis in the management of the pregnancy complicated by rhesus sensitization. Am. J. Obstet. Gynecol. 82:1359, 1961.

Lilly, F., Boyse, E. A. and Old, L. J.: Genetic basis of susceptibility to viral leukemogenesis. Lancet ii:1207, 1964.

Lincoln, P. J. and Dodd, B. E.: The use of low ionic strength solution (LISS) in elution experiments and in combination with papain-treated cells for the titration of various antibodies, including eluted antibody. Vox Sang. 34:221, 1978.

Lisowska, E. and Duk, M.: Effect of modification of amino groups of human erythrocytes on M, N and N$_{v_g}$ blood group specificities. Vox Sang. 28:392, 1975.

Lloyd, K. O., Kabat, E. A. and Licerio, E.: Immunochemical studies on blood groups. Structures and activities of oligosaccharides produced by alkaline degradation of blood group Lewis-a substance. Proposed structure of the carbohydrate chains of human blood-group A, B, H, Le^a, and Le^b substances. Biochemistry 7:2976–90, 1968.

Lockwood, C. M., Rees, A. J., Pearson, T. A., Evans, D. J. Peters, D. K. and Wilson, C. B.: Immunosuppression and plasma exchange in the treatment of Goodpasture's syndrome. Lancet i, 711, 1976.

Loghem, J. J. Van, Hart, M. Van der, Veenhoven-Van Riesz, E., Marga, V. D., Engelfriet, C. P. and Peetoom, F.: Cold auto-agglutinins and hemolysins of anti-I and anti-i specificity. Vox Sang. 7:214–221, 1962.

Lombardo, J. M., Britton, S. J., Hannon, G. and Terry, D.: K$_o$ in a sister and brother, a family study. Abstracts, AABB and ISH Meeting, Washington, p. 59, 1972.

London, I. M.: The metabolism of the erythrocyte. Harvey Lect., 1961.

Longster, G and Giles, C. M.: A new antibody specificity, anti-Rg^a, reacting with a red cell and serum antigen. Vox Sang. 30:175, 1976.

Löw, B. and Messeter, L.: Antiglobulin test in low-ionic strength salt solution for rapid antibody screening and cross-matching. Vox Sang. 26:53, 1974.

Lowenthal, R. M.: Chronic leukemias — treatment by leukapheresis. Exp. Hemat. 5, Suppl. I, p. 73, 1977a.

Lowenthal, R. M.: The clinical value of the continuous-flow blood cell separator. M.D. Thesis, University of Sydney, 1977b.

Lower, R., and Boyle, R.: Philos. Trans. 1 (No. 22): 355, 1866.

Lozner, E. L. and Newhouse, L. R.: Studies on the transmissibility of malaria by plasma transfusion. Am. J. Med. Sci. 206:141, 1943.

Luner, S. J., Sturgeon, P. Azklarek, D. and McQuiston, D. T.: Effects of proteases and neuraminidase on RBC surface charge and agglutination. A kinetic study. Vox Sang. 28:184, 1975.

Lusher, J. M., Zuelzer, W. W. and Parsons, P. J.: Anti-s hemolytic disease: a case report. Transfusion 6:590–591, 1966.

Macdonald, W. B. and Berg, R. B.: Hemolysis of transfused cells during use of the injection (push) technique for blood transfusion. Pediatrics 23:8, 1958.

Macvie, S. I., Morton, J. A. and Pickles, M. M.: The reactions and inheritance of a new blood group antigen, Sd^a. Vox Sang. 13:485–492, 1967.

Madden, H. J., Cleghorn, T. E., Allen, F. H., Jr., Rosenfield, R. E. and Mackeprang, M.: A note on the relatively high frequency of St^a on the red blood cells of orientals, and report of a third example of anti-St^a. Vox Sang. 9:502–504, 1964.

Mainwaring, R. L. and Brueckner, G. G.: Fibrinogen transmitted hepatitis. JAMA 195:437, 1966.

Mainwaring, U. R. and Pickles, M. M.: A further case of anti-Lutheran immunization with some studies on its capacity for human sensitization. J. Clin. Pathol. 1:292–294, 1948.

Maizels, M.: Active cation transport in erythrocytes. Symp. Soc. Exp. Biol. 8:202, 1954.

Mäkelä, O. and Cantell, K.: Destruction of M and N blood group receptors of human red cells by some influenza viruses. Ann. Med. Exp. Fenn. 36:366–374, 1958.

Mallan, M. T., Grimm, W., Hindley, L., Knighton, G., Moulds, M. K. and Moulds, J. J.: The Hall serum: detecting Kn^b, the antithetical allele to Kn^a. Proc. 33rd Ann. Meeting, AABB, Washington, DC, 1980.

Mann, J. D., Cahan, A., Gelb, A. G., Fisher, N., Hamper, J., Tippett, P. Sanger, R. and Race, R. R.: A sex-linked blood group. Lancet i:8–10, 1962.

Marchal, G., Dausset, J. and Colombani, J.: Commun. 8th Congr. Int. Soc. Blood Transfus., Tokyo, 1960.

Marcus, D. M. and Grollman, A. P.: Studies of blood group substances. I. Caprine precipitating antisera to human Le^a and Le^b blood group substances. J. Immunol. 97:867–875, 1966.

Marcus, D. M., Naiki, M. and Kundu, S. K.: Abnormalities in the glycosphingolipid content of human P^k and p erythrocytes. Proc. Nat. Acad. Sci. USA 73:3263, 1976.

Marcus, D. M., Bastani, A., Rosenfield, R. E., and Grollman, A. P.: Studies of blood group substances. II. Hemagglutinating properties of caprine antisera to human Le^a and Le^b blood group substances. Transfusion 7:277–280, 1967.

Marr, A. M. S., Donald, A. S. R., Watkins, W. M. and Morgan, W. T. J.: Molecular and genetic aspects of human blood-group Le^b specificity. Nature 215:1345–1349, 1967.

Marrack, J. R.: The chemistry of antigens and antibodies. London, Medical Research Council, Special Report Series, No. 194, 1938.

Marriott, H. L. and Kekwick, A.: Volume and rate in blood transfusion for the relief of anaemia. Br. Med. J. i;1043, 1940.

Marsh, W. L.: Recent developments relating to the Duffy and Lutheran blood groups. Rec. Adv. Immunohematology. Am. Assoc. Blood Banks, p. 105, 1973.

Marsh, W. L.: Anti-Lu5, and anti-Lu6 and anti-Lu7. Three antibodies defining high frequency antigens related to the Lutheran blood group system. Transfusion, 12:27–34, 1972.

Marsh, W. L.: Anti-i: a cold antibody defining the Ii relationship in human red cells. Br. J. Hematol., 7:200–209, 1961.

Marsh, W. L. and Jenkins, W. J.: Anti-Sp$_1$: The recognition of a new cold auto-antibody. Vox Sang. 15:177, 1968.

Marsh, W. L. and Jenkins, W. J.: Anti-i: a new cold antibody. Nature 188:753, 1960.

Marsh, W. L., Johnson, C. L., Øyen, R., Nichols, M. E., DiNapoli, J., Young, H., Brassel, J., Cusumano, I., Bazaz, G. R., Haber, J. M. and Wolf, C. F. W.: Anti-Sd^x; a "new" auto-agglutinin related to the Sd^a blood group. Transfusion 20; 1–8, 1980.

Marsh, W. L., Johnson, C. L., DiNapoli, J., Øyen, R., Alicea, E., Rao, A. H. and Chandrasekaren, V.: Immune hemolytic anemia caused by auto anti-Sd^x. Proc. 33rd Ann. Meeting, AABB, Washington, DC, 1980.

Marsh, W. L., Thayer, R. S., Deere, W. L., Schmelter, S. E., Freed, P. J., Øyen, R. and Nichols, M. E.: Naturally occurring anti-Kell (anti-K) stimulated by E. coli enterocolitis in a 20-day-old child. Commun. Amer. Assoc. Blood Banks, San Francisco, 1967. See also Transfusion 18: 149, 1978.

Marsh, W. L., Nichols, M. E. and Øyen, R.: unpublished observations, 1974. Cited in March, 1975.

Marsh, W. L., Øyen, R., Nichols, M. E. and Allen, F. H., Jr.: Chronic granulomatous disease and the Kell blood groups. Br. J. Hematol. 29:247, 1975.

Marsh, W. L., Øyen, R., and Allen, F. H.: Kx; a leukocyte and red cell antigen associated with the Kell system. In preparation. 1974. Cited by Race and Sanger, 1975.

Marsh, W. L., Øyen, R. and Nichols, M. E.: Kidd blood group antigens of leukocytes and platelets. Transfusion. 14:378–381, 1974.

Marsh, W. L., Jensen, L. Øyen, R., Stroup, M., Gellerman, M., McMahon, F. J. and Tsitsera, H.: Anti-K13 and the K: −13 phenotype: a blood-group variant related to the Kell system. Vox Sang. 26:34–40, 1974.

Marsh, W. L., Øyen, R. and Allen, F. H., Jr.: Abstract Proc. 26th Ann. Meeting, AABB, Miami Beach, 1973.

Marsh, W. L., Reid, M. E. and Scott, E. P.: Autoantibodies of U blood group specificity in autoimmune hemolytic anemia. Br. J. Hematol. 22:625–629, 1972.

Marsh, W. L., Jensen, L., Decary, F. and Colledge, K.: Water-soluble I blood group substance in the secretions of i adults. Transfusion 12:222–226, 1972.

Marsh, W. L., Nichols, M. E. and Reid, M. E.: The definition of two I antigen components. Vox Sang. 20:209–217, 1971.

Marsh, W. L., Nichols, M. E. and Allen, F. H.: Inhibition of anti-I sera by human milk. Vox Sang. 18:149–154, 1970.

Marshall, J. V.: The Bg antigens and antibodies. Can. J. Med. Techol. 35:26–35, 1973.

Mårtensson, L. and Fudenberg, H. H.: Gm genes and gamma globulin synthesis in the human fetus. J. Immunol. 94:514, 1965.

Masouredis, S. P.: Red cell membrane blood group antigens, in Membrane Structure and Function of Human Blood Cells. Amer. Assoc. Blood Banks, Washington, D.C., 1976.

Masouredis, S. P., Sudora, E. J., Mahan, L. and Victoria, E. J.: Antigen site densities and ultrastructural distribution patterns of red cell Rh antigens. Transfusion 16:94, 1976.

Matson, G. A., Swanson, J., Noades, J., Sanger, R. and Race, R. R.: A "new" antigen and antibody belonging to the P blood group system. Am. J. Hum. Genet. 11:26–34, 1959.

Matson, G. A., Coe, J. and Swanson, J.: Hemolytic transfusion reaction due to anti-Le^a agglutinin. Blood 10:1236–1240, 1955.

Matuhasi, T.: Plasma protein and antibody fractions observed from the serological point of view. Proc. 15th Gen. Assembly Jpn. Med. Congr., Tokyo, 4: 80, 1959.

Matuhasi, T., Kumazawa, H. and Usui, M.: Question of the presence of the so-called cross-reacting antibody. J. Jpn. Soc. Blood. Transf. 6:295, 1960.

Maunsell, K.: Urticarial reactions and desensitization in allergic recipients after serum transfusions. Br. Med. J. ii:236, 1944.

May, J. E., Rosse, W., and Frank, M. M.: Paroxysmal nocturnal hemoglobinuria. Alternate complement pathway mediated lysis induced by magnesium. N. Engl. J. Med. 289:705, 1973.

Mayer, K., Bettigole, R. E., Harris, J. P., et al.: Test in vivo to determine donor compatibility. Transfusion 8:28, 1968.

Mellbye, O. J.: Specificity of natural human agglutinins against red cells modified by trypsin and other agents. Scand. J. Hematol., 6:166, 1969.

Menolasino, N. J., Davidsohn, I. and Lynch, D. E.: A simplified method for the preparation of anti-M and anti-N typing sera. J. Lab. Clin. Med. 44:495, 1954.

Merrild-Hansen, B. and Munk-Andersen, G.: Hemolytic transfusion reaction caused by anti-Le^a. Vox Sang. 2:109–113, 1957.

Metaxas, M. N. and Metaxas-Bühler, M.: Rare genes of the MNSs system affecting the red cell membrane. In Human Blood Groups. Mohn, J. F. et al (eds.). S. Karger, 1977.

Metaxas, M. N. and Metaxas-Bühler, M.: M^k: an apparently silent allele at the MN locus. Nature 202:1123, 1964.

Metaxas, M. N. and Metaxas-Bühler, M.: Studies on the Wright blood group system. Vox Sang. 8:707, 1963.

Metaxas, M. N., Metaxas-Bühler, M. and Edwards, J. H.: MNSs frequencies in 3,895 Swiss blood donors. Vox Sang. 18:385–395, 1970.

Metaxas, M. N., Metaxas-Bühler, M. and Ikin, E. W.: Complexities of the MN locus. Vox Sang. 15:102–117, 1968.

Metaxas, M. N., Metaxas-Bühler, M. and Romanski, J.: Studies on the blood group antigen M^g. I. Frequency of M^g in Switzerland and family studies. Vox Sang. 11:157–169, 1966.

Metaxas, M. N., Matter, M., Metaxas-Bühler, M., Romanski, Y. and Hässig, A.: Frequency of the M^g blood group antigen in Swiss blood donors and its inheritance in several independent families. Proc. 9th Congr. Int. Soc. Blood Transf., Mexico, 1962, 206–209, 1964.

Metaxas, M. N., Metaxas-Bühler, M., Dunsford, I. and Holländer, L.: A further example of anti-Lu^b together with data in support of the Lutheran-secretor linkage in man. Vox Sang. 4:298–307, 1959.

Metaxas-Bühler, M., Cleghorn, T. E., Romanski, J. and Metaxas, M. N.: Studies on the blood group antigen M^g. II. Serology of M^g. Vox Sang. 11:170–183, 1966.

Michael, J. M., Moore, J. A. and Chaplin, H., Jr.: Identification of a C_4 subcomponent on C_3d-coated erythrocytes. Transfusion 16:408, 1976.

Michaelsen, T. E., Frangione, B. and Franklin, E. C.: Primary structure of the "hinge" region of human IgG3. J. Biol. Chem. 252:883, 1977.

Middleton, J. and Crookston, M.: Chido-substance in plasma. Vox Sang. 23:256, 1972.

Middleton, J. and 13 others: Linkage of Chido and HL-A. Tissue Antigens 4:366, 1974.

Miescher, P. A., and Dayer, J. M.: Autoimmune hemolytic anemias. In Textbook of Immunopathology, 2nd Ed. Miescher, P. A. and Müller-Eberhard, H. J., (eds.) Grune & Stratton, 1976.

Milgrom, F.: Studies on blood groups by agglutination of erythrocytic stomatia in gel. In Human Blood Groups. Mohn, J. F. et al. (eds) S. Karger, 1977.

Miller, E. B., Rosenfield, R. E., Vogel, P., Haber, G. and Gibbel, N.: The Lewis blood factors in American Negroes. Am. J. Phys. Anthropol. 12:427–444, 1954.

Miller, L. H., Mason, S. J., Clyde, D. F. and McGinniss, M. H.: The resistance factor to Plasmodium vivax in blacks. The Duffy blood group genotype, FyFy. N. Engl. J. Med. 295:302, 1976.

Miller, L. H., Mason, S. J., Dvorak, J. A., McGinniss, M. H. and Rothman, I. K.: Erythrocyte receptors for (Plasmodium knowlesi) malaria: the Duffy blood group determinants. Science 189:561, 1975.

Mishler, J. M., Janes, A. W., Lowes, B., Farfan, C. and Emerson, P. M.: The utilization of a new strength citrate anticoagulant during centrifugal plateletpheresis. I. Assessment of donor effects. Br. J. Hematol. 34:387, 1976.

Mishler, J. M., Higby, D. J., Rhomberg, W., Nicora, R. W. and Holland, J. F.: Leukapheresis: increased efficiency of collection by the use of hydroxyethyl starch and dexamethasone. In Leucocytes: Separation, Collection and Transfusion, Goldman, J. M. and Lowenthal, R. M. (eds.) Academic Press, 1975.

Mitchison, N. A.: Immunological paralysis in the adult. Proc. R. Soc. Med. 56:937, 1963.

Mitchison, N. A.: Tolerance depending on presence of surviving red cells. In Biological Problems of Grafting. Blackwell Scientific Publications, 1959.

Moghaddam, M., Goldsmith, K. L. G. and Brazier, D. M.: Difficulties encountered in the large-scale production of blood-grouping sera from human citrated plasma. Vox Sang. 30:315, 1976.

Moghaddam, M., Goldsmith, K. L. G. and Kerwick, R. A.: The preparation of blood grouping serum from human citrated plasma. Vox Sang. 20:277, 1971.

Moharram, I.: The blood group factor P in Egypt. Laboratory and Medical Progress 3:1–8, 1942.

Mohn, J. F. and Macvie, S.: Serologic studies on the relationship of the Mi^a and Vw blood group antigens. Unpublished observations, 1967.

Mohn, J. F. and Witebsky, E.: The occurrence of water-soluble Rh substance in body secretions. NY St. J. Med. 48:287, 1948.

Mohn, J. F., Cunningham, R. K. and Bates, J. F.: Quantitative distinctions between subgroups A_1 and A_2. Commun. 14th Congr. Int. Soc. Blood Transf., Helsinki, 1975.

Mohn, J. F., Cunningham, R. K., Pirkola, A., Furuhjelm, U.

and Nevanlinna, H. R.: An inherited blood group A variant in the Finnish population. I. Basic characteristics. Vox Sang. 25:193–211, 1973.

Mohn, J. F., Lambert, R. M., Rosamilia, H. G., Wallace, J., Milne, G. R., Moores, P., Sanger, R. and Race, R. R.: On the relationship of the blood group antigens Mi^a and Vw to the MNSs system. Am. J. Hum. Genet. 10:276–286, 1958.

Mollison, P. L.: Blood Transfusion in Clinical Medicine, 6th Ed. Blackwell Scientific Publications, 1979.

Mollison, P. L.: Blood donation: the transfusion of red cells. In Blood Transfusion in Clinical Medicine, 5th ed. Blackwell Scientific Publications, 1972.

Mollison, P. L.: Blood Transfusion in Clinical Medicine, 5th ed. Blackwell Scientific Publications, 1972.

Mollison, P. L.: Blood Transfusion in Clinical Medicine, 2nd Ed. Blackwell Scientific Publications, 1956.

Mollison, P. L.: The survival of transfused erythrocytes, with special reference to cases of acquired haemolytic anemia. Clin. Sci. 6:137, 1947.

Mollison, P. L. and Thomas, A. R.: Hemolytic potentialities of human blood group antibodies revealed by the use of animal complement. Vox Sang. 4:185, 1959.

Mollison, P. L. and Cutbush, M.: A method of measuring the severity of a series of cases of hemolytic disease of the newborn. Blood 6:777, 1951.

Mollison, P. L. and Cutbush, M.: La maladie hémolytique chez un enfant D^u. Rev. Hématol. 4:608, 1949c.

Mollison, P. L., Frame, M. and Ross, M. E.: Differences between Rh(D) negative subjects in response to Rh(D) antigen. Br. J. Hematol. 19:257, 1970.

Molthan, L.: The new McCoy antigens, McC^c and McC^d. Proc. 33rd Ann. Meeting, AABB, Washington, DC, 1980.

Molthan, L. and Moulds, J.: A new antibody, anti-McC^3 (McCoy) and its relationship to anti-Kn^3 (Knops). Commun., AABB, Chicago, 1975.

Molthan, L. and Crawford, M. C.: Three examples of anti-Lu^b and related data. Transfusion 6:584–589, 1966.

Molthan, L., Crawford, M. N., Marsh, W. L. and Allen, F. H.: Lu9, another new antigen of the Lutheran blood group system. Vox Sang. 24:468–471, 1973.

Molthan, L., Crawford, M. N. and Tippett, P.: Enlargement of the Dombrock blood group system: the finding of anti-Do^b. Vox Sang. 24:382–384, 1973.

Molthan, L., Crawford, M. N., Giles, C. M., Chudnoff, A. and Eichman, M. F.: A new antibody, anti-Yk^a (York), and its relationship to anti-Cs^a (Cost Sterling). Transfusion 9:281, 1969.

Molthan, L., Reidenberg, M. M. and Eichman, M. F.: Positive direct Coombs tests due to cephalothin. N. Engl. J. Med. 277:123, 1967.

Moore, B. P. L.: Proficiency in the detection and titration of blood group antibodies: results of an interlaboratory trial. Can. Med. Assoc. J. 103:1034, 1970.

Moore, H. C. and Mollison, P. L.: Use of a low ionic-strength medium in manual tests for antibody detection. Transfusion 16:291, 1976.

Moore, H. C., Issitt, P. D. and Pavone, B. G.: Successful transfusion of Chido-positive blood to two patients with anti-Chido. Transfusion 15:266, 1975.

Moore, J. A. and Chaplin, H., Jr.: autoimmune hemolytic anemia associated with an IgG cold incomplete antibody. Vox Sang. 24:236, 1973.

Moores, P.: The "Bombay" blood-type in Natal. Abstracts AABB and ISH Meeting. Washington, DC, p. 11. 1972.

Moores, P., Pudifin, D. and Patel, P. L.: Severe hemolytic anemia in an adult associated with anti-T. Transfusion 15:329, 1975.

Moores, P., Botha, M. C. and Brink, S.: Anti-N in the serum of a healthy type MN person — a further example. Amer. J. Clin. Pathol. 54:90, 1970.

Moreau, R., Dausset, J., Bernard, J. and Moullec, J.: Anémie hémolytique acquise avec polyagglutinabilité des hématies par un nouveau facteur présent dans le sérum humain normal (anti-Tn). Bull. Soc. med Hôp. Paris Séance, May 569–587, 1957.

Morell, A., Skvaril, F., Van Loghem, E. and Kleemola, M.: Human IgG subclasses in maternal and fetal serum. Vox Sang. 21:481, 1971.

Moreschi, C.: Neue Tatsachen über die Blutkörperchen Agglutinationen. Zbl. Bakt. 46:49 and 456, 1908.

Morgan, P., Wheeler, C. B. and Bossom, E. L.: Delayed transfusion reaction attributed to anti-Jk^b. Transfusion 7:307, 1967.

Morgan, W. T. J. and Watkins, W. M.: Blood group P$_1$ substance (1) Chemical properties. Proc. 9th Congr. Int. Soc. Blood Transf. Mexico, 1962, 225–229, 1964.

Moriau, M. and 10 others: Hemostasis disorders in open heart surgery with extracorporeal circulation. Importance of the platelet function and the heparin neutralization. Vox Sang. 32:41, 1977.

Morris, R. I., Metzger, A. L., Bluestone, R., and Terasaki, P. I.: HL-A W27 — a clue to the diagnosis and pathogenesis of Reiter's syndrome. N. Engl. J. Med. 290:554–556, 1974a.

Morris, R. I., Metzger, A. L., Bluestone, R. and Terasaki, P. I.: HL-A-W27 — a useful discriminator in the arthropathies of inflammatory bowel disease. N. Engl. J. Med. 290:1117–1119, 1974b.

Morrison, F. S. and Baldini, M.: The favorable effect of ACD on the viability of fresh and stored human platelets. Vox Sang. 12:90, 1967.

Morton, J. A.: The serological reactions of red cells treated with proteolytic enzymes. Ph.D. Thesis, University of London, 1957.

Morton, J. A. and Pickles, M. M.: The proteolytic enzyme test in the detection of incomplete antibodies. J. Clin. Pathol. 4:189, 1951.

Morton, J. A., Pickles, M. M., Sutton, L. and Skov, F.: Identification of further antigens on red cells and lymphocytes. Association of Bg^b with W17 (Te57) and Bg^c with W28 (Da15, Ba*). Vox Sang. 21:141, 1971.

Morton, J. A., Pickles, M. M. and Terry, A. M.: The Sd^a blood group antigen in tissues and body fluids. Vox Sang. 19:472–482, 1970.

Morton, J. A., Pickles, M. M. and Sutton, L.: The correlation of the Bg^a blood group with the HL-A7 leukocyte group: demonstration of antigenic sites on red cells and leukocytes. Vox Sang. 17:536–547, 1969.

Morton, N. E., Mi, M. P. and Yasuda, N.: A study of the S^u alleles in northeastern Brazil. Vox Sang. 11:194–208, 1966.

Moss, W. L.: (1914) Cited by Wiener, A. S.: Blood Groups and Transfusion, 2nd Ed. Charles C Thomas, 1939.

Moss, W. L.: Studies on isoagglutinins and isohemolysins. Bull. Johns Hopkins Hosp. 21:63–70, 1910.

Moulds, J. J., Case, J., Thornton, S., Pulver, V. B. and Moulds, M. K.: Anti-Ce^s: a previously undescribed Rh antibody. Proc. 33rd Ann. Meeting, AABB, Washington, DC, 1980.

Moulds, J. J., Polesky, H. F., Reid, M. and Ellisor, S. S.: Observations on the Gy^a and Hy antigens and the antibodies that define them. Transfusion 15–270, 1975.

Mourant, A. E.: The Distribution of the Human Blood Groups. Blackwell Scientific Publications, 1954.

Mourant, A. E.: A "new" human blood group antigen of frequent occurrence. Nature 158:237, 1946.

Mourant, A. E.: A new rhesus antibody. Nature 155:542, 1945.

Mourant, A. E., Kopec, A. C. and Domaniewska-Sodczak, K.: The Distribution of the Human Blood Groups and Other Biochemical Polymorphisms, 2nd Ed. Oxford University Press, 1976.

Moureau, P.: Les réactions post-transfusionnelles. Rev. Belge Sci. Med. 16:258–300, 1945.

Mueller-Eckhardt, C., and Kretschmer, V.: Autoimmune hemolytic anemias. I. Investigations on immunoglobin type and complement fixation of cell-fixed and eluable autoantibodies. Blut 25:63–76, 1972.

Müller-Eberhard, H. J.: The serum complement system. In Textbook of Immunopathology, 2 Ed. Micocher, P. A., and Müller-Eberhard, H. J. (eds). Vol. 1. Grune & Stratton, 1976.

Müller-Eberhard, H. J.: Complement. Ann. Rev. Biochem. 44:697, 1975.

Müller-Eberhard, H. J.: Chemistry and reaction mechanisms of complement. Advanc. Immunol. 8:1, 1968.

Müller-Eberhard, H. J. and Lepow, I. H.: C'$_1$ esterase effect on activity and physiochemical properties of the fourth component of complement. J. Exp. Med. 121:819, 1965.

Müller-Eberhard, H. J., Hadding, U. and Calcott, M. A.: Current Problems in Complement Research in Immunopathology. 5th International Symposium. Miescher, P. A. and Grabar, P. (eds.). Schwabe, 1967.

Murphy, S. and Gardner, F. H.: Room temperature storage of platelets. Transfusion 16:2, 1976.

Murphy, S., Sayar, S. N. and Gardner, F. H.: Storage of platelet concentrates at 22°C. Blood 35:549, 1970.

Murray, J.: Rh antenatal testing. A suggested nomenclature. Lancet ii:594, 1944.

Murray, J.: A nomenclature of subgroups of the Rh factor. Nature 154:701, 1944.

Murray, J. and Clarke, E. C.: Production of anti-Rh in guinea pigs from human erythrocytes. Nature 169:886–887, 1952.

Murray, J., Race, R. R. and Taylor, G. L.: Serological reactions caused by the rare human gene Rh$_z$. Nature 155:112, 1945.

Murray, R.: Viral hepatitis. Bull. NY Acad. Med. 31:341, 1955.

Mygind, K. and Ahrons, S.: IgG cold agglutinins and first trimester abortion. Vox Sang. 23:552–560, 1973.

Myllylä, G., Furuhjelm, U., Nordling, S., Pirkola, A., Tippett, P., Gavin, J. and Sanger, R.: Persistent mixed field polyagglutinability. Electrokinetic and serological aspects. Vox Sang. 20:7, 1971.

McCreary, J., Vogler, A. L., Sabo, B., Eckstein, E. G. and Smith, T. R.: Another minus-minus phenotype: Bu(a-) Sm-two examples in one family. Transfusion 13:350 (Abstract), 1973.

McCullough, H.: Granulocyte transfusions. In Seminar on Current Technical Topics. AABB, Washington, DC, 1974.

McCune, M. A., Pineda, A. A., Winkelmann, R. K. and Osmundson, P. J.: Controlled study of the therapeutic effect of plasma exchange on scleroderma and Raynaud's phenomenon. Proc. 33rd Ann. Meeting, AABB, Washington, DC, 1980.

McGinnis, M. H. and Goldfinger, D.: Drug reactions due to passively transfused penicillin antibody. Commun. Am. Assoc. Blood Banks, Chicago, 1971.

McIntryre, C., Finigan, L. and Larsen, A. L.: Anti-Co^a implicated in hemolytic disease of the newborn. Transfusion 16:76, 1976.

McNabb, T., Koh, T. Y., Dorrington, K. J., and Painter, R. H.: Structure and function of immunoglobulin domains. V. Binding of immunoglobulin G and fragments to placental membrane preparations. J. Immunol. 117:882, 1976.

Naff, G. B., Pensky, J. and Lepow, I. H.: The macromolecular nature of the first component of human complement. J. Exp. Med. 119:593, 1964.

Naiki, M. and Marcus, D. M.: An immunochemical study of the human blood group P₁, P and Pᵏ glycosphingolipid antigens. Biochemistry 14:4837, 1975.

Naiki, M., Fong, J., Ledeen, R. and Marcus, D. M.: Structure of the human erythrocyte blood group P₁. Biochemistry 14:4831, 1975.

Nakajima, H. and Moulds, J. J.: Doᵃ (Dombrock) blood group antigen in the Japanese. Tests on further population and family studies. Vox Sang. 38:294–296, 1980.

Nakajima, H., Skradski, K. and Moulds, J. J.: Doᵃ (Dombrock) blood group antigen in the Japanese. Vox Sang. 36:103–104, 1979.

Nason, S. G., Vengelen-Tyler, V., Cohen, N., Best, M. and Quirk, J.: A high incidence antibody (Anti-Sc3) in the serum of a Sc:−1,−2 patient. Transfusion 20:531–535, 1980.

Natvig, J. B. and Kunkel, H. G.: Genetic markers of human immunoglobulins: The Gm and Inv systems. Ser. Hemat. 1:66, 1968.

Natvig, J. B., Førre, O. and Michaelsen, T. E.: Restriction of human immune antibodies to heavy chain variable subgroups. Scand. J. Immunol. 5:667, 1976.

Nesmith, L. W. and Davis, J. W.: Hemolytic anemia caused by penicillin. Report of a case in which antipenicillin antibodies cross-reacted with cephalothin sodium. JAMA 203:27, 1968.

Newman, M. M., Hamstra, R. D., and Block, M. H.: Use of banked autologous blood in elective surgery. JAMA 218:861, 1971.

Nicholas, J. W., Jenkins, W. J. and Marsh, W. L.: Human blood chimeras. Brit. Med. J. i;1458, 1957.

Nicholson, G. L., Masouredis, S. P. and Singer, S. J.: Quantitative two-dimensional ultrastructural distribution of Rh₀ (D) antigenic sites on human erythrocyte membranes. Proc. Nat. Acad. Sci. USA 68:1416–1420, 1971.

Nisonoff, A., Hopper, J. E., and Spring, S. B.: The Antibody Molecule. Academic Press, 1975.

Nordhagen, R., Heier Larsen, A. M. and Beckers, D.: Chido, Rogers and C4. Vox Sang. 37:170–178, 1979.

Nordling, S., Sanger, R., Gavin, J., Furuhjelm, U., Myllylá, G. and Metaxas, M. N.: Mᵏ and Mᵍ: some serological and physicochemical observations. Vox Sang. 17:300–302, 1969.

Nugent, M. E., Colledge, K. I. and Marsh, W. L.: Autoimmune hemolytic anemia caused by anti-U. Vox Sang. 20:519–525, 1971.

Nunn, H. D., Giles, C. M. and Dormandy, K. M.: A second example of anti-Ku in a patient who has the rare Kell phenotype, Kᵒ. Vox Sang. 11:611–619, 1966.

Nymand, G., Heron, I., Jensen, K. G., and Lundsgaard, A.: Occurrence of cytotoxic antibodies during pregnancy. Vox Sang. 21:21–29, 1971.

Oberdorfer, C. E., Kahn, B., Moore, V., Zelenski, K., Øyen, R. and Marsh, W. L.: A second example of anti-Fy3 the Duffy blood group system. Transfusion 14:608, 1974.

Ochsner, J. L., Mills, N. L., Leonard, G. L., and Lawson, N.: Fresh autologous blood transfusions with extracorporeal circulation. Ann. Surg. 177:811, 1973.

Ogata, T. and Matuhasi, T.: Further observations on the problems of specific and cross reactivity of blood group antibodies. Proc. 9th Congr. Int. Soc. Blood Transf. Mexico, 1962. Kevger, 1964.

Ogata, T. and Matuhasi, T.: Problems of specific and cross reactivity of blood group antibodies. Proc. 8th Congr. Int. Soc. Blood. Transf. Tokyo, 1960. Kevger, 1962.

Ogata, H., Okubo, Y. and Akabane, T.: Phenotype i associated with congenital cataract in Japanese. Transfusion, 19:166–168, 1979.

Olson, P. R., Cox, C. and McCullough, J.: Laboratory and clinical effects of the infusion of ACD solution during plateletpheresis. Vox Sang. 33:79, 1977.

O'Neill, G. J., Yang, S. Y., Tegoli, J., Berger, R. and DuPont, B.: Chico and Rodgers blood groups are antigenically distinct components of human complement C₄. Nature 273:668, 1978.

Ørjasaeter, H., Kornstad, L., Heier, A. M., Vogt, E., Hagen, P. and Hartmann, O.: A human blood group antigen, Nyᵃ (Nyberg), segregating with the Ns gene complex of the MNSs system. Nature 201:832, 1964.

Ørjasaeter, H., Kornstad, L. and Heier, A.: Studies on the Nyᵃ blood group antigen and antibodies. Vox Sang. 9: 673–683, 1964.

Orlina, A. and Josephson, A.: Comparative viability of blood stored in ACD and CPD. Transfusion 9:62, 1969.

Ottenberg, R.: Studies in isoagglutination. I. Transfusion and the question of intravascular agglutination. J. Exp. Med. 13:425, 1911.

Ottenberg, R. and Epstein, A. A.: Trans. NY Pathol. Soc. 8:187, 1908.

Ottensooser, F. and Silberschmidt, K.: Hemagglutinin anti-N in plant seeds. Nature 172:914, 1953.

Ottensooser, F., Mellone, O. and Biancalana, A.: Fatal transfusion reaction due to the Kell factor. Blood 8:1029, 1953.

Owen, R. D.: Immunogenetic consequences of vascular anastomoses between bovine twins. Science 102:400, 1945.

Parker, A. C., Willis, G., Urbaniak, S. J. and Innes, E. M.: Autoimmune hemolytic anemia with anti-A-autoantibody. Br. Med. J. i:26, 1978.

Parkin, D. M.: Study of a family with unusual ABO phenotypes. Br. J. Hemat. 2:106–110, 1956.

Paterson, J. L. H., Race, R. R. and Taylor, G. L.: A case of human iso-agglutinin anti-M. Br. Med. J. ii:37, 1942.

Pauling, L.: The theory of the structure and process of formation of antibodies. J. Amer. Chem. Soc. 62:2643, 1940.

Payne, R.: The association of febrile transfusion reactions with leuko-agglutinins. Vox Sang. 2:233, 1957.

Payne, R. and Rolfs, M. R.: Fetomaternal leukocyte incompatibility. J. Clin. Invest. 37:1756–1763, 1958.

Payne, R., Tripp, M., Weigle, J., Bodmer, W. and Bodmer, J.: A new leukocyte iso-antigen system in man. Cold Spr. Harb. Symp. Quant. Biol. 29:285–295, 1964.

Peetermans, M. E. and Cole-Dergent, J.: Hemolytic transfusion reaction due to anti-Sdᵃ. Vox Sang. 18:67–70, 1970.

Perham, T. G. M., Caul, E. O., Conway, P. J. and Mott, M. G.: Cytomegalovirus infection in blood donors — a prospective study. Brit J. Hematol. 20:307, 1971.

Perkins, H. A., Payne, R. O., Vyas, G. and Fudenberg, H. H.: Nonhemolytic reactions to blood transfusion and organ transplantation. Proc. 12th Congr. Int. Soc. Blood Transfus., Moscow, 1969.

Perkins, H. A., Payne, R., Ferguson, J. and Wood, M.: Nonhemolytic febrile transfusion reactions. Quantitative effects of blood components with emphasis on isoantigenic incompatibility of leukocytes. Vox. Sang. 11: 578, 1966.

Perrault, R.: Naturally occurring anti-M and anti-N with special case: IgG anti-N in a NN donor. Vox Sang. 24:134, 1973.

Perrault, R.: Low concentration antibodies. VI. Immunogenesis of anti-f. A new look at the Rh system. Upsala·J. Med. Sci. (Suppl) 12, 1972.

Peterson, E. T. and Chisholm, R.: A hemolytic transfusion reaction due to anti-Leᵃ. Proc. 6th Congr. Int. Soc. Blood Transf., 59–62, 1958.

Pettenkofer, H. J., Luboldt, W., Lawonn, H. and Niebuhr,

R.: Über genetische Suppression der Blutgruppen ABO Untersuchungen an einer Familie, bei der die Unterdrückung nicht das Blutgruppenmerkmal B betrifft. Z. ImmunForsch. 120:288–294, 1960.

Petz, L. D. and Garratty, G.: Acquired Immune Hemolytic Anemias. Churchill Livingstone, 1980.

Petz, L. D. and Garratty, G.: Laboratory correlations in immune hemolytic anemias. In Laboratory Diagnosis of Immunologic Disorders. Vyas, G. N., Sites, D. P. and Brecher, G. (eds). Grune & Stratton, 1975.

Petz, L. D., Fink, D., Letsky, E., Fudenberg, H. H. and Müller-Eberhard, H. J.: In vivo metabolism of complement. J. Clin. Invest. 47:2469, 1968.

Pickles, M. M.: Personal communication. Cited by Mollison, P. L., 1979.

Pickles, M. M.: Hemolytic Disease of the Newborn. Blackwell Scientific Publications, 1949.

Pickles, M. M. and Morton, J. A.: The Sd^a blood group. In Human Blood Groups. Mohn, J. F. et al (eds.). S. Karger, 1977.

Pierce, S. R., Hardman, J. T., Steele, S. and Beck, M. L.: Hemolytic disease of the newborn associated with anti-Jk^3. Transfusion 20:189, 1980.

Pinder, L. B., Staveley, J. M., Douglas, R. and Kornstad, L.: Pt^a—a new private antigen. Vox Sang. 7:303–305, 1969.

Pinkerton, P., Tilley, C. and Crookston, M. C.: (1977) Cited by Bird and Wingham, 1977.

Pinkerton, F. J., Mermod, L. E., Liles, B., Jack, J. A. and Noades, J.: The phenotype Jk(a-b-) in the Kidd blood group system. Vox Sang. 4:155–160, 1959.

Pirofsky, B.: Autoimmunization and the Autoimmune Hemolytic Anemias. Williams & Wilkins Co., 1969.

Platelet Transfusion Subcommittee of the Acute Leukemia Task Force: Platelet transfusion procedures. Cancer Chemother. Rep. Part 3, 1:1, 1969.

Plaut, G., Booth, P. B., Giles, C. M. and Mourant, A. E.: A new example of the Rh antibody, anti-C^X. Br. Med. J. i:1215, 1958.

Plaut, G., Ikin, E. W., Mourant, A. E., Sanger, R. and Race, R. R.: A new blood-group antibody, anti-Jk^b. Nature, 171:431, 1953.

Pliam, M. B., McGoon, D. C. and Tarhau, S.: Failure of transfusion of autologous whole blood to reduce banked blood requirements in open heart surgical patients. J. Thorac. Cardiovasc. Surg. 70:338, 1975.

Plischka, H. and Schäfer, E.: A study on the immunoglobulin class of the anti-A$_1$ isoagglutinin. J. Immunol. 108:782, 1972.

Polesky, H. F. and Swanson, J. L.: Studies on the distribution of the blood group antigen Do^a (Dombrock) and the characteristics of anti-Do^a. Transfusion 6:268–270, 1966.

Pollack, W., Ascari, W. Q., Kochesky, R. J., O'Connor, R. R., Ho, T. Y. and Tripodi, D.: Studies on Rh prophylaxis. I. Relationship between doses of anti-Rh and size of antigenic stimulus. Transfusion 11:333, 1971a.

Pollack, W., Ascari, W. Q., Crispen, J. F., O'Connor, R. R. and Ho, T. Y.: Studies on Rh prophylaxis. II. Rh immune prophylaxis after transfusion with Rh-positive blood. Transfusion 11:340, 1971b.

Pollack, W., Hager, H. J., Reckel, R., Toren, D. A. and Singher, H. O.: A study of the forces involved in the second stage of hemagglutination. Transfusion 5:158, 1965.

Polley, M. J. and Mollison, P. L.: The role of complement in the detection of blood group antibodies. Special reference to the antiglobulin test. Transfusion 1:9, 1961.

Polley, M. J., Mollison, P. L. and Soothill, J. F.: The role of 19S gamma globulin blood group antibodies in the antiglobulin reaction. Br. J. Hemat. 8:149, 1962.

Polley, M. J., Adinolfi, M. and Mollison, P. L.: Serological characteristics of anti-A related to type of antibody protein (7Sγ or 19Sγ). Vox Sang. 8:385, 1963.

Pondman, K. W., Rosenfield, R. E., Tallal, L. and Wasserman, L. R.: The specificity of the complement antiglobulin test. Vox Sang. 5:297, 1960.

Porter, R. R.: Hydrolysis of rabbit gamma globulins and antibodies with crystalline papain. Biochem. J. 73:119, 1959.

Potapov, M. I.: Detection of the antigen of the Lewis system, characteristic of the erythrocytes of the secretory group Le(a−b−). Probl. Hemathol. (Moscow). 11:45–49, 1970. (In Russian, with summary in English).

Pretty, H. M., Taliano, V., Fiset, D., Baribeau, G. and Guévin, R.: Another example of Lewis negative Bombay bloods. Vox Sang. 16:179–182, 1969.

Prince, A. M.: Post-transfusion hepatitis: etiology and prevention. In Transfusion and Immunology. Plenary Session Lectures of the 14th Congr. Int. Soc. Blood Transfus., Helsinki, 1975.

Prince, A. M.: An antigen detected in the blood during the incubation period of serum hepatitis. Proc. Nat. Acad. Sci. 60:814, 1968.

Prins, H. K. and Loos, J. A.: Studies on biochemical properties and viability of stored packed cells. In Modern Problems of Blood Preservation. Spielmann, W. and Seidl, S. (eds.). Gustav Fischer, 1970.

Prokop, O. and Uhlenbruck, G.: Human Blood and Serum Groups. Maclaren & Sons, 1969.

Prokop, O. and Rackwitz, A.: Weitere Untersuchungen mit Anti-A$_{hel}$ an Tierblutkörperchen. Acta Biol. Med. Germ. 15:191–192, 1965.

Prokop, O. and Schneider, W.: Das Rheususmosaik R$_1$/--- Dtsch. Z. Gerlichtl. Med. 50:423–428, 1960.

Prokop, O. and Oesterle, P.: Zur Frage der P-Antigenität von Echinokokkenflüssigkeit aus Schweinelebern. Blut 4:157–158, 1958.

Prokop, O., Uhlenbruck, G. and Köhler, W.: A new source of antibody-like substances having anti-blood group specificity. A discussion on the specificity of Helix agglutinins. Vox Sang. 14:321–333, 1968.

Prokop, O., Rackwitz, A. and Schlesinger, D.: A "new" human blood group receptor A$_{hel}$. Tested with saline extracts from Helix hortensis (garden snail). J. Forens. Med. S. Africa 12:108–110, 1965.

Prokop, O., Schlesinger, D. and Rackwitz, A.: Über eine thermostabile "antibody-like substance" (Anti-A$_{hel}$) bei Helix pomatia und deren Herkunft. Z. ImmunForsch. 129:402–412, 1965.

Pruzanski, W., Farid, N., Keystone, E., Armstrong, M. and Greaves, M. F.: The influence of homogeneous cold agglutinins on human B and T lymphocytes. Clin. Immunol. Immunopath. 4:248, 1975.

Puno, C. S. and Allen, F. H. Jr.: Anti-s produced in rabbits. Vox Sang. 16:155–156, 1969.

Purcell, R. H., Feinstone, S. M. and Kapikian, A. Z.: Recent advances in hepatitis A research. In Transmissible Disease and Blood Transfusion, eds T. J. Greenwalt and G. A. Jamieson. Grune & Stratton, New York. (1975)

Race, R. R. and Sanger, R.: Blood Groups in Man, 6th Ed. Blackwell Scientific Publications, Oxford, 1975.

Race, R. R. and Sanger, R.: Blood Groups in Man, 5th Ed. Blackwell Scientific Publications, Oxford, 1968.

Race, R. R. and Sanger, R.: Blood Groups in Man, 4th Ed. Blackwell Scientific Publications, Oxford, 1962.

Race, R. R. and Sanger, R.: The Rh antigen C^u. Heredity 5:285–287, 1951.

Race, R. R., Sanger, R. and Lehane, D.: Quantitative aspects of the blood-group antigen Fy^a. Ann. Eugen. 17:255–266, 1953.

Race, R. R., Sanger, R. and Selwyn, J. G.: A possible

deletion in a human Rh chromosome: a serological and genetical study. Br. J. Exp. Pathol. 32:124, 1951.

Race, R. R., Sanger, R. and Lawler, S. D.: Allelomorphs of the Rh gene C. Heredity 2:237–250, 1948.

Race, R. R., Sanger, R. and Lawler, S. D.: The Rh antigen D^u. Ann. Eugen. 14:171–184, 1948.

Race, R. R., Sanger, R. and Lawler, S. D.: Rh genes allelomorphic to D. Nature 162:292, 1948.

Race, R. R., Taylor, G. L., Boorman, K. E. and Dodd, B. E.: Recognition of Rh genotypes in man. Nature 152:563, 1943.

Ramirez, M. A.: Horse asthma following blood transfusion: report of a case. JAMA 73:985, 1919.

Randazzo, P., Streeter, B. and Nusbacher, J.: A common agglutinin reactive only against bromelin-treated red cells. Commun., AABB, Miami, 1973.

Ratkin, G. A., Osterland, C. K. and Chaplin, H., Jr.: IgG, IgA and IgM cold-reactive immunoglobulin in 19 patients with elevated cold agglutinins. J. Lab. Clin. Med. 82:67, 1973.

Rauner, R. A. and Tanaka, K. R.: Hemolytic transfusion reactions associated with the Kidd antibody (Jk^a). N. Engl. J. Med. 276:1486, 1967.

Rausen, A. R., Rosenfield, R. E., Alter, A. A. et al: A "new" infrequent red cell antigen, Rd (Radin). Transfusion 7:336–342, 1967.

Rawson, A. J. and Abelson, N. M.: Studies of blood group antibodies. VI. The blood group isoantibody activity of γ_{1A} globulin. J. Immunol. 93:192, 1964.

Rawson, A. J. and Abelson, N. M.: Studies of blood group antibodies. III. Observations on the physicochemical properties of isohemagglutinins and isohemolysins. J. Immunol. 85:636, 1960a.

Rawson, A. J. and Abelson, N. M.: Studies of blood group antibodies. IV. Physicochemical differences between iso-anti-A, B and iso-anti-A or iso-anti-B. J. Immunol. 85:640, 1960b.

Reed, T. E. and Moore, B. P. L.: A new variant of blood group A. Vox Sang. 9:363, 1964.

Reepmaker, J.: Relation between polyagglutinability of erythrocytes in vivo and the Hubener-Thomsen-Friedenreich phenomenon. J. Clin. Pathol. 5:266, 1952.

Rege, V. P. et al.: Isolation of serologically active fucose-containing oligosaccharides from human blood-group H substance. Nature 203:360–363, 1964.

Reinsmoen, N., Noreen, H., Friend, P., et al.: Anomalous mixed lymphocyte culture reactivity between HLA-A, B, C, DR identical siblings. Tissue Antigens 13:19, 1979.

Renkonen, K. O.: Studies on hemagglutinins present in seeds of some representatives of the family of Leguminoseae. Ann. Med. Exp. 26:66–72, 1948.

Renton, P. H. and Stratton, F.: Rhesus type D^u. Ann. Eugen. 15:189–209, 1950.

Renton, P. H., Howell, P., Ikin, E. W., Giles, C. M. and Goldsmith, K. L. G.: Anti-Sd^a, a new blood group antibody. Vox Sang. 13:493–501, 1967.

Renwick, J. H. and Lawler, S. D.: Probable linkage between a congenital cataract locus and the Duffy blood group locus. Ann. Hum. Genet. 27:67, 1963.

Reviron, J., Jacquet, A. and Salmon, C.: Un exemple de chromosome "cis-AB." Étude immunologique et génetique du phenotype induit. Nouv. Rev. Franç. Hématol. 8:323, 1968.

Reviron, J., Jacquet, A., Delarue, F., Liberge, G., Salmon, D. and Salmon, C.: Interactions alléliques des gènes de groupes sanguins ABO. Rèsultats préliminaires avec l'anti-B d'un sujet "cis-AB" et étude quantitative avec l'anti-B d'un sujet A₁O. Nouv. Revue Fr. Hématol. 7:425, 1967.

Reynolds, M. V., Vengelen-Tyler, V. and Morel, P. A.: Autoimmune hemolytic anemia associated with auto an-

ti-Gerbich. Proc. 33rd Ann. Meeting, AABB, Washington, DC, November 1980.

Rickard, K. A., Robinson, R. J. and Worlledge, S. M.: Acute acquired hemolytic anemia associated with polyagglutination. Arch. Dis. Childh. 44:102, 1969.

Ring, J. and Messmer, K.: Incidence and severity of anaphylactoid reactions to colloid volume substitutes. Lancet i:466, 1977.

Rochna, E. and Hughes-Jones, N. C.: The use of purified ¹²⁵I-labelled anti-gamma globulin in the determination of the number of D antigen sites on red cells of different phenotypes. Vox Sang. 10:675–686, 1965.

Roelcke, D.: A review: cold agglutination. Antibodies and antigens. Clin. Immunol. Immunopathol. 2:266, 1974.

Roelcke, D., Ebert, W. and Geisen, H. P.: Anti-Pr₃: serological and immunochemical identification of a new anti-Pr subspecificity. Vox Sang. 30:122, 1976.

Roelcke, D., Ebert, W. and Anstee, D. J.: Demonstration of low-titer anti-Pr cold agglutinins. Vox Sang. 27:429, 1974a.

Roelcke, D., Ebert, W. and Feizi, T.: Studies on the specificities of two IgM lambda cold agglutinins. Immunology 27:879, 1974b.

Rogers, M. J., Stiles, P. A. and Wright, J.: A new minus-minus phenotype: three Co(a–b–) individuals in one family. AABB Abstracts, Transfusion 14:508, 1974.

Rohwedder, R. W.: Infección chagásica en dadores de sangre y las probabilidades de transmitirla por medio de la transfusion. Bol. Chile Parasitol. 24:88, 1969.

Romano, E. L., Stolinski, C. and Hughes, N. C.: Distribution and mobility of the A, D and c antigens on human red cell membranes. Studies with a gold-labelled anti-globulin reagent. Br. J. Haematol. 30:507, 1975.

Romans, D. G., Tilley, C. A., Crookston, M. C., Falk, R. E. and Dorrington, K. J.: Conversion of incomplete antibodies to direct agglutinins by mild reduction: evidence for segmental flexibility within the Fc fragment of immunoglobulin G. Proc. Natl. Acad. Sci. USA 74:2531, 1977.

Rood, J. J. van: Leukocyte grouping. Thesis, Leiden, 1962.

Rood, J. J. van, Ernisse, J. G. and Leeuwen, A. van: Leucocyte antibodies in sera from pregnant women. Nature 181:1735–1736, 1958.

Ropars, C., Whylie, S., Cartron, J., Doinel, C., Gerbal, A. and Salmon, C.: Anticorps chez les polystransfusés dirigés contres certaines immunoglobulines IgM. Nouv. Rev. Franç Hématol. 13:459, 1973.

Rosenfield, R. E. and Haber, G. V.: An Rh blood factor, rh₁ (Ce), and its relationship to hr (ce). Am. J. Hum. Genet. 10:474–480, 1958.

Rosenfield, R. E. and Jagathambal: Transfusion therapy for autoimmune hemolytic anemia. Semin. Hematol. 13:311, 1976.

Rosenfield, R. E. and Ohno, G.: Unpublished observations. Cited by Miller et al. 1953.

Rosenfield, R. E. and Vogel, P.: The identification of hemagglutinins with red cells altered with trypsin. Trans. NY Acad. Sci. 13:213, 1951.

Rosenfield, R. E., Schmidt, P. J., Calvo, R. C. and McGinniss, M. H.: Anti-i, a frequent cold agglutinin in infectious mononucleosis. Vox Sang. 10:631, 1965.

Rosenfield, R. E., Allen, F. H., Swisher, S. N. and Kochwa, S.: A review of Rh serology and presentation of a new terminology. Transfusion 2:287–312, 1962.

Rosenfield, R. E., Haber, G. V., Schroeder, R. and Ballard, R.: Problems in Rh typing as revealed by a single Negro family. Am. J. Hum. Genet. 12:147–159, 1960.

Rosenfield, R. E., Haber, G. V., Kissmeyer-Nielsen, F., Jack, J. A., Sanger, R. and Race, R. R.: Ge, a very common red cell antigen. Br. J. Haematol. 6:344, 1960.

Rosenfield, R. E., Vogel, P., Gibbel, N., Sanger, R. and

Race, R. R.: A "new" Rh antibody, anti-f. Brit. Med. J. i:975, 1953.

Rosenfield, R. E., Vogel, P. and Race, R. R.: A further example of the human blood group antibody anti-Fy³. Rev. Hématol. 5:315, 1950.

Rosenthal, M. C. and Schwartz, L.: Reversible agglutination of trypsin-treated erythrocytes by normal human sera. Proc. Soc. Exp. Biol. 76:635, 1951.

Rosse, W. F., Dourmashkin, R. and Humphrey, J. H.: Immune lysis of normal human and paroxysmal nocturnal haemoglobinuria (PNH) red blood cells. III. The membrane defects caused by complement lysis. J. Exp. Med. 123:969, 1966.

Rous, P. and Turner, J. R.: Preservation of living red blood corpuscles in vitro. II. The transfusion of kept cells. J. Exp. Med. 23:219, 1916.

Rowe, A. W.: Preservation of blood by the low glycerol-rapid freeze process. In Red Cell Freezing, A Technical Workshop. Ann. Meeting, AABB, Bal Harbour, Florida, 1973, p. 55.

Rubin, H. and Solomon, A.: Cold agglutinins of anti-i specificity in alcoholic cirrhosis. Vox Sang. 12:227–230, 1967.

Ryder, L. P., Anderson, E. and Svejgaard, A. (eds): HLA and Disease Registry, third report. Munksgaard, 1979.

Sabo, B., McCreary, J., Stroup, M., Smith, D. E. and Weidner, J. G.: Another Kell-related antibody, anti-K19. Vox Sang. 36:97–102, 1979.

Sabo, B., Pancoska, C., Myers, M., Thoreson, S., McCreary, J. and Stroup, M.: Antibodies against two high frequency antigens of the Lutheran system; Lu:2 and Lu:16, made by Lu(a-b-) black females. Proc. 33rd Ann. Meeting, AABB, Washington, DC, 1980.

Sacks, M. S., Weiner, A. S., Jahn, E. F., Spurling, C. L. and Unger, L. J.: Isosensitization to a new blood factor Rh^D with special reference to its clinical importance. Ann. Intern. Med. 51:740–747, 1959.

Salmon, C.: Les phénotypes B faibles B₃, Bₓ, Bₑₗ. Classification pratique proposée. Rev. Franç. Transfus. 19:89, 1976.

Salmon, C.: Données quantitatives et thermodynamiques sur les modifications leucémiques de groupes sanguins ABO. Proc. 10th Congr. Int. Soc. Blood Transf., Stockholm, 337–342, 1964.

Salmon, C.: Étude thermodynamique de l'anticorps anti-B des sujets de phenotype Aₓ. D.Sc. thesis, University of Paris, 1960.

Salmon, C., Reviron, J. and Liberge, G.: Nouvel exemple d'une familie ou le phenotype Aₘ est observé dans 2 générations. Nouw. Revu. Franç. Hématol. 4:359, 1964.

Salmon, C., Schwartzenberg, L. and André, R.: Anémie hémolytique post-transfusionelle chez un sujet A₃ á la suite d'un injection massive de sang A₁. Sang. 30:223, 1959.

Salmon, C., Borin, P. and André, R.: Le groupe sanguin Aₘ dans deux générations d'une meme famille. Rev. Hématol. 13:529, 1958.

Salmon, C., Salmon, D., Liberge, G., André, R., Tippett, P. and Sanger, R.: Un nouvel antigène de groupe sanguin erythrocytaire présent chez 80% des sujets de race blanche. Nouv. Rev. Franç. Hématol. 1:649–661, 1961.

Sanger, R.: An association between the P and Jay systems of blood groups. Nature 176:1163–1164, 1955.

Sanger, R. and Race, R. R.: Subdivisions of the MN blood groups in man. Nature 160:505, 1947.

Sanger, R., Gavin, J., Tippett, P., Teesdale, P. and Eldon, K.: Plant agglutinin for another human blood group. Lancet i:1130, 1971.

Sanger, R., Noades, J., Tippett, P., Race, R. R., Jack, J. A. and Cunningham, C. A.: An Rh antibody specific for V and Rⁱˢ. Nature 186:171, 1960.

Sanger, R., Race, R. R., Greenwalt, T. J. and Sasaki, T.: The S, s and Sᵘ blood group genes in American Negroes. Vox Sang. 5:73–81, 1955.

Sanger, R., Race, R. R. and Jack, J.: The Duffy blood groups of New York Negroes: the phenotype Fy(a-b-). Br. J. Hematol. 1:370, 1955.

Sanger, R., Race, R. R., Rosenfield, R. E., Vogel, P. and Gibbell, N.: Anti-f and the 'new' Rh antigen it defines. Proc. Nat. Acad. Sci. USA 39:824–834, 1953.

Sanger, R., Race, R. R., Walsh, R. J. and Montgomery, C.: An antibody which subdivides the human MN blood groups. Heredity 2:131–139, 1948.

Saravis, C. A.: Some aspects of the serological effect of preservatives on serum proteins. Commun., AABB, Chicago, 1959.

Sausais, L., Krevans, J. R. and Townes, A. S.: Characteristics of a third example of anti-Xgᵃ. Transfusion 4:312 (Abstract), 1964.

Schachter, H., Michaels, M. A., Crookston, M. C., Tilley, C. A. and Crookston, J. H.: A quantitative difference in the activity of blood group A-specific N-acetylgalactosaminyl transferase in serum from A₁ and A₂ human subjects. Biochem. Biophys. Res. Commun. 45:1011, 1971.

Scheffer, H. and Tamaki, H. T.: Anti-Luᵇ and mild hemolytic disease of the newborn. Transfusion 6:497–498, 1966.

Schiff, F. and Boyd, W. C.: Blood Grouping Technic. Interscience Publishers, 1942.

Schiffer, C. A., Aisner, J. and Wiernik, P. H.: Clinical experience with transfusion of cryopreserved platelets. Br. J. Hematol. 34:377, 1976a.

Schiffer, C. A., Buchholz, D. H., Aisner, H., Wolff, J. H. and Wiernik, P. H.: Frozen autologous platelets in the supportive care of patients with leukaemia. Transfusion 16:321, 1976b.

Schiffer, C. A., Lichtenfeld, J. L., Wiernik, P. H., Mardiney, M. and Mehsen, J. J.: Antibody response in patients with acute nonlymphocytic leukemia. Cancer 37:2177, 1976c.

Schlosstein, L. P., Terasaki, I., Bluestone, R. and Pearson, C. M.: High association of an HL-A antigen, W27, with ankylosing spondylitis. N. Engl. J. Med. 288:704–706, 1973.

Schmidt, P. J., Barile, M. F. and McGinniss, M. H.: Mycoplasma (pleuropneumonia-like organism) and blood group I; associations with neoplastic disease. Nature 205:371, 1965.

Schmidt, R., Griffitts, J. J. and Northman, F. F.: A new antibody, anti-Sm, reacting with a high incidence antigen. Transfusion 2:338–340, 1962.

Schultze, H. E. and Heremans, J. F.: Molecular Biology of Human Proteins with Special Reference to Plasma Proteins, Vol. 2. Elsevier, 1966.

Schwarting, G. A., Marcus, D. M. and Metaxas, M.: Identification of sialosylparagloboside as the erythrocyte receptor for an "anti-p" antibody. Vox Sang. 32:257, 1977.

Seaman, M. J., Benson, R., Jones, M. N., Morton, J. A. and Pickles, M. M.: The reactions of the Bennett-Goodspeed group of antibodies with the AutoAnalyzer. Br. J. Hematol. 13:464–473, 1967.

Sears, D., Weed, R. I. and Swisher, S.: Differences in the mechanism of in vitro immune hemolysis related to antibody specificity. J. Clin. Invest. 43:975, 1964.

Serim, N.: Lettres a la rédaction. Phénotype Am avec expression secondaire de l'antigène A dans les hématics. Rev. Franç. Transf. 12:277–280, 1969.

Seyfried, H., Gorska, B., Maj, S., Sylwestrowicz, T., Giles, C. M. and Goldsmith, K. L. G.: Apparent depression of antigens of the Kell blood group system associated with autoimmune acquired hemolytic anemia. Vox Sang. 23:528–536, 1972.

Seyfried, H., Walewska, I. and Werblinska, B.: Unusual inheritance of ABO group in a family with weak B antigens. Vox Sang. 9:268, 1964.

Shanahan, L.: Scianna antigens and antibodies. A new example of Anti-Sc2. A.R.T. Thesis, 1975 (unpublished).

Shapiro, M.: Serology and genetics of a new blood factor: hr^H. J. Forens. Med. 11:52–66, 1964.

Shapiro, M.: Serology and genetics of a new blood factor: hr^3. J. Forens. Med. 7:96–105, 1960.

Shapiro, M.: Blood groups and skin color: their genetics in human anthropology. J. Forensic Med. 1:2, 1953.

Shapiro, M., LeRoux, M. and Brink, S.: Serology and genetics of a new blood factor: hr^B. Haematologia 6:121–128, 1972.

Shattock, S. G.: Chromocyte clumping in acute pneumonia and certain other diseases and the significance of the buffy coat in the shed blood. J. Pathol. 6:303, 1900.

Shattock, S. G.: Chromocyte clumping in acute rheumatism. Br. Med. J. i:1091, 1899.

Shaw, J. F.: HLA typing. Arch. Pathol. Lab. Med. 100:341, 1976.

Shaw, J. F.: Areas of HLA utilization. In HLA Without Tears. American Association of Clinical Pathologists, Chicago, 1975.

Shaw, J. F.: Preliminary screening and tentative identification of HL-A lymphocytotoxic antibodies in a hospital blood bank. Transfusion 13:34, 1973.

Sherman, S. P., and Taswell, H. F.: The need for transfusion of saline-washed red blood cells to patients with paroxysmal nocturnal hemoglobinuria: a myth. Commun. Amer. Assoc. Blood Banks, Atlanta, 1977.

Shields, C. E.: Studies on stored whole blood. II. Use of packed red cells. Transfusion 9:1, 1969a.

Shields, C. E.: Effect of adenine on stored erythrocytes evaluated by autologous and homologous transfusion. Transfusion 9:115, 1969b.

Shields, C. E.: Comparison studies of whole blood stored in ACD and CPD and with adenine. Transfusion 8:1, 1968.

Silvergleid, A. J., Hafleigh, E. B., Harabin, M. A., Wolf, R. M. and Grumet, F. C.: Clinical value of washed-platelet concentrates in patients with nonhemolytic transfusion reactions. Transfusion 17:33, 1977.

Sinclair, M., Buchanan, D. I., Tippett, P. and Sanger, R.: Another antibody related to the Lutheran blood group system (Much.) Vox Sang. 25:156–161, 1973.

Singer, S. J.: Molecular biology of cellular membranes with applications to immunology. In Advances in Immunology, Dixon, F. J. and Kunkel, H. G. (eds). Academic Press, 1974.

Singer, S. J., and Nicolson, G. L.: The fluid mosaic model of the structural cell membranes. Science 175:720, 1972.

Slayter, H. S., Cooper, A. G. and Brown, M. C.: Electron microscopy and physical parameters of human blood group i, A, B, and H antigens. Biochemistry 13:3365, 1974.

Slichter, S. J. and Harker, L. A.: Preparation and storage of platelet concentrates. II. Storage variables influencing platelet viability and function. Br. J. Hematol. 34:403, 1976.

Smerling, M.: S^u in der weissen Bevölkerung (Bericht über Familienuntersuchungen). Beitr. Gericht. Med. 28:237–239, 1971.

Smith, H. W.: The physiology of the renal circulation. Harvey Lect. 35:166, 1940.

Smith, M. I. and Beck, M. L.: The immunoglobulin structure of human anti-M agglutinins. Transfusion 19:472, 1979.

Smith, M. I. and Beck, M. L.: The immunoglobulin class of antibodies with M specificity. Commun., AABB, Atlanta, 1977.

Smith, R. T. and Bridges, R. A.: Immunological unrespon-

siveness in rabbits produced by neonatal injection of defined antigens. J. Exp. Med. 108:227, 1958.

Sneath, J. S. and Sneath, P. H. A.: Transformation of the Lewis groups of human red cells. Nature 176:172, 1955.

Solem, J. H. and Jörgensen, W.: Accidentally transmitted infectious mononucleosis. Acta Med. Scand. 186:433, 1969.

Solomon, J. M.: Behavior of incomplete antibodies in quantitative hemagglutination reactions. Transfusion 4:101, 1964.

Solomon, J. M. and Sturgeon, P.: Quantitative studies of the phenotype A$_{el}$. Vox Sang. 9:476–486, 1964.

Spath, P., Garratty, G. and Petz, L. D.: Studies on the immune response to penicillin and cephalothin in humans. II. Immunohematologic reactions to cephalothin administration. J. Immunol. 107:860, 1971.

Speiser, P.: Ueber die bisher jüngste menschliche Frucht (27 mm/2.2 g), an der bereits die Erbmerkmale A$_1$, M, N, s, Fy(a+), C,c,D,E,e, Jk(a+) im Blut festgestellt werden Konnten. Wien. Klin. Wschr. 71:549–551, 1959.

Speiser, P.: Zur Frage der Vererbbarkeit des irregulaeren Agglutinins Anti-A$_1$ (α_1). Acta Genet. Med. 3:192, 1956.

Speiser, P., Schwarz, J. and Lewkin, D.: Statistiche Ergebnisse von 10,000 Blutgruppen- und Blutfaktorenbestimmungen in der Wiener Bevölkerung 1948 bis 1950. Klin. Med. 6:105, 1951.

Spooner, E. T. C.: The causes of bacterial contamination of blood, serum and plasma in the London Emergency Blood Supply Depots, Nov. 1941-Jan. 1942. Unpublished report to the Medical Research Council, 1942.

Springer, G. F.: Influenza virus vaccine and blood group A-like substances. Transfusion 3:233–236, 1963.

Springer, G. F. and Huprikar, S. V.: On the biochemical and genetic basis of the human blood-group MN specificities. Haematologia 6:81–92, 1972.

Springer, G. F. and Ansell, N. J.: Inactivation of human erythrocyte agglutinogens M and N by influenza viruses and receptor-destroying enzyme. Proc. Nat. Acad. Sci. USA 44:182–189, 1958.

Springer, G. F., Huprikar, S. V. and Tegtmeyer, H.: Biochemical-genetic basis of human blood group MN specificities. Naturwissenschaften 5:274, 1971.

Springer, G. F., Horton, R. E. and Forbes, M.: Origin of anti-human blood group B agglutinins in white leghorn chicks. J. Exp. Med. 110:221–244, 1959.

Staveley, J. M. and Cameron, G. L.: The inhibiting action of hydatid cyst fluid on anti-Tj^a sera. Vox Sang. 3:114–118, 1958.

Stephen, C. R., Martin, R. C. and Bourgeois-Gavardin, M.: Antihistaminic drugs in treatment of nonhemolytic transfusion reactions. JAMA 158:525, 1955.

Stern, K., Goodman, H. S. and Berger, M.: Experimental isoimmunization to hemoantigens in man. J. Immunol. 87:189, 1961.

Stiff, P. J., Murgo, A. J., Wittes, R. E., Clarkson, B. D. and Zaroulis, C. G.: Lekapheresed mononuclear cells (MNC) after chemotherapy: alternative to marrow for autologous transplantation. Proc. 33rd Ann. Meeting, AABB, Washington, DC, 1980.

Stocker, J. W., McKenzie, I. F. C. and Morris, P. J.: IgM activity in human lymphocytotoxic antisera after renal transplantation. Nature 222:483, 1969.

Stoddart, J. C.: Nickel sensitivity as a cause of infusion reactions. Lancet ii:741, 1960.

Stone, B. and Marsh, W. L.: Hemolytic disease of the newborn caused by anti-M. Br. J. Hematol. 5:344, 1959.

Stout, T. D., Moore, B. P. L., Allen, F. H. and Corcoran, P.: A new phenotype—D+G— (Rh: 1,–12). Vox Sang. 8:262–268, 1963.

Strahl, M., Pettenkofer, H. J. and Hasse, W.: A hemolytic transfusion reaction due to anti-M. Vox Sang. 5:34, 1955.

Strange, J. J., Kenworthy, R. J., Webb, A. J. and Giles, C. M.: Wk^a (Weeks), a new antigen in the Kell blood group system. Vox Sang. 27:81–86, 1974.

Stratton, F.: Recent observations on the antiglobulin test. Wadley Med. Bull. 5:182, 1975.

Stratton, F.: Zymosan-coated particles used to prepare anti-Bi^c. Vox Sang. II:232, 1966.

Stratton, F.: The value of fresh serum in the detection and use of anti-Jk^a antibody. Vox Sang. 1:160–167, 1956.

Stratton, F.: Polyagglutinability of red cells. Vox Sang. 4:58, 1954.

Stratton, F.: A new Rh allelomorph. Nature 158:25, 1946.

Stratton, F.: Demonstration of the Rh factor in the blood of a 48 mm. embryo. Nature 152:449, 1943.

Stratton, F. and Rawlinson, V. I.: Observations on the anti-globulin tests. C4 components on erythrocytes Vox. Sang. 31:44. A study performed on batches of serum albumin used as diluents in Rh testing (1976). A report to the International Society of Blood Transfusion/International Committee for Standardization in haematology by their albumin working party. Br. J. Hematol. 32:215, 1976.

Stratton, F. and Diamond, E. R.: The value of a serum and albumin mixture for use in the detection of blood group antigen-antibody reactions. J. Clin. Pathol. 8:218, 1955.

Stratton, F. and Renton, P. H.: Effect of crystalloid solutions prepared in glass bottles on human red cells. Nature 175:722, 1955.

Stratton, F. and Renton, P. H.: Hemolytic disease of the newborn caused by a new Rh antibody, anti-C^x. Br. Med. J. i:962–965, 1954.

Stratton, F., Renton, P. H., and Rawlinson, V. I.: Serologic difference between old and young cells. Lancet ii, 1388, 1960.

Stratton, F., Rawlinson, V. I., Gunson, H. H. and Phillips, P. K.: The role of zeta potential in Rh agglutination. Vox Sang. 24:273, 1973.

Stratton, F., Gunson, H. H. and Rawlinson, V.: Complement fixing antibodies in relation to hemolytic disease of the newborn. Transfusion 5:216, 1965.

Stroup, M.: Personal communication, 1974.

Stroup, M. and MacIlroy, M., Jr.: Five examples of an antibody defining an antigen of high frequency in the Caucasian population. Commun., AABB, San Francisco, 1970.

Stroup, M. and MacIlroy, M.: Evaluation of the albumin antiglobulin technic in antibody detection. Transfusion 5:184, 1965.

Stroup, M., MacIlroy, M., Walker, R. and Aydelotte, J. V.: Evidence that Sutter belongs to the Kell blood group system. Transfusion 5:309–314, 1965.

Strumia, M. M.: Methods of blood preservation in general and preparation and use of red cell suspension. Am. J. Clin. Pathol. 24:260, 1954.

Strumia, M. M., Strumia, P. V. and Eusebi, A. J.: The preservation of blood for transfusion. VII. Effect of adenine and inosine on the adenosine triphosphate and viability of red cells when added to blood stored from 0 to 70 days at 1° C. J. Lab. Clin. Med. 75:244, 1970.

Stuckey, M. A., Osoba, D. and Thomas, J. W.: Hemolytic transfusion reactions. Can. Med. Assoc. J. 90:739, 1964.

Sturgeon, P.: Hematological observations on the anaemia associated with blood type Rh$_{null}$. Blood 36:310–320, 1970.

Sturgeon, P.: The Rh$_o$ variant — D^u. I. Its frequency in a mixed population. Transfusion 2:234, 1962.

Sturgeon, P. and Arcilla, M. B.: Studies on the secretion of blood group substances. I. Observations on the red cell phenotype Le (a+b+x+). Vox Sang. 18:301–322, 1970.

Sturgeon, P., Moore, B. P. L. and Weiner, W.: Notations for two weak A variants: A$_{end}$ and A$_{el}$. Vox Sang. 9:214, 1964.

Sussman, L. N. and Miller, E. B.: Un nouveau facteur sanguin "Vel." Rev. Hematol. 7:368, 1952.

Swanson, J. L.: Laboratory problems associated with leukocyte antibodies. In a seminar on Recent Advances in Immunohematology. AABB, Bal Harbour, Florida, 121–155, 1973.

Swanson, J. and Matson, G. A.: Third example of a human "D-like" antibody or anti-LW. Transfusion 4:257, 1964.

Swanson, J. and Matson, G. A.: Mt^a, a "new" antigen in the MNSs system. Vox Sang. 7:585–590, 1962.

Swanson, J. L., Miller, J., Azar, M. and McCullough, J. J.: Evidence for heterogeneity of LW antigen revealed in family study. Transfusion 14:470–474, 1974.

Swanson, J., Park, B. and McCullough, J.: Kell phenotypes in families of patients with X-linked chronic granulomatous disease. Abstracts, AABB and ISH Meeting, Washington, DC, 1972.

Swanson, J., Olsen, J. and Azar, M. M.: Serological evidence that antibodies of Chido-York-Cs^a specificity are leukocyte antibodies. Fed. Proc. 30:248 Abs., 1971.

Swanson, J., Zweber, M. and Polesky, H. F.: A new public antigenic determinant Gy^a (Gregory). Transfusion 7:304, 1967.

Swanson, J., Polesky, H. F., Tippett, P. and Sanger, R.: A "new" blood group antigen, Do^a. Nature 206:313, 1965.

Szymanski, I. O., Roberts, P. L. and Rosenfield, R. E.: Anti-A autoantibody with severe intravascular hemolysis. N. Engl. J. Med. 294:995, 1976.

Taliano, V., Guévin, R.-M. and Tippett, P.: The genetics of a dominant inhibitor of the Lutheran antigens. Vox Sang. 24:42–47 1973.

Tanner, M. J. A. and Anstee, D. J.: The membrane change in En(a−) human erythrocytes. Biochem. J. 153:271, 1976.

Tanowitz, H. B., Robbins, N. and Leidich, N.: Hemolytic anemia: Associated with severe Mycoplasma pneumoniae pneumonia. N.Y. State J. Med. 78:2231, 1978.

Tate, H., Cunningham, C., McDade, M. G., Tippett, P. A. and Sanger, R.: An Rh gene complex Dc−. Vox Sang. 5:398, 1960.

Taylor, G. L., Race, R. R., Prior, A. M. and Ikin, E. W.: Frequency of the iso-agglutinin x$_1$ in the serum of the subgroups A$_2$ and A$_2$B. J. Pathol. Bacteriol. 54:514–516, 1942.

Tegoli, J., Cortez, M., Jensen, L., and Marsh, W. L.: A new antibody, anti-ILe^{bH}, specific for a determinant formed by the combined action of the I, Le, Se and H gene products. Vox Sang. 21:397–404, 1971.

Tegoli, J., Harris, J. P., Issitt, P. D., and Sanders, C. W.: Anti-IB, an expected "new" antibody detecting a joint product of the I and B genes. Vox Sang. 13:144–157, 1967.

Telischi, M., Behzad, O., Issitt, P. D., and Pavone, B. G.: Hemolytic disease of the newborn due to anti-N. Vox Sang. 31:109, 1976.

Terasaki, P. I., and McClelland J. D.: Microdroplet assay of human serum cytotoxins. Nature 204:998–1000, 1964.

Thomas, E. D.: Bone-marrow transplantation. N. Engl. J. Med. 292:832–837; 292:895, 1975.

Thompson, G. R., Lowenthal, R., and Myant, N. B.: Plasma exchange in the management of homozygous familial hypercholesterolaemia. Lancet i:1208–1211, 1975.

Thompson, P. R., Childers, D. M., and Hatcher, D. E.: Anti-Di^b: first and second examples. Vox Sang. 13:314–318, 1967.

Thomsen, O.: Untersuchungen über die scrologische Gruppendifferenzierung des Organismus. Acta Pathol. Microbiol. Scand. 7:250. Cited by Dausset 1930.

Thomsen, O.: Ein vermehrungsfahiges Agens als Veränderer des isoagglutinatorischen Verhaltens der roten Blukörperchen, eine bisher unbekannte Quelle der Fehibestimmung. Z. Immun.-Forsch. 52:85, 1927.

Thomsen, O., Friedenreich, V., and Worsaae, E.: Über die Möglichkeit des Existenz zweier neues Blutgruppen; auch ein Beitrag zur Beleuchtung sogennantes Untogruppen. Acta Pathol. Microbiol. Scand. 7:157, 1930.

Thomsen, O., and Kettel, K.: Die Stärke der menschlichen Isoagglutinine und entsprechender Blutkörperchenrezeptoren in verschiedenen Lebensaltern. Z. Immun-Forsch. 63:67–93, 1929.

Thomsen, O., and Thisted, A.: Untersuchungen über Isohämolysin in Menschenserum. I. Reaktivierung. Z. Immun.-Forsch. 59:479, 1928a.

Tilley, C. A., Crookston, M. C., Crookston, J. H., Shindman, J. and Schachter, H.: Human blood group A− and H− specified glycosyltransferase levels in the sera of newborn infants and their mothers. Vox Sang. 34:8, 1978.

Tilley, C. A., Crookston, M. C., Haddad, S. A. and Shumak, K. H.: Red blood cell survival studies in patients with anti-Ch^a, anti-Yk^a, anti-Ge and anti-Vel. Transfusion 17:169, 1977.

Tippett, P.: A present view of Rh. Pathologica 64:29, 1972.

Tippett, P.: A case of suppressed Lu^a and Lu^b antigens. Vox Sang. 20:378–380. 1971.

Tippett, P.: Serological Study of the Inheritance of Unusual Rh and Other Blood Group Phenotypes. PhD Thesis, University of London, 1963.

Tippett, P., and Sanger, R.: Observations on subdivisions of the Rh antigen D. Vox Sang. 7:9–13, 1962.

Tippett, P., Sanger, R., Race, R. R., Swanson, J. and Busch, S.: An agglutinin associated with the P and the ABO blood group system. Vox Sang. 10:269–280, 1965.

Tippett, P., Noades, J., Sanger, R., Race, R. R., Sausais, L., Holman, C. A. and Buttimer, R. J.: Further studies of the I antigen and antibody. Vox Sang. 5:107–121, 1960.

Toivanen, P. and Hirvonen, T.: Antigens Duffy, Kell, Kidd, Lutheran and Xg^a on fetal red cells. Vox Sang. 24:372–376, 1973.

Toivanen, P., and Hirvonen, T.: Iso- and heteroagglutinins in human fetal and neonatal sera. Scand. J. Hemat. 6:42–48, 1969.

Toivanen, P., and Hirvonen, T.: Fetal development of red cell antigens K, k, Lu^a, Lu^b, Fy^a, Fy^b, Vel and Xg^a. Scand. J. Hematol. 6:49, 1969.

Tomasi, T. B., Tan, E. M., Solomon, A. and Prendergast, R. A.: Characteristics of an immune system common to certain external secretions. J. Exp. Med. 121:101, 1965.

Tönder, O., and Larsen, B.: A simple method for preparation of antiserum to human gamma-A-globulin. Vox Sang. 18:475, 1970.

Tong, M. J., Stevenson, D., and Gordon, I.: Correlation of e antigen, DNA polymerase activity, and Dane particles in chronic benign and chronic active type B hepatitis infections. J. Inf. Dis. 135:980, 1977.

Tonthat, H., Rochant, H., Henry, A., Leporrier, M. and Dreyfus, B.: A new case of monoclonal IgA kappa cold agglutinin with anti-Pr$_1$ specificity in a patient with persistent HB antigen cirrhosis. Vox Sang. 30:464, 1976.

Toyama, S.: Studies on S-T blood typing system. 1. On the incomplete immune cold T agglutinin. Jpn. J. Leg. Med. 10:105–122, 1956. (In Japanese.)

Truog, P. U., Steiger, L., Contu, G., Galfre, M., Trucco, D., Bernoco, M. et al.: Ankylosing spondylitis (AS): a population and family study using HL-A serology and MLR. In Histocompatibility Testing 1975 (ed. F. Kissmeyer-Nielsen). Munksgaard, 1975, pp. 788–796.

Tsuganezawa, M.: On the anti-T antibody in the goat anti-T immune serum, especially on the incomplete anti-T agglutinin. Jpn. J. Leg. Med. 10:545–552, 1956. (In Japanese.)

Tullis, J. L., Tinch, R. J., Baudanza, P., Gibson, J. G., Diforte, S., Conneely, G. and Murthy, K.: Plateletpheresis in a disposable system. Transfusion II:368, 1971.

Tullis, J. L., Hinman, J., Sproul, M. T. and Nickerson, R. J.: Incidence of post-transfusion hepatitis in previously frozen blood. JAMA 214:719, 1970.

Turner, A. R., MacDonald, R. N. and Cooper, B. A.: Transmission of infectious mononucleosis by transfusion of pre-illness plasma. Ann. Intern. Med. 77:751, 1972.

Uhlenbruck, G. and Krupe, M.: Cryptantigenic N$_{vg}$ receptor in mucoids from Mu/Mu cells. Vox Sang. 10:326, 1965.

Unger, L. J.: A method for detecting Rh$_o$ antibodies in extremely low titer. J. Lab. Clin. Med. 37:825, 1951.

Unger, L. J., and Wiener, A. S.: Some observations on blood factors Rh^A, Rh^B and Rh^C of the Rh-Hr blood group system. Blood 14:522–534, 1959.

Unger, L. J. and Wiener, A. S.: Some observations on the blood factor Rh^A of the Rh-Hr blood group system. Acta Genet. Med. et Gemell. (2nd suppl.) 13–25, 1959.

Unger, L. J., and Wiener, A. S.: Observations on blood factors Rh^A, Rh^{alpha}, Rh^B, and Rh^C. Am. J. Clin. Pathol. 31:95–103, 1959.

Unger, L. J. and Katz, L.: The effect of trypsin on hemagglutinogens determining eight blood group systems. J. Lab. Clin. Med. 39:135, 1952.

Unger, L. J. and Katz, L.: The effect of trypsin on the Duffy factor. J. Lab. Clin. Med. 38:188, 1951.

Unger, L. J., Wiener, A. S. and Katz, L.: Studies on blood factors Rh^A, Rh^B and Rh^C. J. Exp. Med. 110:495–510, 1959.

Unger, L. J., Wiener, A. S., and Sonn, E. B.: Problems in blood grouping in relation to transfusion. Am. J. Clin. Pathol. 16:45, 1946.

Vaerman, J. P. and Heremans, J. F.: Antigenic heterogenicity of human immunoglobulin A proteins. Science 153:647, 1966.

Vale, D. R. and Harris, I. M.: An additional example of autoanti-M. Transfusion 20:440, 1980.

Valeri, C. R.: Circulation and hemostatic effectiveness of platelets stored at 4° C or 22° C: studies in aspirin-treated normal volunteers. Transfusion 16:20, 1976.

Valeri, C. R.: Factors influencing the 24-hour post-transfusion survival and the oxygen transport function of previously frozen red cells preserved with 40% w/v glycerol and frozen at −80° C. Transfusion 14:1, 1974.

Valet, G. and Cooper, N. R.: Isolation and characterization of the proenzyme form of the Clr subunit of the first complement component. J. Immunol. 112:1667, 1974.

Van Der Hart, M. and Van Loghem, J. J.: A further example of anti-Jk^a. Vox Sang. 3:72, 1953.

Van Der Hart, M., Moes, M., Von Der Veer, M. and Van Loghem, J. J.: Ho and Lan — two new blood group antigens. Commun. 8th Congr. Europ. Soc. Hemat., Vienna, 1961.

Van Der Meulen, F. W., Van Der Hart, M., Fleer, A., Von Dem Borne, A. E. G. K., Engelfriet, C. P., and Van Loghem, J. J.: The role of adherence to human mononuclear phagocytes in the destruction of red cells sensitized with non-complement binding IgG antibodies. Br. J. Hematol. 38:541, 1978.

Van Loghem, J. J.: Some comments on autoantibody-induced red cell destruction. Ann. NY Acad. Sci. 124:465, 1965.

Van Loghem, J. J. and Van Der Hart, M.: Varieties of specific auto-antibodies in acquired hemolytic anemia. Vox Sang. 4:2, 1954.

Van Loghem, J. J., Peetoom, F., Van Der Hart, M., Van Der

Veer, M., *et al*.: Serological and immunochemical studies in hemolytic anemia with high-titer cold agglutinins. Vox Sang. 8:33, 1963.

Van Loghem, J. J., Van Der Hart, M., Bok, J. and Brinkerink, P. C.: Two further examples of the antibody anti-Wr^a. Vox Sang. 5:130, 1955a.

Van Loghem, J. J., Van Der Hart, M. and Land, M. E.: Polyagglutinability of red cells as a cause of severe hemolytic transfusion reaction. Vox Sang. 5:125, 1955b.

Van Loghem, J. J., De Raad, H. and Van Hattem, A.: Erythroblastosis foetalis en de bloedgroep Kell. Maadschr. Kindergeneesk. 21:63, 1953a.

Van Oss, C. J., Mohn, J. F. and Cunningham, R. K.: Influence of various physiochemical factors on hemagglutination. Vox Sang. 34:351, 1978.

Van Rood, J. J. and Van Leeuwen, W.: Alloantigens of leukocytes and platelets. *In* Textbook of Immunopathology, 2nd Ed., Miescher, P. A. and Muller-Eberhard, H. J. (eds.) Vol. II. Grune & Stratton, 1976.

Victoria, E. J. Muchmore, E. A., Sudora, E. J., and Masouredis, S. P.: The role of antigen mobility in anti-Rh_0 (D)− induced agglutination. J. Clin. Invest. 56:292, 1975.

Voak, D. and Bowley, C. C.: A detailed serological study on the prediction and diagnosis of ABO haemolytic disease of the newborn (ABO HD). Vox Sang. 17:321, 1969.

Voak, D., Cawley, J. C., Emmines, J. P. and Barker, C. R.: The role of enzymes and albumin in haemagglutination reactions, a serological and ultrastructural study with ferritin-labeled anti-D. Vox Sang. 27:156, 1974.

Voak, D., Anstee, D. and Pardoe, G.: The alpha-galactose specificity of anti-P^k. Vox Sang. 25:263–270, 1973.

Von Dem Borne, A. E., Engelfriet, C. P., Beckers, D., Van Der Kort-Henkes, G., Van Der Giessen, M. and Van Loghem, J. J.: Autoimmune hemolytic anemias. II. Warm hemolysins — serological and immunochemical investigations and ^51Cr studies. Clin. Exp. Immunol. 4:333, 1969.

Von Dungern, E. and Hirszfeld, L.: Ueber Vererbung gruppenspezifischer Strukturen des Blutes. Z. Immun-Forsch 6:284, 1910. (Translation by G. P. Pohlmann, Transfusion, 2:70–74, 1962.)

Vos, G. H.: A study related to the significance of hemolysins observed among aborters, nonaborters and infertility patients. Transfusion 7:40–47, 1967.

Vos, G. H.: The serology of anti-Tj^a-like hemolysins observed in the serum of threatened aborters in Western Australia. Acta Hematol. 35:272–283, 1966.

Vos, G. H.: A comparative observation of the presence of anti-Tj^a-like hemolysins in relation to obstetric history, distribution of the various blood groups and the occurrence of immune anti-A or anti-B hemolysins among aborters and nonaborters. Transfusion 5:327–335, 1965.

Vos, G. H.: Five examples of red cells with the A_x subgroup of blood group A. Vox Sang. 9:160, 1964.

Vos, G. H. and Kirk, R. L.: A "naturally-occurring" anti-E which distinguishes a variant of the E antigen in Australian aborigines. Vox Sang. 7:22–32, 1962.

Vos, G. H., Celano, M. J., Falkowski, F. and Levine, P.: Relationship of a hemolysin resembling anti-Tj^a to threatened abortion in Western Australia. Transfusion 4:87–91, 1964.

Vos, G. H., Vos, D., Kirk, R. L. and Sanger R.: A sample of blood with no detectable Rh antigens. Lancet i:14–15, 1961.

Vries, S. I. De and Smitskamp, H. S.: Hemolytic transfusion reaction due to an anti-Lewis^a agglutinin. Br. Med. J. i:280–281, 1951.

Walker, R. H., Argall, C. I., Steane, E. A., Sasaki, T. T. and Greenwalt, T. J.: Js^b of the Sutter blood group system. Transfusion 3:94–99, 1963.

Walker, R. H., Argall, C. I., Steane, E. A., Sasaki, T. T. and Greenwalt, T. J.: Anti-Js^b, the expected antithetical antibody of the Sutter blood group system. Nature 197:295–296, 1963.

Walker, W. and Bailey, B. M.: Failure to detect Rh-substance in liquor amnii. J. Clin. Pathol. 9:52, 1956.

Wallace, J. and Izatt, M. M.: The Cl^a (Caldwell) antigen: a new and rare human blood group antigen related to the MNSs system. Nature 200:689–690, 1963.

Wallace, J. and Milne, G. R.: A "new" human blood group antigen of rare frequency. Proc. 7th Congr. Int. Soc. Blood Transf., 587–589, 1959.

Wallace, J., Milne, G. R. and Barr, A.: Total screening of blood donations for Australia (hepatitis-associated) antigen and its antibody. Br. Med. J. i:663, 1972.

Waller, M. and Lawler, S. D.: A study of the properties of the Rhesus antibody (Ri) diagnostic for the rheumatoid factor and its application to Gm grouping. Vox Sang. 7:591, 1962.

Walsh, J. H., Purcell, R. H., Morrow, A. G., Chanock, R. H. and Schmidt, P. J.: Post-transfusion hepatitis after open-heart operations. JAMA 211:261, 1970.

Walsh, R. J. and Montgomery, C.: A new human isoagglutinin subdividing the MN blood groups. Nature 160:504, 1947.

Ward, P. A. and McLean, R.: Complement Activity. *In* Bellanti, J. A.: Immunology II. W. B. Saunders Co. 1978.

Warner, W. L.: Red cell preservation and survival determinations in anticoagulant systems. *In* Modern Problems of Blood Preservation. Spielmann, W. and Seidle, S. (eds). Gustav Fischer, 1970.

Watkins, W. M.: Some genetical aspects of the biosynthesis of human blood group substances. Ciba Found. Symp. on Biochemistry of Human Genetics, Churchill, 217, 1959.

Watkins, W. M. and Morgan, W. T. J.: Immunochemical observations on the human blood group P system. J. Immunogenet. 3:15, 1976.

Watkins, W. M. and Morgan, W. T. J.: Blood group P_1 substance (11) Immunological properties. Proc. 9th Congr. Int. Soc. Blood Transf., Mexico, 1962.

Watkins, W. M. and Morgan, W. T. J.: Possible genetical pathways for the biosynthesis of blood group mucopolysaccharides. Vox Sang. 4:97–119, 1959.

Weiner, W. and Vos, G. H.: Serology of acquired hemolytic anemias. Blood 22:606, 1963.

Weiner, W., Gordon, E. G. and Rowe, D.: A Donath-Landsteiner antibody (nonsyphilitic type). Vox Sang. 9:684–697, 1964.

Weiner, W., Sanger, R. and Race, R. R.: A weak form of the blood group antigen A: an inherited character. Proc. 7th Congr. Int. Soc. Blood Transf., 720–725, 1959.

Weiner, W., Tovey, G. H., Gillespie, E. M., Lewis, H. B. M. and Holliday, T. D. S.: Albumin auto-agglutinating property in three sera. A pitfall for the unwary. Vox Sang. 1:279, 1956.

Weiner, W., Battey, D. A., Cleghorn, T. E., Marson, F. G. W. and Meynell, M. J.: Serological findings in a case of hemolytic anemia; with some general observations on the pathogenesis of the syndrome. Br. Med. J. ii:125, 1953.

Wenz, B., Gurlinger, K., O'Toole, A. and Dugan, E.: Leukocyte-poor red cells prepared by microaggregate blood filtration (MABF). Proc. 32nd Ann. Meeting, AABB, Las Vegas, 1979.

West, C. D., Davis, N. C., Forristal, J., Herbst, J. and Spitzer, R.: Antigenic determinants of human β_1c− and β_1g globulins. J. Immunol. 96:650, 1966.

West, C. D., Hong, R. and Holland, N. H.: Immunoglobulin levels from the newborn period to adulthood and in immunoglobin deficiency states. J. Clin. Invest. 41:2054, 1962.

White, W. L., Miller, G. E. and Kaehny, W. D.: Formaldehyde in the pathogenesis of hemodialysis-related anti-

N antibodies. AABB 28th Annual Meeting. Transfusion 17:443, 1975.

Whitehead, V. M.: Paroxysmal nocturnal hemoglobinuria. Can. Med. Assoc. J. 109:961, 1973.

WHO Advances in Viral Hepatitis. Technical Report Series, 602, 1977.

WHO Viral hepatitis, Technical Report Series, 512, 1973.

Wiener, A. S.: Advances in Blood Grouping. Grune & Stratton, 1961.

Wiener, A. S.: Blood Groups and Transfusion, 3rd Ed. Charles C Thomas, 1943.

Wiener, A. S.: Genetic theory of the Rh blood types. Proc. Soc. Exp. Biol. NY, 54:316–319, 1943.

Wiener, A. S.: Hemolytic transfusion reactions. iii. Prevention, with special reference to the Rh and cross-match tests. Am. J. Clin. Pathol. 12:302–311, 1942.

Wiener, A. S. and Ungar, L. J.: Further observations on the blood factors Rh^A, Rh^B, Rh^C and Rh^D. Transfusion 2:230–233, 1962.

Wiener, A. S. and Sonn-Gordon, E. B.: Réaction transfusionnelle hémolytique intra-group due a un hémagglutinogène jusqu'ici non décrit. Rev. Hématol. 2:1–10, 1947.

Wiener, A. S. and Forer, S.: A human serum containing four distinct isoagglutinins. Proc. Soc. Exp. Biol. 47:215, 1941.

Wiener, A. S. and Peters, H. R.: Hemolytic reactions following transfusions of blood of the homologous group, with three cases in which the same agglutinogen was responsible. Ann. Int. Med. 13:2306–2322, 1940.

Wiener, A. S., Gordon, E. B. and Moor-Jankowski, J.: The Lewis blood groups in man; a review with supporting data on non-human primates. I. Forensic Med. 11:67, 1964.

Wiener, A. S., Unger, L. J., Cohen, L. and Feldman, J.: Type-specific cold autoantibodies as a cause of acquired hemolytic anemia and hemolytic transfusion reactions: biologic test with bovine red cells. Ann. Intern. Med. 44:221–240, 1956.

Wiener, A. S., Unger, L. J. and Cohen, L.: Distribution and heredity of blood factor U. Science 119:734–735, 1954.

Wiener, A. S., Unger, L. J. and Gordon, E. B.: Fatal hemolytic transfusion reaction caused by sensitization to a new blood factor, U. JAMA 153:1444–1446, 1953a.

Wiener, A. S., Samwick, A. A., Morrison, H. and Cohen, L.: Studies on immunization in man. II. The blood factor C. Exp. Med. Surg. 11:276, 1953b.

Wiener, A. S., Hurst, J. G., and Sonn-Gordon, E. B.: Studies on the conglutination reaction, with special reference to the nature of conglutinin. J. Exp. Med. 86:267, 1947.

Wilheim, R. F., Nutting, H. M., Devlin, H. B., Jennings, E. R. and Brines, O. A.: Antihistaminics for allergic and pyrogenic transfusion reactions. JAMA 158:529, 1955.

Willoughby, W. F. and Mayer, M. M.: Antibody-complement complexes. Science 150:907, 1965.

Wilson, M. J., Cott, M. E. and Sotus, P. C.: Probable Tn-activation *in utero*. Proc. 33rd Ann. Meeting, AABB, Washington DC, 1980.

Wolf, E.: Untersuchungen zur Definition von Anti-HL-A-Antikörpern in zytotoxischen Schwangerenseren. Z. Immun. Forschg. 142:148–165, 1971.

Wolfe, M. S.: Parasites, other than malaria transmissible by blood transfusion. *In* Transmissible Disease and Blood Transfusion, Greenwalt, T. J. and Jamieson, G. A. (eds.). Grune & Stratton, 1975.

Wood, E. E.: Brucellosis as a hazard of blood transfusion. Br. Med. J. i:27, 1955.

Wood, L. and Beutler, E.: The viability of human blood stored in phosphate adenine media. Transfusion 7:401, 1967.

Woodrow, J. C., Clarke, C. A., Donohof, W. T. A., Finn, R. *et al*: Mechanism of Rh prophylaxis: an experimental study on specificity of immunosuppression. Br. Med. J. 2:57, 1975.

Worlledge, S. M.: Immune drug-induced hemolytic anemias. Semin. Hematol. 6:181, 1969.

Worlledge, S. M. and Dacie, J. V.: Hemolytic and other anemias in infectious mononucleosis. *In* Infectious Mononucleosis, Carter, R. L. and Penman, H. G. (eds.). Blackwell Scientific Publications, 1969.

Worlledge, S. M., Carstairs, K. C. and Dacie, J. V.: Autoimmune hemolytic anemia associated with α-methyldopa therapy. Lancet ii:135, 1966.

Worlledge, S. M. and Rousso, C.: Studies on the serology of paroxysmal cold haemoglobinuria (P.C.H.), with special reference to its relationship with the P blood group system. Vox Sang. 10:293–298, 1965.

Wright, J.: Variations on a theme by Coombs. Can. J. Med. Tech. 29:191, 1967.

Wright, J., Cornwall, S. M. and Matsina, E.: A second example of hemolytic disease of the newborn due to anti-Kp^b. Vox Sang. 10:218–221, 1965.

Wrobel, D. M., Moore, B. P. L., Cornwall, S., Wray, E., Øyen, R. and Marsh, W. L.: A second example of Lu(−6) in the Lutheran system. Vox Sang. 23:205–207, 1972.

Wurzel, H. A., Gottlieb, A. J. and Abelson, N. M.: Immunoglobulin characterization of anti-Tj^a antibodies. AABB Program, Chicago, 103–104, 1971.

Yamaguchi, H., Okubo, Y., Seno, T., Matsushita, K. and Daniels, G. L.: A "new" allele, Kp^c, at the Kell complex locus. Vox Sang. 36:29–30, 1979.

Yamaguchi, H., Okubo, Y. and Tanaka, M.: "Cis AB" bloods found in Japanese families. Jpn. J. Hum. Genet. 15:198, 1970.

Yamaguchi, H., Okubo, Y. and Hazama, F.: Another Japanese A_2B_3 blood-group family with the propositus having O-group father. Proc. Imp. Acad. Japan. 42:517, 1966.

Yamaguchi, H., Okubo, Y. and Hazama, F.: An A_2B_3 phenotype blood showing atypical mode of inheritance Proc. Imp. Acad. Japan 41:316, 1965.

Yaw, P. B., Sentany, M., Link, W. J., Wahle, W. M. and Glover, J. L.: Tumor cells carried through autotransfusion: contraindiction to intraoperative blood recovery? JAMA 231:490, 1975.

Yokoyama, M., Eith, D. T. and Bowman, M.: The first example of auto-anti-Xg^a. Vox Sang. 12:138–139, 1967.

Yokoyama, M. and McCoy, J. E.: Further studies on auto-anti-Xg^a antibody. Vox Sang. 13:15–17, 1967.

Young, L. E.: Blood groups and transfusion reactions. Am. J. Med. 16:885, 1954.

Yunis, J. J. and Yunis, E.: A study of blood group antigens on normoblasts. Proc. 9th Congr. Int. Soc. Blood Transf., Mexico, 1962, 238–243, 1964.

Yunis, J. J. and Yunis, E.: Cell antigens and cell specialization. IV. On the H blood group antigen of human platelets and nucleated cells of the human bone marrow. Blood 24:531–541, 1964.

Yunis, J. J. and Yunis, E.: Cell antigens and cell specialization. I. A study of blood group antigens on normoblasts. Blood 22:53–65, 1963.

Yvart, J., Gerval, R., Carton, J. and Salmon C.: Étude comparée des diverses méthodes de mise en évidence de l'antigène D^u. Rev. Franç. Transfus. 17:201, 1974.

Zak, S. J. and Good, R. A.: Immunochemical studies of human serum gamma globulins. J. Clin. Invest. 38:579, 1959.

Zeitlin, R. A., Sanger, R. and Race, R. R.: Unpublished data. Cited by Race and Sanger, 1958, p. 356.

Zmijewski, C. M. and Fletcher, J. L.: Immunohematology, 2nd Ed. Appleton-Century-Crofts, 1972.

ANSWERS TO QUESTIONS

CHAPTER 1 GENETICS

1. b	10. c	19. b	28. T
2. c	11. c	20. a	29. F
3. a	12. b	21. c	30. F
4. a	13. a	22. b	31. T
5. b	14. c	23. a	32. F
6. a	15. d	24. d	33. T
7. d	16. b	25. d	34. T
8. c	17. d	26. c	35. T
9. b	18. a	27. b	

CHAPTER 2 IMMUNOLOGY

1. a	9. a	17. a, b, d	25. a, d
2. c	10. c	18. d	26. a, b, c, d
3. b	11. c	19. d	27. a, c
4. d	12. d	20. c	28. d
5. b, d, e	13. b, d	21. b, e	29. a
6. a, c	14. c	22. c	30. b
7. a	15. d	23. a, b, c	
8. d	16. b, d	24. a, b, d	

CHAPTER 3 ABO BLOOD GROUP SYSTEM

1. b	6. b	11. c	16. c
2. c	7. b, c	12. b	17. a, c, d
3. a, b, c	8. a	13. b	18. c
4. d	9. b, d	14. c	19. b, d
5. b	10. b, c	15. b	20. b

CHAPTER 4 THE LEWIS BLOOD GROUP SYSTEM

1. c	6. c, d	11. b	16. T
2. a	7. d	12. a, c	17. T
3. a, b, c, e	8. a, d	13. a, c, e	18. F
4. b	9. d	14. d .	19. F
5. c	10. b	15. a	20. T

CHAPTER 5   THE Rh/Hr BLOOD GROUP SYSTEM

1. e

2. b, c, d

3. d

4. a, e

5. a, b, c, d

6. c

7. d

8. a, b, c

9. d

10. b, d

11. a

12. b

13. a, c, d

14. a, d

15.

a R^1r e R^1R^2 i $r''r$ m rr

b R^2r^y f $r'r'$ j R^1R^1 n r^yr''

c R^zR^0 g $r''r''$ k $r'r''$ o R^2r'

d R^1r'' h R^1R^0 l R^2R^2 p $r'r$

16.

a cDe cDe/cde (R^0r) e cDEe cDE/cde (R^2r)

b ce cde/cde (rr) f CcDEe CDe/cDE (R^1R^2)

c CcDEe CDe/cde (R^1r) g Ce Cde/Cde $(r'r')$

d CDe CDe/CDe (R^1R^1) h cDE cDE/cDE (R^2R^2)

17. 1

18. Positive

19. Rh^{ABCd}

20. Transfusion Pregnancy

21. Anti-D

22. Negative

23. G

24. hr′, Rh$_0$, rh″

25. CcDe

CHAPTER 6   THE KELL BLOOD GROUP SYSTEM

1. b

2. b, d

3. e

6. b, d

7. c, d

8. c

11. b, c

12. b, d

13. (a)   k (Cellano)
     (b)   Penney (K3)
     (c)   Js^b K7
     (d)   Peltz K5
     (e)   Js^a

16. F

17. F

18. T

4. b, c

5. a, b, d

9. b

10. a

14. T

15. T

19. T

20. T

21. T

CHAPTER 7   THE DUFFY BLOOD GROUP SYSTEM

1. d

2. b

3. a, b, d

4. c

5. a, d

6. a, b

7. b, d, e

8. a

9. a, b

10. a, b, c

11. b

12. b

13. c

14. b, d, e

15. T

16. F

17. F

18. T

19. T

20. F

CHAPTER 8   THE KIDD BLOOD GROUP SYSTEM

1. c

2. a, c, d

3. a

4. a, c

5. a, b, c

6. b, c, d

7. c, d, e

8. b

9. a

10. b

11. T

12. F

13. T

14. T

15. T

16. F

17. F

18. T

19. T

20. F

CHAPTER 9   THE LUTHERAN BLOOD GROUP SYSTEM

1. b	6. b, c	11. a, b, d	16. T
2. a, b	7. c	12. d	17. T
3. a, b, c	8. b, c	13. T	18. F
4. d	9. b, c	14. T	19. F
5. c	10. a, b	15. F	20. T

CHAPTER 10   THE MNSs BLOOD GROUP SYSTEM

1. c, d	6. c	11. b, c, d	16. T
2. b	7. a, c	12. a, b, c, d	17. T
3. a, b, c	8. a, b, c, d	13. d	18. T
4. d	9. a	14. T	19. F
5. b, c	10. a, b, c	15. F	20. T

CHAPTER 11   THE P BLOOD GROUP SYSTEM

1. a, d	6. a, b, d	11. b, d	16. T
2. b, c	7. b, c, d	12. c	17. F
3. b	8. a, c	13. T	18. F
4. a, b, c	9. a, b, c, d	14. F	19. T
5. b, c	10. a, c	15. T	20. T

CHAPTER 12   THE Ii BLOOD GROUP SYSTEM

1. a, d	6. a, b, c	11. b, d	16. T
2. c	7. a, b, c, d	12. c	17. F
3. d	8. d	13. T	18. F
4. a, c, d	9. a, b, c	14. F	19. T
5. b	10. a, c, d	15. T	20. T

CHAPTER 13   OTHER BLOOD GROUP SYSTEMS

SECTION A: MULTIPLE CHOICE

1. a, c, d	4. a, c, d, e	7. b	10. c
2. c	5. b, d	8. d	
3. a, b	6. a, b, c	9. c	

SECTION B: FILL IN THE BLANKS

11.
a	Saline 20° C	g	Saline 20° C
b	Saline 20° C	h	Indirect antiglobulin test
c	Saline 20° C	i	Saline 20° C
d	Indirect antiglobulin test	j	Saline 20° C
e	Indirect antiglobulin test	k	Indirect antiglobulin test
f	Indirect antiglobulin test	l	Indirect antiglobulin test

12. *ABO, Hh, Sese* (in any order)

13. X

14.

a	B	d	A	g	C	j	C
b	B	e	A	h	C		
c	C	f	A	i	B		

15. H, B, Le^a and Le^b (in any order)

SECTION C: MATCHING ANSWERS

16.

a	Rh/Hr	d	ABO	g	Kidd	j	MNSs
b	Dombrock	e	Duffy	h	Rh/Hr		
c	Kell	f	Cartwright	i	Diego		

SECTION D: TRUE OR FALSE

17.	F	**19.**	T	**21.**	F	**23.**	F
18.	F	**20.**	T	**22.**	T	**24.**	T
						25.	T

CHAPTER 14   THE HLA SYSTEM

1.	b	**6.**	d	**11.**	c	**16.**	T
2.	b	**7.**	b	**12.**	c	**17.**	F
3.	d	**8.**	c	**13.**	F	**18.**	F
4.	a, b, c	**9.**	a, b, c, d	**14.**	T	**19.**	T
5.	c	**10.**	a	**15.**	T	**20.**	T

CHAPTER 15   AUTOIMMUNE HEMOLYTIC ANEMIA

1.	c	**6.**	b	**11.**	a	**16.**	T
2.	d	**7.**	b, c	**12.**	a, b, c	**17.**	F
3.	b	**8.**	b	**13.**	T	**18.**	F
4.	a, b, c, d	**9.**	c	**14.**	T	**19.**	T
5.	a, b, d	**10.**	d	**15.**	F	**20.**	F

CHAPTER 16   HEMOLYTIC DISEASE OF THE NEWBORN

1.	a, c	**6.**	c, d	**11.**	a, b	**16.**	T
2.	a, b, d	**7.**	a, b, c, d	**12.**	c	**17.**	F
3.	d	**8.**	d	**13.**	T	**18.**	T
4.	a, b, c	**9.**	b, c	**14.**	F	**19.**	F
5.	a, c, d	**10.**	b, c, d	**15.**	F	**20.**	T

CHAPTER 17   THE DONATION OF BLOOD

1.	b, c	**6.**	a, c	**11.**	b	**16.**	F
2.	b	**7.**	c	**12.**	d	**17.**	T
3.	d	**8.**	c, d	**13.**	F	**18.**	F
4.	a, b, c	**9.**	e	**14.**	T	**19.**	T
5.	c	**10.**	a	**15.**	T	**20.**	F

CHAPTER 18　BLOOD COMPONENTS

1. b　　　　**3.** d　　　　**5.** c　　　　**7.** d
2. a, b, d　　**4.** b, c, d　　**6.** c, d　　　**8.** a, c

9.　a　Platelet concentrates
　　　b　Leukocyte concentrates (granulocyte
　　　　　concentrates)
　　　c　Leukocyte-poor red blood cells
　　　d　Frozen thawed red blood cells
　　　　　(or washed red blood cells)
　　　e　Fresh frozen plasma (or stored plasma)

　　　f　Human serum albumin
　　　g　Immune serum globulin
　　　h　Cryoprecipitated antihemophilic factor
　　　i　Cryoprecipitated antihemophilic factor
　　　j　Factor IX complex

10.　a　2 to 6° C; 21 days
　　　b　2 to 6° C; 24 hours
　　　c　22° C; 72 hours
　　　d　2 to 6° C; 21 days
　　　e　−80° C; 1 year

　　　f　−18° C or lower; 1 year
　　　g　−18° C or lower; 3 years
　　　h　22° C room temperature; 3 years
　　　i　4° C; 5 years
　　　j　−18° C or lower; 1 year

CHAPTER 19　MATERIALS

1. d　　　　　**6.** c　　　　　　**11.** T　　**16.** F
2. a, c, d　　**7.** d　　　　　　**12.** F　　**17.** F
3. b, c　　　**8.** a, b, c, d　　**13.** F　　**18.** T
4. b, d　　　**9.** b, c　　　　　**14.** T
5. a, b　　　**10.** b　　　　　　**15.** T

CHAPTER 20　QUALITY CONTROL

1. b　　　　**5.** d　　　　　**9.** c　　　　**13.** F
2. d　　　　**6.** a, c, d　　**10.** a, d　　**14.** F
3. b, d　　**7.** b　　　　　**11.** T　　　**15.** T
4. a, c　　**8.** c　　　　　**12.** T

CHAPTER 21　THE CROSSMATCH

1. d　　　　　**6.** a　　　　**11.** d　　**16.** T
2. a, d　　　**7.** b, c　　**12.** c　　**17.** F
3. b, c　　　**8.** a　　　　**13.** F　　**18.** T
4. b, c, d　**9.** c　　　　**14.** F　　**19.** T
5. a, b, c　**10.** d　　　**15.** T　　**20.** F

CHAPTER 22　ANTIBODY IDENTIFICATION AND TITRATION

1. b　　　**4.** a, b, c　　**7.** a, d　　**10.** F
2. b　　　**5.** a, d　　　**8.** F　　　**11.** F
3. d　　　**6.** b, d　　　**9.** T　　　**12.** T

CHAPTER 24   REACTIONS THAT MAY MISLEAD IN THE EXAMINATION OF AGGLUTINATION TESTS

1. a, b, c   4. a, b, c, d   7. T   10. T
2. a, c   5. c   8. F
3. b   6. d   9. T

CHAPTER 25   ADVERSE REACTION TO TRANSFUSION

1. d   4. a, b, d   7. T   10. F
2. a, b, c   5. b   8. T
3. b, c, d   6. c   9. F

Glossary

AAAF (Abbr) Albumin autoagglutinating factor. A condition whereby a patient's serum agglutinates red cells suspended in caprylate-treated albumin but not those suspended in saline. The antibody is directed against sodium caprylate or other fatty-acid salts and not against the albumin itself.

AABB (Abbr) American Association of Blood Banks.

Ab (Abbr) Abbreviation for antibody.

ABO SYSTEM The first and most important family of red cell antigens and antibodies, discovered in 1900 by Karl Landsteiner, which divides the population into four major groups: O, A, B and AB.

ABORTION The termination of pregnancy through natural or unnatural causes before the third month of confinement. See also *Therapeutic abortion.*

ABSORPTION The removal of antibodies from serum by the addition of red cells that possess the corresponding antigen.

ACCURACY A term used to describe the proximity of the "average" value and the "true" value.

ACD (Abbr) Acid citrate dextrose. An anticoagulant composed of citric acid, sodium citrate and dextrose.

ACIDOSIS A pathologic condition resulting from accumulation of acid or loss of base in the body and characterized by increase in hydrogen ion concentration (decrease in pH).

ACQUIRED ANTIGEN An antigen that is not genetically determined and is sometimes transient.

ACRIFLAVINE A yellow coloring agent once used in commercial anti-B antisera.

ADENINE An agent that, when added to ACD or CPD blood, prolongs the maintenance of red cell viability (see text).

ADENOSINE An agent that improves the maintenance of red cell viability and is capable of restoring the ATP content of stored red cells.

ADJUVANT A substance that can increase the specific antibody production to, or the degree of sensitization against, an antigen by increasing its size or length of survival in the circulation.

ADSORPTION The attachment of one substance to the surface of another; in particular, the attachment of antibody to specific receptors on the red cell surface.

Ag (Abbr) Abbreviation for antigen.

AGGLUTINATES Clumps of agglutinated red cells (or any other cells).

AGGLUTINATION The clumping of cells into aggregates, often as a result of antigen-antibody interaction.

AGGLUTININ An antibody that causes agglutination by direct interaction with its corresponding antigen in a saline medium.

ATYPICAL AGGLUTININ An antibody that is occasionally present in the serum of some individuals whose red cells lack the corresponding antigen (also called "irregular agglutinin" or "irregular antibody").

AUTOAGGLUTININ An antibody that reacts with the red cells of the individual in whose serum it was found and that usually agglutinates the red cells of most other individuals also (also called Autoantibody).

AGGLUTINOGEN Another term for red cell antigen.

AHF (Abbr) Antihemophilic factor; factor VIII coagulation factor. A concentrate of this factor is used in the treatment of hemophilia (also called antihemophilic globulin).

AHG (Abbr) Antihuman globulin. See *Antiglobulin reagent.*

AIHA (Abbr) See *Autoimmune hemolytic anemia.*

AIR EMBOLISM Air in the circulation that enters the pulmonary artery and causes a rapid fall in systolic blood pressure. Death can occur as a result of primary respiratory failure from the injection of as little as 40 ml of air in a healthy subject; in critically ill patients, the fatal dose can be considerably less.

ALBUMIN (BOVINE) A colloid used in serologic procedures that enhances agglutination by increasing the dielectric constant of the medium and thus reducing the zeta potential. Prepared from cattle plasma.

ALBUMIN (HUMAN) A fraction of human plasma useful in the treatment of shock, as replacement therapy, after severe burns and in newborn exchange transfusions to assist the binding of unconjugated bilirubin.

ALBUMIN AUTOAGGLUTINATING FACTOR See *AAAF*.

ALDOMET (ALPHA₁-METHYLDOPA) The trade name for a drug commonly used in the treatment of hypertension, which has been implicated as one of the causes of a positive direct antiglobulin test and of autoimmune hemolytic anemia by an unknown mechanism.

ALLELE One of two or more genes that determine alternative characters that are located at the same locus on homologous chromosomes. Also called allelomorph or allelic gene.

ALLELIC GENE See *Allele*.

ALLELOMORPH See *Allele*.

ALLERGIC REACTION A reaction to the transfusion of blood or blood products characterized mainly by hives or wheals (urticaria).

ALLOAGGLUTININ An antibody directed against a species-specific antigen; that is, produced by an individual as a result of antigenic stimulus from another individual of the same species. The term is synonymous with isoagglutinin, although general use of the term alloagglutinin is now preferred.

ALLOANTIBODY See *Alloagglutinin*.

ALLOANTIGEN A constituent of cells or body fluids that can elicit a specific immune response in animals of the same species.

ALLOGRAFT A graft between genetically different members of the same species.

ALLOIMMUNIZATION Formation of antibodies by a member of a species in response to stimulation by an antigen from another member of the same species. Also known as isoimmunization or isosensitization or allosensitization.

ALLOSENSITIZATION See *Alloimmunization*.

ALLOSTERIC REACTION A reaction producing a conformational shift, thus exposing new reactive groups on an antibody molecule.

ALLOTYPES Genetically determined polymorphic variants. The term was first introduced to describe the different antigenic forms of rabbit gamma globulins. It was then extended to include polymorphic variants of plasma proteins in general (e.g.,

haptoglobins, Gc groups) but now includes red cell and white cell polymorphisms.

ALSEVER'S SOLUTION A modified ACD solution used as a suspending medium for test cells.

AMINO ACID Any one of a class of organic compounds containing the amino (NH₂) group and the carboxyl (COOH) group. Amino acids form the chief structure of proteins.

AMNIOTIC FLUID (LIQUOR AMNII) The fluid substance that surrounds the fetus *in utero*.

AMORPH A gene apparently having no product, e.g., a specific antigenic determinant. Sometimes called a silent gene. Also known as an amorphic gene.

ANAMNESTIC RESPONSE A "secondary" response as a result of second or subsequent challenge by a specific antigen. The response is immediate and is associated with an increase in the level of circulating IgG antibody. Also known as the memory response.

ANGSTROM (Å) A unit of measurement equal to 10^{-7} mm.

ANTIBODY A serum protein produced in response to stimulation by a foreign antigen that is capable of reacting specifically with that antigen in an observable way.

ANTICOAGULANT A substance that prevents coagulation or clotting of the blood.

ANTIGEN A substance of high molecular weight that, when introduced parenterally into a "foreign" circulation, is capable of instituting the production of an antibody specific to itself.

ANTIGEN SITES Proteins on the red cell surface responsible for antigenic activity.

ANTIGENIC DETERMINANT The particular site on an antigen molecule that combines with the corresponding antibody.

ANTIGENICITY Potency of a particular substance as an antigen.

ANTIGLOBULIN REAGENT An antiserum used to show agglutination of red cells sensitized with IgG antibody. The reagent is produced in an animal (often a rabbit) in response to the injection of human globulin.

ANTIGLOBULIN TEST (DIRECT) A technique used to detect the *in vivo* sensitization of red cells.

ANTIGLOBULIN TEST (INDIRECT) A serologic procedure used as a pretransfusion test and also as a general test to detect IgG antibodies in serum.

ANTI-HUMAN GLOBULIN See *Antiglobulin reagent*.

ANTITHETICAL Antigens that are the products of allelic genes are said to be antithetical; e.g., Jk^a and Jk^b genes are alleles; Jk^a and Jk^b antigens are antithetical.

APLASTIC ANEMIA A type of anemia caused by the body's inability to produce new red blood cells.

ARACHIS HYPOGAEA A peanut, the extract of which possesses anti-T specificity.

ATYPICAL ANTIBODY An antibody that occurs as an irregular feature of the serum.

AUGMENTATION Enhancement.

AUSTRALIA (Au) ANTIGEN Synonyms, Hepatitis-associated antigen or HAA Hepatitis B antigen (HBA), Hepatitis B surface antigen (HB_sAg).

AUTO Derived from self.

AUTOANTIBODY An antibody that reacts with the red cells of the individual in whose serum it was found and usually reacts with the red cells of most other individuals also. Also called an auto-agglutinin.

AUTOIMMUNE HEMOLYTIC ANEMIA (AIHA) A type of anemia associated with the production of autoantibodies that result in the destruction of the patient's own red cells.

AUTOLOGOUS TRANSFUSION A transfusion of a subject's own red cells collected prior to transfusion. Also known as autotransfusion.

AUTOSOME Any chromosome other than a sex chromosome.

AUTOTRANSFUSION See *Autologous transfusion*.

AVIDITY (OF AN ANTISERUM) A measure of the ability and speed with which an antiserum agglutinates red cells as a property of the combining constant (K).

AZIDE See *Sodium azide*.

BACTERIA Large groups of unicellular microorganisms, existing morphologically as oval or spherical cells (cocci), rods (bacilli), spirals (spirilla) or comma-shaped organisms (vibrios).

BETA GLOBULINS Globulins in the beta globulin portion of plasma.

BILIRUBIN A pigmented breakdown product of hemoglobin, found in bile, serum and occasionally in other body fluids.

BLOCKED CELLS Cells coated with a blocking antibody so that they remain unagglutinated when brought into contact with saline antibody of the same specificity as the blocking antibody.

BLOCKING ANTIBODY An "incomplete" antibody capable of coating the red cell determinant to render it partially or completely blocked and inagglutinable by antibodies of the same specificity.

BLOOD FACTOR An antigenic determinant, or antigen.

BLOOD GROUP Classification of blood according to antigens possessed by the red cells.

BLOOD GROUP ANTIGEN The product of a blood group gene present on the red cell membrane.

BLOOD GROUP SUBSTANCE Soluble antigen capable of neutralizing its specific antibody. The term also applies to an antigen or hapten that has blood group specificity. See also *Group-specific substance*.

BOMBAY GROUP A rare blood type in which the red cells contain no H, A or B substance, and anti-A, anti-B and anti-H are found in the serum. The individual lacks the *H* gene and will type as group O, regardless of which *ABO* genes have been inherited. Classified as O_h.

BROMELIN A proteolytic enzyme prepared from the pineapple, *Ananas sativus*.

BUFFER Any substance or substances in solution that resists changes in pH.

CADAVER BLOOD Blood taken from a donor after death.

CAPILLARY TECHNIQUE A serologic agglutination technique described by Chown that combines serum and red cells in a capillary tube.

CHIMERA An organism whose cells derive from two or more distinct zygote linkages, such as the vascular anastomoses that may occur between twins. In short, possessing a dual population of cells.

CHRISTMAS DISEASE A congenital hemorrhagic diathesis clinically similar to classical hemophilia A, transmitted as a sex-linked recessive and characterized by a deficiency of factor IX coagulation factor (also called Christmas factor), which results in impaired formation of intrinsic thromboplastin. Also called *Hemophilia B*.

CHROMOSOME One of a number of more or less rod-like, dark-staining bodies situated in the nucleus of a cell. The chromosome is distinguishable during mitotic metaphase and is made up of a series of genes in linear arrangement.

CIRCULATORY OVERLOAD Basically, the overloading of the circulation due to the unnecessary transfusion of fluid.

CIS POSITION Being on the same chromosome and within the same cistron.

CISTRON A collection of genes situated so close together that they can have conjoint expression effects when in the *cis* position.

CLONE A group of cells that are homogeneous because they are descendants of a common precursor cell.

CLOSELY LINKED GENES Genes in close proximity on a chromosome so that they are inherited together, usually without crossovers occurring.

CLOTTING The coagulation of blood.

COATED CELLS Cells that are sensitized, though not necessarily blocked, with antibody.

CODOMINANT GENES Two or more allelic genes, each capable of expressing in single dose.

CODON A group of three adjacent bases within a chromosome that controls the positioning of one amino acid on a polypeptide chain.

COLD AGGLUTININ An agglutinin whose optimum temperature of reactivity is in the cold, whose potency decreases rapidly with increase in temperature, and whose reaction at 37° C is negative except in rare circumstances.

COLLOID A substance made up of submicroscopic particles that serves to enhance agglutination. Common colloids in routine blood bank work include bovine albumin and polyvinylpyrrolidone (PVP).

COLLOIDAL SILICA A product of glassware that may agglutinate or lyse red cells in the presence of complement.

COMBINING SITE An antigenic determinant.

COMPATIBILITY TEST A series of procedures used to give an indication of blood group compatibility between the donor and the recipient and to detect irregular antibodies in the recipient's serum.

COMPATIBLE A term used in blood banking to denote that no detectable *in vitro* reaction occurs between the patient's serum and the donor's red cells. The term is not used to denote identical antigenic determinants on the red cells of both donor and recipient; therefore immunization may still follow a "compatible" transfusion.

COMPLEMENT A series of components (mostly beta globulins) present in fresh normal serum that takes part in, or plays a role in, some antigen/antibody interactions. Its activation may result in the lysis of red cells sensitized by hemolysins and in accelerated clearance of red cells from the circulation.

COMPLEMENTOID An "altered" type of complement (usually partly damaged, for example, by heating) that is capable of combining with sensitized red cells without producing the usual lysis and that is also capable of blocking the normal action of complement.

"COMPLETE" ANTIBODY A term that describes an antibody capable of causing agglutination with its corresponding antigen in a saline medium.

COMPOUND ANTIGEN More than one antigen in combination, against which a single antibody appears to be directed. The antigen may be the product of one or more than one gene.

CONCENTRATED RED CELLS Packed red blood cells.

CONGLUTINATION The clumping of sensitized red cells by a substance known as conglutinin, present in normal bovine sera, in the presence of complement. It is sometimes erroneously applied to the clumping effect of human serum or bovine albumin on cells sensitized by "incomplete" Rh antibodies that is independent of complement.

CONSANGUINEOUS Referring to mating between blood relatives.

COOMBS' SERUM Anti-human globulin reagent.

COOMBS' TEST See *Antiglobulin test*.

CORD BLOOD Blood taken from the umbilical vein of a newborn.

CPD (Abbr) Citrate-phosphate-dextrose. An anticoagulant routinely used in blood donations.

CROSS REACTION The reaction of an antibody to an antigen other than the one that originally stimulated its production.

CROSSING OVER The process by which genetic material is exchanged between homologous chromosomes, which can occur during meiosis or mitosis.

CROSSMATCH Another term for compatibility test.

CRYOGLOBULIN Globulin that precipitates from serum at 0 to 4° C.

CRYOPRECIPITATE A term used in the laboratory to refer to concentrated factor VIII coagulation factor, used in the treatment of hemophilia.

DANGEROUS UNIVERSAL DONOR A term now used to describe an individual of blood group O, whose serum may possess sufficient anti-A and anti-B to cause destruction of red cells when transfused into a recipient belonging to another blood group.

DEFIBRINATION The removal of fibrin from plasma to form serum.

DEGLYCEROLIZATION The removal of glycerol from frozen red cells.

DELAYED HEMOLYTIC TRANSFUSION REACTION A rapid increase in antibody concentration and destruction of transfused red cells a few days after transfusion. Usually due to low amounts of antibody undetectable in pretransfusion tests on the recipient, which is stimulated to high titers by the transfusion of red cells possessing the offending antigen.

DELETION The loss of genetic material from a chromosome.

DEPRESSED GENE A gene which, for some reason, is prevented from normal expression.

DETERMINANT See *Antigenic determinant.*

DEXTRAN A plasma expander used to sustain blood volume in patients and used as a substitute for plasma. It is a common cause of rouleaux formation in the recipient.

DEXTROSE A sugar commonly used as a preservative and nutrient for red cells in many anticoagulant solutions.

DIPLOID Possessing a full complement of chromosomes (23 pairs).

DIRECT ANTIGLOBULIN TEST See *Antiglobulin test (Direct).*

DISSEMINATED INTRAVASCULAR COAGULATION The condition that may follow red cell destruction in the blood vessels.

DISULFIDE BONDS The links between antibody molecule chains.

DIZYGOTIC Two zygotes, as in dizygotic twins, meaning from two eggs.

DOLICHOS BIFLORUS A plant, the seed extract of which in solution possesses anti-A$_1$ specificity.

DOMINANT GENE An expressed gene in terms of antigenic product, factor or characteristic whether present in single or double dose (i.e., in the heterozygote or in the homozygote).

DOSAGE A quantitative difference in the strength of the antigen between the homozygote and the heterozygote.

DPG (Abbr) 2,3-Diphosphoglycerate.

DRIFTS A string of apparently agglutinated red cells sometimes seen in tests employing bovine albumin of high concentration. Also known as "comets."

EDTA (Abbr) Ethylenediaminetetraacetic acid. An anticoagulant used in specimens for certain serologic investigations.

ELECTROPHORESIS (OF SERUM) The separation of serum proteins according to their rate of travel when an electric current is passed through a buffer solution. The supporting medium can be Whatman paper, starch or agar gels.

ELUATE In blood banking, the term denotes an antibody solution made by recovery into a fluid medium of antibodies that have been taken up by red cells (i.e., the removal of antibody from the red cells).

ELUTION The process of preparing an eluate.

EMBOLISM See *Air embolism.*

ENHANCEMENT Increase in response.

ENZYME See *Proteolytic enzyme.*

EQUILIBRIUM CONSTANT (K) The measure of the goodness-of-fit of an antibody to its corresponding antigen. When the equilibrium constant is high, the bond between the antigen and the antibody is less easily broken. Also known as combining constant.

ERYTHROBLASTOSIS FETALIS A term once used to describe hemolytic disease of the newborn.

ERYTHROCYTE Red cell.

EXCHANGE TRANSFUSION A transfusion in which the majority of the recipient's blood is replaced.

EXPERIMENTAL ERROR The maximum variation in results obtained by any technique in the hands of an expert.

EXTRAVASCULAR DESTRUCTION The destruction of red cells outside of the blood vessels within the reticuloendothelial system.

Fab FRAGMENT The fragment of the antibody molecule that is capable of antigen binding. Consists of a light chain and part of the heavy chain of the molecule.

FACTOR Synonymous with antigenic determinant. Also used to denote coagulation fractions.

FACTOR I (COAGULATION FACTOR) Fibrinogen.

FACTOR II (COAGULATION FACTOR) Prothrombin.

FACTOR III (COAGULATION FACTOR) Tissue thromboplastin.

FACTOR IV (COAGULATION FACTOR) Calcium.

FACTOR V (COAGULATION FACTOR) Acglobulin, proaccelerin, labile clotting factor.

FACTOR VII (COAGULATION FACTOR) Proconvertin, SPCA, stable clotting factor.

FACTOR VIII (COAGULATION FACTOR) Anti-hemophilic factor. See *AHF*.

FACTOR IX (COAGULATION FACTOR) Plasma thromboplastin component, Christmas factor.

FACTOR X (COAGULATION FACTOR) Stuart-Power factor.

FACTOR XI (COAGULATION FACTOR) Plasma thromboplastin antecedent (PTA).

FACTOR XII (COAGULATION FACTOR) Hageman factor.

FACTOR XIII (COAGULATION FACTOR) Fibrin-stabilizing factor.

FALSE REACTION Any reaction (e.g., agglutination) caused by an "interfering" agent.

Fc FRAGMENT The fragment of the antibody molecule that in certain species can be crystallized. Consists of two pieces of heavy chain.

FEBRILE REACTION A reaction to blood transfusion characterized primarily by elevation of body temperature.

FERTILIZATION The fusion of the male and female sex cells to form a zygote.

FIBRINOGEN A fraction of normal plasma instrumental in the coagulation of red cells (factor I).

FIBRIN-STABILIZING FACTOR Factor XIII coagulation factor.

FICIN A proteolytic enzyme, derived from figs, used in serologic work.

Fy Symbol for the Duffy blood group system.

G6PD DEFICIENCY A deficiency in red cells of glucose-6-phosphate dehydrogenase.

GAMETE A sperm or ovum cell (a sex cell).

GENE One of a number of portions of chromosomal DNA in linear arrangement along a chromosome and coding for the synthesis of a single inherited character.

GENE COMPLEX A group of closely linked genes that are usually inherited and transmitted as a unit.

GENETICS The study of the inheritance and heredity of characteristics based on the original postulations of Gregor Mendel.

GENOTYPE A group of individuals having the same genetic makeup with respect to particular alleles. Also used to denote the genes for a particular trait possessed by an individual.

GLOBULIN A class of proteins to which antibodies belong. They can be separated by electrophoresis into alpha, beta and gamma fractions (see also *Immunoglobulin*).

GLYCEROL A low molecular weight substance used in the freezing of red cells.

GROUP SPECIFIC Blood of the same group as the recipient.

GROUP-SPECIFIC SUBSTANCE A term applied to an antigen or hapten that possesses blood group specificity.

HAGEMAN FACTOR Factor XII coagulation factor.

HALF-LIFE The time taken to decrease to half the original value. For example, the time taken for the potency of an antibody to reduce to half its original strength.

HAPLOID Possessing half the number of chromosomes present in the body (somatic) cells, which is the characteristic state of gametes.

HAPLOTYPE The combination of genetic determinants that leads to a set of antigenic specificities controlled by one chromosome and thus inherited in coupling.

HAPTEN A substance that interacts with the specific antibody combining groups on an antibody molecule but does not stimulate antibody production *in vivo*.

HBAg (Abbr) Hepatitis B antigen; hepatitis-associated antigen; Australia antigen.

HDN (Abbr) Hemolytic disease of the newborn.

HEMATOCRIT A serologic test for the evaluation of the packed cell volume of an individual.

HEMIZYGOUS The genotype of a male for an X-linked trait, because males have only one set of X-linked genes; or the genotype for loci on a monosomic autosome or loci on an autosome whose homologue bears an appropriate deletion.

HEMOCHROMATOSIS Deposition of excess iron in body tissues.

HEMOGLOBIN The oxygen-carrying red pigment of the red blood cells; a term also used for the test or quantitative determination of the hemoglobin content of blood.

HEMOGLOBINURIA The presence of hemoglobin or its derivatives in the urine.

HEMOLYSIN An antibody that, in the presence of complement, is capable of causing hemolysis of red cells.

HEMOLYSIS The breaking down of the red cell membrane, resulting in the liberation of hemoglobin into the plasma.

HEMOLYTIC Causing hemolysis.

HEMOLYTIC ANEMIA Anemia caused by excessive destruction of red cells.

HEMOLYTIC DISEASE OF THE NEW-BORN (HDN) A disease in which fetal red cells are destroyed through the action of maternal antibody.

HEMOLYTIC TRANSFUSION REAC-TION A reaction in which red cells are destroyed *in vivo* after the transfusion of blood.

HEMOPHILIA A A bleeding disorder caused by the lack in the blood of coagulation factor VIII; transmitted by the female to the male as a sex-linked recessive abnormality.

HEMOPHILIA B A hereditary hemorrhagic diathesis due to lack in the blood of coagulation factor IX; transmitted by the female to the male as a sex-linked recessive abnormality. Also called Christmas disease.

HEMOPHILIAC An individual suffering from hemophilia.

HEMORRHAGE Bleeding.

HEMOSIDEROSIS See *Hemochromatosis*.

HEMOSTASIS The arrest of bleeding, including the arrest of the flow of blood within an intact vessel.

HEPARIN An anticoagulant.

HEPATITIS Inflammation of the liver.

HEPATITIS-ASSOCIATED ANTIGEN (HBAg) An antigen of virus-like appearance associated with serum hepatitis. Also known as Australia antigen.

HEREDITARY Inherited, or pertaining to the inheritance of bodily characteristics.

HETEROAGGLUTININS An agglutinin (antibody) directed against antigenic determinants found in another species.

HETEROPHILE ANTIBODIES Antibodies that occur in more than one species of animal and that may be immunologically related to antigens found in plants or microbes.

HETEROSPECIFIC PREGNANCY A pregnancy in which the maternal serum contains anti-A or anti-B antibodies that are incompatible with the fetal red cells.

HETEROTOPIC The transplantation of an accessory organ into an unusual position.

HETEROZYGOUS Having unlike alleles on the corresponding loci of a pair of chromosomes.

HIGH DOSE TOLERANCE See *Immunologic paralysis*.

HIGH-INCIDENCE ANTIGEN An antigen that occurs commonly in the population.

HOMOLOGOUS BLOOD Blood of the same group — usually restricted to mean blood of the same ABO group.

HOMOLOGOUS CHROMOSOMES A pair of chromosomes.

HOMOLOGOUS SERUM JAUNDICE Jaundice or hepatitis caused by direct transfer of a virus contained in transfused human blood or blood products.

HOMOZYGOUS Having like alleles on the corresponding loci of a pair of chromosomes.

HTR (Abbr) Hemolytic transfusion reaction.

HYDROPS FETALIS One form of hemolytic disease of the fetus or newborn in which the fetal tissues retain abnormal quantities of fluid.

HYPERBILIRUBINEMIA Elevated levels of bilirubin in serum.

HYPERIMMUNIZATION Immunization to an unusually high degree.

HYPERTONIC SOLUTION A solution of greater osmotic pressure than blood.

HYPOFIBRINOGENEMIA A decrease (from normal) in plasma fibrinogen level.

HYPOGAMMAGLOBULINEMIA A decrease (from normal) of immunoglobulin levels.

HYPOTONIC SOLUTION A solution of lesser osmotic pressure than blood.

IBERIS AMARA A plant, the seed extract of which in solution has anti-M specificity.

ICTERUS Jaundice.

ICTERUS GRAVIS NEONATORUM Severe jaundice of the newborn — one of the manifestations of hemolytic disease of the newborn.

Ig (Abbr) Immunoglobulin.

IMMUNE ADHERENCE An interaction when complement is fixed to the surface of a cell, and the cell becomes capable of adhering to any other cell that carries the appropriate receptor site.

IMMUNE RESPONSE Any reaction demonstrating specific antibody response to antigenic stimulus.

IMMUNIZATION The process by which an antibody is produced in response to antigenic stimulus.

IMMUNIZED INDIVIDUAL An individual who has produced specific antibody as a result of direct antigenic stimulus.

IMMUNOCYTE A cell that is capable of synthesizing immunoglobulin.

IMMUNOELECTROPHORESIS The identification of proteins separated by agar gel electrophoresis by means of lines of precipitation formed against specific antisera diffusing through the agar under the influence of an electrical current.

IMMUNOGEN Antigen.

IMMUNOGENIC Producing immunity. Antigenic.

IMMUNOGENICITY The ability of an antigen to stimulate antibody production.

IMMUNOGLOBULIN Antibody containing globulins including those proteins without apparent antibody activity that have the same antigenic specificity and are produced by similar cells.

IMMUNOLOGIC ENHANCEMENT Prolongation of the survival of an allograft due to the action of humoral antibody against donor histocompatibility antigens that are lacking in the host.

IMMUNOLOGIC PARALYSIS Absence of immune response after stimulation caused by previous contact with the same antigen in a quantity exceeding that which is required to institute an immune response. Also known as high-dose tolerance.

IMMUNOLOGIC TOLERANCE Absence of normal immunologic response to an antigen.

IMMUNOLOGICALLY COMPETENT CELLS Cells that are capable of producing antibody.

IN VITRO Outside the body.

IN VIVO Inside the body.

INACTIVATION OF SERUM The heating of serum to 56° C for 30 minutes to destroy the heat-labile components of complement.

INCOMPATIBLE A term used in blood banking to indicate a reaction between donor red cells and recipient serum *in vitro*.

INCOMPATIBLE TRANSFUSION Any transfusion that results in an adverse reaction in the patient (including reduced red cell survival).

INCOMPLETE ANTIBODY Any antibody that sensitizes red cells suspended in saline but fails to agglutinate them.

INDIRECT ANTIGLOBULIN TEST See *Antiglobulin test (indirect)*.

INDIRECT COOMBS' TEST See *Antiglobulin test (indirect)*.

INHERITANCE The acquisition of characteristics by transmission of chromosomes and genes from ancestor to descendant.

INHIBITION The prevention of a normal reaction between an antigen and its corresponding antibody, usually because an antigen of the same specificity but from another source is present in the serum.

INHIBITION TECHNIQUE A test that can be either quantitative or qualitative, devised for the detection of group-specific substances by means of their inhibiting effect on the corresponding antibody.

IRREGULAR AGGLUTININ Atypical antibody.

ISOAGGLUTININ An antibody directed against an antigen found in the same species. Now called alloagglutinin.

ISOPHILE ANTIBODY An antibody that reacts with constituents of the red cells that are particular to the red cells used in stimulation yet do not crossreact with antigens present in red cells of another species. (Opposite of heterophile.)

ISOTONIC SOLUTION A solution having the same osmotic pressure as blood.

J CHAIN An extra polypeptide chain present in IgA and IgM molecules.

JAUNDICE Yellowness of the skin due to hyperbilirubinemia.

Jk The symbol for the Kidd blood group system.

K The symbol for the Kell blood group system.

KARYOTYPE An individual's set of chromosomes.

KERNICTERUS Damage and pigmentation of the brain nuclei, particularly of the basal ganglia, associated with severe neonatal jaundice.

KLEIHAUER TECHNIQUE An acid elution method to detect fetal red cells in maternal circulation. Also known as Betke-Kleihauer technique.

LAKED Hemolyzed

Le The symbol for the Lewis blood group system.

LECTIN An extract from seeds that possesses the ability to agglutinate red cells (usually directed against a specific antigen).

LEUKEMIA A disease of the hemopoietic system characterized primarily by an uncontrolled proliferation of leukocytes.

LEUKOCYTE A white cell.

LEUKOPENIA A decrease of leukocytes in peripheral blood.

LINKED GENES Genes that are on the same chromosome and are within measurable distance of one another. Also known as syntenic genes.

LIQUOR AMNII Amniotic fluid.

LOCI Plural of locus.

LOCUS The position on a chromosome occupied by a gene.

LOW-INCIDENCE ANTIGEN An antigen possessed by few members of the population.

Lu The symbol for the Lutheran blood group system.

LW ANTIGEN Landsteiner-Wiener antigen.

LYOPHILIZATION Rapid freezing and dehydration of a biological substance in a high vacuum to prevent chemical breakdown. Also known as freeze-drying.

LYSIS The rupture and breakdown of red cells.

MAJOR CROSSMATCH A compatibility test used to detect the presence of antibody in the recipient's serum (donor's red cells versus recipient's serum).

MEIOSIS Cell division that produces mature sex cells containing half the number of chromosomes possessed by the original cell.

METHYLDOPA See *Aldomet.*

MINOR CROSSMATCH A compatibility test used to detect the presence of antibody in the donor's serum (donor's serum versus recipient's red cells).

MINUS-MINUS PHENOTYPE A phenotype in which the patient's red cells fail to react with all antibodies in a particular system.

MITOSIS Cell division that produces daughter cells with the same number of chromosomes as the original cell. All cell division, with the exception of that which produces sex cells, is mitotic.

MODIFYING GENE A gene that modifies the expression of another gene.

MONOZYGOTIC TWINS Twins derived from a single fertilized egg or zygote.

MOSAIC A mixture of characters produced by a cross-over occurring within the confines of a gene.

MUCOPOLYSACCHARIDE Polysaccharides containing a minor proportion of linked protein or polypeptide.

MULTIPLE BAG UNIT A primary plastic bag containing anticoagulant connected to other bags by means of integral tubing.

MUTATION A change in a gene resulting in the formation of another allele. Allelomorphs are thought to have arisen as a result of mutation.

NATURAL SUBSTANCES Chemical substances in bacteria and plants that resemble blood group antigens.

NATURALLY OCCURRING ANTIBODIES Antibodies that occur without apparent stimulus. Now known as non-red-cell-immune antibodies.

NEONATAL Pertaining to a newborn infant.

NEUTRALIZATION See *Inhibition.*

NOMENCLATURE A terminology; a system of names and naming.

NON-RED-CELL-IMMUNE See *Naturally occurring antibodies.*

NONSECRETOR An individual who does not have water-soluble A, B or H substances in saliva or in other body fluids.

NORMAL SALINE Isotonic saline.

NOTATION A system of symbols used to indicate in brief form more extensive ideas.

NULL PHENOTYPE See *Minus-Minus phenotype.*

OPTIMAL Adjective; the most desirable or satisfactory.

OPTIMUM Noun; the amount or degree of something (e.g., temperature) that is most desirable or satisfactory.

ORTHOTOPIC Transplantation of an organ into its usual position or location.

OVUM The female sex cell.

PACKED CELL VOLUME (PCV) The volume of red cells in a column of blood calculated as a percentage.

PACKED CELLS A donation from which 75 per cent of the plasma has been removed before transfusion. Also known as concentrated red cells or red blood cells.

PANAGGLUTINATION The reaction of red cells, irrespective of blood group, with all human sera.

PANAGGLUTININ An antibody that agglutinates all red cells, irrespective of blood group.

PANEL OF CELLS A set of standard red cells especially selected to detect and identify blood group antibodies.

PAPAIN A proteolytic enzyme commonly used in blood bank tests.

PASSIVE ANTIBODY An antibody injected into an individual to grant temporary immunity against disease, etc.

PCV (Abbr) Packed cell volume.

PERIPHERAL BLOOD Blood in the systemic circulation.

PERITONEAL CAVITY The space between the visceral and parietal layers of the peritoneum.

PHENOTYPE The observed or discernible characteristics of an individual as determined by his genotype and the environment in which he develops. With respect to blood groups, when serologic tests fail to distinguish between two genotypes (such as *AA* and *AO*) which will, however, behave differently as progenitors, such a class of genotype is known as a phenotype.

PHLEBOTOMY The withdrawal of blood from a vein.

PLACENTA The organ on the wall of the uterus to which the embryo is attached by means of the umbilical cord and from which it receives nourishment.

PLACENTAL TRANSFER The exchange of material between mother and fetus.

PLANT AGGLUTININS See *Lectins*.

PLASMA The straw-colored, liquid portion of unclotted blood.

PLASMA THROMBOPLASTIN ANTECEDENT Factor XI coagulation factor.

PLASMA THROMBOPLASTIN COMPONENT Factor IX coagulation factor.

PLASMAPHERESIS A technique whereby blood is removed from a donor, centrifuged and separated, and the packed red cells returned to the donor's circulation. The plasma is then saved and used for purposes such as a laboratory reagent.

POLYAGGLUTINATION The agglutination of red cells by most, but not all, human sera, regardless of blood group.

POLYCYTHEMIA A condition characterized primarily by an increased number of red blood cells.

POLYMORPHISM The existence in a population of more than one alternative phenotype.

POLYPEPTIDE A long chain of amino acids linked by peptide bonds.

POLYSACCHARIDE One of a group of complex carbohydrates of large molecular size.

POLYVINYLPYRROLIDONE (PVP) A synthetic polymer of high molecular weight used as a plasma expander and to enhance agglutination in certain serological tests.

POOL A mixture of serum (or cells) from a number of individuals.

POSITION EFFECT The effect that blood group antigens have upon each other by virtue of the relative position of their genes on the chromosome pair.

POSTNATAL Subsequent to birth.

POTENCY Power or strength.

PRECIPITATION In blood banking, the reaction of soluble antigens with antibody resulting in arcs or flocculation of the complexes in a gel medium.

PRECIPITIN An antibody that reacts with its corresponding antigen to form a precipitate.

PRECURSOR SUBSTANCE A substance in a stage of a process that precedes a later development.

PRENATAL Before birth.

PRIMARY RESPONSE The initial response to a foreign antigen.

PRIVATE ANTIGEN An antigen that occurs rarely in the population.

PROBAND An individual of either sex possessing an unusual trait, which calls an investigator's attention to the family.

PROCONVERTIN Factor VII coagulation factor.

PROPOSITA The female member of a family of unusual characteristic who is the subject of an investigation into related members of the pedigree.

PROPOSITUS Masculine form of proposita.

PROTEIN A complex nitrogenous substance of high molecular weight found in various forms in animals and plants and characteristic of all living matter.

PROTEOLYTIC ENZYME An organic compound that specifically effects the digestion of protein.

PROTHROMBIN Factor II coagulation factor.

PROTOCOL The original record made of the results of a test.

PROZONE A phenomenon in which negative reactions are obtained with low dilutions of an antibody, while a positive reaction is obtained with higher dilutions.

PSEUDOAGGLUTINATION The clumping of cells caused by agents other than antibodies.

PSEUDOMUCINOUS OVARIAN CYST FLUID A fluid from certain ovarian cysts that is rich in blood group substances.

PUBLIC ANTIGEN An antigen possessed by the majority of individuals in the population.

PVP (Abbr) Polyvinylpyrrolidone.

PUTATIVE Reputed, supposed.

PYROGENS Thermostable, filter-passing substances, probably of bacterial origin, that may cause febrile reactions when injected into a recipient.

QUALITY CONTROL A control of all facets of daily work to ensure a high level of performance.

QUANTITATIVE DIFFERENCE See *Dosage*.

REAGENT RED CELLS Red cells used in laboratory testing.

RECESSIVE GENE A gene that gives rise only to its corresponding character when present in "double dose" (i.e., in the homozygote).

RETICULOCYTE A type of immature erythrocyte.

RETICULOENDOTHELIAL SYSTEM The phagocytic cells and the transfer liver cells, spleen and blood-forming cells; the network comprising all the cells that line the blood and lymph vessels of the body.

Rh The symbol for the Rhesus blood group system.

ROULEAUX FORMATION Pseudoagglutination in which red cells give the appearance of stacks of coins.

SALINE An aqueous solution containing sodium chloride.

SALINE ANTIBODY An antibody that reacts with saline-suspended red cells.

SATELLITE BAG A secondary plastic bag connected to a primary bag by means of integral tubing.

SCREENING TEST A test designed for the detection of antibodies. A preliminary test.

SECONDARY RESPONSE A second response to exposure to a foreign antigen, resulting in the production of large amounts of antibody.

SECRETOR An individual who possesses water-soluble A, B or H substances (when appropriate) in saliva and other body fluids.

SECRETORY COMPONENT An additional fragment found in secretory IgA and IgM.

SEDIMENTATION The process of producing a deposit, especially through centrifugation.

SEDIMENTATION RATE The rate at which red cells settle out in anticoagulated blood when left undisturbed.

SEDIMENTATION TEST An agglutination test performed without centrifugation.

SEEDS See *Lectins*.

SEGREGATION According to mendelian law, the appearance of contrasted characters in the offspring of heterozygotes. Also the separation of paired maternal and paternal genes at meiosis in the formation of gametes.

SEMINAL FLUID Semen.

SENSITIZATION (OF AN INDIVIDUAL) Stimulation of an individual by an antigen that renders him or her liable to form antibodies.

SENSITIZATION (OF RED CELLS) The specific attachment of antibody to their antigenic receptors on red cells without agglutination or lysis.

SEQUESTRENE A trademark referring to EDTA and variations of its salts.

SERUM The liquid portion of clotted blood. Plasma from which fibrinogen has been removed.

SEX-LINKED Any characteristic that is inherited by means of one of the sex chromosomes.

SIALIC ACID Any of a family of amino sugars containing nine or more carbon atoms that are nitrogen- and oxygen-substituted acylderivatives of neuaminic acid. It is a component of lipids, polysaccharides and mucoproteins. It is the main substance removed from the red cells by enzyme treatment.

SIBLINGS Children of the same parents; brothers and sisters.

SLIDE TESTS Serologic tests performed on a glass slide.

SODIUM AZIDE A compound, used as a red cell preservative, that inhibits the action of many gram-negative bacteria.

SOLUBLE ANTIGEN Antigen in solution; e.g., blood group substances.

SOMATIC CELLS Body cells as opposed to sex cells.

SPECIES-SPECIFIC Antigens restricted to members of a particular species.

SPECIFICITY The special affinity between an antigen and its corresponding antibody.

SPERM The male gamete or sex cell.

STUART-POWER FACTOR Factor X coagulation factor.

SUBCUTANEOUS Under the skin (but not into a vein).

SUBGROUPS Subdivisions of antigens; often weakened forms.

SUBSTANCES See *Blood group substance.*

SUPPRESSED GENE A gene that is prevented from expression yet that may appear in later generations.

SUPPRESSOR GENE A modifying gene that will completely or partially suppress the expression of another gene.

SURVIVAL STUDIES Studies to determine the *in vivo* survival of transfused material in the circulation.

SYNCOPE A fainting spell.

SYNTENIC GENES Genes known to be on the same chromosome whether or not linkage can be directly measured between them.

TAGGING (OF RED CELLS) The addition of radioactive isotopes to red cells so that the treated cells can be transfused and their survival studied.

TETANY A convulsive response occasionally observed in blood donors, which is thought to be due to hyperventilation.

TETRACYCLINE An antibiotic found to be useful in discouraging the growth of bacteria in blood samples stored at room temperature.

THALASSEMIA A form of hemolytic anemia resulting from hereditary defects in hemoglobin synthesis and characterized by impaired synthesis of one of its polypeptide chains. This results in hypochromic, microcytic erythrocytes.

THALASSEMIA MAJOR The homozygous state in thalassemia, with evidence of clinical illness from early life.

THALASSEMIA MINOR The heterozygous state in thalassemia that may or may not be accompanied by clinical illness.

THERAPEUTIC ABORTION The surgical termination of pregnancy at any time after conception.

THERMAL AMPLITUDE The temperature range within which an antibody reacts.

THROMBOCYTES Platelets.

THROMBOCYTOPENIA Decrease in platelets.

THROMBOPLASTIN A group of substances that increases the rate of conversion of prothrombin to thrombin.

TITER The reciprocal of the highest dilution of antibody giving a 1+ reaction.

TITRATION The test used to determine the strength of an antibody.

TOLERANCE A state of specific nonreactivity to an antigen due to prior exposure to the same antigen under special circumstances.

TOXIC Poisonous.

TRANS POSITION Being on opposite chromosomes, and not necessarily within the same cistron.

TRANSFUSE To perform a transfusion.

TRANSFUSION The introduction into the blood vessel of blood, saline or any other liquid.

TRANSFUSION REACTION Any allergic, febrile or hemolytic state produced in a patient as a result of transfusion.

TRANSFUSIONIST An individual skilled in transfusion therapy.

TRANSLOCATION The transfer of genetic material from one chromosome to another.

TRANSPLACENTAL HEMORRHAGE The exchange of blood between the maternal and fetal circulation or between the fetal and maternal circulation.

TRYPSIN A proteolytic enzyme derived from hog's stomach; used in certain serological investigations.

ULEX EUROPAEUS A plant, the common gorse. An extract of the seeds, in solution, possesses anti-H specificity.

UNIT INHERITANCE The name applied to one of the mendelian laws (see text).

UNIVERSAL DONOR A term once used to denote an individual of blood group O. See *Dangerous universal donor.*

UNIVERSAL RECIPIENT An individual belonging to blood group AB, who can receive blood of any ABO blood group.

URTICARIA Hives or rash (wheals).

VACCINATION The inoculation or ingestion of organisms or antigens to produce immunity to those organisms or antigens in the recipient.

VALENCY The combining capacity of an atom.

VARIANT Different type, usually applied to rarer forms of an antigen.

VENIPUNCTURE Phlebotomy. The puncture of a vein to obtain blood.

VENOUS Pertaining to the veins.

VICIA GRAMINEA A plant; the extract from the seeds, in solution, possesses anti-N specificity.

WARM ANTIBODY An antibody that reacts optimally at 37° C.

WASHING PROCEDURE Successive centrifugation of cells in large volumes of fresh saline to dilute substances in the fluid in which they were originally suspended.

WBC (Abbr) White blood cell; leukocyte.

WHARTON'S JELLY A mucoid connective tissue that makes up the matrix of the umbilical cord.

WHITE CELLS Leukocytes.

X CHROMOSOME The sex-determining factor in ova and in one-half of sperm. The female chromosome.

Y CHROMOSOME The sex-determining factor in sperm which gives rise to male offspring.

ZETA POTENTIAL The electrokinetic potential (see text).

ZYGOTE A fertilized egg cell (ovum).

ANTIGENS IN MAN

No list of human red cell antigens is ever complete, since new antigens are discovered as fast as the lists are compiled. Moreover, many large laboratories have knowledge of private or public antigens that remain unpublished because of insufficient publishable data.

The list presented here is as complete as possible; reference was made to a vast number of published papers and related texts. Of course, some antigens will still have been missed. Compound antigens and antigen variants have also been listed. Frequencies for high- and low-incidence antigens have been given as +99 per cent and −1 per cent, respectively. Exact frequencies in these cases are of interest to the specialist only and are therefore beyond the scope of this book.

It should also be noted that frequencies in almost all cases are approximate, since different studies will often produce different results.

It is hoped the list will be useful to those attemping to find information about the red cell antigens. The year of discovery will help in finding appropriate references, and the frequency will perhaps help when physicians ask that sometimes unanswerable question "How long before I can get blood for my patient?" Those antigens marked with an asterisk (*) are discussed in the main body of the text.

For obvious reasons, the list provides a chance to marvel at the enormous complexity of the blood groups and at the seemingly infinite hospitality of the red cell surface.

A

Antigen (Compound or Variant)	Year of Publication	Blood Group System	Frequency†
A_{xh}^{A1}	1978	ABO	−1%
*A_1	1900	ABO	34%
*A_1Le^b (Seidler) (compound)	1968	Lewis	27%
*A_2 (variant)	1911	ABO	10%
*A_3 (variant)	1936	ABO	−1%
*A_4 (variant; now known as A_x)	1935	ABO	−1%
*A_5 (variant; now known as A_x)	1935	ABO	−1%
*AB (A+B) (compound)	1902	ABO	3%
A_{bantu} (variant; similar to A_x)	1966	ABO	0%‡
A_{el} (variant)	1964	ABO	−1%
A_{end} (variant)	1959	ABO	−1%
A_{finn} (variant; similar to A_{end})	1973	ABO	3%§
A_h (Bombay-like)	1961	ABO	−1%
A_{hel} (A_{HH}; A_{HP})	1965	ABO	45%‖
A_{HH} (A_{hel}; A_{HP})	1965	ABO	45%‖
Ahonen (An^a)	1972	Unrelated; low incidence	−1%
A_{HP} (A_{hel}; A_{HH})	1965	ABO	45%¶
AI (IA) (compound)	1960	Ii	45%
*A_{int} (variant)	1930	ABO	−1%¶
Allen	Unpublished	Unrelated; low incidence	−1%

†In Caucasians, unless otherwise indicated.
‡In South African Bantu 4%.
§In Finns.
‖Recognized by lectin *Helix pomatia*; same reaction with A_1 and A_2 cells.
¶More common in American blacks.

A 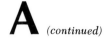 *(continued)*

Antigen (Compound or Variant)	Year of Publication	Blood Group System	Frequency
*A_m *(variant)*	1935	ABO	−1%
A_m^h (O_{Hm}^A)	1965	ABO	−1%
Anuszewska	Unpublished	Unrelated; high incidence	+99%
An^a (Ahonen)	1972	Unrelated; low incidence	−1%
A_o *(variant; now known as A_x)*	1935	ABO	−1%
A^P *(variant)*	1957	ABO	−1%
Armstrong (M^v)	1966	MNS	72%
Armstrong	Unpublished	Unrelated; high incidence	+99%
At^a (August; Augustine)	1967	Unrelated; high incidence	+99%
Au^a (Auberger)	1961	Auberger	82%
Auberger (Au^a)	1961	Auberger	82%
August (At^a; Augustine)	1967	Unrelated; high incidence	+99%
Augustine (At^a; August)	1967	Unrelated; high incidence	+99%
*A_x (A_4; A_5; A_z; A_o)	1935	ABO	−1%
A_z *(variant; now known as A_x)*	1935	ABO	−1%

B

Antigen (Compound or Variant)	Year of Publication	Blood Group System	Frequency
*B	1900	ABO	9%
B_2 *(variant)*	1961	ABO	−1%
B_3 *(variant)*	1955	ABO	−1%
Balkin	Unpublished	Unrelated; low incidence	−1%
Baltzer	Unpublished	Unrelated; low incidence	−1%
Bas (Rh:34)	1972	Rh/Hr	+99%
Batty (By)	1955	Unrelated; low incidence	−1%
Baumler	Unpublished	Unrelated; high incidence	+99%
Be^a (Berrens)	1953	Rh/Hr	−1%
Becker	1951	Unrelated; low incidence	−1%
Begovich	Unpublished	Unrelated; high incidence	+99%
B_{eL}	1979	ABO	1%
Bell	Unpublished	Unrelated; low incidence	−1%
Berrens (Be^a)	1953	Rh/Hr	−1%
Bg^a (DBG)	1967†	Bg	±30%
Bg^b (Ho)	1967†	Bg	−1%
Bg^c (Ot)	1967†	Bg	−1%

†Date of Bg classification.

B *(continued)*

Antigen (Compound or Variant)	Year of Publication	Blood Group System	Frequency
B_h (Bombay-like)	1967	ABO	−1%
BI (IB) (*compound*)	1967	Ii	14%
Bi (Biles)	1961	Unrelated; low incidence	−1%
Big	Unpublished	Unrelated; low incidence	−1%
Biles (Bi)	1961	Unrelated; low incidence	−1%
Bishop (Bp^a)	1964	Unrelated; low incidence	−1%
Black	Unpublished	Unrelated; low incidence	−1%
BLe^b (*compound*)	1972	ABO/Lewis	−1%
B_m (*variant*)	1967	ABO	−1%
B_m^h (O_{Hm}^B)	1965	ABO	−1%
Bøc (K:12)	1973	Kell	+99%
Bonde	1968	Unrelated; low incidence	−1%
Bou (Bout; Bouteille)	Unpublished	Unrelated; high incidence	+99%
Bout (Bou; Bouteille)	Unpublished	Unrelated; high incidence	+99%
Bouteille (Bou; Bout)	Unpublished	Unrelated; high incidence	+99%
Bovet	1968	Unrelated; low incidence	−1%
Box (Bx^a)	1961	Unrelated; low incidence	−1%
Bp^a (Bishop)	1964	Unrelated; low incidence	−1%
Br 726750	1967	Unrelated; low incidence	−1%
Bra (Bradford)	1967	Unrelated; high incidence	+99%
Braden	Unpublished	Unrelated; low incidence	−1%
Bradford (Bra)	1967	Unrelated; high incidence	+99%
Bridgewater	1968	Unrelated; low incidence	−1%
Bruno	Unpublished	Unrelated; high incidence	+99%
Bryant	Unpublished	Unrelated; high incidence	+99%
Bu^a (Burrell; Sc2)	1963	Sciana	−1%
Buckalew	Unpublished	Unrelated; high incidence	+99%
Bultar	Unpublished	Unrelated; high incidence	+99%
Burrell (Bu^a; Sc2)	1963	Sciana	−1%
Burrett (Finlay; Fin)	1955	Unrelated; low incidence	−1%
B_w (*variant*)	1958	ABO	−1%
B_x	1966	ABO	−1%
Bx^a (Box)	1961	Unrelated; low incidence	−1%
By (Batty)	1955	Unrelated; low incidence	−1%

C

Antigen (Compound or Variant)	Year of Publication	Blood Group System	Frequency
C	1920	ABO	59%
°C (rh'; Rh:2)	1941	Rh/Hr	70%
°c (hr'; Rh:4)	1943	Rh/Hr	80%
Cad (Sdᵃ)	1968	Sid	88%
Caldwell (Clᵃ)	1963	MNS	−1%
Car	Unpublished	Unrelated: high incidence	+99%
Carson	Unpublished	Unrelated: low incidence	−1%
°Cartwright (Ytᵃ)	1956	Cartwright	+99%
Cartwright	Unpublished	Unrelated; high incidence	+99%
°CD (G; rhᴳ; Rh:12) (compound)	1958	Rh/Hr	86%
°CE (Rh:22) (compound)	1961	Rh/Hr	1%
°Ce (rhᵢ; Rh:7) (compound)	1958	Rh/Hr	70%
°cE (Rh:27) (compound)	1961	Rh/Hr	30%
°ce (hr; f; Rh:6) (compound)	1953	Rh/Hr	64%
°Cellano (k; K:2)	1949	Kell	+99%
ceˢ (V; hrᵛ; Rh:10)	1955	Rh/Hr	−1%
Ce⁵ (Rh42) (compound)	Unpublished**	Rh/Hr	−
Cᴳ (Rh:21)	1961	Rh/Hr	70%†
Chᵃ (Chido; Gursha)	1967	Chido	+99%
Charles	Unpublished	Unrelated; low incidence	−1%
Chido (Chᵃ; Gursha)	1967	Chido	+99%
Chrᵃ	1955	Unrelated; low incidence	−1%
Cip (Cipriano)	1967	Unrelated; high incidence	+99%
Cipriano (Cip)	1967	Unrelated; high incidence	+99%
Clᵃ (Caldwell)	1963	MNS	−1%
°Claas (KL; K:9)	1968	Kell	+99%
Clements	Unpublished	Unrelated; high incidence	+99%
c-like (Rh:26; Deal)	1964	Rh/Hr	80%
°Coᵃ (Colton)	1967	Colton	+99%
Coates	Unpublished	Unrelated; low incidence	−1%
°Coᵇ	1970	Colton	−1%
°Colton (Coᵃ)	1967	Colton	+99%
Comacho (Rh:32)	1971	Rh/Hr	−1%
Cooper	Unpublished	Unrelated; high incidence	+99%
Coté (Kᵒ-like; K:11)	1971	Kell	+99%
Coté-like (K16)	1974	Kell	+99%
Craig	Unpublished	Unrelated; low incidence	−1%
Cromer (Goᵇ)	1965	?Rh/Hr	+99%
Cross	1967	Unrelated; low incidence	−1%
Csᵃ (Stirling)	1965	Unrelated; high incidence	97%
Cᵘ (variant)	1948	Rh/Hr	−1%
cᵛ (variant)	1948	Rh/Hr	−1%
°Cʷ (rhʷ¹; Rh:8)	1946	Rh/Hr	−1%
Cˣ (rhˣ; Rh:9)	1954	Rh/Hr	−1%

**Reported at AABB Meeting, Washington, 1980.
†Corresponding antibody is capable of reacting with weakest Cᵘ cells.

D

Antigen (Compound or Variant)	Year of Publication	Blood Group System	Frequency
°D (Rh$_0$; Rh:1)	1939	Rh/Hr	85%
Dahl	Unpublished	Unrelated; low incidence	−1%
Davis	Unpublished	Unrelated; high incidence	+99%
D1276	1967	Unrelated; low incidence	−1%
DBG (Donna Bennett Goodspeed; Bg^a)	1967	Bg	±30%
D^{Cor} (Go^a; Gonzalez; Rh:30)	1958	Rh/Hr	−1%
Deal (c-like; Rh:26)	1964	Rh/Hr	80%
°Di^a (Diego)	1955	Diego	−1% †
°Di^b (Luebano)	1967	Diego	+99%
°Diego (Di^a)	1955	Diego	−1% †
°Do^a (Dombrock)	1965	Dombrock	64%
°Do^b	1973	Dombrock	82%
°Dombrock (Do^a)	1965	Dombrock	64%
Donaviesky	1967	Unrelated; low incidence	−1%
Donna (Donna Bennett Goodspeed; DBG; Bg^a)	1967	Bg	±30%
Dp (Dupuy)	1970	Unrelated; high incidence	+99%
Driver	Unpublished	Unrelated; low incidence	−1%
Dropik	1968	Unrelated; low incidence	−1%
°D^u (variant)	1946	Rh/Hr	3% ‡
Duch (Duck)	Unpublished	Unrelated; low incidence	−1%
Duck (Duch)	Unpublished	Unrelated; low incidence	−1%
Duclos (RH:38)	1978	Rh/Hr	+99%
Duffy (Fy^a)	1950	Duffy	65%
Dupuy (Dp)	1970	Unrelated; high incidence	+99%
D^w (Wiel, Rh:23)	1962	Rh/Hr	−1%

† Antigen practically confined to people of Mongolian extraction.
‡ Incidence higher in American Negroes.

E

Antigen (Compound or Variant)	Year of Publication	Blood Group System	Frequency
°E (rh″; Rh:3)	1943	Rh/Hr	30%
°e (hr″; Rh:5)	1945	Rh/Hr	98%
E.Amos	1967	Unrelated; low incidence	−1%
e^i (variant)	1961	Rh/Hr	−1%
El (Eldridge)	1970	Unrelated; high incidence	+99%
Eldridge (El)	1970	Unrelated; high incidence	+99%
°En^a	1965	En	+99%
e^s (VS; Rh:20)	1960	Rh/Hr	−1%
E^T (variant)	1962	Rh/Hr	+99%
E^u (variant)	1950	Rh/Hr	−1%
Evans	1966	Rh/Hr	−1%
Evans (RH:37)	1960	Rh/Hr	−1%
Evelyn	Unpublished	Rh/Hr	−1%
E^w (rh^{w2}; Rh:11)	1955	Rh/Hr	−1%

F

Antigen (Compound or Variant)	Year of Publication	Blood Group System	Frequency
°f (ce; hr; Rh:6) (*compound*)	1953	Rh/Hr	64%
Far	1967	MNS	−1%
Fedor	Unpublished	Unrelated; high incidence	+99%
Fin (Finlay; Burrett)	Unpublished	Unrelated; low incidence	−1%
Finlay (Burrett; Fin)	Unpublished	Unrelated; low incidence	−1%
Fle (Fleming)	1968	Unrelated; high incidence	+99%
Fleming (Fle)	1968	Unrelated; high incidence	+99%
Fr^a	1978	Unrelated	−1%
Frando	Unpublished	Unrelated; high incidence	+99%
French	1968	Unrelated; low incidence	−1%
Fritz (Wr^b)	1971	Wright	+99%
Fuerhart	Unpublished	Unrelated; low incidence	−1%
Fuj (Fujikawa; Junior; Jr^a)	1967	Unrelated; high incidence	+99%
Fujikawa (Fuj; Junior; Jr^a)	1967	Unrelated; high incidence	+99%
Fuller	Unpublished	Unrelated; high incidence	+99%
°Fy^a (Duffy)	1950	Duffy	65%
°Fy^b	1951	Duffy	80%
°Fy3	1971	Duffy	+99%
°Fy4	1973	Duffy	+99%
°Fy5	1973	Duffy	+99%
Fy^x	1965	Duffy	1%

G

Antigen (Compound or Variant)	Year of Publication	Blood Group System	Frequency
°G (rh^G; Rh:12 CD) (*compound*)	1958	Rh/Hr	86%
Gallner	1967	Unrelated; high incidence	+99%
Gambino	Unpublished	Unrelated; low incidence	−1%
Garcia (Rh:32)	1971	Rh/Hr	−1%
°Ge (Gerbich)	1960	Gerbich	+99%
°Gerbich (Ge)	1960	Gerbich	+99%
Gerhany	Unpublished	Unrelated; low incidence	−1%
Geslin	Unpublished	Unrelated; high incidence	+99%
Gf (Griffiths; Gf^a)	1966	Unrelated; low incidence	−1%

G (continued)

Antigen (Compound or Variant)	Year of Publication	Blood Group System	Frequency
Gf^a (Gf; Griffiths)	1966	Unrelated; low incidence	−1%
Gilbraith	Unpublished	Unrelated; low incidence	−1%
Gilfeather (M^g)	1958	MNS	−1%
Gladding	1967	Unrelated; low incidence	−1%
Gn^a (Gonsowski)	1969	Unrelated; high incidence	+99%
Go^a (Gonzalez; D^{Cor}; Rh:30)	1962	Rh/Hr	−1%
Go^b (Cromer)	1965	?Rh/Hr	+99%
Gon	1967	Unrelated; low incidence	−1%
Gonsowski (Gn^a)	1969	Unrelated; high incidence	+99%
Gonzalez (Go^a; D^{Cor}; Rh:30)	1962	Rh/Hr	−1%
Good	1960	Unrelated; low incidence	−1%
Goodspeed (DBG; Bg^a)	1967	Bg	±30%
Gr (Graydon; Vw; Verquist)	1954	MNS	−1%
Graydon (Gr; Vw; Verquist)	1954	MNS	−1%
Green	Unpublished	Unrelated; low incidence	−1%
Gregory (Gy^a)	1966	Unrelated; high incidence	+99%
Griffiths (Gf; Gf^a)	1966	Unrelated; low incidence	−1%
G^u (variant of G)	1971	Rh/Hr	−
Gursha (Chido; Ch^a)	1967	Chido	+99%
Gy^a (Gregory)	1966	Unrelated; high incidence	+99%

H

Antigen (Compound or Variant)	Year of Publication	Blood Group System	Frequency
*H	1948	ABO	+99%
h	Unpublished	Unrelated; high incidence	+99%
Haakestad	Unpublished	Unrelated; low incidence	−1%
Haase	Unpublished	Unrelated; low incidence	−1%
Hamer	Unpublished	Unrelated; high incidence	+99%
Hands	Unpublished	Unrelated; low incidence	−1%
Har (Rh33; R^{oHar}; Hawd)	1971	Rh/Hr	−1%
Harper (Rh32)	1971	Rh/Hr	−1%
Hartley	1968	Unrelated; low incidence	−1%

Table continued on the following page

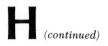 *(continued)*

Antigen (Compound or Variant)	Year of Publication	Blood Group System	Frequency
Hawd (Rh:33; R°ʰᵃʳ; Har)	1971	Rh/Hr	−1%
HD₁ (Pr₁ₕ; Heidelberg; Sp₁)⁻	1969	HD-Pr-Sp	100%
HD₁ (Sp₁; Pr₂d)	1973	HD-Pr-Sp	100%
HDZ (Sp₁; Pr₂)	1969	HD-Pr-Sp	100%
He (Henshaw)	1951	MNS	−1%
Heibel	1968	Unrelated; low incidence	−1%
Heidelberg (HD₁; Pr₁ₕ; Sp₁)	1969	HD-Pr-Sp	100%
Hen (Henry)	1967	Unrelated; high incidence	+99%
Henshaw (He)	1951	MNS	−1%
Hernandez (hrᴴ;Rh:28)	1964	Rh/Hr	−1%
Hey	1974	Unrelated; low incidence	−1%
°HI (IH; IO) *(compound)*	1964	Ii	+99%
Hil (Hill)	1966	MNS	−1%
Hil	Unpublished	Unrelated; low incidence	−1%
Hildebrandt	Unpublished	Unrelated; low incidence	−1%
Hill (Hil)	1966	MNS	−1%
Ho (Bgᵇ)	1963	Bg	2–20%
Hol (Hollister)	1966	Unrelated; low incidence	−1%
Holley (Hy)†	1972	Unrelated; high incidence	+99%
Hollister (Hol)	1966	Unrelated; low incidence	−1%
Holmes	Unpublished	Unrelated; high incidence	+99%
Hov	1973	Unrelated; low incidence	−1%
Hr (Rh:18)	1960	Rh/Hr	+99%
°hr (f; ce; Rh:6) *(compound)*	1953	Rh/Hr	64%
°hr′ (c; Rh:4)	1941	Rh/Hr	80%
°hr″ (e; Rh:5)	1945	Rh/Hr	98%
hrᴮ (Rh:31)	1972	Rh/Hr	−1%
hrᴴ (Rh:28)	1964	Rh/Hr	−1%
Hr⁰ (Rh:17)	1950	Rh/Hr	+99%
hrˢ (Rh:19)	1960	Rh/Hr	97%
hrᵛ (V; ceˢ; Rh:10)	1955	Rh/Hr	−1%
Hᴛ	1961	Unrelated; high incidence	+99%
Htᵃ (Hunt)	1962	Unrelated; low incidence	−1%
Hu (Hunter)	1934	MNS	−1%
Hunt (Htᵃ)	1962	Unrelated; low incidence	−1%
Hunter (Hu)	1934	MNS	−1%
Hutchinson	Unpublished	Unrelated; high incidence	+99%
Hy (Holley)†	1972	Unrelated; high incidence	+99%

†Antigen possibly related to Gy (Gregory).

I

Antigen (Compound or Variant)	Year of Publication	Blood Group System	Frequency
°I	1956	Ii	+99%
°i_1†	1960	Ii	+99%
°i_2	1961	Ii	+99%
IA_1 (*compound*)	1960	Ii	45%
IB (*compound*)	1967	Ii	14%
°I^D (*variant*)	1971	Ii	+99%
°I^F (*variant*)	1971	Ii	+99%
°IH (HI; IO) (*compound*)	1964	Ii	+99%
iH (iO)	1964	Ii	+99%
ILe^{bH} (*compound*)	1971	Ii (Lewis)	72%
In^a	1973	Unrelated; ‡ low incidence	−1%
In^b	1975	Unrelated; ‡ high incidence	−§
°IO (IH; HI) (*compound*)	1964	Ii	+99%
iO (iH) (*compound*)	1964	Ii	+99%
IP_1 (*compound*)	1968	Ii	79%
iP_1 (*compound*)	1968	Ii	79%
I^S (*variant*)	1975	Ii	+99%
I^T (*variant*)	1966	Ii	+99%
$I^T P_1$ (*compound*)	1970	Ii	79%
ILe^{bH} (*compound*)	1971	Lewis	72%

†Amount of i antigen decreases during first 18 months of life.
‡No relationship to any system has been established with tests so far performed.
§Frequency not yet established.

J

Antigen (Compound or Variant)	Year of Publication	Blood Group System	Frequency
Je^a (Jensen)	1972	Unrelated; low incidence	−1%
Jensen (Je^a)	1972	Unrelated; low incidence	−1%
°Jk^a (Kidd)	1951	Kidd	77%
°Jk^b	1953	Kidd	73%
°Jk3	1959	Kidd	+99%
JMH	1977	HTLA; unrelated	+99%
JN (Jn^a)	1967	Unrelated; low incidence	−1%
Jn^a (JN)	1967	Unrelated; low incidence	−1%
Jo^a (Joseph)	1972	Unrelated; high incidence	+99%
Job (Jobbins)	1967	Unrelated; low incidence	−1%
Jobbins (Job)	1967	Unrelated; low incidence	−1%
Joseph (Jo^a)	1972	Unrelated; high incidence	+99%
Jr^a (Junior; Fujikawa; Fuj)	1974	Unrelated; high incidence	+99%
Js^a (Sutter; K:6)	1958	Kell	1%
Js^b (Matthews; K:7)	1963	Kell	+99%
Junior (Jr^a; Fujikawa; Fuj)	1974	Unrelated; high incidence	+99%

K

Antigen (Compound or Variant)	Year of Publication	Blood Group System	Frequency
*K (Kell; K:1)	1946	Kell	9%
*k (Cellano; K:2)	1949	Kell	+99%
*K:1 (K; Kell)	1946	Kell	9%
*K:2 (k; Cellano)	1949	Kell	+99%
*K:3 (Kpᵃ; Penney)	1957	Kell	2%
*K:4 (Kpᵇ; Rautenberg)	1958	Kell	+99%
*K:5 (Kᵒ; Kᵘ; Peltz)	1961	Kell	+99%
*K:6 (Jsᵃ; Sutter)	1958	Kell	1%
*K:7 (Jsᵇ; Matthews)	1963	Kell	+99%
*K:8 (Kʷ)	1965	Kell	5%
*K:9 (Claas; KL)	1968	Kell	+99%
*K:10 (Ulᵃ; Karhula)	1968	Kell	3%
*K:11 (Coté; Kᵒ-like)	1971	Kell	+99%
*K:12 (Bøc)	1973	Kell	+99%
*K:13 (Sgro)	1974	Kell	+99%
*K:14 (San)	1974	Kell	+99%
*K:15 (Kx)	1974	Kell	+99%
*K:16 (Coté-like)	1974	Kell	+99%
*K:17 (Wkᵃ; Weeks)	1974	Kell	−1%
*K:18	1974	Kell	+99%
K:19	1979	Kell	−99%
Kamhuber (Kam)	1966	Unrelated; † low incidence	−1%
*Karhula (Ulᵃ; K:10)	1968	Kell	3%
*Kéll (K; K:1)	1946	Kell	9%
Kelly	1967	Unrelated; high incidence	+99%
Kennedy	Unpublished	?Rh/Hr	−1%
*KL (Claas; K:9)	1968	Kell	+99%
Knᵃ (Knops-Helgeson)	1970	Unrelated; high incidence	+99%
Knops-Helgeson (Knᵃ)	1970	Unrelated; high incidence	+99%
*Kᵒ (Kᵘ; K:5; Peltz)	1961	Kell	+99%
*Kᵒ-like (Coté; K:11)	1971	Kell	+99%
Kollogo	Unpublished	Unrelated; high incidence	+99%
Kosis	Unpublished	Unrelated; high incidence	+99%
*Kpᵃ (Penney; K:3)	1957	Kell	2%
*Kpᵇ (Rautenberg; K:4)	1958	Kell	+99%
Kpᶜ (originally "Levay")	1979	Kell	−1%
*Kᵘ (Kᵒ; K:5; Peltz)	1961	Kell	+99%
*Kʷ (K:8)	1965	Kell	5%
*Kx (K:15)	1974	Kell	+99%

†No relationship to any system has been established with tests so far performed.

L

Antigen (Compound or Variant)	Year of Publication	Blood Group System	Frequency
Lan (Langereis)†	1961	Langereis	+99%
Langereis (Lan)	1961	Langereis	+99%
*Leᵃ (Lewis)	1946	Lewis	22%
*Leᵇ	1946	Lewis	72%
Leᶜ (variant)	1957	Lewis	6%
Leᵈ (variant)	1970	Lewis	2%

†Lan and Soᵃ are thought to be the same antigen.

L *(continued)*

Antigen (Compound or Variant)	Year of Publication	Blood Group System	Frequency
Lee	Unpublished	Unrelated; high incidence	+99%
°Lewis (Le^a)	1946	Lewis	22%
Lewis II (Ls^a; Lw^a)	1963	Unrelated; low incidence	−1%
°Le^x (*variant*)	1949	Lewis	94%
Li^a (Livesey)	1980	?Lutheran	−1%
Lindsay	Unpublished	Unrelated; low incidence	−1%
Livesey (Li^a)	1980	?Lutheran	−1%
Ls^a (Lewis II; Lw^a)	1963	Unrelated; low incidence	−1%
°Lu1 (Lu^a)	1945	Lutheran	8%
°Lu2 (Lu^b)	1956	Lutheran	+99%
°Lu^a (Lu1)	1945	Lutheran	8%
°Lu^b (Lu2)	1956	Lutheran	+99%
°Lu3	1963	Lutheran	+99%
°Lu4	1971	Lutheran	+99%
°Lu5	1972	Lutheran	+99%
°Lu6	1972	Lutheran	+99%
°Lu7	1972	Lutheran	+99%
°Lu8	1972	Lutheran	+99%
°Lu9	1973	Lutheran	2%
°Lu10	1974	Lutheran	1%
°Lu11	1974	Lutheran	+99%
°Lu12	1973	Lutheran	+99%
°Lu13	1973	Lutheran	+99%
°Lu14	1975	Lutheran	2%
Lucy	Unpublished	Unrelated; low incidence	−1%
°Luebano (Di^b)	1967	Diego	+99%
Luke	1965	P	98%
°LW (Rh:25)	1961	Rh/Hr†	+99%
Lw^a (Lewis II; Ls^a)	1963	Unrelated; low incidence	−1%

†Relationship to the Rh/Hr system controversial.

M

Antigen (Compound or Variant)	Year of Publication	Blood Group System	Frequency
°M	1927	MNS	78%
M′	1968	MNS	9%
M$_1$	1960	MNS	4%
M$_2$ (*variant*)	1938	MNS	−
M2443	1967	Unrelated; high incidence	+99%
M^a (M^A) (*variant*)	1966	MNS	78%
Mackin	Unpublished	Unrelated; high incidence	+99%
Mag (Magnard)	1958	Lewis	2%
Magnard (Mag)	1958	Lewis	2%
Man	Unpublished	Unrelated; low incidence	−1%
Mansfield (Peacock)	1967	Unrelated; low incidence	−1%
Mar (Marriot)	1967	Unrelated; low incidence	−1%
Marcus	Unpublished	Unrelated; low incidence	−1%

Table continued on the following page

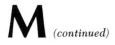
M (continued)

Antigen (Compound or Variant)	Year of Publication	Blood group System	Frequency
Marks	Unpublished	Unrelated; low incidence	−1%
Marriot (Mar)	1967	Unrelated; low incidence	−1%
Martin (Mt^a)	1962	MNS	−1%
Martin	Unpublished	Unrelated; low incidence	−1%
°Matthews (Js^b; K:7)	1963	Kell	+99%
M^c (variant)	1953	MNS	−1%
McAulay	1967	Unrelated; low incidence	−1%
McC^a (McCoy)	1978	Unrelated	98%
McCall	Unpublished	Unrelated; low incidence	−1%
McCoy (McC^a)	1978	Unrelated	98%
McKee	Unpublished	Unrelated; high incidence	+99%
°McLeod (phenotype)	1961	Kell	−1%
M^e (variant)	1961	MNS	78%
M^g (Gilfeather)	1958	MNS	−1%
Mi^a (Miltenberger)	1951	MNS	−1%
Middel	Unpublished	Unrelated; low incidence	−1%
Miltenberger (Mi^a)	1951	MNS	−1%
Miland	Unpublished	Unrelated; low incidence	−1%
Minnie Pearl Davis (MPD)	Unpublished	Unrelated; high incidence	+99%
Mit	1980	?MNSs	−1%
M^k	1968	MNS	−1%
Mo^a (Moen)	1968	Unrelated; low incidence	−1%
Moen (Mo^a)	1968	Unrelated; low incidence	−1%
MPD (Minnie Pearl Davis)	Unpublished	Unrelated; high incidence	+99%
M^r (variant)	1968	MNS	78%
Mt^a (Martin)	1962	MNS	−1%
Mur (Murrell)	1961	MNS	−1%
Murrell (Mur)	1961	MNS	−1%
M^v (Armstrong)	1966	MNS	72%
M^z (variant)	1968	MNS	−1%
MZ443	1967	Unrelated; high incidence	+99%

N

Antigen (Compound or Variant)	Year of Publication	Blood Group System	Frequency
°N	1927	MNS	72%
N$_2$ (variant)	1935	MNS	−1%
N^a (N^A)	1971	MNS	20%†
Ne^a	1981	Unrelated	5%*
Nij^a (Nijhuis)	Unpublished	Unrelated; low incidence	−1%
Nijhuis (Nij^a)	Unpublished	Unrelated; low incidence	−1%
Noble	1968	Unrelated; low incidence	−1%
Ny^a (Nyberg)	1964	MNS	−1%
Nyberg (Ny^a)	1964	MNS	−1%

*In Finns
†In Melanesians

O

Antigen (Compound or Variant)	Year of Publication	Blood Group System	Frequency
°O (*lack of A and B antigens*)	1900	ABO	45%
°O$_h$ (Bombay)	1952	ABO	−1%
O$_{Hm}$ (O$_m^h$) (*para-Bombay*)	1965	ABO	−1%
O$_{Hm}^A$ (A$_m^h$) (*para-Bombay*)	1965	ABO	−1%
O$_{Hm}^B$ (B$_m^h$) (*para-Bombay*)	1967	ABO	−1%
O$_m^h$ (O$_{Hm}$) (*para-Bombay*)	1965	ABO	−1%
Ok^a	1979	Unrelated	+99%
Ola Ware	1967	Unrelated; high incidence	+99%
Or (Orriss)	1964	?MNS	−1%
Orriss (Or)	1964	?MNS	−1%
Ot (Bg^c)	1959	Bg	1–20%

P

Antigen (Compound or Variant)	Year of Publication	Blood Group System	Frequency
°p (P+P$_1$ + P^k; PP$_1$P^k; Tj^a)	1951	P	−1%
°P$_1$	1927	P	79%
°P$_2$	1927†	P	21%
Parra	Unpublished	Unrelated; high incidence	+99%
Pau (Paular)	Unpublished	Unrelated; high incidence	+99%
Paular (Pau)	Unpublished	Unrelated; high incidence	+99%
Pe	1979	Unrelated	−1%
Pea (Pearl)	1968	Unrelated; high incidence	+99%
Peacock (Mansfield)	1967	Unrelated; low incidence	−1%
Pearl (Pea)	1968	Unrelated; high incidence	+99%
°Peltz (K^o; K^u; K:5)	1961	Kell	+99%
°Penney (Kp^a; K:3)	1957	Kell	2%
Perry	Unpublished	Unrelated; high incidence	+99%
Peters (Pt^a)	1969	Unrelated; low incidence	−1%
°P^k	1959	P	−1%
Powell	Unpublished	Unrelated; low incidence	−1%
Pr$_{1h}$ (HD$_1$; Heidelberg; Sp$_1$)	1969	HD-Pr-Sp	100%
Pr$_{1d}$ (HD$_1$; Sp$_1$)	1973	HD-Pr-Sp	100%
Pr$_2$ (HD$_2$; Sp$_1$)	1969	HD-Pr-Sp	100%
Pr$_a$	1971	HD-Pr-Sp	100%
Pr^a (Pritchard)	1968	Unrelated; low incidence	−1%
"Precursor"‡	1969	Unrelated; low incidence	−1%
Pritchard (Pr^a)	1968	Unrelated; low incidence	−1%
Pt^a (Peters)	1969	Unrelated; low incidence	−1%

†Originally called P(−); this classification, P$_2$, was made in 1951.
‡Antibody reacts with apparent specificity with Rh$_{null}$, U-negative and "Bombay cells.

Q

Antigen (Compound or Variant)	Year of Publication	Blood Group System	Frequency
Q	1935	(Antigen now known to be P_1)	

R

Antigen (Compound or Variant)	Year of Publication	Blood Group System	Frequency
Raddon	1968	Unrelated; low incidence	−1%
Radin (Rd; Rd^a)	1967	Unrelated; low incidence	−1%
*Rautenberg (Kp^b; K4)	1958	Kell	+99%
Rb^a (Redelberger)	1978	Unrelated	−1%
Rd (Radin; Rd^a)	1967	Unrelated; low incidence	−1%
Rd^a (Radin; Rd)	1967	Unrelated; low incidence	−1%
Re^a (Reid)	1971	Unrelated; low incidence	−1%
Redelberger (Rb^a)	1978	Unrelated	−1%
Reid (Rd^a)	1971	Unrelated; low incidence	−1%
Reynolds (Rh:32)	1971	Rh/Hr	−1%
Reynolds	Unpublished	Unrelated; high incidence	+99%
*r^G (rh^G; G; CD; Rh12) (compound)	1958	Rh/Hr	86%
*RH (rh_m; Rh29; Total Rh)	1967	Rh/Hr	+99%
*Rh:1 (Rh_o; D)	1939	Rh/Hr	85%
*Rh:2 (rh′; C)	1941	Rh/Hr	70%
*Rh:3 (rh″; E)	1943	Rh/Hr	30%
*Rh:4 (hr′; c)	1941	Rh/Hr	80%
*Rh:5 (hr″; e)	1945	Rh/Hr	98%
*Rh:6 (hr; ce; f)	1953	Rh/Hr	64%
*Rh:7 (rh_i; Ce) (compound)	1958	Rh/Hr	70%
*Rh:8 (rh^{w1}; C^w)	1946	Rh/Hr	1%
*Rh:9 (rh^x; C^x)	1954	Rh/Hr	−1%
*Rh:10 (hr^v; ce^s; V)	1955	Rh/Hr	−1%
*Rh:11 (rh^{w2}; E^w)	1955	Rh/Hr	−1%
*Rh:12 (rh^G; r^G; G; CD) (compound)	1958	Rh/Hr	86%
*Rh:13 (Rh^A)	1957	Rh/Hr	85%
*Rh:14 (Rh^B)	1959	Rh/Hr	85%
*Rh:15 (Rh^C)	1959	Rh/Hr	85%
*Rh:16 (Rh^D)	1959	Rh/Hr	85%
*Rh:17 (Hr_o)	1950	Rh/Hr	+99%
*Rh:18 (Hr)	1960	Rh/Hr	+99%
*Rh:19 (hr^s)	1960	Rh/Hr	97%
*Rh:20 (e^s; VS)	1960	Rh/Hr	−1%
*Rh:21 (C^G)	1961	Rh/Hr	70%
*Rh:22 (CE) (compound)	1961	Rh/Hr	1%
*Rh:23 (Wiel; D^w)	1962	Rh/Hr	−1%
*Rh:24 (E^T)	1962	Rh/Hr	30%
*Rh:25 (LW)	1961	Rh/Hr†	+99%
*Rh:26 (c-like; Deal)	1964	Rh/Hr	80%
*Rh:27 (cE) (compound)	1961	Rh/Hr	30%
*Rh:28 (hr^H)	1964	Rh/Hr	−1%
*Rh:29 (RH; rh_m; total Rh)	1967	Rh/Hr	+99%

†Relationship to Rh/Hr system is controversial.

Antigen (Compound or Variant)	Year of Publication	Blood Group System	Frequency
°Rh:30 (Go^a; Gonzalez; D^{Cor})	1962	Rh/Hr	−1%
°Rh:31 (hr^B)	1968	Rh/Hr	−1%
°Rh:32 ($\overline{\overline{R}}^N$; Troll; Reynolds; Harper; Comacho; Garcia)	1960	Rh/Hr	−1%
°Rh:33 (R^{oHar})	1971	Rh/Hr	−1%
°Rh:34 (Bas; Bastinna)	1972	Rh/Hr	+99%
Rh:35 (1114)	1971	Rh/Hr	−1%
Rh:36 (Berrens, Be^a)	1953	Rh/Hr	−1%
Rh:37 (Evans)	1960	Rh/Hr	−1%
Rh:38 (Duclos)	1978	Rh/Hr	+99%
Rh:39	1979	Rh/Hr	+99%
Rh:40 (Targett)	1979	Rh/Hr	−1%
Rh:41 *(compound)*	Unpublished**	Rh/Hr	—
Rh:42 (Ce^s) *(compound)*	Unpublished**	Rh/Hr	—
°rh' (C; Rh:2)	1941	Rh/Hr	70%
°rh'' (E; Rh:3)	1943	Rh/Hr	30%
°Rh^A (Rh:13)	1957	Rh/Hr	85%
°Rh^B (Rh:14)	1959	Rh/Hr	85%
°Rh^C (Rh:15)	1959	Rh/Hr	85%
°Rh^D (Rh:16)	1959	Rh/Hr	85%
°rh^G (r^G; G; Rh:12; CD) *(compound)*	1958	Rh/Hr	86%
°rh$_i$ (Ce; Rh:7) *(compound)*	1958	Rh/Hr	70%
°rh$_{ii}$ (cE; Rh:27) *(compound)*	1961	Rh/Hr	30%
°rh$_m$ (RH; total Rh; Rh:29)	1967	Rh/Hr	+99%
°Rh$_{mod}$	1971	Rh/Hr	−1%
°Rh$_{null}$	1961	Rh/Hr	−1%
°Rh$_o$ (D; Rh:1)	1939	Rh/Hr	85%
°rh^{w1} (C^w; Rh:8)	1946	Rh/Hr	1%
°rh^{w2} (E^w; Rh:11)	1955	Rh/Hr	−1%
°rh^x (C^x; Rh:9)	1954	Rh/Hr	−1%
Ri^a (Ridley)	1962	MNS	−1%
Rich	1967	Unrelated; low incidence	−1%
Ridley (Ri^a)	1962	MNS	−1%
Rils	Unpublished	Unrelated; low incidence	−1%
Ritter	Unpublished	Unrelated; high incidence	+99%
Rl^a (Rosenlund)	1974	Unrelated; high incidence	+99%
Rm (Romunde)	1954	Unrelated; low incidence	−1%
°$\overline{\overline{R}}^N$ (Rh:32; Troll; Reynolds; Harper; Comacho; Garcia)	1960	Rh/Hr	−1%
Robert	Unpublished	Unrelated; high incidence	+99%
Rogers (Rg^a)	1975	Unrelated; high incidence†	97%
°R^{oHar} (Rh:33)	1971	Rh/Hr	−1%
Romunde (Rm)	1954	Unrelated; low incidence	−1%
Rosebush	Unpublished	Unrelated; high incidence	+99%
Roselund	Unpublished	Unrelated; low incidence	−1%
Roselund (Rl^a)	1974	Unrelated; high incidence	+99%
Rutherford	1968	Unrelated; low incidence	−1%
Ryan	Unpublished	Unrelated; high incidence	+99%

**Reported at AABB Meeting, Washington, 1980.
†Possibly related to HL-A 1,8.

S

Antigen (Compound or Variant)	Year of Publication	Blood Group System	Frequency
°S	1947	MNS	57%
°s	1951	MNS	88%
S₂ (*variant*)	1964	MNS	−
Sadler (Sas)	1969	Unrelated; high incidence	+99%
°San (K:14)	1974	Kell	+99%
Santano	Unpublished	Unrelated; high incidence	+99%
Sas (Sadler)	1969	Unrelated; high incidence	+99%
Sav (Savior)	1967	Unrelated; high incidence	+99%
Savior (Sav)	1967	Unrelated; high incidence	+99%
S^B	1968	MNS	57%
Sc1 (Sm)	1962	Sciana	+99%
Sc2 (Bu^a)	1963	Sciana	−1%
Sch (Schwartz; Swarts)	1968	Unrelated; high incidence	+99%
Schuppenhauer	Unpublished	Unrelated; high incidence	+99%
Schwartz (Swarts; Sch)	1968	Unrelated; high incidence	+99%
Sd^a (Sid)	1967	Sid	88%
Sd^x	1980	Sd	+99%
Seidler (A₁Le^b)	1968	Lewis	27%
Sf^a (Stoltzfus)	1969	Unrelated†	−
Sg (Sgro; K:13)	1974	Kell	+99%
°Sgro (Sg; K:13)	1974	Kell	+99%
Sheerin (Tm)	1965	MNS	25%
Shier	1969	MNS	20%
Sid (Sd^a)	1967	Sid	88%
Simon	Unpublished	Unrelated; high incidence	+99%
Simpson	1968	Unrelated; low incidence	−1%
Sisson	1967	Unrelated; high incidence	+99%
Sj (Stenbar)	1968	MNS	2%
Sk (Skjelbred)	1980	Unrelated	−1%
Skjelbred (Sk)	1980	Unrelated	−1%
SL^a	1980	Unrelated	+99%
Sm (Sc1)	1962	Sciana	+99%
Smith (John Smith)	Unpublished	Unrelated; low incidence	−1%
Snyder	1967	Unrelated; high incidence	+99%
So^a	1967	Unrelated; high incidence	+99%
Sp₁ (Pr₁ₕ; HD₁; Heidelberg)	1968	HD-Pr-Sp	100%
Sp₁ (HD₁; Pr₁ₐ)	1969	HD-Pr-Sp	100%
Sp₁(HD₂; Pr₂)	1969	HD-Pr-Sp	100%
St^a (Stones)	1962	MNS	−1%
Stenbar (Sj)	1968	MNS	2%
Stevenson	Unpublished	Unrelated; low incidence	−1%
Stiarwalt	Unpublished	Unrelated; high incidence	+99%
Stirling (Cs^a)	1965	Unrelated; high incidence	+99%
Stobo	1959	Bg	−1%

S *(continued)*

Antigen (Compound or Variant)	Year of Publication	Blood Group System	Frequency
Stoltzfus (Sfᵃ)	1969	Unrelated†	—
Stones (Stᵃ)	1962	MNS	−1%
Sᵘ	1963	MNS	−1%
Suhany	Unpublished	Unrelated; low incidence	−1%
Sul (Sullivan)	1967	MNS	−1%
Sullivan (Sul)	1967	MNS	−1%
*Sutter (Jsᵃ; K:6)	1958	Kell	1%
Swᵃ (Swann)	1959	Unrelated; low incidence	−1%
Swann (Swᵃ)	1959	Unrelated; low incidence	−1%
Swarts (Schwartz; Sch)	1968	Unrelated; high incidence	+99%

†Possibly an antigen of the white cells.

T

Antigen (Compound or Variant)	Year of Publication	Blood Group System	Frequency
T†	1925	Unrelated; high incidence	+99%
Talbert	Unpublished	Unrelated; high incidence	+99%
Targett (Rh:40)	1979	Rh/Hr	—
Tasich	1968	Unrelated; high incidence	+99%
Tcr‡	1973	Unrelated; low incidence	−1%
Terrano	1967	Unrelated; low incidence	−1%
Terrell	Unpublished	Unrelated; high incidence	+99%
Ters (Tershuur)	1968	Unrelated; high incidence	+99%
Tershuur (Ters)	1968	Unrelated; high incidence	+99%
Thoms	1967	Unrelated; low incidence	−1%
*Tjᵃ (p; PP₁Pᵏ)	1951	P	+99%
Tk†	1972	Unrelated; high incidence	+99%
Tm (Sheerin)	1965	MNS	25%
Tn†	1959	Unrelated; high incidence	+99%
Toᵃ (Torkildsen)	1968	Unrelated; low incidence	−1%
Todd	1967	Unrelated; high incidence	+99%
Torkildsen (Toᵃ)	1968	Unrelated; low incidence	−1%

Table continued on the following page

T *(continued)*

Antigen (Compound or Variant)	Year of Publication	Blood Group System	Frequency
Total Rh (RH; rh$_m$; Rh:29)	1967	Rh/Hr	+99%
Tr^a (Traversu)	1962	Unrelated; low incidence	−1%
Traversu (Tr^a)	1962	Unrelated; low incidence	−1%
Troll (Rh:32)	1971	Rh/Hr	−1%
Truax	Unpublished	Unrelated; high incidence	+99%
Ts (Tsunoi)	1967	Unrelated; low incidence	−1%
Tsunoi (Ts)	1967	Unrelated; low incidence	−1%

†Antigens found on polyagglutinable red cells.
‡Probably the same as Tn.

U

Antigen (Compound or Variant)	Year of Publication	Blood Group System	Frequency
U	1953	MNS	+99%
U11	Unpublished	Unrelated; high incidence	+99%
U^B	1965	MNS	+99%
°Ul^a (Karhula; K:10)	1967	Kell	−1%†

†Up to 5% in certain Finnish isolates.

V

Antigen (Compound or Variant)	Year of Publication	Blood Group System	Frequency
V (ce^s; hr^v; Rh:10)	1955	Rh/Hr	−1%
Ve^a (Vel1; Vel)	1952	Vel	+99%
Vel1 (Ve^a, Vel)	1952	Vel	+99%
Vel2	1968	Vel	+99%
Ven	1952	Unrelated; low incidence	−1%
Vennerra	Unpublished	Unrelated; high incidence	+99%
Verdegoal (Vr; Vr^a)	1958	MNS	−1%
Verweyst (Vw)	1954	MNS	−1%
Vg^a	1981	Unrelated; low incidence	−1%
Vr (Vr^a; Verdegoal)	1958	MNS	−1%
Vr^a (Vr; Verdegoal)	1958	MNS	−1%
Vs (e^s; Rh:20)	1960	Rh/Hr	−1%
V^u (*variant of V*)	1961	Rh/Hr	−
Vw (Verweyst)	1954	MNS	−1%

W

Antigen (Compound or Variant)	Year of Publication	Blood Group System	Frequency
Wade	Unpublished	Unrelated; low incidence	−1%
Waldner	Unpublished	Unrelated; high incidence	+99%
Wallin	Unpublished	Unrelated; high incidence	+99%
Walls	Unpublished	Unrelated; high incidence	+99%
Wb (Webb)	1963	Unrelated; low incidence	−1%
Webb (Wb)	1963	Unrelated; low incidence	−1%
*Weeks (Wkª; K:17)	1974	Kell	−1%
Wetz	1966	Unrelated; low incidence	−1%
Whittle	1967	Unrelated; low incidence	−1%
*Wiel (Dʷ; Rh:23)	1962	Rh/Hr	−1%
Wil (Wilson)	Unpublished	Unrelated; high incidence	+99%
Wilson (Wil)	Unpublished	Unrelated; high incidence	+99%
Wimberley	Unpublished	Unrelated; high incidence	+99%
Winbourne	Unpublished	Unrelated; high incidence	+99%
*Wkª (Weeks; K:17)	1974	Kell	−1%
Woit	Unpublished	Unrelated; high incidence	+99%
Wrª (Wright)	1953	Wright	−1%
Wrᵇ (Fritz)	1971	Wright	+99%
Wright (Wrª)	1953	Wright	−1%
Wu (Wulfsberg)	1966	Unrelated; low incidence	−1%
Wulfsberg (Wu)	1966	Unrelated; low incidence	−1%

X

Antigen (Compound or Variant)	Year of Publication	Blood Group System	Frequency
Xgª	1962	Sex-linked Xg	66% M 89% F

Y

Antigen (Compound or Variant)	Year of Publication	Blood Group System	Frequency
Yahuda (Yh^a)	1968	Unrelated; low incidence	−1%
Yh^a (Yahuda)	1968	Unrelated; low incidence	−1%
Yk^a (York)	1969	Unrelated; high incidence	+99%
York (Yk^a)	1969	Unrelated; high incidence	+99%
Yt^a (Cartwright)	1956	Cartwright	+99%
Yt^b	1964	Cartwright	8%
Yus (Yussef)	1961	Gerbich	+99%
Yussef (Yus)	1961	Gerbich	+99%

Z

Antigen (Compound or Variant)	Year of Publication	Blood Group System	Frequency
Zd	1970	?Rh/Hr	−1%
Zwal	Unpublished	Unrelated; high incidence	+99%

Index